AF671499

Mimics and Red Flags of Multiple Sclerosis

Tomas Uher

Mimics and Red Flags of Multiple Sclerosis

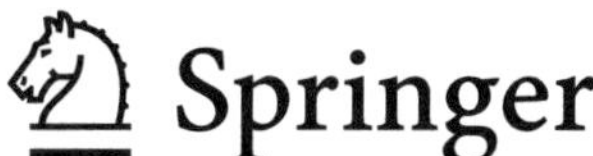

Tomas Uher
Multiple Sclerosis Centre, Neurology
and Centre of Clinical Neuroscience
First Faculty of Medicine Charles University
and General University Hospital in Prague
Prague, Czech Republic

ISBN 978-3-031-98944-5 ISBN 978-3-031-98945-2 (eBook)
https://doi.org/10.1007/978-3-031-98945-2

This Springer imprint is published by the registered company Springer Nature Switzerland AG
The registered company address is: Gewerbestrasse 11, 6330 Cham, Switzerland

"Life is like riding a bicycle. To keep your balance, you must keep moving." (A. Einstein)

I dedicate my work to my patients, colleagues, friends, my family, and all good people. I would also like to express my gratitude to Professor Andrew J. Solomon for his valuable suggestions and for writing the foreword.

This publication was supported by the institutional support of the hospital research RVO-VFN 64165; Czech Ministry of Education—project Cooperatio LF1, research area Neuroscience; and the project National Institute for Neurological Research (Programme EXCELES, ID project No LX22NPO5107)—funded by the European Union—Next Generation EU.

This book has been written entirely by the author. ChatGPT, an AI language model, was utilized solely for correcting English grammar. The content, concepts, and ideas presented in this book remain the original work of the author.

The figures were created with Zoner Photo Studio X.

Foreword

The clinical and radiological heterogeneity of multiple sclerosis (MS) is widely acknowledged, and an accessible, highly sensitive and specific biomarker for MS remains an unmet need in clinical practice. Consequently, accurate diagnosis of MS relies upon clinical acumen that requires a breadth of knowledge for its differential diagnosis. Although MS diagnostic criteria have evolved over the last 60 years, each has relied upon the concept of "no better explanation" as a key element: disorders that may mimic MS must be considered and ruled out in order to diagnose MS.

Advancement in knowledge, particularly over the last decade, has required changes in clinical approaches to MS differential diagnosis. There has been increased recognition of neuroinflammatory disorders that may present with syndromes typical of MS. Newly identified clinical, laboratory, and radiological findings increasingly aid differentiation of these and other disorders from MS. In tandem, data from an expanding spectrum of clinical and radiological presentations previously considered atypical or insufficient for diagnosis challenge the boundaries of MS diagnostic criteria. Importantly, in this context, recent data also increasingly suggest that MS misdiagnosis is prevalent and associated with unnecessary medical risk and morbidity. In some cohorts, misdiagnosis has been identified in approximately one in seven patients who carry a diagnosis of MS. In sum, these recent developments inform optimal and nuanced approaches to MS differential diagnosis that necessitate greater expertise than was required in the past.

Mimics and Red Flags of Multiple Sclerosis by Dr. Tomáš Uher is a new and essential resource that will help inform the clinical care of patients where diagnosis of MS is being considered. This impressive accomplishment systematically and thoughtfully tackles the often daunting breadth of MS differential diagnosis. Comprehensive yet easy to navigate, its practical organization allows readers to quickly find disorders of interest. Each entry is accompanied by an efficient description of key clinical, laboratory, and radiological findings to facilitate accurate diagnosis. These findings are further enriched by a differential diagnosis provided for each disorder. Enhanced figures helpfully highlight MRI features that point to specific diagnoses. Updated data surrounding disease epidemiology, pathobiology, prognosis, and treatment complement diagnostic considerations to further aid clinical care. This exceptionally detailed and thoroughly cited compendium will serve as a principal reference for clinicians navigating MS differential diagnosis in practice for many years to come.

Andrew J. Solomon

Professor and Interim Chair,
Department of Neurological Sciences
and Division Chief, Multiple Sclerosis
The Larner College of Medicine
at The University of Vermont
Burlington, VT, USA

Preface

Multiple sclerosis (MS) is a chronic inflammatory disease of the central nervous system (CNS) presenting with a wide spectrum of clinical and radiological phenotypes. In clinical practice, many patients with MS are initially misdiagnosed with other medical conditions (false-negative diagnosis). Furthermore, patients with various medical conditions are incorrectly diagnosed with MS (false-positive diagnosis). Additionally, in some patients, when an alternative diagnosis is suspected, neither a comprehensive assessment nor observing the disease course over time provides any clues for an alternative diagnosis to MS. The relatively high frequency of MS misdiagnosis is due to the challenging differential diagnosis, which is mainly caused by the following reasons:

- MS has no specific biomarkers, and the diagnosis is made when no other explanations are found for the patient's neurological manifestations (diagnosis per exclusionem).
- The spectrum of alternative diagnoses that mimic MS is very broad.
- MS mimics include several very rare diagnoses, which may be unknown to clinicians owing to their rarity. Diagnosing these conditions may require complex and detailed genetic or metabolic assessments that may not be routinely available.
- There is increasing pressure to diagnose MS early because early treatment initiation is associated with better disease outcomes. However, the growing number of patients seen in practice, decreasing consultation times, and the urgency to start immuno-modulatory treatment (DMT) as soon as possible may lead to limited time for observing the disease course and thorough evaluation by physicians, potentially increasing the risk of misdiagnosis.
- The MS patient population is heterogeneous, and it is possible that a proportion of patients with atypical phenotypes diagnosed with MS have yet undefined or undiscovered diseases. Advances in research may result in discoveries of new diagnoses in the future, like how anti-aquaporine-4 (AQP4) IgG was identified 20 years ago and anti-myelin oligodendrocyte glycoprotein (MOG) IgG approximately 10 years ago.
- Incorrect application of the McDonald diagnostic criteria for MS.
- Geographically variable awareness of MS manifestations among the public and healthcare professionals, along with a shortage of neurologists with adequate

training and limited access to diagnostic equipment in some low- and middle-income countries.

Misdiagnosis of MS is a significant issue because it is associated with potential serious consequences:

- False-Negative Diagnosis: This leads to either late initiation or non-initiation of immunomodulatory treatment, which is associated with poorer prognosis of MS.
- Untargeted Treatment: Misdiagnosis prevents targeted treatment of the underlying medical condition, which may lead to disease progression and worse disease outcomes (e.g., not using enzyme replacement therapy in Fabry disease or biotin supplementation in patients with biotinidase deficiency).
- Missed Genetic Counseling: Patients with unrecognized or late-diagnosed inherited genetic diseases may miss opportunities for genetic counseling, aiding in family planning or prenatal diagnosis.
- Negative Impact of MS Treatments: Some treatments used for MS in patients with alternative diagnoses may have serious adverse effects (e.g., alemtuzumab, dimethyl–fumarate, glatiramer–acetate, interferons, natalizumab or S1P inhibitors in neuromyelitis optica spectrum disorder [NMOSD]; interferons in Susac's syndrome; immunosuppressive drugs in infectious diseases; natalizumab causing progressive multi-focal leukoencephalopathy [PML]; or alemtuzumab triggering autoimmune diseases).
- High Financial Burden: MS treatments are associated with high medical costs [1–7].

Neurologists may not frequently encounter patients with MS who present with atypical clinical courses, imaging findings, or biochemical abnormalities. However, managing these patients—who may have suspected alternative diagnoses to MS—can be extremely time-consuming. This is due to the lack of treatment response and the need for comprehensive assessments to rule out a wide range of potential diagnoses, often resulting in negative findings.

Given the wide range of MS mimickers, it is intellectually challenging to consider all alternative diagnoses and choose a rational diagnostic algorithm that is supported by red flags, rather than resorting to an expensive "fishing expedition" of examining everything. To address these concerns, my goal was to investigate further the differential diagnosis of MS. This investigation resulted in the creation of the book, where I have summarized contemporary knowledge on the manifestations and diagnosis of the most important MS mimickers in a structured manner.

The main aim of this work is to provide an inspiration for alternative diagnoses of MS when managing difficult or atypical cases of patients with potential diagnosis of MS and related demyelinating disorders.

This book has some limitations:

- Scope: The field is vast; therefore, only essential information on the clinical and paraclinical features of various conditions is provided. For a more in-depth understanding of specific diagnoses, consulting specialized literature is recommended.
- Illustrations: Real magnetic resonance scans have been replaced with scan-cartoon hybrid illustrations to enhance clarity and educational value.
- Author's Experience: This work is not based on extensive personal experience with patients diagnosed with the full spectrum of rare MS mimickers. Some of the diagnoses included are known to the author solely from the literature.
- Consequently, this work may contain inaccuracies, particularly when presenting information from non-neurological specialties such as radiology, genetics, and biochemistry. I sincerely apologize for any potential errors and encourage readers to share their feedback (tomas.uher@vfn.cz or tomauher@gmail.com).

Despite these limitations, I hope this work inspires clinicians to carefully consider differential diagnoses in complex cases and proves valuable in their clinical practice.

Prague, Czech Republic Tomas Uher

References

1. Correale J, Solomon AJ, Cohen JA, Banwell BL, Gracia F, Gyang TV, et al. Differential diagnosis of suspected multiple sclerosis: global health considerations. Lancet Neurol. 2024;23(10):1035–49.
2. Solomon AJ, Arrambide G, Brownlee WJ, Flanagan EP, Amato MP, Amezcua L, et al. Differential diagnosis of suspected multiple sclerosis: an updated consensus approach. Lancet Neurol. 2023;22(8):750–68.
3. Zürrer WE, Cannon AE, Ilchenko D, Gaitán MI, Granberg T, Piehl F, et al. Misdiagnosis and underdiagnosis of multiple sclerosis: a systematic review and meta-analysis. Mult Scler. 2024;30(11–12):1409–22.
4. Uher T, Adzima A, Srpova B, Noskova L, Marechal B, Maceski AM, et al. Diagnostic delay of multiple sclerosis: prevalence, determinants and consequences. Mult Scler. 2023;29(11–12):1437–51.
5. Hua LH, Solomon AJ, Tenembaum S, Scalfari A, Rovira À, Rostasy K, et al. Differential diagnosis of suspected multiple sclerosis in pediatric and late-onset populations: a review. JAMA Neurol. 2024.
6. Miller TM. Differential diagnosis of myotonic disorders. Muscle Nerve. 2008;37(3):293–9.
7. Solomon AJ, Pettigrew R, Naismith RT, Chahin S, Krieger S, Weinshenker B. Challenges in multiple sclerosis diagnosis: misunderstanding and misapplication of the McDonald criteria. Mult Scler. 2021;27(2):250–8.

Competing Interests

The author has no competing interests to declare that are relevant to the content of this manuscript.

Contents

Abbreviations

AAG	Autoimmune autonomic ganglionopathy
AAION	Arteritic anterior ischemic optic neuropathy
AAPT	American Academy of Pain Taxonomy
ACE	Angiotensin-converting enzyme
ACPA	Anti-citrullinated protein antibodies
ACR	American College of Rheumatology
AD	Alzheimer disease
ADC	Apparent diffusion coefficient
ADEM	Acute disseminated encephalomyelitis
AE	Autoimmune encephalitis
AHS	Alpers–Huttenlocher disease
ACHR	Acetylcholine receptor
AIDP	Acute inflammatory demyelinating polyneuropathy
AIDS	Acquired immunodeficiency syndrome
Alpha-Gal A	Alpha-galactosidase A
ALS	Amyotrophic lateral sclerosis
ALSP	Adult-onset leukoencephalopathy with axonal spheroids and pigmented glia
AMPAR	α-Amino-3-hydroxy-5-methyl-4-isoxazole propionic acid receptor
AMPH	Amphiphysin
ANA	Antinuclear antibodies
ANCA	Anti-neutrophil cytoplasmic antibodies
ANNA1	Anti-neuronal nuclear antibody type 1 (anti-Hu)
ANNA2	Anti-neuronal nuclear antibody type 2 (anti-Ri)
ANNA3	Anti-neuronal nuclear antibody type 3
anti-Sm	Anti-Smith antibody
anti-SSA	Anti-Sjogren's syndrome A antibody
anti-SSB	Anti-Sjogren's syndrome B antibody
AOA1 and 2	Ataxia with oculomotor apraxia types 1 and 2
aPL	Anti-phospholipid antibodies
ApoB	Apolipoprotein B
APP	Amyloid protein precursor
APS	Antiphospholipid syndrome
APTT	Activated partial thromboplastin time

AQP4	Aquaporin-4
AR	Androgen receptor
ARCA	Autosomal recessive cerebellar ataxia
ARG1	Arginase deficiency
ARSA	Arylsulfatase A
ARSACS	Autosomal recessive spastic ataxia of Charlevoix-Saguenay
ASANN	Autonomic sensory and autonomic neuropathy
Aß42	Amyloid-ß
AT	Ataxia telangiectasia
ATLD	Ataxia telangiectasia-like disorder
ATN1	Atrophin 1
ATP7B	ATPase, copper transporting, beta polypeptide
AV	Arteriovenous
AVED	Ataxia with vitamin E deficiency
B19V	Parvovirus B19
BAEP	Brainstem auditory evoked potentials
BAFF	B cell activating factor
BBE	Bickerstaff brainstem encephalitis
BRAO	Branch retinal artery occlusion
BTD	Biotinidase deficiency
CAA	Cerebral amyloid angiopathy
CADASIL	Cerebral autosomal dominant arteriopathy with subcortical infarcts and leukoencephalopathy
CANVAS	Cerebellar ataxia, neuropathy, vestibular areflexia syndrome
CARASAL	Cathepsin A–related arteriopathy with strokes and leukoencephalopathy
CARASIL	Cerebral autosomal recessive arteriopathy with subcortical infarcts and leukoencephalopathy
cART	Antiretroviral therapy
CASPR2	Contactin-associated protein-like 2
CCPD	Combined central and peripheral demyelination
CD	Celiac disease
CD4	Cluster of differentiation 4 (T-helper lymphocytes)
CDCA	Chenodeoxycholic acid
CIDP	Chronic inflammatory demyelinating polyneuropathy
CIS	Clinically isolated syndrome
CLCN2	Chloride channel protein 2
CLIPPERS	Chronic lymphocytic inflammation with pontine perivascular enhancement responsive to steroids
CMT	Charcot–Marie–Tooth disease
CMV	Cytomegalovirus
CNS	Central nervous system
CoQ10	Coenzyme Q10
COVID-19	Coronavirus disease 2019
CPEO	Chronic progressive external ophthalmoplegia

CPM	Central pontine myelinolysis
CRION	Chronic relapsing inflammatory optic neuropathy
CRMP5	Collapsin response mediator protein 5
CRP	C-reactive protein
CS	Cogan's syndrome
CSF	Cerebrospinal fluid
CSF1R	Colony-stimulating factor 1 receptor
CSS	Churg–Strauss syndrome
CSVD	Cerebral small vessel disease
CT	Computed tomography
CTLA-4	Cytotoxic T-lymphocyte antigen-4
CTX	Cerebrotendinous xanthomatosis
CVS	Central vein sign
CXCL13	C-X-C motif chemokine ligand 13
DAF	Demyelination with autoimmune features
DARS2	Aspartyl-tRNA synthetase 2
DIDMOAD	Diabetes insipidus, diabetes mellitus, optic atrophy, and deafness (Wolfram syndrome)
DIR	Double inversion recovery (MRI sequence)
DIS	Dissemination in space (MS criterion)
DIT	Dissemination in time (MS criterion)
DNA	Deoxyribonucleic acid
DNER	Delta and Notch-like epidermal growth factor-related receptor
DNMT1	DNA methyltransferase 1
DOA	Dominant optic atrophy
DPD-PLUS	Dopamine-responsive dystonia plus
DPPX	Dipeptidyl-peptidase-like protein 6 (autoantibody target)
DRD	Dopa-responsive dystonia
DRD2	Dopamine receptor 2
DRPLA	Dentatorubral-pallidoluysian atrophy
DSA	Digital subtraction angiography
DSC	Dynamic susceptibility contrast
dsDNA	Anti-double stranded deoxyribonucleic acid
DTI	Diffusion tensor imaging
DWI	Diffusion-weighted imaging
EA	Early antigen
EBNA	Nuclear antigen
EBV	Epstein–Barr virus
ECD	Erdheim–Chester disease
ECG	Electrocardiogram
EDSS	Expanded Disability Status Scale
EEG	Electroencephalogram
ELISA	Enzyme-linked immunosorbent assay
EMA	Anti-endomysial antibodies
EMG	Electromyography

ENA	Extractable nuclear antigen
ESR	Erythrocyte sedimentation rate
ESSDAI	EULAR Sjögren's syndrome disease activity index
EULAR	European League Against Rheumatism
FAT-SAT	Fat saturation
FDG-PET	18-Fludeoxyglucose positron emission tomography
FLAIR	Fluid-attenuated inversion recovery
FLAMES	FLAIR-hyperintense lesions in anti-MOG-associated encephalitis with seizures
FMR1	Fragile X mental retardation 1 gene
FND	Functional neurological disorder
FRDA	Friedreich's ataxia
FTA-ABS	GQ1b+A121:B133
FXS	Fragile X syndrome
FXTAS	Fragile X–associated tremor/ataxia syndrome
GABA-A-R	Gamma-aminobutyric acid type A receptor
GABA-B-R	Gamma-aminobutyric acid type B receptor
GAD65	Glutamic acid decarboxylase 65
GAM	Granulocyte activation markers
Gb3	Globotriaosylceramide
GBS	Guillain–Barré syndrome
GCIPL	Ganglion cell–inner plexiform layer
GCL	Ganglion cell layer
GCS	Glasgow Coma Scale
GFAP	Glial fibrillary acidic protein
GLA	α-Galactosidase A
GLUT1	Glucose transporter type 1 (deficiency syndrome)
GlyR	Glycine receptor
GNACHR	Ganglionic acetylcholine receptor
GP1AB	Glycoprotein Ib Platelet Subunit Alpha
GPA	Granulomatosis with polyangiitis
GPL	IgG phospholipid units
GQ1b	Ganglioside Q1b antibody
GRE	Gradient echo
HAND	HIV-associated neurocognitive disorder
HaNDL	Headache with neurological deficits and lymphocytosis
HAV	Hepatitis A virus
HBV	Hepatitis B virus
HCV	Hepatitis C virus
HES	Hyper-eosinophilic syndrome
HEV	Hepatitis E virus
HHH	Hyperornithinemia-Hyperammonemia-Homocitrullinuria
HHV-6	Human herpesvirus 6
HHV-7	Human herpesvirus 7
HIT	Head impulse test

HIV	Human immunodeficiency virus
HLA	Human leukocyte antigen
HLA-B51	Human leukocyte antigen-B51
HLH	Hemophagocytic lymphohistiocytosis
HSP	Hereditary spastic paraplegia
HSV	Herpes simplex virus
HTLV-1	Human T-lymphotropic virus type 1
IATM	Idiopathic acute transverse myelitis
IBD	Inflammatory bowel disease
IDH	Isocitrate dehydrogenase
IF	Intrathecal fraction
IFN-**A**	Interferon-alpha
Ig	Immunoglobulin
IgG4-RD	Immunoglobulin G4-related disease
Ig-LON5	Immunoglobulin-like domain containing, cell adhesion molecule 5
IL-2	Interleukin-2
IL-6	Interleukin-6
IPND	International Panel for NMO Diagnosis
IRIS	Immune reconstitution inflammatory syndrome
JAK	Janus kinase inhibitor
JCV	John Cunningham virus
JXG	Juvenile xanthogranuloma
KCTD16	Potassium channel tetramerization domain-containing protein 16
KFLC	Kappa free light chains
KLHL11	Kelch-like protein 11
KSS	Kearns–Sayre syndrome
LBSL	Leukoencephalopathy with brainstem and spinal cord involvement and lactate elevation
LDH	Lactate dehydrogenase
LDL-C	Low-density lipoprotein cholesterol
L-DOPA	Levodopa
LEMS	Lambert Eaton syndrome
LETM	Longitudinally extensive transverse myelitis
LGI1	Leucine-rich glioma inactivated 1
LHON	Leber's hereditary optic neuropathy
LCH	Langerhans cell histiocytosis
LMNB1	Lamin B1
LOMS	Late-onset multiple sclerosis
LRP4	Low-density lipoprotein receptor-related protein 4
LS	Leigh's syndrome
LSPFD	Lysosomal storage and peroxisomal function disorders
LUZP4	Leucine zipper protein 4
MAG	Myelin-associated glycoprotein
MAP1B	Microtubule-associated protein 1B
MAT	Microscopic agglutination test

MBP	Myelin basic protein
MCP	Middle cerebellar peduncles
MD	Mitochondrial disorder
MDS	Mitochondrial depletion syndrome
MELAS	Mitochondrial encephalomyopathy, lactic acidosis, and stroke-like episodes
MEP	Motor evoked potentials
MERRF	Myoclonic epilepsy with ragged-red fibers
MFS	Miller Fisher syndrome
MG	Myasthenia gravis
MGLUR1	Metabotropic glutamate receptor 1
MGLUR5	Metabotropic glutamate receptor 5
MGUS	Monoclonal gammopathy of undetermined significance
MILS	Maternally inherited Leigh syndrome
MIMODS	Mitochondrial multiple organ dysfunction syndrome
MIRAS	Mitochondrial recessive ataxia syndrome
MM	Moyamoya disease and syndrome
MNGIE	Mitochondrial neurogastrointestinal encephalomyopathy
mNGS	Metagenomic next-generation sequencing
MOG	Myelin oligodendrocyte glycoprotein
MOGAD	Myelin oligodendrocyte glycoprotein antibody-associated disease
MPA	Microscopic polyangiitis
MPAN	Mitochondrial membrane protein–associated neurodegeneration
MPL	IgM phospholipid units
MR	Magnetic resonance
MRA	Magnetic resonance angiography
MRI	Magnetic resonance imaging
MRS	Magnetic resonance spectroscopy
MRZ	Measles, rubella, zoster reaction
MS	Multiple sclerosis
MSA	Multiple system atrophy
mtDNA	Mitochondrial DNA
MTHFR	Methylenetetrahydrofolate reductase
MTTP	Microsomal triglyceride transfer protein
MUSK	Muscle-specific kinase
N2O	Nitrous oxide
NAA	N-acetylaspartate
NAAS	Neuronal acetylcholine receptor antibody-associated syndrome
NAION	Non-arteritic anterior ischemic optic neuropathy
NARP	Neuropathy, ataxia, and retinitis pigmentosa
NBD	Neuro-Behçet's disease
NF155	Neurofascin 155
NFL	Neurofilament light chain
NGS	Next-generation sequencing
NK	Natural killer

NMDAR	N-methyl-D-aspartate receptor
NMO	Neuromyelitis optica
NMOSD	Neuromyelitis optica spectrum disorder
NOACS	Non-vitamin K oral anticoagulants
NPION	Non-arteritic posterior ischemic optic neuropathy
NPSLE	Neuropsychiatric complications of systemic lupus erythematosus
NS1	Non-structural protein 1
NSAIDs	Non-steroidal anti-inflammatory drugs
NSCLC	Non-small cell lung cancer
NSE	Neuron-specific enolase
NTZ	Natalizumab
OCB	Oligoclonal bands
OCT	Optical coherence tomography
OSP-39	Outer surface protein 39
P/Q VGCC	P/Q-type voltage-gated calcium channel
P5CS	Delta-1-pyrroline-5-carboxylate synthetase
PACNS	Primary angiitis of the central nervous system
PADMAL	Pontine autosomal dominant microangiopathy with leukoencephalopathy
PCA1 and 2	Purkinje cell antibody type 1 and 2
PCA-TR	Purkinje cell antibody–related
PCGE	Cerebral punctate and curvilinear gadolinium enhancements
PCNSL	Primary central nervous system lymphoma
PCR	Polymerase chain reaction
PDE	Phosphodiesterase
PDH	Pyruvate dehydrogenase
PERM	Progressive encephalomyelitis with rigidity and myoclonus
PFO	Patent foramen ovale
PCH	Pontocerebellar hypoplasia
PIRA	Progression independent of relapse activity
PLES	Posterior leukoencephalopathy syndrome
PLS	Primary lateral sclerosis
PMA	Progressive muscular atrophy
PML	Progressive multifocal leukoencephalopathy
PML-IRIS	Progressive multifocal leukoencephalopathy-associated immune reconstitution inflammatory syndrome
POLG	DNA polymerase gamma
POMS	Pediatric-onset multiple sclerosis
PPMS	Primary progressive multiple sclerosis
PRES	Posterior reversible encephalopathy syndrome
PRE-SCI	Posterior reversible encephalopathy syndrome with spinal cord involvement
PRLs	Paramagnetic rim lesions
PS	Pearson syndrome

PSEN1 and 2	Presenilin-1 and 2
PWI	Perfusion-weighted imaging
QSM	Quantitative susceptibility mapping
RAPD	Relative afferent pupillary defect
rCBV	Relative cerebral blood volume
RCVS	Reversible cerebral vasoconstriction syndrome
RDD	Rosai–Dorfman disease
REM	Rapid eye movement (sleep phase)
RINR	Recurrent idiopathic neuroretinitis
RIS	Radiologically isolated syndrome
RNA	Ribonucleic acid
RNFL	Retinal nerve fiber layer
RPR	Rapid plasma reagin
RRMS	Relapsing-remitting multiple sclerosis
rtPA	Recombinant tissue plasminogen activator
RVCL-S	Retinal vasculopathy with cerebral leukoencephalopathy and systemic manifestations
S100	S100 protein
S1P	Sphingosine-1-phosphate
SACD	Subacute combined degeneration of the spinal cord
SANDO	Sensory ataxic neuropathy, dysarthria, and ophthalmoparesis
SARS-CoV-2	Severe acute respiratory syndrome coronavirus 2
SBMA	Spinal and bulbar muscular atrophy (Kennedy's disease)
SCAN1	Spinocerebellar ataxia with axonal neuropathy type 1
SCLC	Small cell lung cancer
SELs	Slowly evolving lesions
SIADH	Syndrome of inappropriate antidiuretic hormone secretion
SICCA	Sjögren's International Collaborative Clinical Alliance
SICRET syndrome	Retinocochleocerebral vasculopathy, small infarctions of cochlear, retinal, and encephalic tissue syndrome
SjS	Sjogren syndrome
SLAM	Signaling lymphocytic activation molecule
SLE	Systemic lupus erythematosus
SMA	Spinal muscular atrophy
SMA-4	Spinal muscular atrophy type 4
SMN1 and 2	Survival motor neuron 1 and 2
SNAPS	Synaptic-associated proteins
SOX1	SRY-box transcription factor 1
SPECT	Single-photon emission computed tomography
SPG	Spastic paraplegia gene
SPMS	Secondary progressive multiple sclerosis
SPOAN	Spastic paraplegia, optic atrophy, and neuropathy
SSA/RO	Sjögren's syndrome-related antigen A (Ro)
SSB/LA	Sjögren's syndrome-related antigen B (La)

SSEP	Somatosensory evoked potentials
SSPE	Subacute sclerosing panencephalitis
STIR	Short tau inversion recovery
STRIVE-1	Standards for Reporting Vascular Changes on Neuroimaging 1
SuS	Susac's syndrome
SWI	Susceptibility-weighted imaging (MRI sequence)
T. pallidum	Treponema pallidum
T. whipplei	Tropheryma whipplei
TAI	Traumatic axonal injury
TG2	Anti-transglutaminase 2
TIA	Transient ischemic attack
TNF	Tumor necrosis factor
TPO	Thyroid peroxidase
TPPA	Treponema pallidum particle agglutination assay
TRIM46	Tripartite motif-containing protein 46
tRNA	Transfer ribonucleic acid
TSH	Thyroid-stimulating hormone
TTPA	Alpha-tocopherol transfer protein
UCH-L1	Ubiquitin carboxy-terminal hydrolase L1
VCA	Viral capsid antigen
VDRL	Venereal disease research laboratory
VEP	Visual evoked potentials
VGKC	Voltage-gated potassium channel
VLA-4	Very late antigen 4
VLDR	Very low-density lipoprotein receptor
VZV	Varicella-zoster virus
WD	Whipple disease
WE	Wernicke's encephalopathy
WES	Whole exome sequencing
X-ALD	X-linked adrenoleukodystrophy
XP	Xeroderma pigmentosum

1 Multiple Sclerosis (MS)

1.1 Epidemiology

- Incidence 2.1/100.000/year (globally).
- Prevalence:
  - 44.0/100.000 (globally)
  - 143/100.000 (Europe)
  - 117/100.000 (Americas)
  - 33/100.000 (E. Mediterranean)
  - >9/100.000 (Africa, Southeast Asia, Western Pacific)
- Female/male ratio 2–3/1, but this ratio increases [1, 2].

1.2 Etiology and Definition

- An immune-mediated disease of the central nervous system (CNS) is triggered by a neuroinflammatory autoimmune response to self-antigens in individuals with a genetic predisposition. The disease is marked by demyelination, inflammation, lesion formation, and neurodegeneration. It is believed that the progressive neurodegeneration of the CNS primarily results from neuroinflammation rather than being an independent process. Additionally, a peripheral immune response targeting the CNS is considered crucial in the early stages of disease progression. Conversely, immune pathophysiological processes within the CNS become predominant at the later, progressive phases of the disease [3–6].
- MS does not result from a single-gene defect. Instead, multiple genes with incomplete penetrance are associated with an increased risk of developing the disease. The majority of the susceptibility loci for MS are shared with other autoimmune disorders. Additionally, the associated genetic loci have only a modest influence on the risk of developing MS. Therefore, prominent family history is atypical for MS [7, 8].

T. Uher, *Mimics and Red Flags of Multiple Sclerosis*,
https://doi.org/10.1007/978-3-031-98945-2_1

- The most important environmental risk factors include Epstein–Barr virus (EBV) infection, decreased sunlight exposure, low vitamin D levels, smoking, obesity, psychological stress, unhealthy diet, or gut microbiome abnormalities [9].

1.3 Clinical Features

- The clinical presentation of MS includes a wide range of neurological signs and symptoms resulting from focal and diffuse damage to the brain and spinal cord. These neurological presentations are not specific to MS, making diagnosis based solely on clinical criteria very challenging or nearly impossible. They include mostly the following manifestations:
  - Muscle weakness (paresis) and spasticity
  - Cerebellar syndrome with ataxia, tremor, abnormalities in stance and gait
  - Dysarthria, dysphagia, nystagmus, peripheral facial palsy, diplopia, internuclear ophthalmoplegia, or other cranial nerve involvements
  - Sensory symptoms such as paresthesias (numbness), hypesthesia (loss of sensation), dysesthesia, or neuropathic pain
  - Bowel and bladder dysfunction, including retention, incontinence, or urgency
  - Walking difficulties, usually of multifactorial etiology
  - Fatigue, cognitive impairment, and affective disorders [10–12]
  - Visual dysfunction is primarily due to optic neuritis (only rarely associated with lesions in the occipital lobe). Retrobulbar optic neuritis in MS is characterized by
    - Often the first clinical manifestation of MS (25%)
    - Occurs during disease in the majority of patients (50–70%)
    - Typically mild to moderate
    - Unilateral involvement (95%)
    - Subacute onset (Progression to the nadir over 1 week)
    - Pain
      - Worse on eye movements or mild periocular (90%)
      - Eye discomfort (92%)
      - Worsening of eye movement (70%)
      - Eye pain before vision loss (40%)
    - Contrast sensitivity loss (Often not fully recover)
    - High-contrast visual acuity loss
      - Usually mild at nadir (>6/60) (67%)
      - Rarely no perception of light (3%)
      - Often full recovery (after 12 months; >6/12; 90%)
    - Visual field loss (Diffuse [37%], central [29%])
    - Abnormal color vision (dyschromatopsia)
    - Positive relative afferent pupillary deficit (RAPD)
    - Positive symptoms (photopsia)
      - Rare but may occur due to ephaptic transmission between optic nerve axons

    - Flashes of lights, geometric patterns, or shimmering edges or borders around such patterns or scotomas.
    - More frequent in retinal pathologies
  - Infrequent mild disc edema (36%)
  - Optic disc pallor
    - Mainly in the temporal quadrants
    - Often, even when excellent clinical recovery
  - Good recovery
    - Usually prompt response to corticosteroids
    - Initial rapid, then a slow improvement continuing up to 6–12 months (>90%) [13–16]
- The Expanded Disability Status Scale (EDSS) quantifies neurological signs and symptoms in MS and is used for monitoring clinical disease activity [12].
- Rare manifestations of MS (but considered as red flags) include, for example
  - Anterior or pan-uveitis
  - Headache
  - Hearing loss
  - Insidious cognitive decline
  - Onset before the age of 11 years or after 50 years
  - Optic neuritis with normal brain and spinal cord magnetic resonance imaging (MRI)
  - Painless visual loss
  - Paroxysmal dysarthria and ataxia
  - Recurrent or stereotyped deficits
  - Progressive or recurrent myelopathy without other neurological deficits
  - Seizures
  - Selective dorsal column involvement
  - Severe optic neuritis (acuity of 20/200 or worse) [11, 17, 18]
- The comprehensive list of clinical red flags is provided in the chapter titled “Clinical Red Flags” of MS.

1.4 Disease Course

- The mean age of symptom onset is 32 years [1, 19].
- Onset before the age of 11 years, defined as pediatric-onset MS (POMS), is rare and considered a red flag. Similarly, late-onset MS (LOMS), characterized by disease onset in patients over the age of 50, is also relatively rare and regarded as a red flag [11, 18].
- The clinical course of MS can follow several distinct disease patterns:
  - Radiologically Isolated Syndrome (RIS): This stage presents MS-typical findings on brain MRI, but there are no clinical signs or symptoms suggestive of MS. RIS is associated with a significantly increased risk of developing MS [20].
  - Clinically Isolated Syndrome (CIS): This stage refers to the first clinical episode suggestive of MS. According to the McDonald criteria from 2017 [21],

some patients with enhanced lesions on brain MRI or positive oligoclonal bands may already be diagnosed with MS at this stage.
- Relapsing-Remitting MS (RRMS): The most common disease pattern accounting for 80% of cases. It is characterized by clinical attacks (relapses) of new neurological symptoms, followed by remissions. Clinical manifestations during the relapse last for at least 24 hours occur in the absence of fever, infection, or other causes (such as heat sensitivity or pseudo-relapse), and they are separated from a prior relapse by at least 30 days. During relapses, patients typically experience clinical deterioration over several days, remain at a nadir for a week or two, and then gradually recover over the following weeks, achieving either partial or full recovery [22]. Although paroxysmal neurological symptoms, such as trigeminal neuralgia, Lhermitte's phenomenon, tonic spasm, or seizure do not last at least 24 hours, they should be sufficient for fulfillment of MS diagnostic criteria [23].
- Secondary Progressive MS (SPMS): This follows relapsing-remitting MS and typically occurs in the later stages of the disease. It is marked by severe neurological disability, an absence or very low frequency of relapses, progressive disability, and poor response to immuno-modulatory treatments.
- Primary Progressive MS (PPMS): Characterized by a progression of disability from the onset of symptoms, without early relapses or remissions. This type of MS has a poor response to most immuno-modulatory treatments. Progressive-relapsing MS (PRMS): This rarest subtype is associated with the worst prognosis. It is characterized by a steady progression of disability from the onset of symptoms, accompanied by occasional relapses. However, this subtype is considered to overlap with other disease courses and is therefore no longer used in current terminology [22].

1.5 Brain Imaging

- Lesions (are of focal hyperintensity/hypointensity) in the CNS represent a heterogeneous and dynamic group of focal brain pathologies, ranging from edema and inflammation to demyelination, gliosis, and axonal loss.
- Lesions' location:
  - Lesions are distributed mildly asymmetrically between hemispheres.
  - Periventricular white matter:
    - Lesions abut (touch) the lateral ventricles without a band of normal-appearing white matter between the ventricle and the lesion.
    - Periventricular lesions are often perpendicular to the lateral ventricles have a calloso-striatal orientation and form wedge-shaped hyperintensities with a broad base toward the lateral ventricle ("Dawson's fingers").
    - The following T2 lesions are not considered as periventricular
      - Lesions in deep gray matter (e.g., amygdala, caudate, putamen, hippocampus, hypothalamus, nucleus accumbens, globus pallidus, thalamus, subthalamus, and epithalamus). However, high-resolution MRI scanners frequently reveal focal lesions in the deep gray matter as well.
      - Lesions touching the third ventricle or the cerebral aqueduct.

    - Lesions touching the fourth ventricle are considered as infratentorial, not periventricular.
    - Lesions in deep and paraventricular white matter (these lesions are close to the ventricles but do not abut them).
  - Linear plate-like lesions parallel to the lateral ventricles ("periventricular banding" or "halo") are not typical for MS and are more commonly associated with cerebral small vessel disease (CSVD).
  - Similarly, long lesions that parallel the long axis of the corpus callosum (which may progress into pencil-thin peri-ependymal lesions) and occur in NMOSD are not typical for MS.
  - Periventricular lesions must be distinguished from enlarged perivascular spaces (Virchow-Robin spaces), which have signal intensity like cerebrospinal fluid (CSF)—appearing hyperintese on T2-weighted images but hypointense on fluid-attenuated inversion recovery (FLAIR) images.
- Juxtacortical and cortical lesions:
  - T2-hyperintense lesions touching the cortex (without a band of normal-appearing white matter between the cortical gray matter and the lesion) or intracortical lesions.
  - Juxtacortical and cortical lesions are common; however, most of these lesions remain undetected on standard MRI.
  - Leukocortical lesions are most visible, but intracortical and especially subpial lesions (located along the subpial surface) are more prevalent. Subpial lesions are associated with inflammation in the adjacent meninges.
  - Juxtacortical lesions typically involve the subcortical arcuate U-fibers, which are short association fibers connecting adjacent gyri within the subcortical white matter. These lesions can occur in all brain lobes, including the cerebellum. U-fibers are typically spared in cerebrovascular diseases due to their rich blood supply.
  - Large cortical lesions and large white matter lesions extending into the superficial cortical layers are atypical for MS.
- Infra-tentorial:
  - Lesions are most often located in the pons and cerebellum, less frequently in the mesencephalon (midbrain) and medulla oblongata.
  - They are typically adjacent to the inner or outer CSF borders.
  - Midbrain (mesencephalon):
    - Frequently lesions in the cerebral peduncles and near the periaqueductal gray matter.
  - Pons:
    - Typical for MS are lesions adjacent to inner or outer CSF borders, such as lesions touching the cisterns or the floor of the fourth ventricle (often affecting the medial longitudinal fasciculus), lesions at the pontine surface, or at the trigeminal nerve entry zone.
    - Atypical for MS are lesions (often symmetric) in the central pons along the transverse pontine fibers, which lie in the vascular border zone and are often of vascular origin.
  - Oblongata:
    - Typical uni- or bilateral lesions are located paramedially.

  - Cerebellum:
    - Frequently lesions in the cerebellar hemispheres.
    - Also frequently seen in the medial cerebellar peduncles and less commonly in the superior cerebellar peduncles.
- Other Typical Locations:
  - Optic nerve: short T2 lesions; in acute optic neuritis, these may also show contrast enhancement and optic nerve swelling.
  - Temporal lobe: Focal lesions, particularly in the inferior temporal lobe adjacent to the temporal horn of the lateral ventricle.
  - Trigone of the lateral ventricle: An area of the lateral ventricle at the confluence of the occipital and temporal horns, where the choroid plexus may be enlarged [21, 24–26].

- Lesions' appearance:
  - Round to ovoid in shape.
  - The lesions typically range in size from 3 mm to 16–20 mm in diameter along the long axis. Punctate lesions smaller than 3 mm should not be considered when assessing MRI criteria.
  - Tumefactive lesions larger than 20 mm are rare.
  - Cortical lesions have a curvilinear shape (specific to MS), or they can be oval or wedge-like.
  - Infratentorial lesions present as discrete subpial "linings" along the periphery of the brainstem, follow nerve root entry zones, or have a round to ovoid shape if located centrally in the brainstem or cerebellum [21, 24, 25].
- Lesions' signal on MRI:
  - Lesions show a hyperintense signal on T2-weighted images.
  - Some T2 hyperintense lesions appear hypointense on spin-echo T1-weighted imaging. There are two types of T1-hypointense lesions:
    A. New lesions that disappear within 6–12 months, likely due to remyelination or resolution of edema.
    B. T1-hypointense lesions that persist beyond 12 months, referred to as "black holes," which represent areas of permanent focal axonal loss. The presence of black holes may have negative prognostic value for future disability progression [27, 28].
  - The majority of acute MS lesions do not exhibit restricted diffusion on diffusion-weighted imaging (DWI) and apparent diffusion coefficient (ADC) maps. However, approximately 14% may show restricted diffusion at the lesions' edge (periphery) over a period of several days to 2–3 weeks, with significant restriction occurring within the first 7 days of lesion formation. In these cases, restricted diffusion can precede contrast enhancement, potentially resembling ischemic lesions. In contrast, acute ischemic lesions typically show contrast enhancement later, during the days to weeks following the onset of infarction [29–31].
- Contrast Enhancement:
  - The presence of contrast-enhancing lesions on T1 postcontrast images indicate acute inflammation with blood-brain barrier breakdown. Enhancement in MS persists only 2–8 weeks (typically 3–4 weeks).

  - Similar to T2 lesions, the enhancing lesion should have a long axis of at least 3 mm.
  - Contrast enhancement typically follows a nodular pattern (68%). Larger lesions may exhibit an open-ring (horseshoe) pattern of enhancement (23%). The closed-ring pattern is less common and usually observed in tumors or abscesses. The open-ring pattern is generally open towards the side that abuts the ventricles or cortical gray matter [24, 25, 32, 33].
  - Leptomeningeal enhancement on post-contrast T1 images (greater than 5 minutes after contrast administration) is rare and serves as a red flag for the diagnosis of MS.
  - In contrast, focal leptomeningeal enhancement seen on post-contrast FLAIR images (15 minutes after contrast administration) is relatively common, indicating focal meningeal inflammation, and is more pronounced in advanced disease stages [34, 35].
  - Punctate or miliary contrast enhancement is atypical for MS.
  - Spontaneous T1 hyperintense signal (without the application of contrast agent) may indicate calcification, hemorrhage, or melanin.
  - Occasionally, focal increased T1 signal on post-contrast images may be attributed to flow artifacts from vessels or capillary telangiectasia [24].
- Perilesional changes:
  - Typically, there is either no or only minimal vasogenic edema and mass effect [24, 25].
- Evolution over time:
  - Extremely frequent occurrence of asymptomatic (clinically silent) new and newly enlarging lesions.
  - Lesions may enlarge, shrink, or remain stable over time, but it is extremely rare for them to completely disappear.
  - However, some lesions in certain MS mimickers may completely resolve, which can serve as a red flag for the diagnosis of MS [24, 36].
- Brain atrophy:
  - Increased rate of whole-brain and regional brain volume loss, which mildly correlates with neurological disability. The highest rate of brain atrophy is observed in the thalamus, corpus callosum, cortical gray matter, and cerebellum [37–40].
- Central vein sign (CVS):
  - MS pathology typically occurs around veins and venules.
  - Therefore, the CVS is observed in most patients with MS (>80%).
  - CVS is defined as a thin hypointense line or small dot (<2 mm) running partially or entirely, but centrally, through a lesion that is at least 3 mm in diameter and not confluent.
  - CVS is less frequently observed in cortical gray matter compared to white matter lesions.
  - A cut-off of >50% in patients with less than ten white matter lesion, or the presence of at least six lesions with CVS can be used to diagnose MS in specific situations [24, 41–46].

- Paramagnetic rim lesions (PRLs)
  - Chronic active lesions contain iron-enriched macrophages and microglia at the lesion edges.
  - The paramagnetic properties of iron deposits at the edges of these lesions can be visualized as a hypointense partial or complete rim on susceptibility-weighted imaging (SWI), quantitative susceptibility mapping (QSM), or T2*-weighted images.
  - While the majority of PRLs slowly expand, a minority may shrink.
  - Occur in about 40% of patients.
  - PRLs are highly specific for MS, and presence of one or more PRLs can be used to diagnose MS in specific situations. They can also aid in differential diagnosis, particularly when used in conjunction with the CVS.
  - Associated with a higher disease burden.
- Slowly evolving lesions (SELs):
  - Occur 10 times more frequently than PRLs.
  - A proportion of SELs can also be classified as PRLs.
  - Reflect chronic inflammation and neuronal tissue loss.
  - Have greater T1 hypointense volume and are more likely to develop into persistent black holes compared to non-SEL lesions.
  - Although more common in advanced stages of the disease, they can also occur in early disease and are associated with a higher disease burden.
  - The majority of PRLs can also be classified as SELs.
  - Chronic lesions identified as both PRL and SEL are associated with the most severe brain tissue damage [25, 46–48].
- Brain imaging red flags:
  - Rarely, a patient with advanced neurological disability may exhibit a relatively small lesion burden in the CNS. Sometimes, this could be explained by microstructural tissue damage and predominant cortical neuronal loss, which are challenging to detect using conventional imaging techniques [49, 50].
  - A comprehensive list is provided in the chapter titled "Imaging Red Flags and Key Features in the Differential Diagnosis of Multiple Sclerosis."

1.6 Spinal Cord Imaging

- The vast majority of patients with MS (80–85%) have spinal cord lesions. Compared to brain lesions, these are more often symptomatic than asymptomatic.
- Lesions' location:
  - Lesions tend to align with the long axis of the cord and most often affect the white and gray matter of the cervical and upper thoracic spine.
  - They involve less than 50% of the axial cord area.
  - Lesions are typically located in the peripheral dorsal and/or lateral spinal cord and usually reach the outer surface of the cord.

  - However, lesions can also be found in the anterior white matter and central gray matter, although lesions strictly located in the gray matter are uncommon.
- Lesions appearance:
  - Typically, T2-hyperintense and T1-hypointense or isointense.
  - Usually small (but >3 mm in diameter), short (one to two spinal segments) lesions.
  - Circumscribed (well-demarcated).
  - Cigarette-shaped on sagittal images and wedge-shaped on axial images.
  - Long lesions are extremely rare in MS, and when present, they usually result from the coalescence of adjacent lesions.
  - A proportion of patients exhibit not only focal but also diffuse spinal cord lesions, making it difficult to distinguish them from artifacts. The origin of diffuse spinal cord lesions remains unclear, with several hypotheses proposed, including the transition of focal lesions to diffuse lesions as the disease progresses. Diffuse spinal cord lesions are not included in the current MS diagnostic criteria due to their low specificity and limited reliability in lesion detection.
- Contrast enhancement:
  - Acute lesions may occasionally show contrast enhancement (mostly nodular, less frequently open-ring or closed-ring), but this is less common compared to acute lesions in the brain.
- Perilesional changes:
  - Acute spinal cord lesions may be accompanied by mild edema and an increase in regional spinal cord volume.
  - Perifocal edema is typically less pronounced relative to lesion size compared to tumors.
- Evolution over time:
  - Lesions may enlarge, shrink, or remain stable over time, but they very rarely disappear completely.
- Spinal cord atrophy:
  - Many patients with MS exhibit spinal cord atrophy, which correlates with disability. The rate of spinal cord volume loss is typically faster than that of the brain.
- Spinal cord imaging red flags:
  - Spinal cord imaging appears to be less useful for the differential diagnosis of MS in children compared to adults [24, 51–54].
  - The comprehensive list is provided in the chapter titled "Imaging Red Flags and Key Features in the Differential Diagnosis of Multiple Sclerosis" (Fig. 1.1).

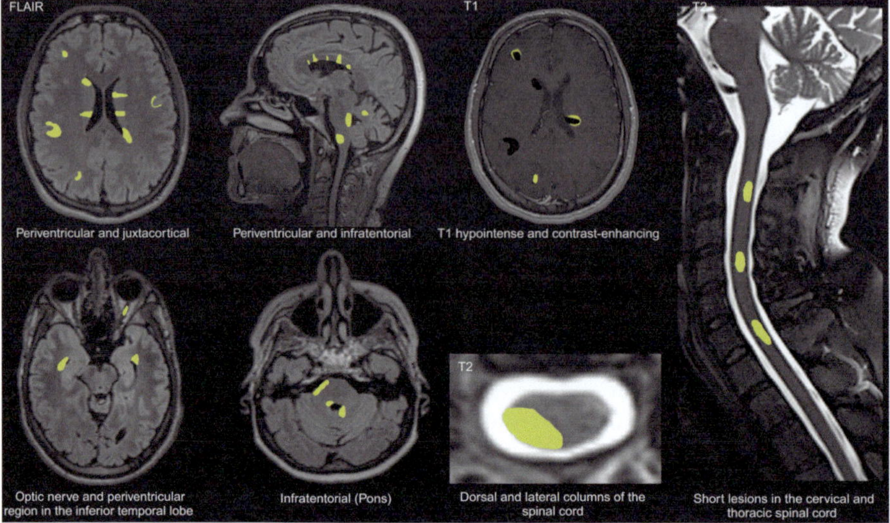

Fig. 1.1 Typical location and appearance of lesions in multiple sclerosis (MS)

1.7 Blood Work

- Routine testing typically yields normal results.
- Higher concentrations of low-density lipoprotein cholesterol (LDL-C) are associated with slightly higher disability, lesion burden, and brain atrophy [55].
- All patients with MS are EBV antibody seropositive [56].
- Higher concentrations of neurofilament light chain, an unspecific marker of neuroaxonal loss, are associated with increased clinical and radiological disease activity. These levels typically decrease following treatment intervention, but they are, in general, not useful in differentiating MS from other conditions [57–59].

1.8 Examination of CSF

- Concentrations of lactate and glucose are normal.
- Elevated protein concentration is infrequent (10%) and usually mild.
- Similarly, a mildly increased albumin quotient is relatively rare and associated with a higher rate of brain atrophy and elevated levels of neurofilament light chain, indicating greater neuroaxonal loss [60–63].
- Normal cytology (80–85%) or mild mononuclear pleocytosis (<50 cells/mm^3) (15–20%), typically without neutrophils and eosinophils [62–65].

- CSF-restricted oligoclonal immunoglobulin G (IgG) bands (OCB) are almost always present (>90–95% of continental European patients; lower frequency in Asian, African, and South American patients) and persist over time regardless of clinical disease activity and treatment [63, 66–68].
- Disease-modifying treatments for MS may decrease protein concentration, pleocytosis, albumin quotient, and IgG index, and they may reduce the occurrence of CSF-restricted OCB, although the latter is rare. Notably, around 10% of patients on natalizumab experienced a disappearance of CSF-restricted OCB positivity [68–70].

1.9 Kappa Free Light Chain

- Kappa free light chains (KFLC) are small immunoglobulin fragments that reflect and quantify B-cell activity. The KFLC index and intrathecal fraction (IF), measures of intrathecal production of free kappa chains, have been suggested as alternatives to CSF-restricted OCB for diagnosing MS.
- The automated, easy-to-perform, reliable, and standardized analysis of this quantitative measure may provide an advantage over the relatively unstandardized and time-consuming qualitative assessment of OCB.
- Although the combined analysis of both CSF-restricted OCB and the KFLC index or IF does not appear to improve diagnostic performance, it does enhance the specificity of MS diagnosis, which may be particularly important for the differential diagnosis of MS in patients with atypical phenotypes [71–73].
- The following cut-offs have been proposed for diagnosing MS:
  - McDonald 2024 criteria: KFLC index >6.1 [75]
  - Other suggested cut-offs included KFLC index >8.92 and KFLC IF >67.3% for typical MS cases; and KFLC index >11.56 and KFLC IF >67.9% for atypical MS cases [72]
- Many authors suggest that the KFLC index or IF could be used in clinical practice as alternatives to OCB for diagnosing MS [72, 74]. KFLC index is included in the new McDonald 2024 diagnostic criteria for MS and can substitute CSF-restricted OCB in diagnosis of MS [46].
- It is important to note that increased KFLC index and IF may be observed not only in MS but also in other conditions such as viral encephalitis, neuroborreliosis, syphilis, anti-N-methyl-D-aspartate receptor (NMDAR)-encephalitis, primary angiitis of the CNS (PACNS), amyotrophic lateral sclerosis (ALS), non-inflammatory polyneuropathy, or stroke [76].

1.10 Fundoscopy

- Fundoscopy may show papillitis and a hyperemic optic disc with blurred margins or normal findings. Optic disc pallor, especially in the temporal region, is commonly observed after optic neuritis, even in cases where there is near-complete clinical recovery [14, 77].

1.11 OCT

- Optical coherence tomography (OCT) measures the unmyelinated axons in the eye and can reflect the overall neural degeneration in MS.
- In acute optic neuritis, the peripapillary retinal nerve fiber layer (RNFL) thickness may be normal or slightly increased, depending on the extent of optic disc edema.
- Optic neuritis often (75%) leads to permanent neuroaxonal injury, quantified as thinning of the RNFL and macular ganglion cell-inner plexiform layer (GCIPL) layers of the inner retina. Most patients with acute optic neuritis experience a loss of 10–20 μm in RNFL thickness within 3–6 months after the onset of optic neuritis. Abnormal OCT supporting optic nerve involvement is defined as an inter-eye difference of at least 6 μm in peripapillary RNFL thickness or at least 4 μm in composite macular GCIPL thickness, with no better alternative explanation. Optic nerve involvement identified by OCT represents the fifth anatomical location that can be used for the diagnosis of MS.
- In chronic stages, progressive thinning of the RNFL (in average by 46%) and the GCIPL is frequently found.
- The extent of RNFL and GCIPL thinning predicts long-term visual impairment and correlates with disability and brain atrophy.
- RNFL thickness is also reduced in the eyes without previous optic neuritis and is associated with optic radiation damage (in average by 26–28%).
- The greatest reductions in RNFL are observed in the temporal quadrants.
- This can be explained by the combination of several factors that make the temporal quadrant of the optic disc particularly susceptible to damage in MS.
  - The temporal quadrant of the optic disc contains axons from the macular region, including those within the papillomacular bundle. This bundle carries a high density of small-caliber axons that project to the parvocellular layers of the lateral geniculate nucleus, which are more vulnerable to damage from demyelinating processes.
  - The demyelinating lesions in MS often affect the smaller, more delicate axons, which are concentrated in the temporal quadrant.
  - The temporal part of the optic nerve and its associated fibers have a higher metabolic demand and are more susceptible to ischemic damage.
  - Since the temporal RNFL is associated with the central visual field, its damage is more likely to be symptomatic and noticed clinically.
- However, this preferential loss of axons in the temporal quadrant of the RNFL is not entirely specific to MS [14, 46, 77–80].

1.12 Electrophysiological Studies

- Visual evoked potentials (VEP)
  - Delayed P100 latency present in 42–100% of patients with MS and in 77–100% of those during optic neuritis.

  - During acute optic neuritis, there is typically a delay in the latency of wave P100 as well as a reduction in amplitude. As the patient recovers from optic neuritis, the amplitude often improves, but the latency usually remains elevated.
  - Therefore, typically seen an increase in P100 latency (>115 ms) without a decrease in amplitude, which is typical for demyelinating optic neuropathy in MS. A marked or disproportionally reduced amplitude suggesting concurrent axonal injury is infrequent in MS (red flag), as the amplitude is usually normal or only mildly reduced.
  - VEP may help detect subtle subclinical optic nerve injury or confirm a history of previous clinical or subclinical optic neuritis. Therefore, delayed latencies are commonly present not only in the eye affected by optic neuritis but also in the contralateral, non-optic neuritis eye of patients with MS, likely due to subclinical demyelination.
  - It has been suggested to include optic nerve pathology, as assessed by VEP, as a fifth region in the current dissemination in space (DIS) criteria. Abnormal VEP supporting optic nerve involvement is defined as a delayed latency (or asymmetric inter-ocular latencies) 2.5 standard deviations greater than the mean for both absolute peak P100 latency and inter-ocular latency, whose exact numerical measures depend on technical and methodological factors, and are also dependent on centre oand device. Optic nerve involvement identified by VEP represents the fifth anatomical location that can be used for the diagnosis of MS [13, 46, 78, 81].
- Brainstem auditory evoked potentials (BAEP)
  - May be used to detect clinical and subclinical pathology in the auditory pathways, including the auditory nerve and brainstem. However, its sensitivity for detecting brainstem involvement is relatively low [81].
- Somatosensory evoked potentials (SSEP)
  - Evaluate mostly dorsal columns and the thalamo-cortical sensory system. Their value lies in detecting of pathology in symptomatic patients with normal imaging (for example increased latencies of upper thoracic response, P14 wave from the brainstem or cortical response).
  - They have also a value in predicting of future disability.
  - Although, the spinal cord MRI is the more sensitive marker of the spinal involvement, SSEP are more closely associated with disability [81, 82].
- MEP (Motor-evoked potentials)
  - Evaluate the corticospinal tract. Increased central motor conduction time is correlated with EDSS and predict future disability [81].
- Conduction studies and electromyography (EMG):
  - Small proportion of the examined nerves (14.2–16.5%) show subtle subclinical pathological findings without evidence of small-fiber pathology [83, 84]. However, marked peripheral neuropathy is atypical for MS and is considered as a red flag [11].

1.13 Diagnosis of Relapsing-Remitting MS

- There is no single specific biomarker for MS, and diagnosis relies on integration of clinical, imaging, and laboratory findings.
- It is crucial to emphasize that the original McDonald diagnostic criteria were not designed to differentiate MS from other conditions but rather to identify MS or a high likelihood of the disease in patients with a typical CIS, once other diagnoses have been considered unlikely. It should be emphasized, however, that the newest 2024 McDonald diagnostic criteria also aim, at least partially, to assist in the differential diagnosis.
- The McDonald 2024 diagnostic criteria are based on several key principles.

1. Identification of a syndrome "typical" of MS-related demyelination:
   - Presence of one of a limited number of syndromes typical for an MS-related demyelinating attack or relapse including uni-lateral optic neuritis, focal supratentorial syndrome, focal brainstem syndrome, cerebellar syndrome, or partial myelitis.
   - The McDonald criteria were validated only in patients presenting with the aforementioned syndrome. Therefore, their application in patients with other clinical presentations must be undertaken with great caution. However, according to the 2024 McDonald criteria, MS can also be diagnosed in patients with RIS (without clinical manifestations) or in those with neurological symptoms that do not constitute a clear typical attack or progressive disability (e.g., paroxysmal symptoms or other non-specific neurological signs), provided that dissemination in space and time is demonstrated (see details below).
2. Objective clinical or paraclinical evidence of CNS involvement:
   - Examples: a presence of RAPD, delayed P100 latency on VEP or optic nerve lesion in a patient with optic neuritis; or a presence of internuclear ophthalmoplegia or brainstem lesion in patient with diplopia; or a detection of a hemisensory level or spinal cord lesion or abnormal somatosensory evoked potentials in a patient with sensory or motor symptoms suggestive of myelitis.
   - In contrast, in patients with neurological symptoms (such as visual loss) but a normal neurological examination and not corresponding MRI or other paraclinical findings, caution is warranted before making a diagnosis of MS. Applying the McDonald criteria without objective evidence reduces their specificity for MS.
3. Demonstration of dissemination in space (DIS), indicating a multi-focal CNS process, can be demonstrated by
   A. One or more T2-hyperintense lesions in two or more of five MS-typical areas of the CNS: optic nerve, periventricular, cortical/juxtacortical, and infratentorial brain regions, and the spinal cord. Both symptomatic and asymptomatic MRI lesions are considered.
   B. In patients with a typical clinical presentation or steady disability progression for at least 12 months, the presence of one or more T2-hyperintense lesions in at least four of the five MS-typical CNS regions is sufficient to establish the diagnosis of MS.
   C. In patients with PPMS, the presence of two spinal cord lesions is sufficient to establish DIS. In other words, a second spinal cord lesion can substitute

for an additional brain anatomical location in patients with primary progressive disease.

D. An additional clinical attack affecting a different CNS site is no longer sufficient to demonstrate DIS under the 2024 McDonald diagnostic criteria.

4. Demonstration of dissemination in time (DIT) can be demonstrated by
   A. An additional clinical attack occurring at least 30 days after the previous relapse. Care should be taken when accepting symptoms that are based solely on patient-reported subjective changes, especially in the absence of objective evidence of a current or past attack.
   B. The simultaneous presence of gadolinium-enhancing and non-enhancing lesions.
   C. Occurrence of a new T2-hyperintense or gadolinium-enhancing lesion on follow-up MRI, with reference to a baseline scan, irrespective of the timing of the baseline MRI.
   D. Presence of two or more CSF-restricted OCB or positive KFLC index.
   E. However, under the 2024 McDonald criteria, DIT is no longer a mandatory requirement for diagnosing MS.
5. "No better explanation" other than MS
   - Many different disorders may fulfill the diagnostic criteria for MS; therefore, careful attention to red flags is essential before confirming an MS diagnosis. Having detailed knowledge of the numerous red flags associated with disorders that can mimic MS is challenging, sometimes making it difficult to avoid misdiagnosing MS. Therefore, the diagnosis of MS should be periodically reassessed.
   - The threshold for additional testing and a detailed search for red flags should be low, particularly in situations where
     - Clinical and imaging evidence supporting a diagnosis of MS is insufficient.
     - There are clinical or paraclinical features atypical of MS.
     - Primary progressive MS is being considered.
     - In patients with disease onset at age 50 or older, and in those with significant vascular risk factors (e.g., hypertension, smoking, diabetes, dyslipidaemia), it is strongly recommended to confirm the diagnosis by demonstrating a spinal cord lesion, CSF positivity, or the presence of the CVS [11, 18, 21, 46, 85, 86].

1.14 Diagnosis of Radiologically Isolated Syndrome (RIS)

- According to the McDonald 2024 criteria, in patients with incidental discovery of MS typical CNS white matter lesions or patients with non-specific manifestations can be diagnosed MS. Diagnosis of MS can be diagnosed in patients with RIS, who fulfill DIS and DIT (lesion activity or simultaneous presence contrast-enhancing and non-enhancing lesions); or fulfill DIS and have positive CSF-restricted OCB or positive KFLC index; or fulfil DIS and have at least 6 lesions with CVS. To remind again, DIS according to the McDonald 2024 criteria can be diagnosed in patients with typical lesions in two of the five regions (i.e., optic nerve, intracortical or juxtacortical, periventricular, infratentorial, and spinal cord), regardless of whether these lesions are symptomatic. For reference, the previous RIS criteria are summarised below [46].

- 2009 criteria (more strict Okuda criteria):
  - For dissemination in space is required at least three of the four features
    - Nine or more (T2-hyperintense) lesions or one contrast-enhancing lesion in the brain
    - Three periventricular lesions
    - One juxtacortical lesion
    - One infratentorial or spinal lesion
  - For dissemination in time is required at one of the two features:
    - One contrast-enhancing lesion 3 months after baseline
    - One new T2-hyperintense lesion at follow-up MRI [20]
- 2023 criteria:
  - Some asymptomatic individuals might exhibit only one or two of the four disseminations in space (DIS) criteria but still have lesions highly suggestive of MS. Therefore, updated criteria have been developed.
  - For dissemination in space is required
    - Presence of one or more T2-hyperintense lesions (ovoid, well circumscribed; ≥3 mm in length) in one or more of four areas of the CNS: periventricular, cortical or juxtacortical, and infra-tentorial brain regions, and the spinal cord (optic nerve involvement is not considered yet).
  - In addition, is required at least two of the three features:
    - Spinal cord lesion
    - CSF-restricted OCB
    - Occurrence of new T2-hyperintense or contrast-enhancing lesions
- If patients who met the previous (2019 and 2023) criteria experienced a clinical relapse, they could be diagnosed with MS [87].

1.15 Diagnosis of Clinically Isolated Syndrome (CIS)

- CIS refers to a first episode of neurological symptoms suggestive of CNS demyelination, lasting at least 24 h and occurring in the absence of fever or infection. However, this episode does not yet fulfil the diagnostic criteria for MS [21, 46].

1.16 Diagnosis of Primary Progressive MS (PPMS)

- Clinical requirements:
  - Patients demonstrate steady increase of objectively documented neurological disability, independent of relapses, over a period of at least 12 months (assessed either retrospectively or prospectively). Fluctuations, periods of stability, and superimposed relapses are acceptable.
- Paraclinical requirements:
  - The 2024 McDonald criteria for diagnosing PPMS are the same as those for RRMS. The only exception is that the presence of a second spinal cord lesion can substitute for an additional brain anatomical location [21, 46].

1.17 The McDonald 2024 Diagnostic Criteria

- The new diagnostic criteria for MS are expected to enhance specificity and allow for earlier diagnosis. The major advances include:
  - The optic nerve is now recognised as a fifth anatomical location. Optic nerve involvement can be demonstrated by MRI, OCT, or VEP. In addition, the criteria for demonstrating dissemination in space have been revised (Table 1.1).
  - The CVS and PRLs are not required for diagnosis but can support the diagnosis of MS in specific situations.
  - Demonstration of dissemination in time is no longer essential for diagnosis of MS in all patients.
  - The KFLC index is interchangeable with CSF-restricted OCB and can substitute for OCB for diagnosis of MS.
  - In patients with RIS or non-specific clinical presentations, fulfilling DIS together with DIT, positive CSF, or the presence of CVS is sufficient for diagnosing MS.
  - The 2024 McDonald criteria provide a unified framework for the diagnosis of both relapsing- and progressive-onset MS, as well as paediatric- and adult-onset MS [46].
  - A summary of potential scenarios for diagnosing MS using the 2024 McDonald criteria is provided in Table 1.1.

Table 1.1 Summary of potential scenarios for diagnosing MS using the 2024 McDonald criteria [46]

Clinical onset	Brain MRI lesions located	Additional requirements 1	Additional requirements 2	Diagnosis of MS
Typical, suggestive of MS	Lesions in 4–5 CNS sites (out of 5[a]) → DIS+	–	–	Yes[f]
	Lesions in 2–3 CNS sites (out of 5[a]) → DIS+	Presence of DIT[b] or positive CSF[c] or positive CVS[d]	–	Yes[f]
	Lesion in 1 CNS site (out of 5[a]) → DIS–	Presence of DIT[b] or positive CSF[c]	Positive CVS[d] or positive PRLs[e]	Yes[f]
RIS or atypical presentation	Lesions in ≥2 CNS sites (out of 5[a]) → DIS+	Presence of DIT[b] or positive CSF[c] or positive CVS[d]	–	Yes

Note: The same diagnostic algorithm applies to patients with primary progressive MS, with the only exception that the presence of a second spinal cord lesion can substitute for an additional brain anatomical site

Legend: *CNS* central nervous system; *CVS* central vein sign; *DIT* dissemination in time; *DIS* dissemination in space; *MS* multiple sclerosis; *PRLs* paramagnetic rim lesion; + positive; – negative

[a]Five anatomical locations typically affected in MS include the optic nerve, intracortical or juxtacortical regions, periventricular region, infratentorial region, and spinal cord.

[b]DIT (dissemination in time) can be demonstrated by:
Occurrence of a new clinical relapse
New active lesion (new or contrast-enhancing) on MRI
Simultaneous presence of contrast-enhancing and non-enhancing lesions

[c]Positive cerebrospinal fluid (CSF):
≥2 CSF-restricted oligoclonal bands (OCB) or
Elevated kappa free light chain (KFLC) index

[d]Positive CVS:
≥6 lesions with a central vein sign (CVS) or
≥5 lesions with CVS in patients with <10 white matter lesions

[e]Positive PRLs:
≥1 lesion with paramagnetic rim

[f]Patients with a typical clinical presentation suggestive of MS, but who do not fulfill the paraclinical diagnostic criteria, can be diagnosed with clinically isolated syndrome (CIS)

1.18 Treatment

- Currently, there is no cure for MS. Available treatments primarily aim to prevent or reduce neuroinflammation.
- High-dose corticosteroids and in some cases, plasmapheresis are used for management of acute relapses.
- Long-term therapy to prevent disease activity includes a variety of immune therapies with specific mechanisms and targets. At present, new immuno-modulatory (disease-modifying) treatments are the most effective options for managing MS. However, a significant challenge is that most therapies are effective mainly during the early stages of the disease, with limited impact on the later, progressive phases. Most MS therapies significantly alter the survival and trafficking of

immune cells (alemtuzumab; anti-CD20 drugs; cladribine; dimethyl fumarate; glatiramer acetate; interferon-beta; natalizumab; S1P inhibitors; teriflunomide). In addition, cytostatic therapies such as cyclophosphamide, mitoxantrone, or azathioprine are rarely used as off-label immunosuppressive treatment, usually for patients not indicated or responding to established disease-modifying treatment.
- In addition, a wide range of symptomatic drugs including analgesics, spasmolytics, anti-spastics, antidepressants, or anxiolytics is used for relief of various symptoms associated with CNS dysfunction [10, 88].
- Finally, psychotherapy, aerobic and anaerobic exercises, rehabilitation, physiotherapy, and ergotherapy are important elements of successful and comprehensive care for MS patients [89].
- Early initiation of effective immunomodulatory treatment is associated with better prognosis [90–93].
- A detailed description of the mechanisms of action of various drugs and treatment strategies is beyond the scope of this publication.

1.19 Prognosis

- On average, MS is associated with a lifespan that is 5–10 years shorter than that in the general population. However, this gap is narrowing owing to advancements in treatment and care [94].

References

1. Walton C, King R, Rechtman L, Kaye W, Leray E, Marrie RA, et al. Rising prevalence of multiple sclerosis worldwide: insights from the Atlas of MS, third edition. Mult Scler. 2020;26(14):1816–21.
2. Koch-Henriksen N, Sørensen PS. The changing demographic pattern of multiple sclerosis epidemiology. Lancet Neurol. 2010;9(5):520–32.
3. Mahad DH, Trapp BD, Lassmann H. Pathological mechanisms in progressive multiple sclerosis. Lancet Neurol. 2015;14(2):183–93.
4. Hemmer B, Kerschensteiner M, Korn T. Role of the innate and adaptive immune responses in the course of multiple sclerosis. Lancet Neurol. 2015;14(4):406–19.
5. Weiner HL. The challenge of multiple sclerosis: how do we cure a chronic heterogeneous disease? Ann Neurol. 2009;65(3):239–48.
6. Baecher-Allan C, Kaskow BJ, Weiner HL. Multiple sclerosis: mechanisms and immunotherapy. Neuron. 2018;97(4):742–68.
7. International Multiple Sclerosis Genetics C, Beecham AH, Patsopoulos NA, Xifara DK, Davis MF, Kemppinen A, et al. Analysis of immune-related loci identifies 48 new susceptibility variants for multiple sclerosis. Nat Genet. 2013;45(11):1353–60.
8. International Multiple Sclerosis Genetics C, Hafler DA, Compston A, Sawcer S, Lander ES, Daly MJ, et al. Risk alleles for multiple sclerosis identified by a genomewide study. N Engl J Med. 2007;357(9):851–62.
9. Olsson T, Barcellos LF, Alfredsson L. Interactions between genetic, lifestyle and environmental risk factors for multiple sclerosis. Nat Rev Neurol. 2017;13(1):25–36.
10. Jakimovski D, Bittner S, Zivadinov R, Morrow SA, Benedict RH, Zipp F, et al. Multiple sclerosis. Lancet. 2024;403(10422):183–202.

11. Solomon AJ, Arrambide G, Brownlee WJ, Flanagan EP, Amato MP, Amezcua L, et al. Differential diagnosis of suspected multiple sclerosis: an updated consensus approach. Lancet Neurol. 2023;22(8):750–68.
12. Kurtzke JF. Rating neurologic impairment in multiple sclerosis: an expanded disability status scale (EDSS). Neurology. 1983;33(11):1444–52.
13. Vidal-Jordana A, Rovira A, Arrambide G, Otero-Romero S, Río J, Comabella M, et al. Optic nerve topography in multiple sclerosis diagnosis: the utility of visual evoked potentials. Neurology. 2021;96(4):e482–e90.
14. Toosy AT, Mason DF, Miller DH. Optic neuritis. Lancet Neurol. 2014;13(1):83–99.
15. Bennett JL, Costello F, Chen JJ, Petzold A, Biousse V, Newman NJ, et al. Optic neuritis and autoimmune optic neuropathies: advances in diagnosis and treatment. Lancet Neurol. 2023;22(1):89–100.
16. Petzold A, Fraser CL, Abegg M, Alroughani R, Alshowaeir D, Alvarenga R, et al. Diagnosis and classification of optic neuritis. Lancet Neurol. 2022;21(12):1120–34.
17. Miller DH, Weinshenker BG, Filippi M, Banwell BL, Cohen JA, Freedman MS, et al. Differential diagnosis of suspected multiple sclerosis: a consensus approach. Mult Scler. 2008;14(9):1157–74.
18. Hua LH, Solomon AJ, Tenembaum S, Scalfari A, Rovira À, Rostasy K, et al. Differential diagnosis of suspected multiple sclerosis in pediatric and late-onset populations: a review. JAMA Neurol. 2024;
19. Romero-Pinel L, Bau L, Matas E, León I, Muñoz-Vendrell A, Arroyo P, et al. The age at onset of relapsing-remitting multiple sclerosis has increased over the last five decades. Mult Scler Relat Disord. 2022;68:104103.
20. Okuda DT, Mowry EM, Beheshtian A, Waubant E, Baranzini SE, Goodin DS, et al. Incidental MRI anomalies suggestive of multiple sclerosis: the radiologically isolated syndrome. Neurology. 2009;72(9):800–5.
21. Thompson AJ, Banwell BL, Barkhof F, Carroll WM, Coetzee T, Comi G, et al. Diagnosis of multiple sclerosis: 2017 revisions of the McDonald criteria. Lancet Neurol. 2018;17(2):162–73.
22. Lublin FD, Reingold SC, Cohen JA, Cutter GR, Sorensen PS, Thompson AJ, et al. Defining the clinical course of multiple sclerosis: the 2013 revisions. Neurology. 2014;83(3):278–86.
23. Heward KD, Roy-Hewitson C, Solomon AJ. Multiple sclerosis presenting with paroxysmal symptoms: patients at the limitations of current diagnostic criteria. Mult Scler. 2024;30(11–12):1566–70.
24. Filippi M, Preziosa P, Banwell BL, Barkhof F, Ciccarelli O, De Stefano N, et al. Assessment of lesions on magnetic resonance imaging in multiple sclerosis: practical guidelines. Brain. 2019;142(7):1858–75.
25. Wattjes MP, Ciccarelli O, Reich DS, Banwell B, de Stefano N, Enzinger C, et al. 2021 MAGNIMS-CMSC-NAIMS consensus recommendations on the use of MRI in patients with multiple sclerosis. Lancet Neurol. 2021;20(8):653–70.
26. Bouman PM, Steenwijk MD, Pouwels PJW, Schoonheim MM, Barkhof F, Jonkman LE, et al. Histopathology-validated recommendations for cortical lesion imaging in multiple sclerosis. Brain. 2020;143(10):2988–97.
27. Trapp BD, Peterson J, Ransohoff RM, Rudick R, Mörk S, Bö L. Axonal transection in the lesions of multiple sclerosis. N Engl J Med. 1998;338(5):278–85.
28. Barkhof F, McGowan JC, van Waesberghe JH, Grossman RI. Hypointense multiple sclerosis lesions on T1-weighted spin echo magnetic resonance images: their contribution in understanding multiple sclerosis evolution. J Neurol Neurosurg Psychiatry. 1998;64 Suppl 1:S77–9.
29. Hyland M, Bermel RA, Cohen JA. Restricted diffusion preceding gadolinium enhancement in large or tumefactive demyelinating lesions. Neurol Clin Pract. 2013;3(1):15–21.
30. Abou Zeid N, Pirko I, Erickson B, Weigand SD, Thomsen KM, Scheithauer B, et al. Diffusion-weighted imaging characteristics of biopsy-proven demyelinating brain lesions. Neurology. 2012;78(21):1655–62.

31. Eisele P, Szabo K, Griebe M, Rossmanith C, Förster A, Hennerici M, et al. Reduced diffusion in a subset of acute MS lesions: a serial multiparametric MRI study. AJNR Am J Neuroradiol. 2012;33(7):1369–73.
32. Guttmann CR, Ahn SS, Hsu L, Kikinis R, Jolesz FA. The evolution of multiple sclerosis lesions on serial MR. AJNR Am J Neuroradiol. 1995;16(7):1481–91.
33. He J, Grossman RI, Ge Y, Mannon LJ. Enhancing patterns in multiple sclerosis: evolution and persistence. AJNR Am J Neuroradiol. 2001;22(4):664–9.
34. Absinta M, Vuolo L, Rao A, Nair G, Sati P, Cortese IC, et al. Gadolinium-based MRI characterization of leptomeningeal inflammation in multiple sclerosis. Neurology. 2015;85(1):18–28.
35. Zivadinov R, Ramasamy DP, Vaneckova M, Gandhi S, Chandra A, Hagemeier J, et al. Leptomeningeal contrast enhancement is associated with progression of cortical atrophy in MS: a retrospective, pilot, observational longitudinal study. Mult Scler. 2017;23(10):1336–45.
36. Sechi E, Krecke KN, Messina SA, Buciuc M, Pittock SJ, Chen JJ, et al. Comparison of MRI lesion evolution in different central nervous system demyelinating disorders. Neurology. 2021;97(11):e1097–e109.
37. Uher T, Krasensky J, Malpas C, Bergsland N, Dwyer MG, Kubala Havrdova E, et al. Evolution of brain volume loss rates in early stages of multiple sclerosis. Neurol Neuroimmunol Neuroinflamm. 2021;8(3)
38. Uher T, Vaneckova M, Krasensky J, Sobisek L, Tyblova M, Volna J, et al. Pathological cut-offs of global and regional brain volume loss in multiple sclerosis. Mult Scler J. 2019;25(4):541–53.
39. Uher T. Clinical relevance of brain atrophy measures in multiple sclerosis. 1st ed. Prague: Karolinum; 2023.
40. Sastre-Garriga J, Pareto D, Battaglini M, Rocca MA, Ciccarelli O, Enzinger C, et al. MAGNIMS consensus recommendations on the use of brain and spinal cord atrophy measures in clinical practice. Nat Rev Neurol. 2020;16(3):171–82.
41. Solomon AJ. Progress towards a diagnostic biomarker for MS: central vein sign. Mult Scler. 2020;26(4):394–6.
42. Cagol A, Cortese R, Barakovic M, Schaedelin S, Ruberte E, Absinta M, et al. Diagnostic performance of cortical lesions and the central vein sign in multiple sclerosis. JAMA Neurol. 2024;81(2):143–53.
43. Sinnecker T, Clarke MA, Meier D, Enzinger C, Calabrese M, De Stefano N, et al. Evaluation of the central vein sign as a diagnostic imaging biomarker in multiple sclerosis. JAMA Neurol. 2019;76(12):1446–56.
44. Sati P, Oh J, Constable RT, Evangelou N, Guttmann CR, Henry RG, et al. The central vein sign and its clinical evaluation for the diagnosis of multiple sclerosis: a consensus statement from the North American Imaging in Multiple Sclerosis Cooperative. Nat Rev Neurol. 2016;12(12):714–22.
45. Maggi P, Absinta M, Grammatico M, Vuolo L, Emmi G, Carlucci G, et al. Central vein sign differentiates Multiple Sclerosis from central nervous system inflammatory vasculopathies. Ann Neurol. 2018;83(2):283–94.
46. Calvi A, Clarke MA, Prados F, Chard D, Ciccarelli O, Alberich M, et al. Relationship between paramagnetic rim lesions and slowly expanding lesions in multiple sclerosis. Mult Scler. 2023;29(3):352–62.
47. Elliott C, Rudko DA, Arnold DL, Fetco D, Elkady AM, Araujo D, et al. Lesion-level correspondence and longitudinal properties of paramagnetic rim and slowly expanding lesions in multiple sclerosis. Mult Scler. 2023;29(6):680–90.
48. Meaton I, Altokhis A, Allen CM, Clarke MA, Sinnecker T, Meier D, et al. Paramagnetic rims are a promising diagnostic imaging biomarker in multiple sclerosis. Mult Scler. 2022;28(14):2212–20.
49. Takewaki D, Lin Y, Sato W, Ono H, Nakamura M, Araki M, et al. Normal brain imaging accompanies neuroimmunologically justified, autoimmune encephalomyelitis. Neurol Neuroimmunol Neuroinflamm. 2018;5(3):e456.

50. Trapp BD, Vignos M, Dudman J, Chang A, Fisher E, Staugaitis SM, et al. Cortical neuronal densities and cerebral white matter demyelination in multiple sclerosis: a retrospective study. Lancet Neurol. 2018;17(10):870–84.
51. Ciccarelli O, Cohen JA, Reingold SC, Weinshenker BG. Spinal cord involvement in multiple sclerosis and neuromyelitis optica spectrum disorders. Lancet Neurol. 2019;18(2):185–97.
52. Andelova M, Uher T, Krasensky J, Sobisek L, Kusova E, Srpova B, et al. Additive effect of spinal cord volume, diffuse and focal cord pathology on disability in multiple sclerosis. Front Neurol. 2019;10
53. Andelova M, Vodehnalova K, Krasensky J, Hardubejova E, Hrnciarova T, Srpova B, et al. Brainstem lesions are associated with diffuse spinal cord involvement in early multiple sclerosis. BMC Neurol. 2022;22(1):270.
54. Lukas C, Sombekke MH, Bellenberg B, Hahn HK, Popescu V, Bendfeldt K, et al. Relevance of spinal cord abnormalities to clinical disability in multiple sclerosis: MR imaging findings in a large cohort of patients. Radiology. 2013;269(2):542–52.
55. Lorincz B, Jury EC, Vrablik M, Ramanathan M, Uher T. The role of cholesterol metabolism in multiple sclerosis: from molecular pathophysiology to radiological and clinical disease activity. Autoimmun Rev. 2022;21(6):103088.
56. Bjornevik K, Cortese M, Healy BC, Kuhle J, Mina MJ, Leng Y, et al. Longitudinal analysis reveals high prevalence of Epstein-Barr virus associated with multiple sclerosis. Science. 2022;375(6578):296–301.
57. Uher T, Havrdova EK, Benkert P, Bergsland N, Krasensky J, Srpova B, et al. Measurement of neurofilaments improves stratification of future disease activity in early multiple sclerosis. Mult Scler. 2021;27(13):2001–13.
58. Uher T, Schaedelin S, Srpova B, Barro C, Bergsland N, Dwyer M, et al. Monitoring of radiologic disease activity by serum neurofilaments in MS. Neurol Neuroimmunol Neuroinflamm. 2020;7(4)
59. Benkert P, Meier S, Schaedelin S, Manouchehrinia A, Yaldizli Ö, Maceski A, et al. Serum neurofilament light chain for individual prognostication of disease activity in people with multiple sclerosis: a retrospective modelling and validation study. Lancet Neurol. 2022;21(3):246–57.
60. Uher T, Horakova D, Tyblova M, Zeman D, Krasulova E, Mrazova K, et al. Increased albumin quotient (QAlb) in patients after first clinical event suggestive of multiple sclerosis is associated with development of brain atrophy and greater disability 48 months later. Mult Scler. 2016;22(6):770–81.
61. Uher T, McComb M, Galkin S, Srpova B, Oechtering J, Barro C, et al. Neurofilament levels are associated with blood-brain barrier integrity, lymphocyte extravasation, and risk factors following the first demyelinating event in multiple sclerosis. Mult Scler. 2021;27(2):220–31.
62. Stangel M, Fredrikson S, Meinl E, Petzold A, Stüve O, Tumani H. The utility of cerebrospinal fluid analysis in patients with multiple sclerosis. Nat Rev Neurol. 2013;9(5):267–76.
63. Deisenhammer F, Zetterberg H, Fitzner B, Zettl UK. The cerebrospinal fluid in multiple sclerosis. Front Immunol. 2019;10:726.
64. Zeman D, Adam P, Kalistová H, Sobek O, Anděl J, Anděl M. Cerebrospinal fluid cytologic findings in multiple sclerosis. A comparison between patient subgroups. Acta Cytol. 2001;45(1):51–9.
65. Vlad B, Reichen I, Neidhart S, Hilty M, Lekaditi D, Heuer C, et al. Basic CSF parameters and MRZ reaction help in differentiating MOG antibody-associated autoimmune disease versus multiple sclerosis. Front Immunol. 2023;14:1237149.
66. Franciotta D, Salvetti M, Lolli F, Serafini B, Aloisi F. B cells and multiple sclerosis. Lancet Neurol. 2008;7(9):852–8.
67. Lechner-Scott J, Spencer B, de Malmanche T, Attia J, Fitzgerald M, Trojano M, et al. The frequency of CSF oligoclonal banding in multiple sclerosis increases with latitude. Mult Scler. 2012;18(7):974–82.
68. Ganapathy Subramanian R, Horakova D, Vaneckova M, Lorincz B, Krasensky J, Kubala Havrdova E, et al. Natalizumab induces changes of cerebrospinal fluid measures in multiple sclerosis. Diagnostics (Basel). 2021;11(12)

69. Schlüter M, Oswald E, Winklmeier S, Meinl I, Havla J, Eichhorn P, et al. Effects of Natalizumab therapy on intrathecal immunoglobulin G production indicate targeting of plasmablasts. Neurol Neuroimmunol Neuroinflamm. 2021;8(5)
70. Harrer A, Tumani H, Niendorf S, Lauda F, Geis C, Weishaupt A, et al. Cerebrospinal fluid parameters of B cell-related activity in patients with active disease during natalizumab therapy. Mult Scler. 2013;19(9):1209–12.
71. Rosenstein I, Rasch S, Axelsson M, Novakova L, Blennow K, Zetterberg H, et al. Kappa free light chain index as a diagnostic biomarker in multiple sclerosis: a real-world investigation. J Neurochem. 2021;159(3):618–28.
72. Levraut M, Laurent-Chabalier S, Ayrignac X, Bigaut K, Rival M, Squalli S, et al. Kappa free light chain biomarkers are efficient for the diagnosis of multiple sclerosis: a large multicenter cohort study. Neurol Neuroimmunol Neuroinflamm. 2023;10(1)
73. Reiber H, Zeman D, Kušnierová P, Mundwiler E, Bernasconi L. Diagnostic relevance of free light chains in cerebrospinal fluid – the hyperbolic reference range for reliable data interpretation in quotient diagrams. Clin Chim Acta. 2019;497:153–62.
74. Arrambide G, Espejo C, Carbonell-Mirabent P, Dieli-Crimi R, Rodríguez-Barranco M, Castillo M, et al. The kappa free light chain index and oligoclonal bands have a similar role in the McDonald criteria. Brain. 2022;145(11):3931–42.
75. Montalban X. et al. Diagnosis of multiple sclerosis: 2024 revisions of the McDonald criteria. Lancet Neurol. 2025;24(10):850–65. https://doi.org/10.1016/S1474-4422(25)00270-4.
76. Konen FF, Schwenkenbecher P, Jendretzky KF, Gingele S, Witte T, Sühs KW, et al. Kappa free light chains in cerebrospinal fluid in inflammatory and non-inflammatory neurological diseases. Brain Sci. 2022;12(4)
77. Suh A, Hampel G, Vinjamuri A, Ong J, Kamran SA, Waisberg E, et al. Oculomics analysis in multiple sclerosis: current ophthalmic clinical and imaging biomarkers. Eye (Lond). 2024;38:2701.
78. Bennett JL. Optic neuritis. Continuum (Minneap Minn). 2019;25(5):1236–64.
79. Evangelou N, Konz D, Esiri MM, Smith S, Palace J, Matthews PM. Size-selective neuronal changes in the anterior optic pathways suggest a differential susceptibility to injury in multiple sclerosis. Brain. 2001;124(Pt 9):1813–20.
80. Frohman EM, Fujimoto JG, Frohman TC, Calabresi PA, Cutter G, Balcer LJ. Optical coherence tomography: a window into the mechanisms of multiple sclerosis. Nat Clin Pract Neurol. 2008;4(12):664–75.
81. Habek M, Adamec I, Barun B, Crnošija L, Gabelić T, Krbot SM. Clinical neurophysiology of multiple sclerosis. Adv Exp Med Biol. 2017;958:129–39.
82. Wuschek A, Bussas M, El Husseini M, Harabacz L, Pineker V, Pongratz V, et al. Somatosensory evoked potentials and magnetic resonance imaging of the central nervous system in early multiple sclerosis. J Neurol. 2023;270(2):824–30.
83. Gartzen K, Katzarava Z, Diener HC, Putzki N. Peripheral nervous system involvement in multiple sclerosis. Eur J Neurol. 2011;18(5):789–91.
84. Anlar O, Tombul T, Kisli M. Peripheral sensory and motor abnormalities in patients with multiple sclerosis. Electromyogr Clin Neurophysiol. 2003;43(6):349–51.
85. Solomon AJ, Pettigrew R, Naismith RT, Chahin S, Krieger S, Weinshenker B. Challenges in multiple sclerosis diagnosis: misunderstanding and misapplication of the McDonald criteria. Mult Scler. 2021;27(2):250–8.
86. Solomon AJ. Diagnosis, differential diagnosis, and misdiagnosis of multiple sclerosis. Continuum (Minneap Minn). 2019;25(3):611–35.
87. Lebrun-Frenay C, Kantarci O, Siva A, Azevedo CJ, Makhani N, Pelletier D, et al. Radiologically isolated syndrome. Lancet Neurol. 2023;22(11):1075–86.
88. Wiendl H, Gold R, Berger T, Derfuss T, Linker R, Mäurer M, et al. Multiple Sclerosis Therapy Consensus Group (MSTCG): position statement on disease-modifying therapies for multiple sclerosis (white paper). Ther Adv Neurol Disord. 2021;14:17562864211039648.
89. Brown TR, Kraft GH. Exercise and rehabilitation for individuals with multiple sclerosis. Phys Med Rehabil Clin N Am. 2005;16(2):513–55.

90. Uher T, Adzima A, Srpova B, Noskova L, Marechal B, Maceski AM, et al. Diagnostic delay of multiple sclerosis: prevalence, determinants and consequences. Mult Scler. 2023;29(11–12):1437–51.
91. Cobo-Calvo A, Tur C, Otero-Romero S, Carbonell-Mirabent P, Ruiz M, Pappolla A, et al. Association of very early treatment Initiation with the risk of long-term disability in patients with a first demyelinating event. Neurology. 2023;101(13):e1280–e92.
92. Brown JWL, Coles A, Horakova D, Havrdova E, Izquierdo G, Prat A, et al. Association of initial disease-modifying therapy with later conversion to secondary progressive multiple sclerosis. JAMA. 2019;321(2):175–87.
93. He A, Merkel B, Brown JWL, Zhovits Ryerson L, Kister I, Malpas CB, et al. Timing of high-efficacy therapy for multiple sclerosis: a retrospective observational cohort study. Lancet Neurol. 2020;19(4):307–16.
94. Lunde HMB, Assmus J, Myhr KM, Bø L, Grytten N. Survival and cause of death in multiple sclerosis: a 60-year longitudinal population study. J Neurol Neurosurg Psychiatry. 2017;88(8):621–5.

2 Autoimmune Demyelinating Diseases of Central Nervous System (CNS)

2.1 Acute Disseminated Encephalomyelitis (ADEM)

2.1.1 Epidemiology

- Incidence 0.1–0.9/100.000/year [1, 2].
- The occurrence is highest in winter and spring, likely owing to the increased prevalence of community infections.
- Most commonly seen in children; although, adults can also be affected.
- Median age of symptom onset is 5–8 years.
- Males are slightly more frequently affected [2, 3].

2.1.2 Etiology and Definition

- Demyelinating disorder of the central nervous system (CNS), which is typically preceded by an infection (50–85%) or less commonly by vaccination (5%) within days or weeks (mean delay 14 days; range 1–60 days). The presence of preceding infection or vaccination is not required for diagnosis.
- It is hypothesized that infectious microorganisms, sharing epitopes similar to myelin-associated peptides, trigger an autoimmune perivenular demyelination through molecular mimicry.
- In general, remyelination of demyelinating lesions is more robust than that in multiple sclerosis (MS) [1–4].
- High proportion (40–57%) of children with ADEM have positive anti-myelin oligodendrocyte glycoprotein (anti-MOG) immunoglobulin G (IgG) antibodies in the serum [5, 6].

T. Uher, *Mimics and Red Flags of Multiple Sclerosis*,
https://doi.org/10.1007/978-3-031-98945-2_2

2.1.3 Clinical Features

- Neurological manifestations depend on the lesion location and burden.
- Diagnosis of ADEM requires the presence of polyfocal CNS symptoms and encephalopathy.
- In contrast to MS, patients with ADEM often present with encephalopathy characterized by behavioral changes and altered consciousness that cannot be attributed to fever or seizures. Both only rarely occur in MS, particularly in the fulminant variant of MS.
- Clinical manifestations may also encompass brainstem symptoms, optic neuritis (can be bilateral), transverse myelitis, and atypical symptoms such as fever, seizures, or meningism.
- Children and adults with ADEM exhibit similar clinical manifestations [7].
- Peripheral nervous system involvement, mainly polyradiculoneuropathy, may occur in some patients, a feature not typically observed in MS [8].
- Some patients may have prodromal symptoms (malaise and headache) [1, 3].
- Systemic involvement, such as cardiac complications are rare [9].

2.1.4 Disease Course

- Acute or subacute symptoms onset.
- Symptoms reach their nadir within 3 days, which is atypical for MS [2, 10].
- There are various subtypes of the course
- Monophasic
  - In the vast majority of cases.
  - Without new clinical or magnetic resonance imaging (MRI) activity 3 months after the disease onset.
  - Worsening of symptoms, recurrence of initial symptoms, or the occurrence of new symptoms within 3 months of disease onset are not classifies as relapses [1, 2, 10, 11].
- Relapsing
  - Very rare (1–20%) [12].
  - New clinical and MRI activity is considered a relapse only if it occurs more than 3 months after disease onset; otherwise, it is considered as disease activity associated with the initial presentation of ADEM.
  - Relapses in adults are often associated with a future diagnosis of MS or neuromyelitis optica spectrum disorder (NMOSD) [13].
  - Children who test positive for anti-MOG IgG antibodies have a higher risk of relapse (30% within 2 years) compared to those who test negative. High and persisting levels of anti-MOG IgG are associated with relapsing disease, whereas lower titers are more commonly associated with monophasic ADEM [6].

- There are different patterns of relapsing ADEM
  1. Recurrent ADEM (RDEM)
     - The new symptoms resemble those at the disease onset.
  2. Multiphasic ADEM (MDEM)
     - Associated with new and different clinical and MRI manifestations.
     - Often associated with anti-MOG IgG antibodies.
     - Most common in small children (<9 years); only rarely in adults.
  3. ADEM followed by optic neuritis (ADEM-ON)
     - Optic neuritis occurs >3 months after the disease onset.
     - Often associated with anti-MOG IgG antibodies.
  4. ADEM-MS
     - A rare variant of ADEM representing the initial manifestation of MS.
  5. ADEM-NMOSD
     - A rare variant of ADEM representing the initial manifestation of NMOSD [1, 2, 6, 11, 12].

2.1.5 Brain Imaging

- Lesions' location
  - MRI during the first days of the disease may be normal [14], but later it becomes pathologic.
  - Bilateral, asymmetrically distributed multi-focal lesions in both white matter (mainly juxtacortical and deep), gray matter (basal ganglia or thalamus), and cortical gray–white matter junction.
  - The infra-tentorial region (cerebellum and brainstem) is also frequently affected.
  - There is relative sparing of periventricular white matter (or infrequent involvement) and the absence of ovoid lesions perpendicular to the edges of the lateral ventricles.
  - Lesions in the optic nerves and corpus callosum usually do not occur.
  - However, U-fibers (short association fibers connecting adjacent gyri in the cortex) are frequently involved, as seen in MS.
  - Children more often exhibit MRI lesions in the deep gray matter, whereas adults more commonly have lesions in the white matter.
  - Anti-MOG IgG-positive children may rarely exhibit a leukodystrophy-like pattern.
  - Intracortical pathology including microglial aggregates, subpial microglial activation, diffuse meningeal inflammation, and demyelination is probably responsible for encephalopathy [7, 11, 15, 16].
- Lesions' appearance
  - Large tumefactive (>1–2 cm in diameter) or less frequently punctate T2 hyperintense lesions.

  - Flocculent or patchy with poorly defined margins (MS are lesions more sharply defined).
  - Although, T1 hypointensities are commonly seen in MS, they are rare in ADEM, which is associated with relative axonal sparing.
  - Acutely might be peripheral (not central) restricted diffusion, which is associated with a worse prognosis or only signs of vasogenic edema.
- Contrast enhancement (30%)
  - Irregular, punctate, ring, incomplete ring, or peripheral.
  - All lesions appear to be of a similar pathological age; therefore, vast majority of lesions may exhibit contrast enhancement, which is highly atypical for MS.
  - However, simultaneous enhancement of all lesions in ADEM is rare; therefore, in such cases, alternative diagnoses such as sarcoidosis, neoplasms, or CNS lymphoma must always be excluded [5, 10, 17–19].
- Perilesional changes
  - Surrounding edema.
  - Weaker mass effect than would be expected for the size of the lesion.
  - Rare cases may be complicated by severe brain edema and raised intracranial pressure requiring neurosurgical decompression [2, 20, 21].
- Evolution over time
  - During clinical improvement, MRI may show progression, indicating a lag between clinical symptoms and MRI pathology recovery [2].
  - Follow-up imaging usually shows partial or complete resolution of lesion load without development of new lesions [10, 18].
  - In contrast, in MS, complete resolution of lesions is atypical, and the occurrence of new lesions is very frequent [22].
- Differential diagnosis from MS based on imaging findings
  - Algorithm to discriminate between ADEM and MS at the time of the clinical disease onset is based on the presence of the three features
    1. two or more periventricular lesions
    2. presence of black holes (T1 hypo-intense lesions) and
    3. absence of a bilateral lesion pattern.
  - If at least two of these three features are present, MS is more likely to be diagnosis [2, 20, 21].

2.1.6 Spinal Cord Imaging

- The frequency of cord lesions is not well described, but it is likely not rare.
- Lesions are commonly large, longitudinally extensive transverse myelitis (LETM), and with edema.
- Contrast enhancement is variable [2, 5, 10] (Fig. 2.1).

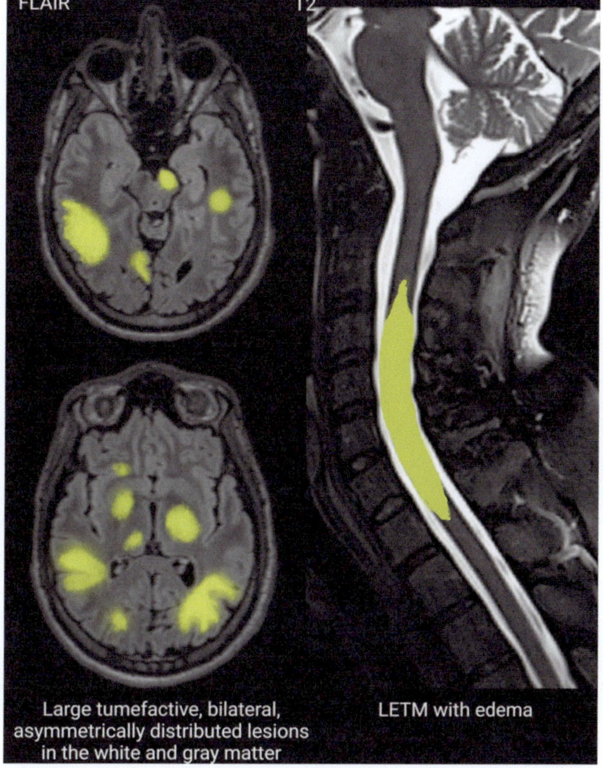

Fig. 2.1 MRI characteristics of acute disseminated encephalomyelitis (ADEM)

2.1.7 Blood Work

- Leukocytosis, elevated C-reactive protein (CRP) or erythrocyte sedimentation rate (ESR) resembling findings in infectious meningo-encephalitis is observed in 50% of the children [7].
- Children are commonly positive for anti-MOG IgG antibodies [1, 5, 6, 11].
- Anti-MOG IgG antibodies are rarely positive exclusively in cerebrospinal fluid (CSF) (4–7%). For more details, see the chapter "Myelin oligodendrocyte glycoprotein antibody disease") [23].

2.1.8 Examination of CSF

- Elevated concentration of protein (23–66%)
- Mononuclear pleocytosis (range 0–270/μL; usually <100/μL) (28–86%).
- Very high pleocytosis might indicate rather infectious meningo-encephalitis.
- CSF-restricted oligoclonal bands (OCB) are typically absent or positive only transiently (10–30%) [2, 3, 18].

2.1.9 Electrophysiology

- Electroencephalogram (EEG) may show epileptic activity (10–30%) [24].
- Nerve conduction studies may rarely show signs of peripheral neuropathy [8].

2.1.10 Diagnosis

- There is no good biomarker of ADEM; therefore, the diagnosis relies on the clinical presentation, typical MRI findings, and the exclusion of alternative diagnoses.
- It can be difficult to distinguish ADEM from an atypical first presentation of relapsing-remitting MS with tumefactive lesions [10].
- Neuropathology is rarely necessary for excluding other diagnoses [1, 2].
- The consensus diagnostic criteria for ADEM are available only for children [25].
- A significant proportion of children (8.5%) [26] and adults (35%) [27], initially diagnosed with ADEM, are later re-diagnosed with MS owing to the occurrence of multiple relapses beyond 3 months. In patients experiencing three or more relapses, alternative diagnoses such as MS, NMOSD, or myelin oligodendrocyte glycoprotein antibody-associated disease (MOGAD) are more likely [10].

2.1.11 Differential Diagnosis

- Acute hypertensive encephalopathy and posterior reversible encephalopathy syndrome (PRES); anti-NMDAR encephalitis; Anti-phospholipid syndrome; Autoimmune-mediated vasculitis; Behçet's disease; CNS lymphoma; CNS vasculitis, chronic lymphocytic inflammation with pontine perivascular enhancement responsive to steroids (CLIPPERS); Fabry disease; genetic/metabolic disorders and leukodystrophies; gliomatosis cerebri; hemophagocytic lymphohistiocytosis; mitochondrial encephalopathy, lactic acidosis, and stroke-like episodes (MELAS); MOGAD; MS; NMOSD; sarcoidosis; or scleroderma.
- The stroke-like onset, symmetrical involvement, or progressive disease course observed in these mimics may suggest a diagnosis other than ADEM [1, 2].

2.1.12 Treatment and Prognosis

- Corticosteroids or plasmapheris PLEX and intravenous immunoglobulin in non-responders [10].
- Often good recovery during several months; no or minimal residual deficit in majority of cases (80%); mortality in children is low (1–5%) [2, 3, 28].
- Children with anti-MOG IgG antibodies have more favorable outcomes than those who are anti-MOG IgG-negative [5].
- Children have more favorable outcomes compared to adults [7].
- Recurrent ADEM has worse outcomes compared to monophasic ADEM [1].

2.2 Acute Hemorrhagic Leukoencephalitis (AHLE)

2.2.1 Synonyms

- Hurst's acute necrotizing hemorrhagic leukoencephalitis; Hurst's disease [29]

2.2.2 Epidemiology

- Very rare disease of unknown prevalence.
- Occurs in children and adults [10, 30–32].

2.2.3 Etiology and Definition

- Considered as a fulminant hemorrhagic (catastrophic) form of ADEM.
- Histopathology shows fibrinoid vascular necrosis and microhemorrhages with perivenous demyelination and meningitis [10, 31, 33].

2.2.4 Clinical Features

- Monophasic, fulminant, and severe encephalopathy with multi-focal CNS symptoms, leading to death within one week of onset.
- Similarly to ADEM, often preceded by a vaccination or infection [10, 29].

2.2.5 Brain and Spinal Cord Imaging

- Similar findings as in severe ADEM, but with hemorrhages into the demyelinating lesions [10] (Fig. 2.2).

2.2.6 Blood Work

- Routine blood tests are normal.

2.2.7 Examination of CSF

- Commonly elevated concentration of protein and mononuclear pleocytosis
- CSF-restricted OCB are usually negative [31, 34].

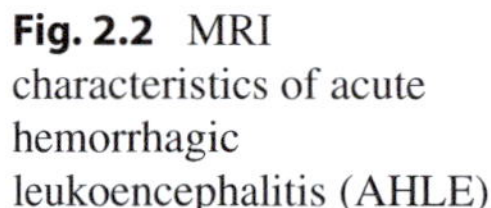

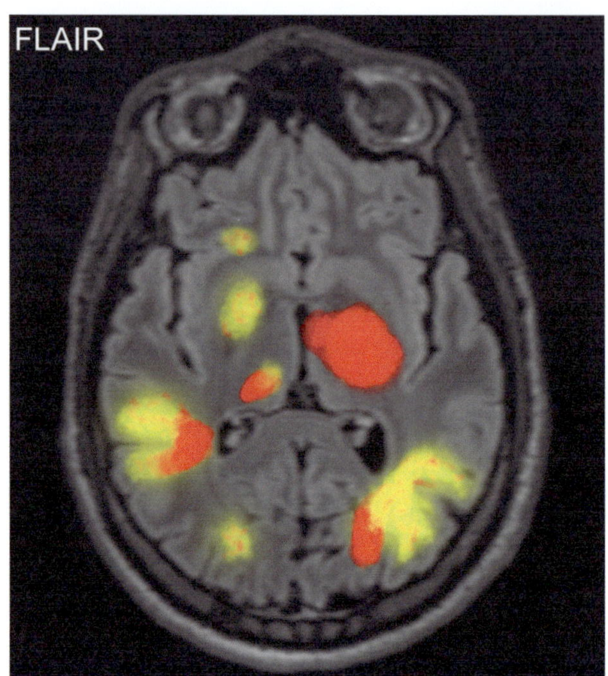

Fig. 2.2 MRI characteristics of acute hemorrhagic leukoencephalitis (AHLE)

2.2.8 Diagnosis

- Based on fulminant clinical course and imaging features.

2.2.9 Differential Diagnosis

- Often misdiagnosed as viral encephalitis [10, 34].

2.2.10 Treatment and Prognosis

- Corticosteroids, intravenous immunoglobulins, cyclophosphamide, and plasmapheresis.
- Cranial decompression may be required.
- Although the disease is fatal for the majority of patients within a few days, cases of full recovery have been reported [10, 30, 31, 34].

2.3 Autoimmune Glial Fibrillary Acidic Protein (GFAP) Astrocytopathy

2.3.1 Epidemiology

- Prevalence 0.6/100.000 (USA), but the disease is likely underdiagnosed.
- Female/male ratio 1/1; without racial preference.
- Children are affected in only 10% of cases [35].

2.3.2 Etiology and Definition

- GFAP is the primary filament protein found in astrocytes and serves as a crucial component of the cytoskeleton involved in various astrocyte functions.
- There are several potential mechanisms underlying GFAP astrocytopathy:

  A. An acquired inflammatory astrocytopathy affecting the CNS. The exact cause of the disorder is unclear, but about 20% of affected patients also have other autoimmune diseases [36].
  B. Approximately 25% of patients have a coexisting neoplasm, most often mature ovarian teratoma (75%), less frequently other cancers [36–39].
  C. Some cases may occur in the context of dysregulated T-cell immunity following immuno-modulatory treatment for autoimmunity or cancer, such as checkpoint inhibitor therapy or anti-CD25 therapy with daclizumab [36–40].
  D. Remains unclear whether infections may trigger GFAP autoimmunity [36].

2.3.3 Clinical Features

- The onset of clinical disease is often preceded by flu-like symptoms, including rhinorrhea, sore throat, fever, and cough (30–40%) or herpetic infection.
- Almost all patients (94%) with anti-GFAP IgG positivity in the CSF exhibit at least one of the following corticosteroid-responsive manifestations: meningitis, encephalitis, or myelitis.
- Meningo-encephalitis (55%)
  - Delirium (60%), meningeal syndrome (60%), tremor (40%), psychiatric symptoms (30%), or [drug-resistant] seizures (20%).
- Myelopathy (5%)
  - Usually occurs in combination with meningo-encephalitis as meningo-encephalo-myelitis.
  - Sensory and mild motor symptoms, rather than severe paresis as observed in NMOSD or several other disorders.
- Meningo-encephalo-myelitis (40%)
  - Combination of meningo-encephalitis and myelopathy [36, 37, 41].
- Ocular involvement

  - Optic neuritis is rare.
  - However, the number of patients exhibits an optic neuropathy due to venous inflammation with retinal venular leakage on fluorescein angiography and optic disc edema.
  - Visual symptoms are typically mild but may vary from asymptomatic bilateral optic disc edema (60%) to severe bilateral visual loss (usually corticosteroids-responsive; however, treatment-unresponsive cases may occur).
  - Frequently, painless blurred vision (30%).
  - Ocular pathology is associated with a higher risk of relapses [37, 38, 43].
- Other Clinical Features
  - Ataxia (40%), other movement disorders (chorea, myoclonus, and tremor), peripheral neuropathy (<5%), or dysautonomia (20%) [36, 37, 41].

2.3.4 Disease Course

- The median age of symptom onset is 44–50 years (range, 8–103 years).
- Subacute or insidious disease onset.
- Relapsing-remitting (20%) or monophasic disease course (80%) [36, 37, 41].

2.3.5 Brain Imaging

- Normal imaging findings are rare.
- Often small T2 hyperintense lesions in subcortical white matter, basal ganglia, hypothalamus, brainstem, or cerebellum (50%).
- A few patients may exhibit a high lesion load with leukodystrophy-like pattern.
- Contrast enhancement if frequent (66%) and specific.
  - A typical linear, radial perivascular pattern of enhancement in the deep white matter, particularly in GFAP-enriched periventricular regions around the lateral ventricles, is often present (>50%) (Fig. 2.3).
  - Additionally, leptomeningeal, punctate, serpentine, and ependymal enhancement or a radial pattern of enhancement in the cerebellum may be observed.
  - Similar findings can be seen sometimes in patients with sarcoidosis or lymphomatoid granulomatosis, which is a very rare Epstein-Barr virus (EBV)-driven lymphoproliferative disease [36, 37, 41, 44, 45].

2.3.6 Spinal Cord Imaging

- Spinal cord involvement (>40%).
- Centrally located longitudinally extensive transverse myelitis (LETM) (80%). The spinal cord lesions tend to be more subtle and blurred compared with those seen in NMOSD or MOGAD cases.
- Sometimes enhancement is observed around the central spinal canal, which is the GFAP-enriched region [37, 44, 45].

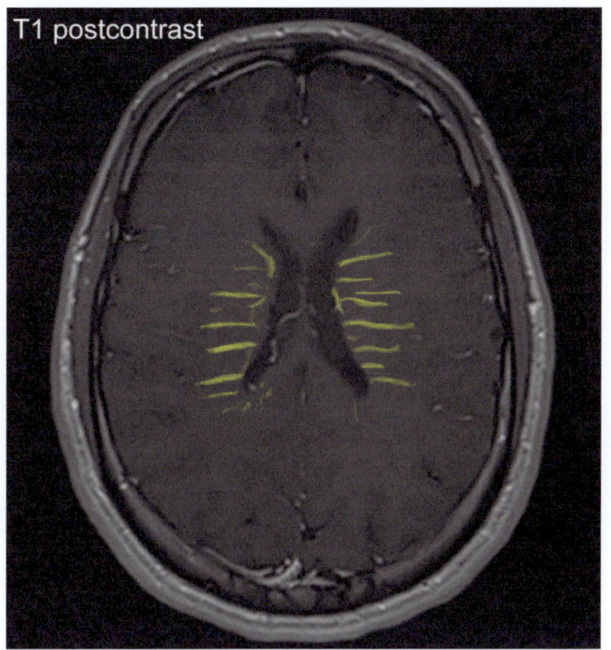

Fig. 2.3 Linear, radial perivascular pattern of enhancement in the deep white matter in glial fibrillary acidic protein (GFAP) astrocytopathy

2.3.7 Blood Work

- Anti-GFAP IgG antibodies may be detected in serum and CSF or exclusively in the CSF. However, the detection of anti-GFAP IgG in serum is often transient and less specific compared to detection in CSF, since it may also occur in conditions such as traumatic brain injury, brain tumors, autism, lead exposure, or diabetes [36, 37, 44].
- The coexistence of anti-GFAP IgG with anti-aquaporin-4 (AQP4) IgG, anti-N-methyl-D-aspartate receptor (NMDAR) IgG, or anti-myelin oligodendrocyte glycoprotein (MOG) IgG autoantibodies may occur. These patients typically exhibit a phenotype like those with only anti-GFAP IgG positivity. However, some patients with coexisting anti-AQP4 IgG positivity may also have concomitant NMOSD. Patients with coexisting anti-NMDAR IgG positivity tend to display a phenotype more resembling NMDAR encephalitis [36].
- Non-neural autoantibodies such as anti-nuclear antibodies (ANA), Sjogren's syndrome antigen A (Ro/SS-A), or double-stranded DNA (dsDNA) antibodies are frequently detected (75%) [43].

2.3.8 Examination of CSF

- Positive anti-GFAP IgG antibodies (100%).
  - Detected by combination of indirect immunofluorescence assay, cell-based assay, or Western blot.

- Elevated concentration of protein (80%).
- Pleocytosis (lymphocyte-predominant; mean 80 cells/mm3) (90%).
- CSF-restricted OCB (50%) [36, 37, 44].

2.3.9 OCT

- Optical coherence tomography (OCT) shows the retinal nerve fiber layer (RNFL) thickening [36].

2.3.10 Electrophysiology

- Visual evoked potentials (VEP) show an axonal optic neuropathy with irreversible damage, similar to those in NMOSD [42].

2.3.11 Diagnosis

- There are no established diagnostic criteria for GFAP astrocytopathy, and many questions regarding diagnosis remain unanswered [44].
- Diagnosis is currently based on a combination of clinical and imaging phenotype along with the detection of IgG reactive with GFAP in the CSF (higher positive predictive value compared to serum testing). However, it is important to emphasize that GFAP IgG positivity may occasionally occur in other diagnoses such as astrocytoma [37, 44].

2.3.12 Differential Diagnosis

- NMOSD and MOGAD
  - Longitudinally extensive myelitis and severe, bilateral visual symptoms with optic disc edema that are unresponsive to treatment may resemble NMOSD or MOGAD. Therefore, GFAP astrocytopathy should be considered in patients who test negative for anti-AQP4 and anti-MOG IgG antibodies. Optic disc edema occurs in some patients with NMOSD (5–33%) and in the majority of patients with MOGAD (80%).
- Idiopathic intracranial hypertension
  - Although patients with GFAP astrocytopathy might experience blurred vision and optic disc edema, their CSF opening pressure is normal.
- MS
  - Visual loss in MS is usually associated with pain and is neither severe nor bilateral [42].

2.3.13 Treatment and Prognosis

- Corticosteroids, mycophenolate mofetil, azathioprine, cyclophosphamide, or anti-CD20 therapies.
- Patients with relapsing-remitting course require long-term treatment.
- If diagnosed and treated early, the prognosis is generally favorable for the majority of patients [37].

2.4 Baló Concentric Sclerosis

2.4.1 Epidemiology

- A very rare disease of unknow prevalence.
- Female/male ratio 2/1.
- More frequent in Asia [46, 47].

2.4.2 Etiology and Definition

- Inflammatory demyelinating disease of CNS with alternating rings of demyelination and relatively preserved myelin [10].
- Can be associated with MS, seropositive NMOSD but also with cerebral autosomal dominant arteriopathy with bubcortical infarcts and leukoencephalopathy (CADASIL), progressive multifocal leukoencephalopathy (PML), herpetic neuroinfections, or hepatitis C (HCV) [47, 48].
- Hypothesized that focal neuro-inflammation, accompanied by extensive production of nitric oxide and oxygen radicals, can lead to impaired mitochondrial function. This, in turn, may trigger histotoxic hypoxia, resulting in the destruction of myelin sheaths and partial axonal damage. The concentric lesion grows through radial expansion around an inactive core. At the expanding lesions' edge, sublethal tissue injury may induce tissue preconditioning, which is a physiological response aimed at halting plaque growth. However, in aggressive lesions, the zone of protected preconditioned tissue may become overwhelmed, leading to new demyelination. Repeated occurrences of this process may result in the concentric pattern of lesions, characterized by demyelinated and preserved myelinated layers [49].
- The association between Baló lesions and MS is not clear. Baló lesions may occur during the clinical course of otherwise typical relapsing-remitting MS. Therefore, there is ongoing discussion regarding whether Balo's concentric sclerosis is a rare variant of MS (which is the most common view), a distinct disease, or merely an unspecific pattern of brain injury associated with various demyelinating diseases [47, 48].

2.4.3 Clinical Features

- Variable focal neurological deficits, including optic neuritis in some cases [50].
- Common symptoms associated with any intracerebral mass lesions, including encephalopathy, headache, incontinence, seizures, and other focal deficits [47]

2.4.4 Disease Course

- The age of symptom onset is comparable to that of MS (median, 34–38 years; range 3–62 years) [47, 48].
- Course is monophasic (50%), relapsing-remitting course (50%) [48], or very rarely asymptomatic [51].

2.4.5 Brain Imaging

- Lesions' location
  - White matter, basal ganglia, pons, and cerebellum
  - Lesions are multifocal or single.
  - Patients with a Baló or Baló-like lesion have frequently (55%) also other focal lesions typical for MS, but only a third of the patients exhibit MRI pattern typical for MS.
  - Baló lesions spare cortical U-fibers [47, 52].
- Lesions' appearance
  - Often large (tumefactive) onion-like lesions in white matter consisting of ≥2 concentric rings (lamellae) of alternating T2 hyper- and hypo-intensity and surrounding a so-called storm center of T2 hyperintensity.
  - "Baló-like lesions" have also ≥2 alternating bands of signal intensity on non-T2 weighted images or have atypical radiologic features (layered alternating bands or mosaic patterns) with biopsy evidence of alternating bands of demyelination and relatively preserved myelin [47, 48].
  - Large Baló-type lesions are very rare, but small concentric bands of demyelinated and myelinated layers might be observed in fulminant active lesions of other demyelinating diseases [53].
  - Sometimes restricted diffusion in the outer ring [54] (Fig. 2.4).
- Contrast enhancement
  - Peripheral ring, concentric or patchy enhancement pattern (67%).
- Perilesional changes
  - Edema is minimal [47].
- Evolution over time
  - Baló lesions may occur de novo or in patients with preexisting diagnosis of MS [48].

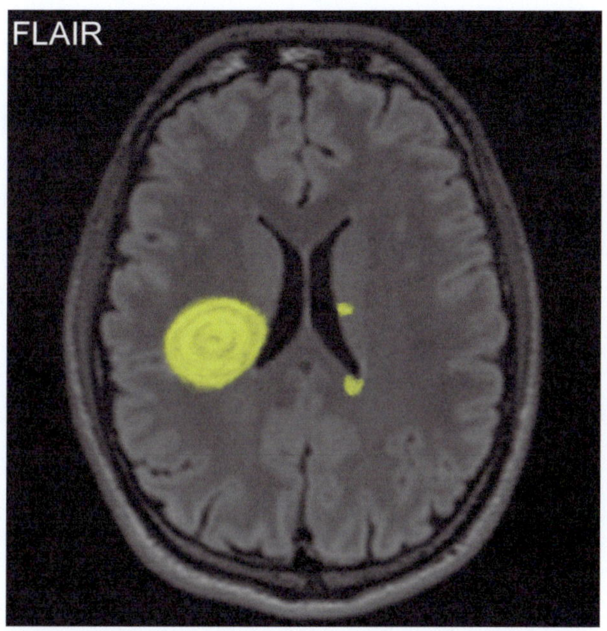

Fig. 2.4 Tumefactive, onion-like lesions in the white matter in Baló concentric sclerosis

- Initially is often restricted diffusion followed by a T2 hypo-intense ring and later by evolution of contrast enhancement suggesting the primary brain tissue injury with a subsequent disruption of the blood–brain barrier [48].
- Over time, some lesions keep the onion-like patter even after 1 year of follow-up [55], other lesions may lose their typical pattern and transform to the tumefactive demyelinating lesion, or large plaque [56].

- Associated findings
  - Baló lesions do not have increased uptake on 18-fluorodeoxyglucose on positron emission tomography (FDG-PET), unlike other acute demyelinating lesions or high-grade tumors, which can help with differential diagnosis [57].
  - 7 Tesla MRI may show microhemorrhages in Baló lesions [58].

2.4.6 Spinal Cord Imaging

- Rarely large edematous spinal cord lesions.
- Patients diagnosed with MS can later develop Baló lesions; therefore, patients may exhibit findings typical of MS [59].

2.4.7 Blood Work

- Routine blood tests are normal including negative anti-AQP4 or anti-MOG IgG antibodies [48].

2.4.8 Examination of CSF

- Elevated protein concertation (41–67%).
- Mild pleocytosis (range 6–27 cells/mm^3) (25–28%) [48, 60].
- Elevated IgG index (25%).
- CSF-restricted OCB (34%), but in half of cases disappear over time [60].

2.4.9 Diagnosis

- Based on MRI findings.
- The majority of the patients do not have a diagnosis of CNS demyelinating disease at disease onset [48].

2.4.10 Differential Diagnosis

- Can be mistaken for a brain tumor (glioblastoma multiforme or primary CNS lymphoma), brain abscess, or tumefactive demyelination, and some patients undergo a brain biopsy to exclude alternative diagnosis [47].
- Acute symptom onset in some patients may mimic a vascular event [61].

2.4.11 Treatment and Prognosis

- Data are scarce, and no randomized trials are available.
- Used corticosteroids, cyclophosphamide, intravenous Immunoglobulins, or plasmapheresis [47].
- Alemtuzumab showed no benefit in patients with high levels of disability [62].
- If fulfilled diagnostic criteria for MS, consider MS disease-modifying therapies.
- According to some authors, many patients with isolated Baló lesions have a better prognosis than those with coexisting typical MS lesions. Therefore, adopting a watch-and-wait approach in these patients might be reasonable [47].
- The prognosis varies widely, ranging from a benign course to fulminant disease resulting in death, which occurs in approximately 10–14% of cases [47, 48].
- Marked clinical improvement or full recovery from the initial attack is observed in 83% of treated patients [52].

2.5 Combined Central and Peripheral Demyelination

2.5.1 Synonyms

- MS with peripheral neuropathy; Chronic inflammatory demyelinating polyneuropathy (CIDP) with central demyelination

2.5.2 Epidemiology

- Rare condition.

2.5.3 Etiology and Definition

- It is not considered as a simple combination of MS and CIDP.
- The combined central and peripheral demyelination (CCPD) is probably heterogeneous disease.
- The pathogenesis is unknown; however, it is hypothesized that autoreactive lymphocytes and/or antibodies targeting specific peripheral and central nervous system epitopes may cross the blood–brain and blood–nerve barriers, simultaneously triggering an inflammatory process.
- Some patients have antibodies to neurofascin-155 (NF155), a protein expressed on both central and peripheral myelin. These patients typically exhibit a relapsing disease course and respond well to intravenous immunoglobulin.

2.5.4 Clinical Features

- Involvement of both the central and peripheral nervous system can occur, with either primary peripheral or primary central nervous system manifestations.
- CNS involvement may include retrobulbar neuritis, encephalopathy, or other manifestations also observed in patients with MS.
- Peripheral nervous system involvement may include myeloradiculoneuropathy, cranial neuropathy, length-dependent peripheral neuropathy, or pseudo-Guillain-Barré syndrome.

2.5.5 Disease Course

- Disease onset is often preceded by infection (10–85%).
- Monophasic (30%) or relapsing and progressive (70%) disease course.
- Relapsing-remitting course (42%), mainly due to CNS involvement (often occurrence of new spinal cord lesions).
- PNS involvement symptoms usually progress insidiously.
- PNS and CNS involvement is simultaneous or rapidly subsequent (71%), CNS precedes peripheral involvement (19%), or peripheral system precedes CNS involvement (10%).
- Simultaneous onset of central and peripheral involvement is associated with greater disability and increased lesion load in brain and spinal cord compared with a temporally separated onset.

2.5.6 Brain Imaging

- Approximately half of the patients meet the dissemination in space criteria according to the McDonald 2010 diagnostic criteria.

2.5.7 Spinal Cord Imaging

- Often LETM.

2.5.8 Blood Work

- Routine testing typically yields normal results.
- Some patients have positive IgG or IgM antibodies to NF155.
- Described rare cases of patients with CCPD and positive anti-MOG Ig.

2.5.9 Examination of CSF

- Commonly elevated concentration of protein (74%).
- Mild mononuclear pleocytosis (58%).
- CSF-restricted OCB are not frequent (16%) and may disappear or change to a mirror pattern (corresponding OCB) in around 29% of cases.

2.5.10 OCT

- Patients with CIDP have subtle RNFL thinning primarily observed in the temporal quadrants.

2.5.11 Electrophysiology

- Nerve conduction studies show demyelinative features (75%), conduction block (42%), or only pure axonal neuropathy (26%)
- Visual evoked potentials (VEP) often show prolonged latencies (50–64%)

2.5.12 Diagnosis

- The current diagnostic criteria for MS and CIDP may not fully capture the broad spectrum of combined phenotypes seen in CCPD, making these criteria potentially too restrictive.

- For instance, only 74% of patients meet the diagnostic criteria for CIDP, and only 50% fulfill the dissemination-in-space criterion required for an MS diagnosis.

2.5.13 Differential Diagnosis

- MS and CIDP or other conditions affecting peripheral nervous system.

2.5.14 Treatment and Prognosis

- Clinically active patients are often refractory to high-dose corticosteroids and intravenous Immunoglobulins treatment. In such cases, plasmapheresis and anti-CD20 therapy may be considered as alternative options.
- Patients with CCPD who are positive for NF155 antibodies generally respond better to intravenous Immunoglobulins and plasmapheresis, showing more favorable outcomes.
- While Natalizumab is effective in treating CNS pathology, it frequently exacerbates peripheral symptoms.
- Overall, treatment responses are typically partial and most effective during the early stages of the disease, leading to poor outcomes for most patients (>70%) [63–67].

2.6 Idiopathic Acute Transverse Myelitis

2.6.1 Epidemiology

- Incidence 0.86/100.000/year.
- Prevalence 7.9/100.000 [68].
- Idiopathic acute transverse myelitis (IATM) represents 16.5% of acute myelopathy syndromes [69].
- Advances in imaging and laboratory assessments have improved the ability to identify the specific cause of myelopathy in patients previously diagnosed with IATM. Therefore, the incidence of IATM is expected to decrease in the future [70].

2.6.2 Etiology and Definition

- Immune-mediated myelopathy of undetermined etiology [70, 71].
- Up to 70% of patients previously diagnosed with IATM have an alternative specific cause of myelopathy. The most common alternative cause is MS [72].
- Therefore, the IATM is considered a diagnosis of exclusion following a comprehensive evaluation for a wide range of alternative diagnoses [70, 72, 73].

2.6.3 Clinical Features

- Diagnostic criteria of IATM proposed by the Transverse Myelitis Consortium Working Group in 2002 include
  - Sensory, motor, or autonomic dysfunction caused by the spinal cord pathology.
  - Signs and symptoms are bilateral, often asymmetric.
  - There is a sensory level on the trunk.
  - Clinical nadir is between 4 hours and 21 days after disease onset.
    - Spinal cord strokes, functional neurological disorders, traumatic myelopathies, and sometimes NMOSD and MOGAD are frequently associated with acute symptom onset (minutes/hours). On the other hand, inflammatory myelopathies typically progress over days.
  - There is imaging (contrast enhancement on MRI) or biochemical (positive CSF-restricted OCB or IgG index) evidence of inflammation.
  - Alternative diagnoses must be excluded [71].
- The IATM diagnostic criteria were published many years ago, before discovery of anti-AQP4 IgG, anti-MOG IgG, or advanced MRI sequences. Therefore, revisions to the criteria are needed [72].
- Patient presenting with unilateral neurological deficits or lacking a sensory level on the trunk is not diagnosed with IATM but rather with partial acute transverse myelitis.
- Patients meeting the clinical criteria for IATM but lacking evidence of inflammation (as indicated by normal MRI and CSF findings; 15.2% of patients) [74] are not diagnosed with IATM but are instead classified as having possible IAMT [71].

2.6.4 Brain Imaging

- Normal.

2.6.5 Spinal Cord Imaging

- MRI is frequently normal (22.5–50%); in these patients, the pathology on follow-up MRI occurs only rarely.
- Typically, central T2 hyperintense lesion extending over >2 segments, involving >2/3 of the cross-sectional area of the spinal cord.
- The thoracic spinal cord is most frequently affected.
- Lesions are usually longer compared to those seen in MS, with 32.4% of patients presenting with longitudinally extensive transverse myelitis (LETM).
- Lesions may exhibit edema with a focal expansion of cord volume (50%).
- Often exhibit contrast enhancement with variable patterns, including diffuse, heterogeneous, or peripheral enhancement (37–74%). Enhancement is more commonly observed in the subacute stage than in the acute stage [74–78] (Fig. 2.5).

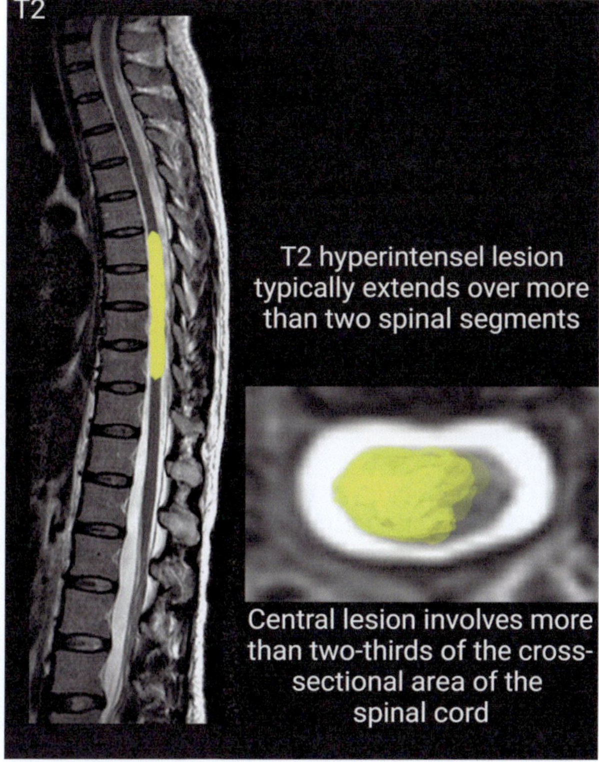

Fig. 2.5 MRI characteristics of idiopathic acute transverse myelitis

2.6.6 Blood Work

- Normal.

2.6.7 Examination of CSF

- Concentrations of glucose and protein are usually normal.
- Pleocytosis (23–62%).
- Elevated IgG index (20%).
- CSF-restricted OCB are present in
  - 17–18.5% of patients with definite and possible IATM.
  - 62% of patients with partial acute transverse myelitis with or without brain lesions [69, 74, 79, 80].

2.6.8 Diagnosis

- See "Clinical features."
- Can be challenging and should only be made after a comprehensive evaluation and exclusion of specific etiologies of myelopathy [70].
- Uncertain diagnosis is better than premature labeling [81].

2.6.9 Differential Diagnosis

- Rarely does the first demyelinating event of MS present as a definite or possible case of IATM [74, 82, 83].
- Factors associated with higher risk of "conversion" to MS
  - Young age.
  - Sensory symptoms.
  - Greater disability at disease onset.
  - CSF-restricted OCB (conversion rate is 33.3%).
  - Short spinal cord lesions (<2 segments).
  - Partial acute transverse myelitis and presence of brain lesions (conversion rate 44–93%).
- Factors associated with lower risk of "conversion" to MS
  - Absence of OCB with a normal IgG index (conversion rate 0%).
  - Absence of CSF-restricted OCB (conversion rate 2%).
  - Definite and possible IATM (conversion rate 10–13%).
  - LETM [74, 80, 82–86].
- In general, myelopathies associated with systemic inflammatory diseases affecting only the CNS, such as isolated spinal sarcoidosis; vascular spinal cord disorders, such as spinal dural AV fistulas; paraneoplastic syndromes; or systemic vasculitis associated with spinal cord involvement are often challenging to diagnose.

2.6.10 Treatment and Prognosis

- High-dose corticosteroids and plasmapheresis [70, 74].
- Poor outcome in 10–35% of patients [74, 81, 82].
- Risk factors associated with a poor outcome include: back pain, severe neurological deficits, motor deficit at disease onset, symptom progression within 24 hours, relapse occurrence, sphincter dysfunction, spinal shock, and LETM [69, 75].

2.7 Marburg's Variant of Multiple Sclerosis

2.7.1 Epidemiology

- Rare variant of MS with an unknown prevalence.

2.7.2 Etiology and Definition

- Fulminant malignant form of MS [10].

2.7.3 Clinical Features

- Common symptoms include seizures, headaches, vomiting, bilateral optic neuritis, cognitive deficit, apraxia, aphasia, and hemi- or quadri-paresis.
- Typically, there is no confusion or decreased consciousness, as seen in conditions such as ADEM or other encephalopathies.

2.7.4 Disease Course

- Acute and severe.
- Monophasic rapidly progressing (stepwise or continuous) disease [10, 87].

2.7.5 Brain Imaging

- Lesions' location
  - Distribution of lesions typical for MS (predominantly white matter).
  - Lesions resembles those in MS but are more destructive.
  - Usually do not extend into gray matter as in ADEM.
  - An involvement of cortical gray matter is limited compared to MS.
- Lesions' appearance
  - T2 hyperintense lesions are ill-defined and substantially larger than in MS (tumefactive).
- Contrast enhancement
  - Enhancement (mostly ring-like) of only a proportion of lesions suggests varying lesion "ages," supporting the diagnosis of Marburg's MS rather than ADEM.
- Perilesional changes
  - Often severe perilesional edema resembling ADEM.
  - Schilder's disease may mimic Marburg's MS, but it is associated with only one or two large lesions without marked perifocal edema.

- Evolution over time
  - Rapid progression of lesion activity (new or enlarging lesions) over time, which distinguishes it from ADEM, where MRI findings remain stable or regress over time [10, 87–89].

2.7.6 Spinal Cord Imaging

- The cord might also be affected, like what is observed in MS [10].

2.7.7 Blood Work

- Routine blood tests are normal.

2.7.8 Examination of CSF

- CSF is normal or shows an elevated concentration of protein.
- CSF-restricted OCB are usually absent [10, 87–89].

2.7.9 Diagnosis

- Is based on fulminant disease course and imaging.

2.7.10 Treatment and Prognosis

- Although current treatment strategies have improved patient prognosis, severe disability and mortality rates remain high, often attributed to extensive brainstem involvement.
- Corticosteroids and plasmapheresis frequently yield unsatisfactory results. Mitoxantrone, cyclophosphamide, or anti-CD20 therapy has shown more promising outcomes in some cases. The effectiveness of current disease-modifying treatments remains unknown [10, 87–90].

2.8 Myelin Oligodendrocyte Glycoprotein Antibody-Associated Disease (MOGAD)

2.8.1 Epidemiology

- Prevalence 2.0 (1.1–3.4)/100.000.
- Incidence 0.34 (0.1–0.5)/100.000/year (both likely underestimated).

- Approximately two to three times more prevalent than seropositive NMOSD and 50 times less frequent than MS.
- Individuals of all ages can be affected, but the incidence is higher in children.
- All geographical regions are equally affected [11, 91].

2.8.2 Etiology and Definition

- It is hypothesized that insufficiently developed tolerance towards oligodendrocyte glycoprotein (MOG) is associated with the persistence of MOG autoreactive T cells that have evaded elimination in the thymus. Consequently, autoantibodies targeting MOG, along with activated immune cells in the peripheral blood, may cross the blood–brain barrier during relapses (the outside-in model) [92].
- The pathogenesis includes antibody-dependent and antibody-independent immunopathological processes, such as complement deposition, inflammatory CD4-predominant T-cell infiltrates, granulocytosis, astrogliosis, microglial activation, moderate axonal loss, and the preservation of oligodendrocyte precursors. Complement activation is not considered as the initial mechanism, as is suggested in NMOSD [93].

2.8.3 Disease Course

- The disease presents either as monophasic or relapsing, with relapses being assessed solely based on clinical manifestations rather than MRI activity.
- Relapses tend to occur more frequently during the early stages of the disease and following corticosteroid reduction or cessation. Some patients may experience clusters of early relapses.
- Although the first relapse can manifest after several years, the median time to the initial relapse is approximately 10–15 months [11, 94].
- Clinical disease progression independent of relapsing activity (PIRA) is typically not observed in MOGAD, unlike in MS.
- Clinical manifestations primarily include optic neuritis, myelitis, and brain involvement, such as ADEM, cerebral cortical encephalitis, and brainstem or cerebellar syndromes.
- Children with MOGAD most often present with ADEM, whereas adults usually experience optic neuritis, myelitis, or brainstem syndrome [11].

2.8.4 Optic Neuritis (Clinical and Imaging Features)

- Occurs in around 35% of children and 55–60% of adults with MOGAD.
- MOGAD is the cause of optic neuritis in
  - 50% of children (especially <11 years of age) [95].

  - 5% of adults.
  - 39% of adults with severe optic disc edema [96, 97].
- Clinical features
  - Monophasic or recurrent.
  - Isolated, or combined with ADEM, myelitis, or other CNS symptoms [11].
  - Bilateral optic nerve involvement (31–84%) is twice as common in MOGAD compared to NMOSD and almost 10 times more prevalent than in MS, where it occurs in only 5% of cases.
  - Often results in severe visual acuity loss, which can include central vision, similar to the presentation observed in NMOSD.
  - Color vision loss and severe retro-orbital pain can also be present.
  - Relative afferent pupillary defect (RAPD) typically tests positive, except of cases with bilateral involvement or prior contralateral pathology [11].
  - Typically, there is a rapid and complete recovery, especially following corticosteroid treatment [11, 98, 99].
  - Severe headache, occasionally misdiagnosed as migraine, may precede the onset of visual deficits. The pain arises from pronounced intra-orbital and peri-optic inflammation, involving the meninges and nociceptive fibers surrounding the optic nerve [100].
- Fundoscopy
  - Often severe disc swelling, sometimes accompanied by hemorrhages (45–95%). This presentation is uncommon in NMOSD and extremely rare in MS [99].
- Optic nerve imaging
  - MRI findings of the optic nerve in MOGAD may display similarities and distinctive features compared to NMOSD or MS.
  - A high frequency of longitudinally extensive optic nerve lesions, a characteristic shared with NMOSD but exceedingly rare in MS.
  - Optic nerve lesions (often with contrast enhancement) may occur in the orbital, canalicular, or intracranial portions, a characteristic shared with NMOSD and MS.
  - Optic sheath involvement is typical in MOGAD, whereas it is exceptionally rare in NMOSD.
  - The involvement of the chiasm is observed only in NMOSD. In MOGAD, when chiasmal involvement is present, it results from the spread of longitudinally extensive lesions from the optic nerve into the chiasm.
  - Optic nerve edema is frequently present in MOGAD and NMOSD, whereas it is less commonly observed in MS.
  - Dedicated MRI sequences are essential for achieving optimal sensitivity in detecting optic nerve pathology (for example, short-tau inversion-recovery [STIR], fat-suppressed spin-echo [FAT-SAT], 3D double inversion-recovery [DIR], fat-suppressed post-contrast T1) [11, 97, 98].

2.8.5 Transverse Myelitis (Clinical and Imaging Features)

- Occurs in around 10% of children and 25–30% of adults with MOGAD.
- Clinical features
  - Isolated or combined with ADEM or optic neuritis.
  - Simultaneous clinical or MRI brain or optic nerve involvement during myelitis is often in MOGAD and MS but infrequent in NMOSD [11, 101].
  - Recurrent transverse myelitis without relapses involving other CNS regions is rare [102].
  - Although myelitis typically presents as moderate to severe at its nadir (50% of cases have EDSS>4.0) [103], the recovery from relapses is generally favorable. Occasionally, despite achieving satisfactory motor recovery, individuals may experience persistent sphincter and sexual dysfunction. This pattern is characteristic of MOGAD but is rare in seropositive NMOSD or MS patients [101, 104].
  - During relapses, bowel and bladder dysfunction can be severe, a characteristic feature of MOGAD and NMOSD but not commonly observed in MS [11, 101, 104].
  - Painful spasms and neuropathic pain are more commonly associated with seropositive NMOSD myelitis than with MOGAD or MS [11].
- Spinal cord imaging
  - Lesions' location
    - Vast majority of patients with myelitis have spinal cord lesions, but 10% of patients have normal cord imaging at disease onset. In these cases, imaging is recommended to repeat after 1–2 weeks [105].
    - Involvement of the cervical, thoracic, and lumbar spinal cord is equally common. In contrast, MS predominantly affects the cervical cord, whereas NMOSD commonly affects mostly the cervical and thoracic spinal cord [101].
    - 26–40% of patients demonstrate involvement of the conus medullaris, a frequency much higher than that observed in NMOSD (6%) or MS (1.3%) [106].
    - On axial planes, lesions are predominantly centrally located (66–75%) or confined to the gray matter (30–50%), leading to the characteristic H-sign (28%), which is not commonly seen in NMOSD (8%) or MS (0%). Occasionally, an asymptomatic dilatation of central spinal canal (hydrosyringomyelia) may resemble the H-sign on imaging.
    - Only 20–25% of lesions are found in the white matter.
    - Typically involve more than 50% of the cross-sectional area of the spinal cord [11, 101, 107].
  - Lesions' appearance
    - Most often longitudinally extensive transverse myelitis (LETM) (76%); however, some patients may have only (single or multiple) short spinal cord lesions (15–24%) as typically seen in MS or combined LETM and

short cord lesions (48%) [101]. LETM is extremely rare in MS, and long spinal cord lesions observed in advanced stages of MS are often a result of fusion of multiple short lesions over time [11, 108].
    - T2 hyperintense lesions often have ill-defined borders (typically well-defined in MS).
    - Bright spotty lesions, characterized by markedly increased focal T2 signal similar to or higher than CSF and corresponding hypo-intense signal on T1 images, are typical findings in NMOSD. However, they are not observed in MOGAD or MS, which aids in the differential diagnosis of LETM cases [107, 109].
- Contrast enhancement (71%)
    - Less pronounced (subtle or missing) than in NMOSD.
    - Heterogeneous enhancement with blurred margins ("cloud-like"), well-defined nodular enhancement, or leptomeningeal (arachnoid mater and pia mater) enhancement.
    - Sometimes also observed thickening and contrast enhancement of the dorsal nerve roots of spinal cord or cauda equina.
    - The leptomeningeal enhancement is common in MOGAD but rarely seen in MS or NMOSD [11, 101, 107, 110].
- Perilesional changes
    - Cord edema usually less pronounced than in NMOSD [11, 107].
- Evolution over time
    - Following treatment or spontaneously, spinal cord lesions often reduce in size or resolve completely (especially smaller lesions; may represent rather edema than true demyelination), which is atypical for both NMOSD and MS [101].
    - The new clinically silent spinal cord lesions are rare (as in NMOSD) but may occur.
    - Due to the relatively high lesion dynamics (new and disappearing lesions), it is recommended to perform re-baseline imaging after a few weeks.
    - However, slowly progressive myelopathy, which is frequently seen in MS, is very rare in MOGAD [111].
- Associated findings
    - Spinal cord atrophy may occur in severe cases [103].

2.8.6 ADEM (Clinical and Imaging Features)

- The most common manifestation in children under 10 years of age, representing half of all ADEM cases in this age group. Children diagnosed with ADEM who test positive for anti-MOG IgG antibodies are typically 2–3 years younger than seronegative children [11, 112].
- ADEM is rare in other demyelinating disorders such as MS and NMOSD. In adults, ADEM is only seldomly associated with MOGAD in adults (5.6%) and MS in children [113].

- Clinical features
  - Typically preceded by infection with fewer; mainly respiratory [114].
  - Complete recovery is frequent (70%) [94, 112]; however, in rare cases, it may be associated with a poor outcome [11].
  - Relapses are frequent in seropositive cases (38%) but rare in seronegative cases (3%), with a median time to the first relapse of 4.7 months [112, 113].
- Brain and spinal cord imaging (for details, see the chapter on ADEM).

2.8.7 Cerebral Cortical Encephalitis

- In only 6.7% of patients with MOGAD but not observed in NMOSD or MS.
- Clinical features
  - Fever, headache, somnolence, encephalopathy, seizures (focal, generalized, or status epilepticus), rarely, life-threatening rise of intracranial pressure [11, 115].
  - Diencephalic syndrome and narcolepsy as sometimes seen in NMOSD do not occur [11, 116], but area postrema syndrome may rarely occur in MOGAD [117].
- Brain imaging
  - Fluid-attenuated inversion recovery (FLAIR)-hyperintense lesions in anti-MOG associated encephalitis with seizures (FLAMES) is subtype of MOGAD.
  - Usually unilateral, less frequently bilateral T2 hyperintense cortical lesions with increased signal on DIR sequences.
  - Additionally, sulcal FLAIR hyperintensities and leptomeningeal contrast enhancement are commonly observed, often with minimal to no cortical involvement [11, 118].

2.8.8 Brain Parenchymal Manifestations

- Clinical features
  - Monofocal or polyfocal neurological deficits depending on extent and location of brain pathology. Rare cases of cranial neuropathy and aseptic meningitis have also been reported.
- Brain imaging
  - Imaging findings in MOGAD are variable, lacking pathognomonic features and often exhibiting similarities with ADEM, NMOSD, or to a lesser extent MS [11, 94, 112, 115, 119].
  - Patients with optic or brain symptoms may have clinically silent spinal cord lesions and vice versa, 33–50% patients with myelitis have clinically silent brain or optic nerve lesions [101].

- Lesions' location
  - At disease onset often normal findings on brain MRI (47–68%) [120]. In the MS, only 8–16% of patients who subsequently fulfill criteria for MS has negative initial imaging [97].
  - Often uni- or bilateral lesions, typically in deep gray matter (thalamus, basal ganglia), but also in deep white matter, cerebellum, and brainstem.
  - Relatively often (20%), large diffuse T2 lesions are observed in the brainstem (midbrain, pons, or medulla), with 40% of these cases being asymptomatic.
  - Also, large poorly demarcated uni- or bilateral lesions in the middle cerebellar peduncles are typical for MOGAD but atypical for MS and NMOSD and may help in differential diagnosis [11, 94, 112, 115, 119].
  - Cerebral encephalitis can be associated with cortical lesions, which are also visible on FLAIR (see above) [118].
  - Rarely present lesions in area postrema and mesencephalon similarly as in NMOSD [117] but diencephalic lesions around third ventricle, and periependymal lining surrounding ventricles, which are typical for NMOSD are absent [11, 94, 115, 119, 121].
- Lesions' appearance
  - Lesions tend to be low in number but often large tumefactive.
  - Tumefactive lesions in MOGAD are more common than in NMOSD (22% vs. 5%).
  - Typically, ill-defined (fluffy/poorly demarcated) and well-demarcated lesions are infrequent.
  - Leukodystrophy-like pattern may occur [11, 112, 115, 119, 122].
  - Persistent T1 hypo-intense lesions are typical for MS or NMOSD but rare in MOGAD [119].
  - Proportion of lesions with central vein sign (CVS) is low.
  - Smoldering lesions are not observed [94].
- Contrast Enhancement
  - Subtle "cloud-like," linear, nodular, or perivascular pattern.
  - Or may be leptomeningeal around brainstem or cortex.
  - Usually not an ovoid open ring as seen in MS [11, 115, 120].
- Perilesional changes
  - Lesions typically do not exhibit pronounced edema or a mass effect [11, 112, 115, 119]. However, rarely tumefactive lesions in children may be associated with a marked edema, mass effect, and life-threatening brain herniation [123, 124].
- Evolution over time
  - The occurrence of new clinically silent brain lesions is rare (<4–10%), but strongly predictive for future clinical relapses [111, 125].
  - Lesion resolution, including tumefactive lesions, is more frequent than in MS or NMOSD [122, 126] (Fig. 2.6).

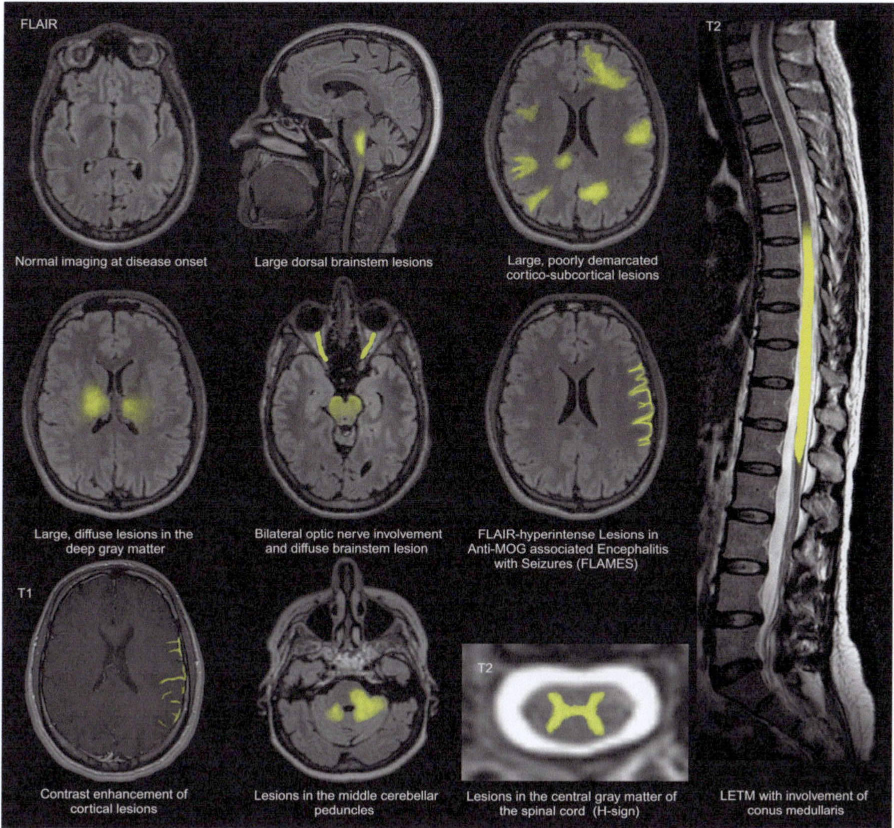

Fig. 2.6 MRI characteristics of myelin oligodendrocyte glycoprotein antibody-associated disease (MOGAD)

2.8.9 Blood Work

- Who should be tested
  - Considering the low frequency of anti-MOG IgG positivity among patients fulfilling diagnostic criteria for MS (0.3–2.5%) [127, 128] and the fact that many seropositive cases are false-positive (even when used highly specific and sensitive assays), screening for anti-MOG IgG should be performed only in patients with suspected MOGAD.
  - Anti-MOG IgG positivity is infrequent in adults with a first demyelinating event suggestive of MS. However, it was suggested to evaluate anti-MOG IgG in patients with optic neuritis and absence of CSF-restricted OCB, LETM, or negative MRI [129].
  - More than 50% of children under 11 years of age with acute demyelinating event of CNS has positive anti-MOG IgG, hence screening of this population is advised [11].

  - Clear positive anti-MOG IgG titers are rarely found in healthy controls or in patients with other neurological diseases. Seropositivity alone does not meet criteria for MOGAD, and future research is needed to show whether such individuals are at higher risk of developing MOGAD in the future [11, 95, 127].
- Dual positivity
  - In contrast to NMOSD, MOGAD does not exhibit a strong association with other autoimmune disorders or positivity for various autoantibodies [130].
  - Positivity of anti-MOG and anti-aquaporin-4 (AQP4) IgG is uncommon, and when it does occur, levels of antibodies against AQP4 are typically high while anti-MOG IgG levels are low. Such patients are diagnosed with NMOSD. Therefore, individuals who test positive for anti-AQP4 IgG should not undergo testing for anti-MOG IgG. Conversely, patients exhibiting clinical symptoms indicative of NMOSD but testing negative for anti-AQP4 IgG should be evaluated for anti-MOG IgG [11, 131].
  - Rarely patients with MOGAD may test positive for anti-NMDAR IgG (4–7.5%) owing to history of NMDAR encephalitis or overlap syndrome with features of MOGAD and NMDA encephalitis [11, 132].
- Interpretation
  - Testing for anti-MOG IgG demonstrates higher sensitivity in serum compared to CSF. It is strongly recommended to employ live cell-based assays, which offer higher sensitivity, or fixed cell-based assays, which have lower sensitivity rather than enzyme-linked immunosorbent assay (ELISA). In fixed assays, clear positivity is evident in titers above 1:100, whereas titers above 1:10 are considered indicative of low positivity. Higher titers of anti-MOG IgG are correlated with a higher positive predictive value of MOGAD [11, 95, 112, 133].
  - It is recommended to carefully interpretate positive anti-MOG IgG results (especially those with low titers) in patients with atypical features for MOGAD. In these cases, a false positivity is probable [11].
  - High titers of anti-MOG IgG at disease onset do not predict future disease activity or recovery. However, persistently high titers are associated with an elevated risk of future relapse [11].
  - MOGAD is associated with elevated serum tau but not glial fibrillary acidic protein (GFAP) and neurofilament light chain (NfL) levels in relapses. In contrast, NMOSD patients have increased serum NfL and GFAP levels in relapses. MS patients have increased only serum NfL levels during relapses [134, 135].
  - Very small proportion of MS patients may have low titers of anti-MOG IgG [91].
- Timing of Testing
  - Serum testing during the relapse, before, or 3 months after treatment initiation may increase a chance of positive result [11].
  - Anti-MOG IgG titers usually decline over time but may remain positive over years.
  - Disappearance of anti-MOG IgG occurs in 25% (most within 1 year) and predicts lower risk of relapse.
  - In contrast, seroconversion from negativity to positivity is extremely rare [94].

2.8.10 Examination of CSF

- Mildly elevated concentration of protein (30%).
- Mild pleocytosis (>5 cells/mm^3) (50%).
  - Among these, a subset of patients (<12%) has marked pleocytosis (>100 cells/mm^3).
  - Pleocytosis tends to be more pronounced during relapses compared to remission periods, and it is more prevalent in patients diagnosed with ADEM or myelitis than those with optic neuritis.
- CSF-restricted OCB are not common (20%).
  - In some patients, positivity of CSF-restricted OCB is only transient.
  - Although, presence of CSF-restricted OCB does not exclude diagnosis of MS it strongly favors it.
- MRZ reaction (a polyspecific, intrathecal humoral immune response directed against three neurotropic viruses: measles, rubella, and varicella zoster) is absent in MOGAD but positive in MS [133, 136].
- Only proportion (40–70%) of patients with positive anti-MOG IgG in blood exhibit anti-MOG IgG also in CSF [11, 137].
- A small percentage of seronegative patients (3–5%) displays anti-MOG IgG only in CSF. Hence, supplementary CSF testing for anti-MOG IgG can be utilized in certain patients to support the diagnosis of MOGAD [11, 137, 138].

2.8.11 OCT

- The optic neuritis often involves the orbital portion of the optic nerve and is longitudinally extensive. This leads to more significant disc swelling and thickening of the retinal nerve fiber layer (RNFL) compared to optic neuritis in MS. This characteristic can aid in distinguishing optic neuritis in MOGAD from that in MS. A RNFL cut-off value of 175 μm has high specificity (96%), albeit a low sensitivity (45%) for diagnosing of MOGAD [139].
- As disease progresses, OCT shows reduction of RNFL thickness in all segments, but this is diagnostically unspecific and very similar to findings in NMOSD patients [98].
- Majority of MOGAD patients have abnormal OCT despite recovering vision after an optic neuritis [140].
- Differences in OCT findings between MOGAD and NMOSD:
  - RNFL thinning in MOGAD tends to be less severe and more diffuse compared to NMOSD. However, MOGAD is associated with more frequent relapses, so retinal pathology over the course of the disease is often comparable between these two conditions.
  - RNFL thinning in MOGAD may stabilize or improve over time, particularly with appropriate immunosuppressive therapy. In contrast, progressive RNFL thinning is more common in NMOSD, especially in patients with recurrent optic neuritis.
  - MOGAD may be associated with peripapillary retinal hemorrhages or retinal vasculitis, which are typically not observed in NMOSD.

  - Ganglion cell-inner plexiform layer (GCIPL) thinning and reduced superficial vascular plexus density are more severe in MOGAD than in NMOSD [140, 141].

2.8.12 Electrophysiology

- MOGAD is rarely (3%) associated with peripheral neuropathy [142].
- Patients with visual deficit usually show prolonged VEP latencies [140].

2.8.13 Diagnosis

- Patients with the typical clinical phenotype and clear positive anti-MOG IgG measured by fixed or live cell-based assay can be diagnosed with MOGAD.
- Patients with typical clinical phenotype (optic neuritis, myelitis, ADEM, cerebral monofocal or polyfocal deficits, brainstem or cerebellar deficits, cerebral cortical encephalitis often with seizures), but
  - Low positive titers measured by fixed or live cell-based assay,
  - Positive serum results from fixed cell-based assay without known titer, or
  - Seronegative patients with clear positive anti-MOG IgG in CSF are required to have anti-AQP4 IgG seronegativity and additional ≥1 of the supporting features such as:
    - Bilateral simultaneous clinical involvement (in case of optic neuritis)
    - Longitudinal optic nerve involvement (>50% length of the optic nerve) (in case of optic neuritis)
    - Perineural optic sheath enhancement (in case of optic neuritis)
    - Optic disc edema (in case of optic neuritis)
    - LETM (in case of myelitis)
    - Central cord lesion or H-sign (in case of myelitis)
    - Spinal conus lesion (in case of myelitis)
    - Multiple ill-defined T2 lesions in supra- and/or infratentorial whita matter (in case of brain, brainstem, or cerebral syndrome)
    - Deep gray matter involvement (in case of brain, brainstem, or cerebral syndrome)
    - Ill-defined T2-hyperintensity involving pons, middle cerebellar peduncle or medulla (in case of brain, brainstem, or cerebral syndrome)
    - Cortical lesion with or without lesional and overlying meningeal enhancement (in case of brain, brainstem, or cerebral syndrome)
- Patients should be diagnosed with MOGAD only after alternative diagnoses have been excluded [11, 143, 144].

2.8.14 Differential Diagnosis

- Number of patients (33%) fulfill diagnostic criteria for MS [145].

- NMOSD, MS, ADEM, small vessel vasculitis, NMDAR encephalitis (may overlap with MOGAD), systemic lupus erythematosus (SLE), tuberculosis, borreliosis, syphilis, sarcoidosis, Behçet's disease, Leber hereditary optic neuropathy (LHON), CNS lymphoma, gliomatosis cerebri, PRES, PML, and other CNS infections [107].

2.8.15 Treatment and Prognosis

- Acute treatments include corticosteroids or plasmapheresis, immuno-adsorption, and intravenous Immunoglobulins for patients who do not respond to corticosteroids [146].
- Long-term maintenance immunotherapy is usually initiated after a second relapse of MOGAD. The maintenance treatment is subject of debate and has been extrapolated from NMOSD studies, which is not ideal considering differences in pathophysiology between both diseases [147, 148].
- 50% of patients have monophasic disease and may not require long-term immunosuppression, but it is difficult to identify those who will have either monophasic or relapsing phenotype [146, 148].
- Patients who become seronegative (25%) are more likely to have monophasic disease [113, 114, 146].
- Tumefactive MOGAD is not associated with worse prognosis [122].

2.9 Neuromyelitis Optica Spectrum Disorders (NMOSD)

2.9.1 Synonyms

- Devic disease

2.9.2 Definition

- Neuromyelitis optica (NMO) is defined by simultaneous or consecutive acute relapses of optic neuritis and transverse myelitis.
- Some patients present only with optic neuritis or with transverse myelitis, others may have cerebral, diencephalic or brainstem involvement. Therefore, the term NMOSD has been introduced [91, 149, 150].
- The forthcoming, not yet finalized 2025 International Panel on NMO Diagnosis (IPND) consensus criteria for NMOSD suggest distinguishing NMO spectrum disease in seropositive individuals from NMO spectrum syndrome in those who are seronegative for anti-aquaporin-4 (AQP4) IgG [202].

2.9.3 Epidemiology

- Incidence 0.04–0.73/100.000/years (worldwide).
- Incidence 0.2 (0.02–0.5)/100.000/years (Europe; only seropositive cases).
- Prevalence 1.2 (0.3–10)/100.000 (worldwide).

- Occurs worldwide but has a significantly higher incidence among non-white populations, particularly those of Afro-Caribbean, African, and Asian ethnicity.
- Female/male ratio 9–10:1 (seropositive cases) and 3:1 (seronegative cases).
- Most NMOSD cases are seropositive, with 80% testing positive for AQP4 IgG (later in the text, information about seropositive NMOSD patients is provided).
- Prevalence of MOGAD is probably higher compared to seropositive NMOSD patients, not only in children, but also in adults, and in Asian and non-Asian populations. There is no evidence for an association between incidence and increasing latitude as seen in MS [121, 149, 151, 152].

2.9.4 Etiology

- An inflammatory disorder of the CNS, primarily characterized as an autoimmune astrocytopathy. However, it also causes secondary damage to oligodendrocytes and neurons due to astrocyte pathology.
- In most cases (80%), the disorder is caused by pathogenic IgG autoantibodies against aquaporin-4 (anti-AQP4), which target the most abundant water channel in the CNS.
- Genetic and/or environmental factors likely play a role in the pathogenesis. Risk factors for the disease include vitamin D deficiency, smoking, a low number of infections in early life, and certain human leukocyte antigen (HLA) haplotypes [121, 149].

2.9.5 Clinical Features

- Simultaneous or consecutive isolated acute relapses of optic neuritis and transverse myelitis. However, the clinical spectrum is broader than initially thought and can also include, although less commonly, supratentorial and brainstem encephalitis.
- Mild corticospinal relapses with a good recovery can occur in NMOSD, although severe symptoms and residual deficit are more typical.

A. Transverse myelitis
   - Initial symptom (47%)
   - Motor and sensory manifestations
   - Often with pain (neuropathic, painful paroxysmal tonic spasms, neuropathic pruritus, spasticity-associated, dysesthesia, and hyperalgesia/allodynia).
   - Recovery rate of relapses decreases over time. Overall, incomplete recovery from myelitis is high (>80%).
   - Residual severe sensory and motor deficits after relapse is more common in NMOSD than MOGAD or MS. However, severe residual sphincter dysfunction is more typical for MOGAD due to its common involvement of the spinal conus.

- Partial transverse myelitis, such as cases with uni-lateral involvement, especially when not associated with longitudinally extensive transverse myelitis (LETM) on MRI, represents a red flag. In such instances, MS or other diagnoses should be considered.

B. Optic neuritis
- Initial symptom (45%)
- Visual deficits, including blurred vision, decreased visual acuity, visual field defects (scotomas), phosphenes, color desaturation, and a positive relative afferent pupillary defect (RAPD) in cases with uni-lateral or asymmetrical involvement.
- Optic neuritis is typically severe, and complete visual field loss during relapse is more frequent in NMOSD and MOGAD than in MS.
- Often preceded or accompanied by ocular and/or retrobulbar pain, which can be worsened by eye movements.
- Non-central scotomas (altitudinal, quadrant, three-quadrant, hemianopsia, or bitemporal hemianopsia) are observed in 25% of patients with seropositive NMOSD. For MS are typically central scotomas.
- Optic neuritis can be unilateral or bilateral (simultaneous or rapidly sequential). Contralateral optic neuritis may occur within a few days or weeks. From a long-term perspective, both eyes are almost always affected. Therefore, both eyes must be examined, as one eye may be affected asymptomatically. Bilateral optic neuritis is most common in MOGAD, less common in NMOSD, and rare in MS.
- Although optic disc swelling (papilledema) may occur (5–33%), it is more severe and more frequently observed in MOGAD (80%). The same holds true for retinal hemorrhages, which usually occur only in MOGAD and not in NMOSD or MS.
- Recovery rate of relapses decreases over time. Overall, incomplete recovery from optic neuritis is high (66%).
- Simultaneous optic neuritis with transverse myelitis is rare (4.4%).

C. Brainstem encephalitis
- Often, the dorsal medulla oblongata is affected, leading to area postrema syndrome, characterized by intractable acute or subacute nausea, vomiting, and/or hiccups. Area postrema syndrom is much less common in anti-AQP4-negative and MOGAD patients. It can be diagnosed if there is evidence of involvement of the area postrema on MRI or if symptoms persist for more than 48 hours despite a negative MRI. Diagnosis also requires a lack of complete resolution of symptoms after symptomatic therapy and the exclusion of alternative diagnosis.
- Oculomotor disturbances, other cranial nerves deficits, cerebellar syndrome with ataxia, and other brainstem syndromes may occur.

D. Only very rarely present diencephalic lesions causing hypersomnolence/ narcolepsy or a syndrome of inadequate antidiuretic hormone secretion (SIADH)

E. Encephalitis
- Cerebral symptoms are more common in children.

- Headache, cognitive deficit, and psychiatric symptoms.
- Motor and sensory deficits due to hemispheric white matter lesions.
- Seizures are very rare (more frequent in MOGAD).

F. Extra-CNS complications (because AQP4 receptors are expressed also outside the CNS)
- Myositis
- Internal otitis
- Gastritis
- Vitamin B12 deficiency
- Comorbid autoimmune disorders are present in 25–40% of NMOSD seropositive patients. They include SLE, Sjögren's syndrome, myasthenia gravis, anti-phospholipid syndrome, rheumatoid arthritis, celiac disease, or rarely NMDAR encephalitis.
- Their presence may alter the clinical presentation of NMOSD [11, 121, 149, 151].

2.9.6 Disease Course

- Symptom onset usually occurs in adulthood, but NMOSD can also affect older individuals (20–28% have disease onset >60 years) or, rarely, children.
- A median age of disease onset around 40 years of age.
- Monophasic disease may occur, particularly in anti-AQP4 IgG negative patients.
- AQP4-IgG positive patients experience a relapsing course, with a median time to the second relapse being 9 months (ranging from 1 month to more than a decade).
- A new relapse should occur >4 weeks after the onset of the previous attack.
- Relapses are frequently preceded by infections (20–30%).
- Myelitis and optic neuritis may occur simultaneously or, more commonly, successively.
- Atypical disease courses include
  - Accumulation of neurological disability is primarily driven by acute clinical relapses rather than progression independent of relapsing activity (PIRA), which is often seen in MS. Although NMOSD may be associated with mild progression independent of relapses, significant PIRA is a red flag for NMOSD, and alternative diagnosis such as MS should be considered.
  - Time to relapse nadir <4 hours is atypical (consider vascular etiology).
  - Continual worsening for >4 weeks from relapse onset (consider sarcoidosis, neoplasm, etc.) [11, 121, 149–151, 153].

2.9.7 Optic Nerve Imaging

- Required dedicated sequences for optic nerve imaging.
- Longitudinally extensive optic nerve T2 hyperintense or T1 contrast-enhancing lesions (≥ half of the length of the optic nerve or involving optic chiasm). In MS, short optic nerve lesions occur.

- Optic nerve edema is infrequent but may occur (however, it is common in MOGAD and very rare in MS).
- Predominantly affect the posterior portions of the optic nerve and often also optic chiasm.
- Contrary to NMOSD, lesions in MS affect the anterior part of the optic nerve, are not longitudinal extensive and do not affect optic chiasm.
- MOGAD is more frequently associated with involvement of the anterior portion of the optic nerve, although posterior lesions, with or without the extension into the chiasm, may rarely also occur. In addition, enhancement of the perineural optic nerve sheath strongly favors MOGAD over NMOSD or MS.
- Simultaneous bilateral optic nerve involvement at disease onset may occur (15%). Although, it is less common than in MOGAD, significantly more common than in MS, where bilateral optic lesions are very rare [97, 149, 150].

2.9.8 Brain Imaging

- Majority of patients do not have typical imaging features.
- Lesions' location and appearance
  A. Normal findings (52%; at disease onset).
  B. Non-specific asymptomatic T2 lesions in white matter are relatively often.
  C. NMOSD-typical white matter lesions are located in circumventricular organs and tend to be longitudinally extensive. They occur in around 7% of patients with NMOSD but usually not present in MS; they include
     - Dorsal medulla oblongata (especially in area postrema and the solitary tract).
       - Either small localized, bilateral, or contiguous with an upper cervical spinal cord lesion.
       - Rarely may occur also in MOGAD or MS.
     - Periependymal surface of the fourth ventricle in the brainstem and cerebellum.
     - Dentate region of the cerebellum.
     - Periependymal surface of the third ventricle, thalamus, and hypothalamus.
     - Periaqueductal involvement may lead to aqueductal stenosis and obstructive hydrocephalus.
     - Extensive periependymal involvement around the lateral ventricle; often with contrast enhancement.
     - Large, confluent (uni-lateral or bilateral) subcortical or deep white matter lesion; often with cloud-like contrast enhancement (3%).
     - Long corticospinal tract lesions, uni-lateral or bilateral, contiguously involving internal capsule and cerebral peduncle.
     - Long (1/2 of the length of the corpus callosum or greater), diffuse, heterogeneous, or edematous corpus callosum lesions.

D. MS-typical MRI lesions
    - Such as Dawson fingers or periventricular lesions located in the inferior temporal lobe lesions are extremally rare.
    - The presence of lesions fulfilling diagnostic MRI criteria for MS does not exclude diagnosis of NMOSD but considered as a red flag.
    - Only a minority of patients meet the Barkhoff's criteria for MRI diagnosis of MS at disease onset, although 16–40% do so later in the disease course.
    - Cortical lesions are very rare (only around 3%; especially in acute stages; often reversible) (but often in MS and MOGAD with seizures).
    - Central vein sign may occur but is much less frequent than in MS.

- Contrast enhancement
  - Around 60% (64.6% seropositive; 55.6% seronegative) of patients during an acute (<1 month from relapse onset) relapse (optic neuritis and/or LETM) show enhancing brain lesions.
  - Different patterns of enhancement include cloud-like (patchy, with blurred margins); pencil-thin (linear periependymal); leptomeningeal; perivascular; enhancement of the brainstem, hypothalamus, and corticospinal tract lesions; and enhancement of optic nerves and optic chiasm.
  - Isolated nodular (shown only on post-contrast T1, but not on T2-weighted images), ring and open-ring enhancement is typical for MS, and they are rarely seen in NMOSD.
  - Enhancement is associated with higher relapse rate in the future.
- Evolution over time
  - The occurrence of asymptomatic CNS lesions may be observed in <10–20% of cases during the relapse-free period, which is more common than in MOGAD (<4–10%) but much less common than in MS.
  - Optic nerve, spinal cord, or brain lesions may occur successively during the single relapse.
  - Complete resolution or size reduction of brain lesions is significantly less common in NMOSD and MS than in MOGAD.
- Other remarks
  - Clinically silent lesions less likely as compared to MS.
  - Occasionally observed restricted diffusion of large or symptomatic callosal lesions during an acute relapse [122, 126, 149–151, 154–156].

2.9.9 Spinal Cord Imaging

- Lesions' location
  - Rarely normal findings in patients with spinal manifestations (in these patients should be repeated antibody testing to exclude false positivity).
  - Cervical cord lesions often extend into the brainstem.
  - Lesions primarily occur in the gray matter (>70% of the lesion volume), whereas in MS, they primarily occur in the white matter. Sometimes there is

exclusive involvement of gray matter, with "H-shaped" T2 hyperintensity on axial images called the "H-sign." This sign is even more typical for MOGAD but is atypical for MS.
  - Lesions in the lumbar segments and conus are more typical for MOGAD than for NMOSD or MS.
  - Involvement of the entire spinal cord may occasionally be present in NMOSD, similarly to MOGAD, but this is not seen in MS.
- Lesions' appearance
  - Typically, transverse myelitis with T2 hyperintense lesions comprising >50% of cross-sectional area.
  - Typically, longitudinally extensive lesions (lesion ≥3 contiguous complete vertebral segments) or focal atrophy in patients with a history of acute myelitis.
  - Short cord lesions may be present in combination with LETM or occur exclusively in 10–18% of NMOSD cases. Moreover, 7–14% of initial and 8% of subsequent relapses of myelitis in NMOSD are not associated with the LETM. Absence of LETM can be also caused by fragmentation of longitudinally extensive lesion.
  - However, occurrence of short new lesions during a relapse is more typical for MOGAD (50% sometime through disease course) and MS than for NMOSD. It is important to note that short lesions may represent still evolving (if MRI is performed too early) or already resolving (if MRI is performed too late after occurrence of relapse) LETM. Therefore, short myelitis lesions do not rule out NMOSD.
  - Sometime lesion edema, necrosis, or cavitations with hypo-intense signal on T1-weighed images. Edema of acute lesions is common in NMOSD, though it may also be present in MOGAD or MS.
  - Typical bright spotty lesions (with markedly increased T2 signal).
- Contrast enhancement
  - Common, but not required for diagnosis.
  - Ring-shaped (as in MS), patchy or irregular.
  - This ring-shaped enhancement (often elongated in NMOSD) occurs almost only in patients with NMOSD and MS, aiding in the differential diagnosis from other myelopathies. Notably, NMOSD is typically associated with LETM, whereas MS generally presents with short spinal cord lesions.
  - May persist >1 months but no longer than 3 months.
  - Occasionally present leptomeningeal enhancement.
  - Rarely, spinal nerve root enhancement or myeloradiculitis can occur. This may also be observed, albeit very rarely, in MOGAD and pediatric MS. Therefore, alternative diagnoses beyond NMOSD should be considered.
- Evolution over time
  - Complete resolution or volume reduction of spinal cord T2 lesions is significantly less common in NMOSD and MS than in MOGAD.
  - The new clinically silent spinal cord lesions during remission-free periods are not frequent (as in MOGAD) but can occur.

  - If new lesions occur during immunomodulatory treatment, they are typically nonspecific. However, if they display characteristics typical of NMOSD, they may indicate an upcoming relapse within the next few weeks to months.
  - Lesions may progress to cystic cavitation.
- Associated findings
  - In advanced stages observed sharply demarcated longitudinally extensive cord atrophy with or without T2 signal changes [106, 126, 149, 151, 157] (Fig. 2.7).

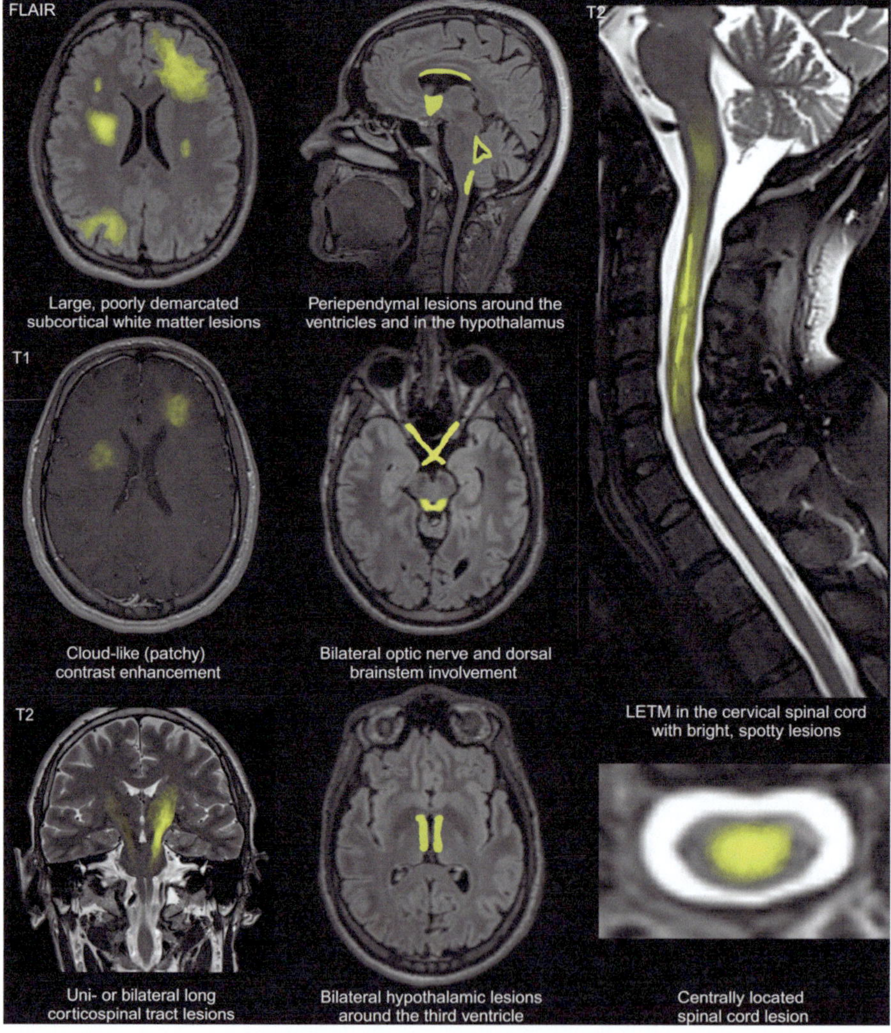

Fig. 2.7 MRI characteristics of neuromyelitis optica spectrum disorders (NMOSD)

2.9.10 Imaging Red Flags for NMOSD

- Brain lesions perpendicular to lateral ventricles (Dawson fingers) or adjacent to lateral ventricle in the inferior temporal lobe, or juxtacortical lesions involving subcortical U-fibers, or cortical lesions (consider MS).
- Absence of LETM.
- Spinal lesions located predominantly in the peripheral spinal cord, white matter, or diffuse, indistinct signal changes (consider MS).
- Lesions with persistent (>3 months) contrast enhancement or persistent contrast enhancement despite immunotherapy (consider other diagnosis than MS or NMOSD such as tumor, lymphoma, or vascular malformation).
- Brain linear perivascular radial contrast enhancement (consider anti-glial fibrillary acidic protein (GFAP) IgG-associated astrocytopathy, sarcoidosis, vasculitis, or lymphoma)[121, 150].

2.9.11 Blood Work

- Presence of anti-AQP4 IgG (80%; seropositive NMOSD)
- Seropositivity may occur years before the clinical onset of the disease. In these cases, patients should be closely monitored, but a diagnosis of NMOSD cannot be made at that stage.
- Who should be tested
  - Although anti-AQP4 IgG are highly specific for NMOSD, they should be evaluated only in suspected cases to avoid false positivity and false-positive diagnosis of NMOSD.
- How to test
  - It is recommended to use the best available detection method (cell-based assay); ELISA is not recommended and if obtained, result should be confirmed by live cell-based assay.
  - Live cell-based assay has a higher sensitivity than commercial formalin fixed cell-based assays; however, live cell-based assay often not available routinely. Live cell-based assay is the reference standard for diagnostic antibody testing. However, positive fixed cell-based assay result does not require confirmation by live cell-based assay.
- When to test
  - AQP4-IgG should be tested before treatment initiation or weeks-months after high-dose corticosteroids or plasmapheresis.
  - Confirmation of positive test results is generally recommended and mandatory if any red flags are present.
  - Advised retesting seronegative patients with suspected NMOSD during acute relapses and/or treatment-free intervals. In case of doubts, live cell-based assay should be used.
- Monitoring of anti-AQP4 IgG levels for prediction of future relapse is not recommended because
  - The levels vary significantly between timepoints and patients.
  - Titers increase only shortly before attack onset.

  - Rising antibody levels do not always lead to relapse.
  - Some relapses occur without a significant rise in titers, especially in patients under immunosuppression [121, 149, 158, 202].
- Double seronegative NMOSD patients (without anti-AQP4 and anti-MOG IgG)
  - Careful consideration of alternative diagnoses is recommended.
  - It is still unclear whether this subgroup of patients should be considered a single disease or a heterogeneous group with different demyelinating conditions. According to the forthcoming, not yet finalized 2025 IPND consensus criteria for NMOSD, double-seronegative patients will be classified as having NMO spectrum clinical syndrome [202].

2.9.12 Examination of CSF

- Elevated concentration of protein.
  - More frequently pronounced than in MS.
  - Albumin quotient is elevated in 50% and highly elevated in 25% of patients with NMOSD and MOGAD. In MS is the elevation less frequent (10%) and almost always only mild ($<12 \times 10^{-3}$).
- Some patients with NMOSD and MOGAD exhibit increased lactate concentrations during attacks, a phenomenon not seen in MS. However, lactate levels in these conditions are generally much lower than those in bacterial meningitis.
- Lymphocytic pleocytosis
  - Can be normal cytology, especially in patients with isolated optic neuritis or in remission.
  - Most patients show pleocytosis, often with more than 50 cells/mm^3. Such high pleocytosis is rare in MS.
  - Similarly to MOGAD, can sometimes be found >100 cells/mm^3, particularly in patients with acute myelitis.
  - Neutrophils are present in 50% of NMOSD and MOGAD patients, but never in higher proportions in patients with MS.
  - Eosinophils are present in 10% of cases in NMOSD but never seen in MS and only very rarely found in MOGAD.
- CSF-restricted OCB are present in a small proportion of patients (<10–20%). Their positivity may be only transient during acute relapse and such positivity does not exclude diagnosis of NMOSD.
- The Measles-Rubella-Zoster (MRZ) reaction is always negative in NMOSD and MOGAD but is positive in around 70% of MS patients.
- In general, most CSF alterations are more common during acute myelitis than optic neuritis.
- Testing of anti-AQP4 IgG in the CSF may aid in the very rare cases in which nonspecific coexisting serum antibodies mask a weak anti-AQP4 IgG signal or if testing is performed shortly after PLEX [121, 149, 158, 159].
- It has been shown that granulocyte activation markers (GAM) in CSF and adhesion molecules, measured within 21 days of the onset of clinical relapse, are higher in NMOSD and can differentiate NMOSD from MS with high specificity (76–100%) and sensitivity (87–100%) [160].

2.9.13 Laboratory Red Flags for NMOSD

- Isolated anti-AQP4 IgG positivity only in the CSF but not in the serum. It can be rarely true positive if evaluated shortly after PLEX, therefore recommended retesting or using an alternative assay.
- Anti-AQP4 IgM and/or IgA positivity, but IgG negativity is not sufficient for making a diagnosis of seropositive NMOSD.
- Double positivity for anti-AQP4 and anti-MOG IgG is extremely rare; therefore, retesting is recommended.
- Positive CSF-restricted OCB or Measles-Rubella-Varicella-Zoster (MRZ) reaction are typical for MS but atypical for NMOSD [121, 150].

2.9.14 OCT

- More severe thinning of the retinal nerve fiber layer (RNFL) and ganglion cell/inner plexiform layer (GCIPL) than is seen in MS optic neuritis.
- Greater RNFL atrophy, especially in non-temporal quadrants than in MS.
- In contrast to MS, clinically unaffected eyes in NMOSD have usually normal OCT findings.
- A single relapse of optic neuritis in MOGAD typically causes less severe damage than in NMOSD. However, MOGAD is associated with more frequent relapses, so retinal thinning over the course of the disease is comparable between the two conditions.
- Visual outcomes after optic neuritis are better in patients with MOGAD than in those with NMOSD despite similar severity of macular GCIPL thinning.
- Although OCT aids in differential diagnosis, its utility for reliably distinguishing NMOSD from MOGAD and MS, particularly in patients with advanced disease stages, is still limited [121, 139, 149].

2.9.15 Electrophysiological Studies

- VEP frequently show prolonged P100 latencies (42%).
- Additionally, reduced amplitudes are commonly present, suggesting axonal damage or even a complete lack of response. This is commonly seen in NMOSD and MOGAD but rarely in MS [149, 161].
- Both, OCT and VEP may be used to confirm optic nerve involvement [202].

2.9.16 Diagnosis

- Originally, the revised diagnostic criteria from 2006 required for diagnosis of NMO combination of optic neuritis, acute myelitis, and at least two of three supportive criteria including LETM on spinal cord MRI, brain lesions on MRI non-diagnostic for MS, or NMO-IgG seropositivity [162].

- In 2007 introduced the term NMOSD including [163]
  - A. AQP4-IgG-seropositive patients with limited or inaugural forms of NMO (e.g., first-attack LETM or recurrent or bilateral optic neuritis) at high risk for future attacks.
  - B. The cerebral, diencephalic, and brainstem lesions that occur in a minority of patients with otherwise typical NMO.
  - C. AQP4-IgG-seropositive patients with coexisting other autoimmune disorders such as systemic lupus erythematosus or Sjögren's syndrome.
  - D. Potentially also the patients diagnosed with opticospinal MS representing an MS phenotype occurring mostly in Asia and distinguished from Western MS.
- The revised NMOSD diagnostic criteria for adults proposed by the International Panel for NMO Diagnosis (IPND) were published in 2015 [150]
- Diagnostic criteria for NMOSD with AQP4-IgG positivity include
  1. At least 1 core clinical characteristic (see below).
  2. Positive anti-AQP4 IgG.
  3. Exclusion of alternative diagnoses.
- Diagnostic criteria for NMOSD without anti-AQP4 IgG positivity (or with unknown anti-AQP4 IgG status)
  1. At least two core clinical characteristics (during the one or more attacks) and meeting all of the following requirements
     - A. At least one core clinical characteristic must be
       - optic neuritis.
       - acute myelitis with LETM.
       - or area postrema syndrome.
     - B. Dissemination in space (≥2 different core clinical characteristics).
     - C. Fulfillment of additional MRI requirements, as applicable.
  2. Negative anti-AQP4 IgG.
  3. Exclusion of alternative diagnoses.
- Core clinical characteristics
  1. Optic neuritis.
  2. Acute myelitis.
  3. Area postrema syndrome (hiccups, nausea or vomiting).
  4. Acute brainstem syndrome.
  5. Symptomatic narcolepsy or acute diencephalic clinical syndrome with NMOSD-typical diencephalic MRI lesions.
  6. Symptomatic cerebral syndrome with NMOSD-typical brain lesions
- Additional MRI requirements for NMOSD without anti-AQP4 IgG and NMOSD with unknown anti-AQP4 IgG status
  1. Acute optic neuritis
     - A. with normal findings or only non-specific WM lesions, or
     - B. with optic nerve T2-hyperintense lesion or T1 gadolinium enhancing lesion extending over >1/2 optic nerve length or involving optic chiasm.

2. Acute myelitis
   A. with LETM on spinal cord MRI or
   B. with ≥3 contiguous segments of focal spinal cord atrophy in patients with history compatible with acute myelitis.
3. Area postrema syndrome with dorsal medulla/area postrema lesions.
4. Acute brainstem syndrome with periependymal brainstem lesions [150].

- The forthcoming IPND 2025 consensus criteria will redefine NMOSD to better reflect recent biomarker and clinical discoveries. The revision will distinguish AQP4-IgG positive NMOSD as a distinct disease entity, separate from seronegative cases. Diagnosis of NMO spectrum disease will require detection of AQP4-IgG antibodies using the live cell-based assay as the reference standard, together with one or two core clinical characteristics depending on presentation. Newly recognized core clinical characteristics will include also acute brainstem or cerebellar syndrome. The panel also highlights paroxysmal tonic spasms and neuropathic pruritus as features that should prompt evaluation for AQP4-IgG. The term "disease" will formally replace "disorder" in NMOSD nomenclature for seropositive cases, emphasizing its defined immunopathological basis. Patients without detectable antibodies will be classified as having NMO spectrum syndrome, acknowledging biological heterogeneity and ongoing diagnostic uncertainty. The new diagnostic criteria will be applied to both children and adults [202].

2.9.17 Differential Diagnosis

- NMOSD is sometime misdiagnosed as MS or MOGAD [164, 165] and number of patients (5–42%) fulfill diagnostic criteria for MS [166, 167] (Tables 2.1, 2.2, 2.3, and 2.4).

Table 2.1 Differences in clinical and imaging characteristics of optic neuritis among patients with MS, anti-AQP4 IgG positive NMOSD and MOGAD

Characteristic		MS	NMOSD	MOGAD
Clinical features	Simultaneous bilateral optic neuritis	Extremely rare (<5%)	May be present (17–82%, less frequent than in MOGAD)	Frequent (31–84%)
	Visual acuity deficit at nadir	Mild-moderately impaired	Moderate-severely impaired	Moderate-severely impaired
	Relapse-related vision loss recovery	Typically, favorable	Maybe be poor	Typically, favorable
	Associated with headache	Extremely rare (<5%)	May be present (28–50%)	Frequent (73–92%)

(continued)

Table 2.1 (continued)

Characteristic		MS	NMOSD	MOGAD
Fundoscopy at nadir	Optic disc swelling	May be present, but only rarely moderate-severe (11–14%)	May be present (7–52%)	Extremely frequent moderate swelling (45–92%)
	Optic disc hemorrhage	Extremely rare	Infrequent	Infrequent
OCT	RNFL thinning	Often, particularly in temporal quadrants	Severe and global	Global, but less severe than in NMOSD patients with same number of optic relapses
MRI (Lesions' location)	Orbital optic nerve lesion	Frequent	Frequent	Frequent/Extremely frequent
	Canalicular optic nerve lesion	Infrequent	Frequent	Frequent
	Intracranial optic nerve lesion	May be present	Frequent	Frequent
	Optic sheath involvement	Not reported	Extremely rare	May be present
	Chiasmal involvement	Extremely rare	May be present (can be present in isolation)	Infrequent (as an extension from longitudinally extensive lesion)
	Optic tract involvement	Extremely rare	Infrequent	Extremely rare
MRI (Lesions' appearance)	Optic nerve T2 hyperintensity	Extremely frequent	Extremely frequent	Extremely frequent
	Longitudinally extensive (>50% of length) optic nerve involvement	Extremely rare	Frequent	Frequent/extremely frequent
	Optic nerve edematous appearance	May be present	Extremely frequent	Extremely frequent
	Optic nerve head swelling on MRI	Extremely rare	Infrequent	May be present
	Optic nerve gadolinium enhancement	Extremely frequent	Extremely frequent	Extremely frequent

Adopted from Banwell et al. 2023 [11] and modified [126, 149–151, 154–157, 169–172]
Extremely rare: <5%; Infrequent: 5–20%; May be present: 21–50%; Frequent: 50–80%; Extremely frequent: >80%).

Table 2.2 Differences in clinical and imaging characteristics of myelitis among patients with MS, anti-AQP4 IgG positive NMOSD and MOGAD

Characteristic		MS	NMOSD	MOGAD
Clinical features	Simultaneous brain or optic nerve (clinical or radiological) involvement	Extremely frequent	Infrequent	May be present/ frequent
	Severity of symptoms at nadir	Mild to moderate	Severe	Moderate to severe
	Relapse-related motor deficit recovery	Very good	Moderate to poor	Very good
	Relapse-related severe bladder dysfunction	Infrequent	Frequent	Frequent
	Residual severe bladder dysfunction despite good motor function	Infrequent	Infrequent	May be present
	Painful tonic spasms	Infrequent	May be present	Extremely rare
	Progressive myelopathy	May be present	Not reported	Not reported
MRI (Lesions' location)	Multiple lesions	Frequent	Infrequent	Frequent
	Normal MRI in acute stage	Extremely rare	Extremely rare	Initially 10%; later around 5%
	Spinal segments involvement	Cervical > thoracic	Cervical – thoracic	Cervical-thoracic-lumbar (equally common)
	Conus involvement	Rare	Rare/Infrequent	May be present/ Frequent
	Axial distribution of lesions	Frequent peripherally located wedge-shaped lesions; most often in dorsal and lateral columns; <50% of axial cord area	Frequent central GM and WM involvement; isolated involvement of GM (H-sign) is infrequent; >50% of axial cord area	Frequent central GM and WM involvement; or only GM (H-sign); >50% of axial cord area

(continued)

Table 2.2 (continued)

Characteristic		MS	NMOSD	MOGAD
MRI (Lesions' appearance)	Length of T2-lesions	LETM: Extremely rare (<3%); Short lesions: Extremely frequent	LETM: Extremely frequent; Short lesions: Infrequent (10–18%)	LETM: Frequent/ extremely frequent; Short lesions: may be present (15–24%)
	Lesion borders	Typically, well-defined	Often ill-defined	Often ill-defined
	T1 hypointensity	Rare	Frequent in acute lesions, uncommon in chronic stage	Rare
	Cord swelling	May be present mild edema	Frequent/may be present	May be present (less pronounced than in NMOSD)
	Bright spotty lesions	Extremely rare	May be present	Extremely rare
	Lesion enhancement in acute phase	Frequent: Nodular; less frequently open-ring or closed-ring (80%)	Frequent (90%): Irregular, patchy or ring-like (lens-shaped)	May be present/ frequent; No clear pattern (50%); may be also present lepto-meningeal
	Lesions complete resolution after treatment	Infrequent	Infrequent	Frequent (50–80%)

Adopted from Banwell et al. 2023 [11] and modified [101, 126, 149–151, 154–157, 169, 170, 173, 174]

- NMOSD must be considered in all patients with acute transverse myelitis, optic neuritis, encephalitis, or brainstem encephalitis.
- Mimics of NMOSD include mainly the following diagnoses (adopted from Jarius et al., 2023) [121]
- Non-infectious inflammatory diseases
  - Relapsing and progressive MS, MOGAD; sarcoidosis; Behçet's disease; Sjögren's syndrome (may coexist with NMOSD); SLE (may coexist with NMOSD); Sharp syndrome, overlap syndromes; systemic vasculitis; primary CNS vasculitis; anti-NMDAR encephalitis; anti-GFAP associated encephalomyelitis; paraneoplastic neurological syndromes (e.g., anti-CV2/CRMP5, anti-GAD65, anti-Hu, anti-Ri, antiamphiphysin, and, in patients with a diencephalic syndrome, anti-Ma2/Ta-IgG, anti-IgLON5 encephalitis); para-/postinfectious myelitis; para-/postvaccinal myelitis; IgG4-related disease; Susac's syndrome; CLIPPERS; ADEM.

Table 2.3 Differences in clinical and imaging characteristics of brain involvement among patients with MS, anti-AQP4 IgG positive NMOSD and MOGAD

Characteristic		MS	NMOSD	MOGAD
Clinical features	ADEM	Infrequent in children, Extremely rare in adults	Extremely rare	Frequent in children; Extremely rare in adults
	Cerebral cortex encephalitis with seizures	Not reported	Not reported	Infrequent
	Diencephalic syndrome/ narcolepsy	Not reported	May be present/ frequent	Extremely rare
	Area postrema syndrome	Extremely rare (only case reports)	May be present/ frequent	Extremely rare/ infrequent
	Brainstem/ cerebellar involvement	Frequent/ extremely frequent	May be present	May be present
MRI (Lesions' location)	Typical brain *regions*	Periventricular and juxta-cortical WM; Corpus callosum; Brainstem and cerebellum; Inferior temporal lobe WM	Periependymal lining surrounding the ventricular system; Area Postrema; Diencephalic lesions surrounding third ventricle	Deep/sub-cortical brain WM; Deep GM (thalami, basal ganglia); Cortical GM; Brainstem and cerebellum
MRI (Lesions' appearance)	Lesion's morphology	Multifocal ovoid/ round, well-demarcated lesions; Dawson´s fingers; U-fiber lesions; Central venule sign Smoldering/ slowly evolving lesions	Can be normal MRI; or lesions: nonspecific; large confluent; peri-ependymal around circum-ventricular organs and tend to be longitudinally extensive; linear in medulla; or along corticospinal tracts	Can be normal MRI or Fluffy/ poorly demarcated lesions; can occur leukodystrophy-like pattern
	T1 hypointense lesions	Frequent	May be present	Extremely rare
	Enhancement patterns	Ovoid-nodular most frequent 2/3; Open-ring 1/3; Close-ring is rare/infrequent	Patchy/"cloud-like"; Pencil-thin pattern of the ependymal surface of lateral ventricles	Nonspecific; Leptomeningeal around brainstem; Cortical (linear) leptomeningeal

(continued)

Table 2.3 (continued)

Characteristic		MS	NMOSD	MOGAD
Lesions' evolution	Partial or complete resolution of T2 lesions	Extremely rare	May be present	Frequent
	Occurrence of asymptomatic new or enlarging lesions	Frequent	Infrequent (in relapse-free period); May be present during relapses	Rare/Infrequent

Adopted from Banwell et al. 2023 [11] and modified [126, 149–151, 154–157, 169, 170]

Table 2.4 Differences in laboratory characteristics among patients with MS, anti-AQP4 IgG positive NMOSD and MOGAD [11, 126, 149–151, 154–157, 169, 170, 172, 174]

Characteristic		MS	NMOSD	MOGAD
CSF	Glucose level	Normal	Normal	Normal
	Lactate level	Normal	Can be mild increase of concentration during relapse	Can be mild increase of concentration during relapse
	Concentration of protein	Normal or only mild elevation 10%	Elevation (50%) Marked elevation 25%	Mild elevation (30%)
	Pleocytosis (>5 cells/μL)	20–30%	>50%	>50%
	Pleocytosis (>50 cells/μL)	Rare	20–50%	12–50%
	Presence of neutrophils	Absent (or only a very small number)	50%	50%
	Presence of eosinophils	Absent	10%	Absent
	CSF – restricted OCB (pattern II or III)	80–95%; typically, permanent	<20%; can be only transient	20%; can be only transient
	MRZ reaction	Positive (70%)	Negative	Negative
Blood	Anti-AQP4 IgG	Negative	Positive in blood (80% seropositive, 20% seronegative)	Negative
	Anti-MOG IgG	Negative	Negative	Positive in blood; both in blood and CSF; or rarely only in CSF (3–5%)

- Infectious diseases
  - Viral myelitis (e.g., varicella zoster virus (VZV); enteroviruses; herpes simplex virus (HSV); cytomegalovirus (CMV); EBV; West Nile virus; human immunodeficiency virus (HIV); human T-lymphotropic virus (HTVL 1/2); tick-borne encephalitis virus; poliovirus); tuberculosis; syphilis; Lyme neuroborreliosis; Bartonella henselae; other rare infections.
- Vascular diseases
  - Spinal cord infarction; spinal dural arteriovenous fistula; Anterior/posterior ischemic (including non-arteritic) optic neuropathy; sinus thrombosis; CADASIL.
- Neoplastic diseases
  - CNS lymphoma; intramedullary tumors (e.g., ependymoma and astrocytoma, hemangioblastoma, rarely others).
- Genetic and metabolic diseases
  - E.g., vitamin B12; folate; vitamin E; copper or biotinidase deficiencies; Leber's hereditary optic neuropathy (LHON); leukodystrophies (including Alexander disease).
- Other diseases
  - Idiopathic intracranial hypertension (bilateral papilledema); traumatic spinal cord injury; compressive myelopathy; etc.
- Presence of anti-AQP4 IgG in patients with paraneoplastic neurological syndromes does not per se exclude a paraneoplastic nature of NMOSD.
- In contrast, alternative diagnosis must be carefully excluded, especially in patients with seronegative NMOSD. Biochemical screening for alternative diagnoses should include ANA, extractable nuclear antigen (ENA), anti-ds-DNA-antibodies, c/p antineutrophil cytoplasmic antibody (ANCA), cardiolipin antibodies, hypovitaminoses, other metabolic disorders, infections, autoimmune encephalitis, and neoplastic and paraneoplastic disorders (anti-collapsin response-mediator protein-5 [CRMP5/CV2] antibody-associated optic neuropathy and myelopathy or anti-Ma-associated diencephalic syndrome) [121].
- Anti-AQP4 IgG are almost always negative in patients with connective tissue disorders, who do not have typical symptoms of NMOSD [149].

2.9.18 Treatment

- High-dose corticosteroids and plasmapheresis or immunoadsorption are used for acute relapses.
- Anti-CD20 terapies, inebilizumab, satralizumab, eculizumab, ravalizumab, azathioprine or mycophenolate mofetil are used chronically to achieve long-term stabilization [121, 149, 151, 168].

2.9.19 Prognosis

- NMOSD has previously been associated with a poor prognosis, but with new treatments, it can often be relatively well-controlled. However, untreated, or late-treated patients frequently develop severe neurological disabilities, primarily due to incomplete recovery from relapses.
- Respiratory insufficiency caused by brainstem or high cervical lesions and urosepsis due to bladder dysfunction are the most common causes of death [121, 149, 151, 168].

2.10 Post- and Para-Infectious Myelitis and Optic Neuritis

- It arises from an immune-mediated response to an infectious agent, most commonly viral, less frequently bacterial, or fungal, during the recovery phase. Diagnosis typically occurs in patients with a history of infection or vaccination within 4 weeks preceding the clinical presentation of myelitis.
- Para-infectious etiology accounts for up to 40% of transverse myelitis cases in children and 6–45% in adults.
- Distinguishing between infectious and post-infectious myelitis and optic neuritis can pose a challenge.
- MRI findings often lack specificity, typically presenting long T2 hyperintensity with mild edema and frequently contrast enhancement.
- Leptomeningeal and/or nerve root enhancement may also be present in some cases [76].

2.11 Schilder's Disease

2.11.1 Synonym

- Myelinoclastic diffuse sclerosis; Encephalitis periaxialis diffusa.

2.11.2 Epidemiology

- A very rare disorder of unknown prevalence that primarily affects children, though it can also occur in older adults [10, 175].

2.11.3 Etiology and Definition

- Remains unclear whether it represents a distinct demyelinating disease or an atypical variant of MS. Although the pathology of Schilder's disease mirrors that of MS [176], the distinct immunological profile suggests that Schilder's disease and MS are likely separate entities [177].

- The diagnosis of Schilder's disease has occasionally been incorrectly applied to certain patients with leukodystrophies [10].

2.11.4 Clinical Features

- Depend on size and location of the lesions, but usually include encephalopathy (with or without seizures), deafness, cortical blindness or other focal neurological deficits.
- Similarly to ADEM, symptoms onset is frequently preceded by an infectious illness and prodromal symptoms such as headache, malaise, or fever.
- The peripheral nervous system remains unaffected.

2.11.5 Disease Course

- Subacute symptoms onset.
- Most commonly monophasic (less relapsing or chronic progressive) [176, 178].

2.11.6 Brain Imaging

- Lesions' location
  - Single, or frequently two or more large lesions (additional small lesions typical of MS are usually absent).
  - Bilateral and roughly symmetrical lesions, though they are sometime asymmetric or rarely even unilateral.
  - Mostly fronto-parietal white matter involvement, including the centrum semiovale and the corpus callosum.
  - Cortical gray matter, cerebellum and brainstem are typically spared.
- Lesions' appearance
  - Large T2 hyperintense tumefactive lesions with at least 30 × 20 mm in size in two of three dimensions.
  - Confluent demyelinating lesions, occasionally seen in chronic stages, may resemble leukodystrophies.
  - Restricted diffusion may occur in the acute stages.
- Contrast enhancement
  - Can be discrete open-ring enhancement.
- Perilesional changes
  - Only mild edema [175, 176, 178] (Fig. 2.8).

2.11.7 Spinal Cord Imaging

- Spinal cord is typically spared, cord lesions are present only rarely [177].

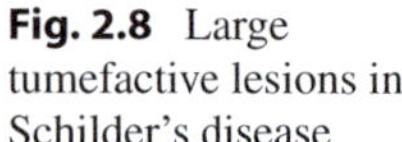

Fig. 2.8 Large tumefactive lesions in Schilder's disease

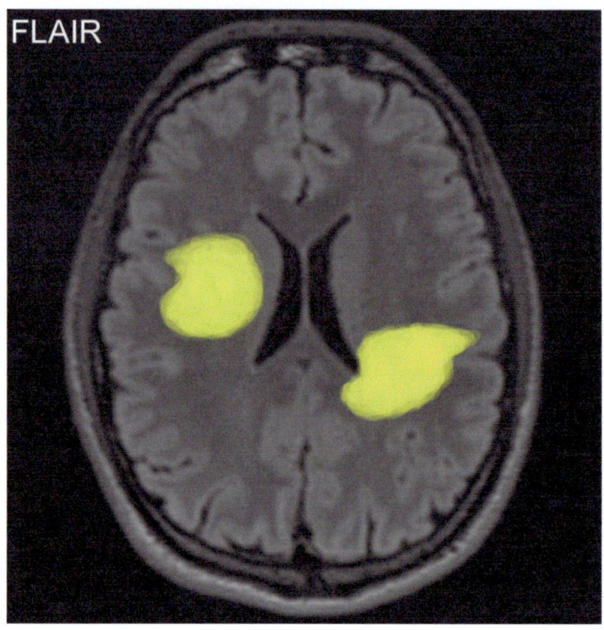

2.11.8 Blood Work

- Routine blood tests are normal, without metabolic abnormalities suggesting leukodystrophies [10].

2.11.9 Examination of CSF

- Normal concentration of lactate.
- Elevated concentration of protein (44%).
- Mild pleocytosis (21%) or normal cytology (79%).
- CSF-restricted OCB are present only sometime (20%).
- Measles-Rubella-Zoster (MRZ) reaction is negative.
- Markedly increased concentration of myelin basic protein (MBP) [10, 175, 178].

2.11.10 Diagnosis

- Based on imaging and absence of peripheral nervous system pathology and metabolic abnormalities [10, 175, 178].

2.11.11 Differential Diagnosis

- Distinguishing between Schilder's disease and tumefactive demyelination, Marburg variant of MS, tumefactive MS, ADEM, NMOSD, MOGAD or neoplasm may be challenging [10].

2.11.12 Treatment and Prognosis

- Recommendations are solely based on case reports, which have documented the use of corticosteroids, intravenous immunoglobulins, and anti-CD20 therapy [178].

2.12 Solitary Sclerosis

2.12.1 Epidemiology

- Rare disorder of unknown prevalence [179–181].

2.12.2 Etiology and Definition

- Inflammatory demyelinating disorder with a single focal lesion in the white matter of the brain or spinal cord, causing progressive upper motor neuron syndrome.
- Around 13% of patients have a first-degree relative with MS [181], leading some authors to regard this condition as a localized manifestation of primary progressive MS, without meeting the criterion for spatial dissemination [182].
- The biopsy shows demyelinating origin of the lesions [10, 181].
- There is a clinical-radiological paradox concerning the presence of a single lesion and the subsequent development of a progressive MS course. In this context, some authors hypothesize either diffuse involvement of the CNS akin to MS, whereas others underscore the potential significance of the solitary lesions' strategic location [181].

2.12.3 Clinical Features

- Spastic (face-sparing) hemiparesis, less often monoparesis, quadriparesis, or paraparesis.
- Other less frequent manifestations may include bowel/bladder dysfunction, sensory loss or ataxia [181, 183].

2.12.4 Disease Course

- The symptoms onset is typically insidious resembling the primary progressive MS. Only a minority of cases experience acute or subacute myelopathy at disease onset, followed by incomplete remission.
- Disability is slowly progressive without any relapses [181, 183].
- The mean age of onset is 50 years of age (range, 23–71) [179–181].

2.12.5 Brain and Spinal Cord Imaging

- The strategically located single lesion usually affects the corticospinal tracts in:
  - Ventral or lateral columns, or central part of upper cervical cord (most common location).
  - Ventral cervico-medullary junction.
  - Ventral brainstem (pons-mesencephalic junction).
  - Rarely thoracic cord or motor tracts in periventricular white matter [179–184].
- In addition to strategically located solitary lesions, some patients (27%) may also exhibit non-specific T2 hyperintensitis in brain white matter. These lesions tend to be asymmetric and lack mass effect.
- Spinal cord lesion is typically short (<3 vertebral segments).
- Temporary contrast enhancement of the solitary lesion is rare (7%) [181] (Fig. 2.9).

2.12.6 Blood Work

- Normal.

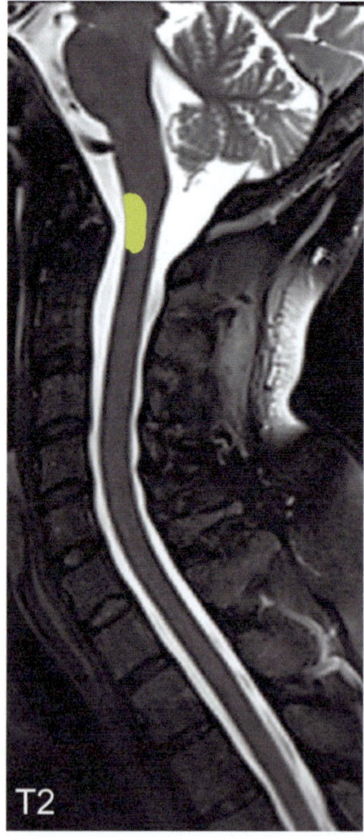

Fig. 2.9 Strategically located single lesion affecting the corticospinal tracts in solitary sclerosis

2.12.7 Examination of CSF

- Mildly elevated concentration of protein (50%).
- Mild pleocytosis is rare (8%) [179].
- CSF-restricted OCB (65%).
- Elevated IgG index and/or CSF-restricted OCB (74%) [180, 181, 183, 185].
- Neurofilament light chain levels in blood and CSF are usually normal [180].

2.12.8 Electrophysiology

- VEP are usually normal [181], but some patients might have prolonged latencies [186].
- May be present impaired somatosensory evoked potentials within central proprioceptive pathways (33%) [181].

2.12.9 Diagnosis

- Required the presence of progressive motor deficit lasting at least one year, along with a single, strategically located CNS inflammatory demyelinating lesion [182].

2.12.10 Differential Diagnosis

- Presence of CSF-restricted OCB and normal neurofilament light chain (NfL) levels might help to distinguish solitary sclerosis from primary lateral sclerosis and amyotrophic lateral sclerosis (ALS) [175].
- Brain FDG-PET scans in patients with primary lateral sclerosis reveal the presence of the "stripe sign," attributed to hypometabolism in the primary motor cortex. This sign is not observed in patients with solitary sclerosis [187].
- Some patients may eventually meet the diagnostic criteria for MS over time. Therefore, MS should be considered in the differential diagnosis, even in the absence of spatial dissemination [188].

2.12.11 Treatment and Prognosis

- Case studies reported improvement after 4-aminopyridine and poor response to high-dose corticosteroids [180, 181, 184].
- The response to disease-modifying or immunosuppressive therapy is poor [181].

2.13 Tumefactive Multiple Sclerosis

2.13.1 Epidemiology

- Prevalence 1.4–8.2/100 MS patients [189–192].

2.13.2 Etiology and Definition

- Uncommon variant of MS, characterized by tumefactive demyelinating lesions.
- There is no consensus regarding the definition of these lesions, but they are usually defined as those larger than 20 mm in diameter.
- Tumefactive demyelination might occur also in association with other conditions such as NMOSD, MOGAD, ADEM, Marburg disease, Schilder's Disease, Balo's concentric sclerosis but also HIV, SLE, Sjogren's syndrome, Behçet's disease, or some drugs such as tacrolimus [10, 16, 193].
- In case of MS, newly occurred tumefactive demyelinating lesions might also occur as a rebound phenomenon after treatment cessation [194].
- Biopsy in tumefactive MS shows hypercellular lesions with confluent demyelination, abundant foamy macrophages containing myelin debris, reactive astrogliosis, relative axonal preservation and variable perivascular, and parenchymal lymphocytic inflammation [192].

2.13.3 Clinical Features

- Usually, polysymptomatic disease onset.
- Neurological deficit depends on the character, size, and location of the lesions.
- Patients might sometime experience seizures, aphasia, apraxia, headache, speech, or cognitive deficit. These atypical symptoms for MS may be explained by the involvement of cortical gray matter and/or by the presence of edema.
- The disease course is usually relapsing remitting, less frequently monophasic.
- Symptoms onset is typically in second to fourth decade of life, rarely in children and elderly patients [10, 16, 191, 195, 196].

2.13.4 Brain Imaging

- There are several typical imaging features, but none are pathognomic.
- Lesions' location
  - Mostly in subcortical white matter of the frontal lobe > parietal lobe > corpus callosum > periventricular > occipital lobe > temporal lobe.
  - Rare in cerebellum, deep and cortical gray matter, and brainstem.

  - Single tumefactive lesion (24%).
  - Multiple lesions (tumefactive combined with non-tumefactive) (76%).
  - Lesion may spread across the corpus callosum in a "butterfly" configuration and simulate an infiltrative astrocytoma or lymphoma (7–12%).
- Lesions' appearance
  - T2 hyperintense lesions larger than 20 mm in diameter (most often within 50 mm; median 40 mm).
  - Well-defined margins (73%), or less frequently diffuse character (38%).
  - T1-weighed imaging show iso-intense (2%), mild/moderately hypo-intense (33%), or markedly hypo-intense (65%) signal.
- Contrast enhancement (81–95%)
  - Almost always exhibits enhancement, which is often atypical.
  - Close-ring (more common) or open-ring (less common; typically, closed towards gray matter) (51–65%); less common heterogeneous (40–50%); homogeneous (10%); diffuse; fluffy/cotton ball; concentric; nodular or punctiform/punctate enhancement.
  - May show ring-shaped restriction of diffusion at the periphery with an area of central hypo-intensity on diffusion-weighted imaging (DWI). Only rarely can central restricted diffusion occur in demyelinating lesions with an intense inflammatory core, which may mimic a brain abscess.
  - Only rarely seen enhancement after 6 months (2%).
- Perilesional changes
  - Edema (77%); mild (59%) or moderate/marked (41%).
  - Mass effect (45%); mild (64%) or moderate/marked (36%).
  - Compared to tumors or abscesses, tumefactive lesions exhibit relatively low mass effect and edema for their size.
  - May be present a perilesional T1- and T2-hypointense ring, corresponding with the area of contrast enhancement on post-contrast T1 images (30.5–48%).
- Evolution over time
  - Most MS patients with tumefactive demyelination have a typical course of MS; only a small number of patients have relapsing tumefactive demyelination.
  - Often seen significant reduction of lesion volume following corticosteroids, typically within 12 weeks.
  - Recommended follow-up imaging after 1.5–6 months [10, 16, 52, 191–193, 196–199] (Fig. 2.10).

2.13.5 Spinal Cord Imaging

- Often present lesions typical for MS (40–50%) [191].

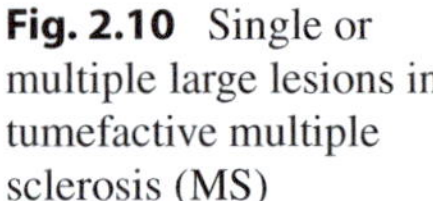

Fig. 2.10 Single or multiple large lesions in tumefactive multiple sclerosis (MS)

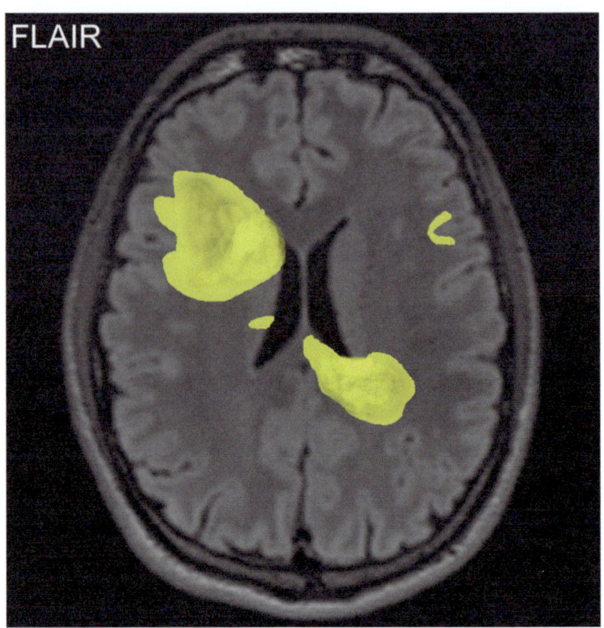

2.13.6 Examination of CSF

- Slightly elevated concentrations of protein (57%).
- Mild pleocytosis (43%).
- Patients with a single tumefactive demyelinating lesion at disease onset less frequently exhibit CSF-restricted OCB compared to typical MS patients (52% vs. 90–95% in MS).
- Patients with multiple lesions (including tumefactive lesion/s) have more often positive CSF-restricted OCB (86%) compared to those with single tumefactive lesions (around 30%).
- Elevated concentration of myelin basic protein (67%) [189, 191, 192, 195, 196].

2.13.7 Diagnosis

- Based on McDonald 2017 criteria and imaging characteristics [182].
- The decision of when to biopsy a tumefactive lesion to exclude alternative diagnoses can be challenging [10, 16]. Histopathological examination may also pose challenges, and misinterpretations of biopsy findings are common.
- This is driven by some similar histopathological features shared by MS and neoplastic lesions such as hypercellularity, presence of atypical reactive astrocytes or mitotic figures. Around one-third of biopsies are originally misdiagnosed, with astrocytoma being the most often misdiagnosed (more often low-grade than high-grade gliomas) [192].

2.13.8 Differential Diagnosis

- A tumefactive lesion (particularly if single) must be distinguished from other demyelinating disease, neoplasm, abscess, ischemia, or infection.
- Serial MRI typically shows a decrease in the size of demyelinating lesions, while neoplasms tend to increase in volume.
- Hypodensity on brain computed tomography (CT), corresponding to areas of contrast enhancement, occurrs more frequently in demyelinating lesions than in neoplasms (93% vs. 4%), may also aid in diagnosis.
- In tumefactive demyelination the changes on DWI evolve rapidly (from few days to couple of weeks), which is usually not seen in patients with neoplasms or abscesses, where the findings on DWI are more stable over time.
- Metastases and high-grade gliomas exhibit variable findings on DWI, which depend on factors such as the specific part of the lesion, their histology, and tumor cellularity.
- Abscesses show central rather than peripheral restriction of diffusivity.
- Majority of acute demyelinating lesions exhibit not only temporary restricted diffusion but also simultaneous contrast enhancement, distinguishing them from acute ischemic lesions usually showing only restricted diffusion.
- In some cases, MR spectroscopy and FDG-PET could aid in the differential diagnosis [10, 16, 52, 192, 197, 200, 201].
- The presence of a peripheral T2-hypointense rim, T1-hypointensity, diffusion restriction (particularly in an arc pattern), ring enhancement, and a Baló-like or cystic appearance favors tumefactive MS over MOGAD and NMOSD.
- Diffusion restriction of tumefactive lesions is more frequent in NMOSD than in MOGAD (67% vs. 26%) [122].

2.13.9 Treatment and Prognosis

- Same as that used in MS.
- The short-term outcome is often more severe than in typical MS relapse, with a slower recovery and a higher risk of residual deficits, but long-term prognosis is comparable with that of a typical MS [196].

References

1. Otallah S. Acute disseminated encephalomyelitis in children and adults: a focused review emphasizing new developments. Mult Scler. 2021;27(8):1153–60.
2. Paolilo RB, Deiva K, Neuteboom R, Rostásy K, Lim M. Acute disseminated encephalomyelitis: current perspectives. Children (Basel, Switzerland). 2020;7(11).
3. Koelman DL, Mateen FJ. Acute disseminated encephalomyelitis: current controversies in diagnosis and outcome. J Neurol. 2015;262(9):2013–24.
4. Nishiyama M, Nagase H, Tomioka K, Tanaka T, Yamaguchi H, Ishida Y, et al. Clinical time course of pediatric acute disseminated encephalomyelitis. Brain Dev. 2019;41(6):531–7.

5. Baumann M, Sahin K, Lechner C, Hennes EM, Schanda K, Mader S, et al. Clinical and neuroradiological differences of paediatric acute disseminating encephalomyelitis with and without antibodies to the myelin oligodendrocyte glycoprotein. J Neurol Neurosurg Psychiatry. 2015;86(3):265–72.
6. Hennes EM, Baumann M, Schanda K, Anlar B, Bajer-Kornek B, Blaschek A, et al. Prognostic relevance of MOG antibodies in children with an acquired demyelinating syndrome. Neurology. 2017;89(9):900–8.
7. Ketelslegers IA, Visser IE, Neuteboom RF, Boon M, Catsman-Berrevoets CE, Hintzen RQ. Disease course and outcome of acute disseminated encephalomyelitis is more severe in adults than in children. Mult Scler. 2011;17(4):441–8.
8. Marchioni E, Ravaglia S, Piccolo G, Furione M, Zardini E, Franciotta D, et al. Postinfectious inflammatory disorders: subgroups based on prospective follow-up. Neurology. 2005;65(7):1057–65.
9. Lademann H, Bertsche A, Petzold A, Zack F, Büttner A, Däbritz J, et al. Acute disseminated encephalomyelitis with seizures and myocarditis: a fatal triad. Medicina (Kaunas, Lithuania). 2020;56(6).
10. Hardy TA, Reddel SW, Barnett MH, Palace J, Lucchinetti CF, Weinshenker BG. Atypical inflammatory demyelinating syndromes of the CNS. Lancet Neurol. 2016;15(9):967–81.
11. Banwell B, Bennett JL, Marignier R, Kim HJ, Brilot F, Flanagan EP, et al. Diagnosis of myelin oligodendrocyte glycoprotein antibody-associated disease: international MOGAD Panel proposed criteria. Lancet Neurol. 2023;22(3):268–82.
12. Cole J, Evans E, Mwangi M, Mar S. Acute disseminated encephalomyelitis in children: an updated review based on current diagnostic criteria. Pediatr Neurol. 2019;100:26–34.
13. Koelman DL, Chahin S, Mar SS, Venkatesan A, Hoganson GM, Yeshokumar AK, et al. Acute disseminated encephalomyelitis in 228 patients: a retrospective, multicenter US study. Neurology. 2016;86(22):2085–93.
14. Wong YYM, van Pelt ED, Ketelslegers IA, Catsman-Berrevoets CE, Hintzen RQ, Neuteboom RF. Evolution of MRI abnormalities in paediatric acute disseminated encephalomyelitis. Eur J Paediatr Neurol. 2017;21(2):300–4.
15. Pohl D, Alper G, Van Haren K, Kornberg AJ, Lucchinetti CF, Tenembaum S, et al. Acute disseminated encephalomyelitis: updates on an inflammatory CNS syndrome. Neurology. 2016;87(9 Suppl 2):S38–45.
16. Hardy TA, Chataway J. Tumefactive demyelination: an approach to diagnosis and management. J Neurol Neurosurg Psychiatry. 2013;84(9):1047–53.
17. Marin SE, Callen DJ. The magnetic resonance imaging appearance of monophasic acute disseminated encephalomyelitis: an update post application of the 2007 consensus criteria. Neuroimaging Clin N Am. 2013;23(2):245–66.
18. Dale RC, de Sousa C, Chong WK, Cox TC, Harding B, Neville BG. Acute disseminated encephalomyelitis, multiphasic disseminated encephalomyelitis and multiple sclerosis in children. Brain. 2000;123(Pt 12):2407–22.
19. Tenembaum S, Chamoles N, Fejerman N. Acute disseminated encephalomyelitis: a long-term follow-up study of 84 pediatric patients. Neurology. 2002;59(8):1224–31.
20. Callen DJ, Shroff MM, Branson HM, Li DK, Lotze T, Stephens D, et al. Role of MRI in the differentiation of ADEM from MS in children. Neurology. 2009;72(11):968–73.
21. Ketelslegers IA, Neuteboom RF, Boon M, Catsman-Berrevoets CE, Hintzen RQ. A comparison of MRI criteria for diagnosing pediatric ADEM and MS. Neurology. 2010;74(18):1412–5.
22. Uher T, Havrdova E, Sobisek L, Krasensky J, Vaneckova M, Seidl Z, et al. Is no evidence of disease activity an achievable goal in MS patients on intramuscular interferon beta-1a treatment over long-term follow-up? Mult Scler. 2017;23(2):242–52.
23. Mariotto S, Gajofatto A, Batzu L, Delogu R, Sechi G, Leoni S, et al. Relevance of antibodies to myelin oligodendrocyte glycoprotein in CSF of seronegative cases. Neurology. 2019;93(20):e1867–e72.
24. Boesen MS, Blinkenberg M, Koch-Henriksen N, Thygesen LC, Uldall PV, Magyari M, et al. Implications of the International Paediatric Multiple Sclerosis Study Group consensus crite-

ria for paediatric acute disseminated encephalomyelitis: a nationwide validation study. Dev Med Child Neurol. 2018;60(11):1123–31.
25. Krupp LB, Banwell B, Tenembaum S. Consensus definitions proposed for pediatric multiple sclerosis and related disorders. Neurology. 2007;68(16 Suppl 2):S7–12.
26. Peche SS, Alshekhlee A, Kelly J, Lenox J, Mar S. A long-term follow-up study using IPMSSG criteria in children with CNS demyelination. Pediatr Neurol. 2013;49(5):329–34.
27. Schwarz S, Mohr A, Knauth M, Wildemann B, Storch-Hagenlocher B. Acute disseminated encephalomyelitis: a follow-up study of 40 adult patients. Neurology. 2001;56(10):1313–8.
28. Menge T, Hemmer B, Nessler S, Wiendl H, Neuhaus O, Hartung HP, et al. Acute disseminated encephalomyelitis: an update. Arch Neurol. 2005;62(11):1673–80.
29. Hurst AE. Acute hemorrhagic leukoencephalitis: a previously undefined entity. Med J Aust. 1941;1:6.
30. Markus R, Brew BJ, Turner J, Pell M. Successful outcome with aggressive treatment of acute haemorrhagic leukoencephalitis. 1997;63(4):551–2.
31. Manzano GS, McEntire CRS, Martinez-Lage M, Mateen FJ, Hutto SK. Acute disseminated encephalomyelitis and acute hemorrhagic Leukoencephalitis following COVID-19: systematic review and meta-synthesis. Neurol Neuroimmunol Neuroinflamm. 2021;8(6).
32. Alsaid HM, Atawneh MAA, Abukhalaf S, Daoud A, Hamadah A, Gharaibeh K. Acute hemorrhagic Leukoencephalitis - a rare but fatal form of acute disseminated encephalomyelitis - complicated by brain herniation: a case report and literature review. Am J Case Rep. 2022;23:e935636.
33. Robinson CA, Adiele RC, Tham M, Lucchinetti CF, Popescu BF. Early and widespread injury of astrocytes in the absence of demyelination in acute haemorrhagic leukoencephalitis. Acta Neuropathol Commun. 2014;2:52.
34. Klein CJ, Wijdicks EF, Earnest FT. Full recovery after acute hemorrhagic leukoencephalitis (Hurst's disease). J Neurol. 2000;247(12):977–9.
35. Dubey D, Pittock SJ, Kelly CR, McKeon A, Lopez-Chiriboga AS, Lennon VA, et al. Autoimmune encephalitis epidemiology and a comparison to infectious encephalitis. Ann Neurol. 2018;83(1):166–77.
36. Flanagan EP, Hinson SR, Lennon VA, Fang B, Aksamit AJ, Morris PP, et al. Glial fibrillary acidic protein immunoglobulin G as biomarker of autoimmune astrocytopathy: analysis of 102 patients. Ann Neurol. 2017;81(2):298–309.
37. Kunchok A, Zekeridou A, McKeon A. Autoimmune glial fibrillary acidic protein astrocytopathy. Curr Opin Neurol. 2019;32(3):452–8.
38. Dubey D, Hinson SR, Jolliffe EA, Zekeridou A, Flanagan EP, Pittock SJ, et al. Autoimmune GFAP astrocytopathy: prospective evaluation of 90 patients in 1 year. J Neuroimmunol. 2018;321:157–63.
39. Luessi F, Engel S, Spreer A, Bittner S, Zipp F. GFAPalpha IgG-associated encephalitis upon daclizumab treatment of MS. Neurol Neuroimmunol Neuroinflamm. 2018;5(5):e481.
40. Fang B, McKeon A, Hinson SR, Kryzer TJ, Pittock SJ, Aksamit AJ, et al. Autoimmune glial fibrillary acidic protein Astrocytopathy: a novel Meningoencephalomyelitis. JAMA Neurol. 2016;73(11):1297–307.
41. Chen JJ, Aksamit AJ, McKeon A, Pittock SJ, Weinshenker BG, Leavitt JA, et al. Optic disc edema in glial fibrillary acidic protein autoantibody-positive meningoencephalitis. J Neuroophthalmol. 2018;38(3):276–81.
42. Greco G, Masciocchi S, Diamanti L, Bini P, Vegezzi E, Marchioni E, et al. Visual system involvement in glial fibrillary acidic protein Astrocytopathy: two case reports and a systematic literature review. Neurol Neuroimmunol Neuroinflamm. 2023;10(5).
43. Long Y, Liang J, Xu H, Huang Q, Yang J, Gao C, et al. Autoimmune glial fibrillary acidic protein astrocytopathy in Chinese patients: a retrospective study. Eur J Neurol. 2018;25(3):477–83.
44. Shan F, Long Y, Qiu W. Autoimmune glial fibrillary acidic protein astrocytopathy: a review of the literature. Front Immunol. 2018;9:2802.

45. Sechi E, Morris PP, McKeon A, Pittock SJ, Hinson SR, Weinshenker BG, et al. Glial fibrillary acidic protein IgG related myelitis: characterisation and comparison with aquaporin-4-IgG myelitis. J Neurol Neurosurg Psychiatry. 2019;90(4):488–90.
46. Tabira T. Concentric sclerosis (Balo). Nihon Rinsho. 1994;52(11):2971–5.
47. Hardy TA, Miller DH. Balo's concentric sclerosis. Lancet Neurol. 2014;13(7):740–6.
48. Jolliffe EA, Guo Y, Hardy TA, Morris PP, Flanagan EP, Lucchinetti CF, et al. Clinical and radiologic features, pathology, and treatment of Balo concentric sclerosis. Neurology. 2021;97(4):e414–e22.
49. Stadelmann C, Ludwin S, Tabira T, Guseo A, Lucchinetti CF, Leel-Ossy L, et al. Tissue preconditioning may explain concentric lesions in Balo's type of multiple sclerosis. Brain. 2005;128(Pt 5):979–87.
50. Hulcombe JE, Bradfield JM, Tannenberg AE, Pender MP. Balo's concentric sclerosis in a woman from Papua New Guinea. J Clin Neurosci. 1999;6(1):46–8.
51. Shankar SK, Rao TV, Srivastav VK, Narula S, Asha T, Das S. Balo's concentric sclerosis: a variant of multiple sclerosis associated with oligodendroglioma. Neurosurgery. 1989;25(6):982–6.
52. Wallner-Blazek M, Rovira A, Fillipp M, Rocca MA, Miller DH, Schmierer K, et al. Atypical idiopathic inflammatory demyelinating lesions: prognostic implications and relation to multiple sclerosis. J Neurol. 2013;260(8):2016–22.
53. Barnett MH, Prineas JW. Relapsing and remitting multiple sclerosis: pathology of the newly forming lesion. Ann Neurol. 2004;55(4):458–68.
54. Kavanagh EC, Heran MK, Fenton DM, Lapointe JS, Nugent RA, Graeb DA. Diffusion-weighted imaging findings in Balo concentric sclerosis. Br J Radiol. 2006;79(943):e28–31.
55. Ng SH, Ko SF, Cheung YC, Wong HF, Wan YL. MRI features of Balo's concentric sclerosis. Br J Radiol. 1999;72(856):400–3.
56. Kastrup O, Stude P, Limmroth V. Balo's concentric sclerosis. Evolution of active demyelination demonstrated by serial contrast-enhanced MRI. J Neurol. 2002;249(7):811–4.
57. Bolcaen J, Acou M, Mertens K, Hallaert G, Van den Broecke C, Achten E, et al. Structural and metabolic features of two different variants of multiple sclerosis: a PET/MRI study. J Neuroimaging. 2013;23(3):431–6.
58. Berghoff M, Schlamann MU, Maderwald S, Grams AE, Kaps M, Ladd ME, et al. 7 tesla MRI demonstrates vascular pathology in Balo's concentric sclerosis. Mult Scler. 2013;19(1):120–2.
59. Kreft KL, Mellema SJ, Hintzen RQ. Spinal cord involvement in Balo's concentric sclerosis. J Neurol Sci. 2009;279(1–2):114–7.
60. Jarius S, Wurthwein C, Behrens JR, Wanner J, Haas J, Paul F, et al. Balo's concentric sclerosis is immunologically distinct from multiple sclerosis: results from retrospective analysis of almost 150 lumbar punctures. J Neuroinflammation. 2018;15(1):22.
61. Mowry EM, Woo JH, Ances BM. Balo's concentric sclerosis presenting as a stroke-like syndrome. Nat Clin Pract Neurol. 2007;3(6):349–54.
62. Brown JW, Coles AJ, Jones JL. First use of alemtuzumab in Balo's concentric sclerosis: a case report. Mult Scler. 2013;19(12):1673–5.
63. Ogata H, Matsuse D, Yamasaki R, Kawamura N, Matsushita T, Yonekawa T, et al. A nationwide survey of combined central and peripheral demyelination in Japan. J Neurol Neurosurg Psychiatry. 2016;87(1):29–36.
64. Puthenparampil M, Terrin A, Federle L, Gizzi M, Perini P, Gallo P. Acute simultaneous development of brain tumour-like lesion and demyelinating polyneuropathy in a patient with chronic relapsing myelitis. Mult Scler. 2018;24(4):546–50.
65. Ingwersen J, Graf J, Kluge J, Weise M, Dietrich M, Lee JI, et al. CNS involvement in chronic inflammatory demyelinating polyneuropathy: subtle retinal changes in optical coherence tomography. Neurol Neuroimmunol Neuroinflamm. 2022;9(1).
66. Cortese A, Franciotta D, Alfonsi E, Visigalli N, Zardini E, Diamanti L, et al. Combined central and peripheral demyelination: clinical features, diagnostic findings, and treatment. J Neurol Sci. 2016;363:182–7.

67. Papadopoulou M, Tzanetakos D, Moschovos C, Korona A, Vartzelis G, Voudris K, et al. Combined central and peripheral demyelination (CCPD) associated with MOG antibodies: report of four new cases and narrative review of the literature. J Clin Med. 2024;13(12).
68. Sechi E, Shosha E, Williams JP, Pittock SJ, Weinshenker BG, Keegan BM, et al. Aquaporin-4 and MOG autoantibody discovery in idiopathic transverse myelitis epidemiology. Neurology. 2019;93(4):e414–e20.
69. de Seze J, Lanctin C, Lebrun C, Malikova I, Papeix C, Wiertlewski S, et al. Idiopathic acute transverse myelitis: application of the recent diagnostic criteria. Neurology. 2005;65(12):1950–3.
70. Lopez Chiriboga S, Flanagan EP. Myelitis and other autoimmune myelopathies. Continuum (Minneap Minn). 2021;27(1):62–92.
71. Proposed diagnostic criteria and nosology of acute transverse myelitis. Neurology. 2002;59(4):499–505.
72. Zalewski NL, Flanagan EP, Keegan BM. Evaluation of idiopathic transverse myelitis revealing specific myelopathy diagnoses. Neurology. 2018;90(2):e96–e102.
73. Barreras P, Fitzgerald KC, Mealy MA, Jimenez JA, Becker D, Newsome SD, et al. Clinical biomarkers differentiate myelitis from vascular and other causes of myelopathy. Neurology. 2018;90(1):e12–21.
74. Cobo Calvo A, Mañé Martínez MA, Alentorn-Palau A, Bruna Escuer J, Romero Pinel L, Martínez-Yélamos S. Idiopathic acute transverse myelitis: outcome and conversion to multiple sclerosis in a large series. BMC Neurol. 2013;13:135.
75. al Deeb SM, Yaqub BA, Bruyn GW, Biary NM. Acute transverse myelitis. A localized form of postinfectious encephalomyelitis. Brain. 1997;120(Pt 7):1115–22.
76. Goh C, Desmond PM, Phal PM. MRI in transverse myelitis. JMRI. 2014;40(6):1267–79.
77. Harzheim M, Schlegel U, Urbach H, Klockgether T, Schmidt S. Discriminatory features of acute transverse myelitis: a retrospective analysis of 45 patients. J Neurol Sci. 2004;217(2):217–23.
78. Choi KH, Lee KS, Chung SO, Park JM, Kim YJ, Kim HS, et al. Idiopathic transverse myelitis: MR characteristics. AJNR Am J Neuroradiol. 1996;17(6):1151–60.
79. Alvarenga MP, Thuler LC, Neto SP, Vasconcelos CC, Camargo SG, Alvarenga MP, et al. The clinical course of idiopathic acute transverse myelitis in patients from Rio de Janeiro. J Neurol. 2010;257(6):992–8.
80. Young J, Quinn S, Hurrell M, Taylor B. Clinically isolated acute transverse myelitis: prognostic features and incidence. Mult Scler. 2009;15(11):1295–302.
81. Mariano R, Flanagan EP, Weinshenker BG, Palace J. A practical approach to the diagnosis of spinal cord lesions. Pract Neurol. 2018;18(3):187–200.
82. Li R, Qiu W, Lu Z, Dai Y, Wu A, Long Y, et al. Acute transverse myelitis in demyelinating diseases among the Chinese. J Neurol. 2011;258(12):2206–13.
83. Scott TF, Kassab SL, Singh S. Acute partial transverse myelitis with normal cerebral magnetic resonance imaging: transition rate to clinically definite multiple sclerosis. Mult Scler. 2005;11(4):373–7.
84. Perumal J, Zabad R, Caon C, MacKenzie M, Tselis A, Bao F, et al. Acute transverse myelitis with normal brain MRI : long-term risk of MS. J Neurol. 2008;255(1):89–93.
85. Ruet A, Deloire MS, Ouallet JC, Molinier S, Brochet B. Predictive factors for multiple sclerosis in patients with clinically isolated spinal cord syndrome. Mult Scler. 2011;17(3):312–8.
86. Sellner J, Lüthi N, Bühler R, Gebhardt A, Findling O, Greeve I, et al. Acute partial transverse myelitis: risk factors for conversion to multiple sclerosis. Eur J Neurol. 2008;15(4):398–405.
87. Suzuki M, Kawasaki H, Masaki K, Suzuki SO, Terada T, Tsuchida T, et al. An autopsy case of the Marburg variant of multiple sclerosis (acute multiple sclerosis). Intern Med. 2013;52(16):1825–32.
88. Capet N, Levraut M, Delourme A, Thomel-Rocchi O, Bourg V, Cabre P, et al. Marburg multiple sclerosis variant: complete remission with very early administration of mitoxantrone-A case report. Neurol Ther. 2022;11(1):507–13.

89. Manuel A, Vasudevan MC. A case of Marburg's variant of multiple sclerosis successfully treated with IVIg and Mitoxantrone. Ann Indian Acad Neurol. 2021;24(1):92–4.
90. Jeffery DR, Lefkowitz DS, Crittenden JP. Treatment of Marburg variant multiple sclerosis with mitoxantrone. J Neuroimaging. 2004;14(1):58–62.
91. O'Connell K, Hamilton-Shield A, Woodhall M, Messina S, Mariano R, Waters P, et al. Prevalence and incidence of neuromyelitis optica spectrum disorder, aquaporin-4 antibody-positive NMOSD and MOG antibody-positive disease in Oxfordshire, UK. J Neurol Neurosurg Psychiatry. 2020;91(10):1126–8.
92. Corbali O, Chitnis T. Pathophysiology of myelin oligodendrocyte glycoprotein antibody disease. Front Neurol. 2023;14:1137998.
93. Hoftberger R, Guo Y, Flanagan EP, Lopez-Chiriboga AS, Endmayr V, Hochmeister S, et al. The pathology of central nervous system inflammatory demyelinating disease accompanying myelin oligodendrocyte glycoprotein autoantibody. Acta Neuropathol. 2020;139(5):875–92.
94. Waters P, Fadda G, Woodhall M, O'Mahony J, Brown RA, Castro DA, et al. Serial anti-myelin oligodendrocyte glycoprotein antibody analyses and outcomes in children with demyelinating syndromes. JAMA Neurol. 2020;77(1):82–93.
95. Reindl M, Waters P. Myelin oligodendrocyte glycoprotein antibodies in neurological disease. Nat Rev Neurol. 2019;15(2):89–102.
96. Hassan MB, Stern C, Flanagan EP, Pittock SJ, Kunchok A, Foster RC, et al. Population-based incidence of optic neuritis in the era of Aquaporin-4 and myelin oligodendrocyte glycoprotein antibodies. Am J Ophthalmol. 2020;220:110–4.
97. Ramanathan S, Prelog K, Barnes EH, Tantsis EM, Reddel SW, Henderson AP, et al. Radiological differentiation of optic neuritis with myelin oligodendrocyte glycoprotein antibodies, aquaporin-4 antibodies, and multiple sclerosis. Mult Scler. 2016;22(4):470–82.
98. Bennett JL, Costello F, Chen JJ, Petzold A, Biousse V, Newman NJ, et al. Optic neuritis and autoimmune optic neuropathies: advances in diagnosis and treatment. Lancet Neurol. 2023;22(1):89–100.
99. Chen JJ, Flanagan EP, Jitprapaikulsan J, Lopez-Chiriboga ASS, Fryer JP, Leavitt JA, et al. Myelin oligodendrocyte glycoprotein antibody-positive optic neuritis: clinical characteristics, radiologic clues, and outcome. Am J Ophthalmol. 2018;195:8–15.
100. Asseyer S, Hamblin J, Messina S, Mariano R, Siebert N, Everett R, et al. Prodromal headache in MOG-antibody positive optic neuritis. Mult Scler Relat Disord. 2020;40:101965.
101. Mariano R, Messina S, Kumar K, Kuker W, Leite MI, Palace J. Comparison of clinical outcomes of transverse myelitis among adults with myelin oligodendrocyte glycoprotein antibody vs Aquaporin-4 antibody disease. JAMA Netw Open. 2019;2(10):e1912732.
102. Jitprapaikulsan J, Lopez Chiriboga AS, Flanagan EP, Fryer JP, McKeon A, Weinshenker BG, et al. Novel glial targets and recurrent longitudinally extensive transverse myelitis. JAMA Neurol. 2018;75(7):892–5.
103. Mariano R, Messina S, Roca-Fernandez A, Leite MI, Kong Y, Palace JA. Quantitative spinal cord MRI in MOG-antibody disease, neuromyelitis optica and multiple sclerosis. Brain. 2021;144(1):198–212.
104. Jurynczyk M, Messina S, Woodhall MR, Raza N, Everett R, Roca-Fernandez A, et al. Clinical presentation and prognosis in MOG-antibody disease: a UK study. Brain. 2017;140(12):3128–38.
105. Sechi E, Krecke KN, Pittock SJ, Dubey D, Lopez-Chiriboga AS, Kunchok A, et al. Frequency and characteristics of MRI-negative myelitis associated with MOG autoantibodies. Mult Scler. 2021;27(2):303–8.
106. Etemadifar M, Salari M, Kargaran PK, Sigari AA, Nouri H, Etemadifar F, et al. Conus medullaris involvement in demyelinating disorders of the CNS: a comparative study. Mult Scler Relat Disord. 2021;54:103127.
107. Shahriari M, Sotirchos ES, Newsome SD, Yousem DM. MOGAD: how it differs from and resembles other neuroinflammatory disorders. AJR Am J Roentgenol. 2021;216(4):1031–9.

108. Asnafi S, Morris PP, Sechi E, Pittock SJ, Weinshenker BG, Palace J, et al. The frequency of longitudinally extensive transverse myelitis in MS: a population-based study. Mult Scler Relat Disord. 2020;37:101487.
109. Hyun JW, Lee HL, Park J, Kim J, Min JH, Kim BJ, et al. Brighter spotty lesions on spinal MRI help differentiate AQP4 antibody-positive NMOSD from MOGAD. Mult Scler. 2022;28(6):989–92.
110. Rinaldi S, Davies A, Fehmi J, Beadnall HN, Wang J, Hardy TA, et al. Overlapping central and peripheral nervous system syndromes in MOG antibody-associated disorders. Neurol Neuroimmunol Neuroinflamm. 2021;8(1).
111. Camera V, Holm-Mercer L, Ali AAH, Messina S, Horvat T, Kuker W, et al. Frequency of new silent MRI lesions in myelin oligodendrocyte glycoprotein antibody disease and Aquaporin-4 antibody neuromyelitis optica spectrum disorder. JAMA Netw Open. 2021;4(12):e2137833.
112. Armangue T, Olive-Cirera G, Martinez-Hernandez E, Sepulveda M, Ruiz-Garcia R, Munoz-Batista M, et al. Associations of paediatric demyelinating and encephalitic syndromes with myelin oligodendrocyte glycoprotein antibodies: a multicentre observational study. Lancet Neurol. 2020;19(3):234–46.
113. Cobo-Calvo A, Ruiz A, Rollot F, Arrambide G, Deschamps R, Maillart E, et al. Clinical features and risk of relapse in children and adults with myelin oligodendrocyte glycoprotein antibody-associated disease. Ann Neurol. 2021;89(1):30–41.
114. Lopez-Chiriboga AS, Majed M, Fryer J, Dubey D, McKeon A, Flanagan EP, et al. Association of MOG-IgG serostatus with relapse after acute disseminated encephalomyelitis and proposed diagnostic criteria for MOG-IgG-associated disorders. JAMA Neurol. 2018;75(11):1355–63.
115. Wegener-Panzer A, Cleaveland R, Wendel EM, Baumann M, Bertolini A, Hausler M, et al. Clinical and imaging features of children with autoimmune encephalitis and MOG antibodies. Neurol Neuroimmunol Neuroinflamm. 2020;7(4).
116. Suzuki K, Nakamura T, Hashimoto K, Miyamoto M, Komagamine T, Nagashima T, et al. Hypothermia, hypotension, hypersomnia, and obesity associated with hypothalamic lesions in a patient positive for the anti-aquaporin 4 antibody: a case report and literature review. Arch Neurol. 2012;69(10):1355–9.
117. Kunchok A, Krecke KN, Flanagan EP, Jitprapaikulsan J, Lopez-Chiriboga AS, Chen JJ, et al. Does area postrema syndrome occur in myelin oligodendrocyte glycoprotein-IgG-associated disorders (MOGAD)? Neurology. 2020;94(2):85–8.
118. Jain K, Cherian A, Thomas B. FLAMES: A novel burning entity in MOG IgG associated disease. Mult Scler Relat Disord. 2021;49:102759.
119. Jurynczyk M, Geraldes R, Probert F, Woodhall MR, Waters P, Tackley G, et al. Distinct brain imaging characteristics of autoantibody-mediated CNS conditions and multiple sclerosis. Brain. 2017;140(3):617–27.
120. Cobo-Calvo A, Ruiz A, Maillart E, Audoin B, Zephir H, Bourre B, et al. Clinical spectrum and prognostic value of CNS MOG autoimmunity in adults: the MOGADOR study. Neurology. 2018;90(21):e1858–e69.
121. Jarius S, Aktas O, Ayzenberg I, Bellmann-Strobl J, Berthele A, Giglhuber K, et al. Update on the diagnosis and treatment of neuromyelits optica spectrum disorders (NMOSD) - revised recommendations of the Neuromyelitis Optica Study Group (NEMOS). Part I: Diagnosis and differential diagnosis. J Neurol. 2023;270(7):3341–68.
122. Cacciaguerra L, Morris P, Tobin WO, Chen JJ, Banks SA, Elsbernd P, et al. Tumefactive demyelination in MOG Ab-associated disease, multiple sclerosis, and AQP-4-IgG-positive neuromyelitis optica spectrum disorder. Neurology. 2023;100(13):e1418–e32.
123. Sinha S, Banwell B, Tucker A, Storm PB, Huh J, Lang SS. Hemicraniectomy and externalized ventricular drain placement in a pediatric patient with myelin oligodendrocyte glycoprotein-associated tumefactive demyelinating disease. Childs Nerv Syst. 2022;38(1):185–9.
124. Uzura Y, Takeuchi H, Ashida S, Fujii C, Shishido-Hara Y, Inaba T, et al. A tumefactive anti-MOG antibody associated disorder heralding central nervous system B-cell lymphoma: case report on diagnostic challenge. J Neuroimmunol. 2022;365:577823.

125. Fadda G, Banwell B, Waters P, Marrie RA, Yeh EA, O'Mahony J, et al. Silent new brain MRI lesions in children with MOG-antibody associated disease. Ann Neurol. 2021;89(2):408–13.
126. Sechi E, Krecke KN, Messina SA, Buciuc M, Pittock SJ, Chen JJ, et al. Comparison of MRI lesion evolution in different central nervous system demyelinating disorders. Neurology. 2021;97(11):e1097–e109.
127. Sechi E, Buciuc M, Pittock SJ, Chen JJ, Fryer JP, Jenkins SM, et al. Positive predictive value of myelin oligodendrocyte glycoprotein autoantibody testing. JAMA Neurol. 2021;78(6):741–6.
128. Cobo-Calvo A, d'Indy H, Ruiz A, Collongues N, Kremer L, Durand-Dubief F, et al. Frequency of myelin oligodendrocyte glycoprotein antibody in multiple sclerosis: a multicenter cross-sectional study. Neurol Neuroimmunol Neuroinflamm. 2020;7(2).
129. Villacieros-Alvarez J, Espejo C, Arrambide G, Castillo M, Carbonell-Mirabent P, Rodriguez M, et al. MOG antibodies in adults with a first demyelinating event suggestive of multiple sclerosis. Ann Neurol. 2023;95:116.
130. Longbrake E. Myelin oligodendrocyte glycoprotein-associated disorders. Continuum (Minneap Minn). 2022;28(4):1171–93.
131. Kunchok A, Chen JJ, McKeon A, Mills JR, Flanagan EP, Pittock SJ. Coexistence of myelin oligodendrocyte glycoprotein and Aquaporin-4 antibodies in adult and pediatric patients. JAMA Neurol. 2020;77(2):257–9.
132. Martinez-Hernandez E, Guasp M, Garcia-Serra A, Maudes E, Arino H, Sepulveda M, et al. Clinical significance of anti-NMDAR concurrent with glial or neuronal surface antibodies. Neurology. 2020;94(22):e2302–e10.
133. Reindl M, Schanda K, Woodhall M, Tea F, Ramanathan S, Sagen J, et al. International multicenter examination of MOG antibody assays. Neurol Neuroimmunol Neuroinflamm. 2020;7(2).
134. Kim H, Lee EJ, Kim S, Choi LK, Kim K, Kim HW, et al. Serum biomarkers in myelin oligodendrocyte glycoprotein antibody-associated disease. Neurol Neuroimmunol Neuroinflamm. 2020;7(3).
135. Barro C, Healy BC, Liu Y, Saxena S, Paul A, Polgar-Turcsanyi M, et al. Serum GFAP and NfL levels differentiate subsequent progression and disease activity in patients with progressive multiple sclerosis. Neurol Neuroimmunol Neuroinflamm. 2023;10(1):e200052.
136. Jarius S, Lechner C, Wendel EM, Baumann M, Breu M, Schimmel M, et al. Cerebrospinal fluid findings in patients with myelin oligodendrocyte glycoprotein (MOG) antibodies. Part 2: results from 108 lumbar punctures in 80 pediatric patients. J Neuroinflammation. 2020;17(1):262.
137. Carta S, Cobo Calvo Á, Armangué T, Saiz A, Lechner C, Rostásy K, et al. Significance of myelin oligodendrocyte glycoprotein antibodies in CSF: a retrospective multicenter study. Neurology. 2023;100(11):e1095–e108.
138. Kwon YN, Kim B, Kim JS, Mo H, Choi K, Oh SI, et al. Myelin oligodendrocyte glycoprotein-immunoglobulin G in the CSF: clinical implication of testing and association with disability. Neurol Neuroimmunol Neuroinflamm. 2022;9(1).
139. Chen JJ, Sotirchos ES, Henderson AD, Vasileiou ES, Flanagan EP, Bhatti MT, et al. OCT retinal nerve fiber layer thickness differentiates acute optic neuritis from MOG antibody-associated disease and Multiple Sclerosis: RNFL thickening in acute optic neuritis from MOGAD vs MS. Mult Scler Relat Disord. 2022;58:103525.
140. Roca-Fernández A, Camera V, Loncarevic-Whitaker G, Messina S, Mariano R, Vincent A, et al. The use of OCT in good visual acuity MOGAD and AQP4-NMOSD patients; with and without optic neuritis. Mult Scler J Exp Transl Clin. 2021;7(4):20552173211066446.
141. Lang Y, Kwapong WR, Kong L, Shi Z, Wang X, Du Q, et al. Retinal structural and microvascular changes in myelin oligodendrocyte glycoprotein antibody disease and neuromyelitis optica spectrum disorder: an OCT/OCTA study. Front Immunol. 2023;14:1029124.
142. Dinoto A, Licciardi NM, Reindl M, Chiodega V, Schanda K, Carta S, et al. Peripheral neuropathy and MOG-IgG: a clinical and neuropathological retrospective study. Mult Scler Relat Disord. 2022;68:104214.

143. Cortese R, Prados Carrasco F, Tur C, Bianchi A, Brownlee W, De Angelis F, et al. Differentiating multiple sclerosis from AQP4-Neuromyelitis Optica Spectrum disorder and MOG-antibody disease with imaging. Neurology. 2023;100(3):e308–e23.
144. Geraldes R, Arrambide G, Banwell B, Rovira À, Cortese R, Lassmann H, et al. The influence of MOGAD on diagnosis of multiple sclerosis using MRI. Nat Rev Neurol. 2024;20(10):620–35.
145. Jarius S, Ruprecht K, Kleiter I, Borisow N, Asgari N, Pitarokoili K, et al. MOG-IgG in NMO and related disorders: a multicenter study of 50 patients. Part 2: epidemiology, clinical presentation, radiological and laboratory features, treatment responses, and long-term outcome. J Neuroinflammation. 2016;13(1):280.
146. Al-Ani A, Chen JJ, Costello F. Myelin oligodendrocyte glycoprotein antibody-associated disease (MOGAD): current understanding and challenges. J Neurol. 2023;270(8):4132–50.
147. Whittam DH, Karthikeayan V, Gibbons E, Kneen R, Chandratre S, Ciccarelli O, et al. Treatment of MOG antibody associated disorders: results of an international survey. J Neurol. 2020;267(12):3565–77.
148. Chen JJ, Flanagan EP, Bhatti MT, Tisavipat N, Jamali S, Kunchok A, et al. Details and outcomes of a large cohort of MOG-IgG associated optic neuritis. Mult Scler Relat Disord. 2022;68:104237.
149. Jarius S, Paul F, Weinshenker BG, Levy M, Kim HJ, Wildemann B. Neuromyelitis optica. Nat Rev Dis Primers. 2020;6(1):85.
150. Wingerchuk DM, Banwell B, Bennett JL, Cabre P, Carroll W, Chitnis T, et al. International consensus diagnostic criteria for neuromyelitis optica spectrum disorders. Neurology. 2015;85(2):177–89.
151. Jarius S, Ruprecht K, Wildemann B, Kuempfel T, Ringelstein M, Geis C, et al. Contrasting disease patterns in seropositive and seronegative neuromyelitis optica: a multicentre study of 175 patients. J Neuroinflammation. 2012;9:14.
152. Papp V, Magyari M, Aktas O, Berger T, Broadley SA, Cabre P, et al. Worldwide incidence and prevalence of neuromyelitis optica: a systematic review. Neurology. 2021;96(2):59–77.
153. Kappos L, Wolinsky JS, Giovannoni G, Arnold DL, Wang Q, Bernasconi C, et al. Contribution of relapse-independent progression vs relapse-associated worsening to overall confirmed disability accumulation in typical relapsing multiple sclerosis in a pooled analysis of 2 randomized clinical trials. JAMA Neurol. 2020;77(9):1132–40.
154. Sinnecker T, Dörr J, Pfueller CF, Harms L, Ruprecht K, Jarius S, et al. Distinct lesion morphology at 7-T MRI differentiates neuromyelitis optica from multiple sclerosis. Neurology. 2012;79(7):708–14.
155. Pittock SJ, Lennon VA, Krecke K, Wingerchuk DM, Lucchinetti CF, Weinshenker BG. Brain abnormalities in neuromyelitis optica. Arch Neurol. 2006;63(3):390–6.
156. Orman G, Wang KY, Pekcevik Y, Thompson CB, Mealy M, Levy M, et al. Enhancing brain lesions during acute optic neuritis and/or longitudinally extensive transverse myelitis may portend a higher relapse rate in neuromyelitis optica spectrum disorders. AJNR Am J Neuroradiol. 2017;38(5):949–53.
157. Juryńczyk M, Tackley G, Kong Y, Geraldes R, Matthews L, Woodhall M, et al. Brain lesion distribution criteria distinguish MS from AQP4-antibody NMOSD and MOG-antibody disease. J Neurol Neurosurg Psychiatry. 2017;88(2):132–6.
158. Papadopoulos MC, Verkman AS. Aquaporin 4 and neuromyelitis optica. Lancet Neurol. 2012;11(6):535–44.
159. Jarius S, Eichhorn P, Franciotta D, Petereit HF, Akman-Demir G, Wick M, et al. The MRZ reaction as a highly specific marker of multiple sclerosis: re-evaluation and structured review of the literature. J Neurol. 2017;264(3):453–66.
160. Leppert D, Watanabe M, Schaedelin S, Piehl F, Furlan R, Gastaldi M, et al. Granulocyte activation markers in cerebrospinal fluid differentiate acute neuromyelitis spectrum disorder from multiple sclerosis. J Neurol Neurosurg Psychiatry. 2023;94(9):726–37.
161. Ringelstein M, Kleiter I, Ayzenberg I, Borisow N, Paul F, Ruprecht K, et al. Visual evoked potentials in neuromyelitis optica and its spectrum disorders. Mult Scler. 2014;20(5):617–20.

162. Wingerchuk DM, Lennon VA, Pittock SJ, Lucchinetti CF, Weinshenker BG. Revised diagnostic criteria for neuromyelitis optica. Neurology. 2006;66(10):1485–9.
163. Wingerchuk DM, Lennon VA, Lucchinetti CF, Pittock SJ, Weinshenker BG. The spectrum of neuromyelitis optica. Lancet Neurol. 2007;6(9):805–15.
164. Gahlen A, Trampe AK, Haupeltshofer S, Ringelstein M, Aktas O, Berthele A, et al. Aquaporin-4 antibodies in patients treated with natalizumab for suspected MS. Neurol Neuroimmunol Neuroinflamm. 2017;4(4):e363.
165. Kira J, Itoyama Y, Kikuchi S, Hao Q, Kurosawa T, Nagato K, et al. Fingolimod (FTY720) therapy in Japanese patients with relapsing multiple sclerosis over 12 months: results of a phase 2 observational extension. BMC Neurol. 2014;14:21.
166. Kim HJ, Paul F, Lana-Peixoto MA, Tenembaum S, Asgari N, Palace J, et al. MRI characteristics of neuromyelitis optica spectrum disorder: an international update. Neurology. 2015;84(11):1165–73.
167. Matthews L, Marasco R, Jenkinson M, Küker W, Luppe S, Leite MI, et al. Distinction of seropositive NMO spectrum disorder and MS brain lesion distribution. Neurology. 2013;80(14):1330–7.
168. Kümpfel T, Giglhuber K, Aktas O, Ayzenberg I, Bellmann-Strobl J, Häußler V, et al. Update on the diagnosis and treatment of neuromyelitis optica spectrum disorders (NMOSD) - revised recommendations of the Neuromyelitis Optica Study Group (NEMOS). Part II: Attack therapy and long-term management. J Neurol. 2024;271(1):141–76.
169. Filippi M, Preziosa P, Banwell BL, Barkhof F, Ciccarelli O, De Stefano N, et al. Assessment of lesions on magnetic resonance imaging in multiple sclerosis: practical guidelines. Brain. 2019;142(7):1858–75.
170. Wattjes MP, Ciccarelli O, Reich DS, Banwell B, de Stefano N, Enzinger C, et al. 2021 MAGNIMS-CMSC-NAIMS consensus recommendations on the use of MRI in patients with multiple sclerosis. Lancet Neurol. 2021;20(8):653–70.
171. Toosy AT, Mason DF, Miller DH. Optic neuritis. Lancet Neurol. 2014;13(1):83–99.
172. Jeyakumar N, Lerch M, Dale RC, Ramanathan S. MOG antibody-associated optic neuritis. Eye (Lond). 2024;38(12):2289–301.
173. Dubey D, Pittock SJ, Krecke KN, Morris PP, Sechi E, Zalewski NL, et al. Clinical, radiologic, and prognostic features of myelitis associated with myelin oligodendrocyte glycoprotein autoantibody. JAMA Neurol. 2019;76(3):301–9.
174. Fadda G, Flanagan EP, Cacciaguerra L, Jitprapaikulsan J, Solla P, Zara P, et al. Myelitis features and outcomes in CNS demyelinating disorders: comparison between multiple sclerosis, MOGAD, and AQP4-IgG-positive NMOSD. Front Neurol. 2022;13:1011579.
175. Miyamoto N, Kagohashi M, Nishioka K, Fujishima K, Kitada T, Tomita Y, et al. An autopsy case of Schilder's variant of multiple sclerosis (Schilder's disease). Eur Neurol. 2006;55(2):103–7.
176. Poser CM, Goutieres F, Carpentier MA, Aicardi J. Schilder's myelinoclastic diffuse sclerosis. Pediatrics. 1986;77(1):107–12.
177. Jarius S, Haas J, Paul F, Wildemann B. Myelinoclastic diffuse sclerosis (Schilder's disease) is immunologically distinct from multiple sclerosis: results from retrospective analysis of 92 lumbar punctures. J Neuroinflammation. 2019;16(1):51.
178. Poser S, Luer W, Bruhn H, Frahm J, Bruck Y, Felgenhauer K. Acute demyelinating disease. Classification and non-invasive diagnosis. Acta Neurol Scand. 1992;86(6):579–85.
179. Schmalstieg WF, Keegan BM, Weinshenker BG. Solitary sclerosis: progressive myelopathy from solitary demyelinating lesion. Neurology. 2012;78(8):540–4.
180. Giacopuzzi Grigoli E, Cinnante C, Doneddu PE, Calcagno N, Lenti S, Ciammola A, et al. Progressive motor neuron syndromes with single CNS lesions and CSF oligoclonal bands: never forget solitary sclerosis! Neurol Sci. 2022;43(12):6951–4.
181. Keegan BM, Kaufmann TJ, Weinshenker BG, Kantarci OH, Schmalstieg WF, Paz Soldan MM, et al. Progressive solitary sclerosis: gradual motor impairment from a single CNS demyelinating lesion. Neurology. 2016;87(16):1713–9.

182. Thompson AJ, Banwell BL, Barkhof F, Carroll WM, Coetzee T, Comi G, et al. Diagnosis of multiple sclerosis: 2017 revisions of the McDonald criteria. Lancet Neurol. 2018;17(2):162–73.
183. Weinshenker BG, Gilbert JJ, Ebers GC. Some clinical and pathologic observations on chronic myelopathy: a variant of multiple sclerosis. J Neurol Neurosurg Psychiatry. 1990;53(2):146–9.
184. Cohen M, Lebrun C, Ayrignac X, Labauge P, Assouad R. Solitary sclerosis: experience from three French tertiary care centres. Mult Scler. 2015;21(9):1216.
185. Barakat B, Messina S, Nayak S, Kassa R, Sechi E, Flanagan EP, et al. Cerebrospinal fluid evaluation in patients with progressive motor impairment due to critical central nervous system demyelinating lesions. Mult Scler J Exp Transl Clin. 2022;8(1):20552173211052159.
186. Ayrignac X, Carra-Dalliere C, Homeyer P, Labauge P. Solitary sclerosis: progressive myelopathy from solitary demyelinating lesion. A new entity? Acta Neurol Belg. 2013;113(4):533–4.
187. Claassen DO, Josephs KA, Peller PJ. The stripe of primary lateral sclerosis: focal primary motor cortex hypometabolism seen on fluorodeoxyglucose F18 positron emission tomography. Arch Neurol. 2010;67(1):122–5.
188. Lebrun C, Cohen M, Mondot L, Ayrignac X, Labauge P. A case report of solitary sclerosis: this is really multiple sclerosis. Neurol Ther. 2017;6(2):259–63.
189. Fereidan-Esfahani M, Decker PA, Eckel Passow JE, Lucchinetti CF, Flanagan EP, Tobin WO. Population-based incidence and clinico-radiological characteristics of tumefactive demyelination in Olmsted County, Minnesota, United States. Eur J Neurol. 2022;29(3):782–9.
190. Frederick MC, Cameron MH. Tumefactive demyelinating lesions in multiple sclerosis and associated disorders. Curr Neurol Neurosci Rep. 2016;16(3):26.
191. Villarreal JV, Abraham MJ, Acevedo JAG, Rai PK, Thottempudi N, Fang X, et al. Tumefactive multiple sclerosis (TMS): a case series of this challenging variant of MS. Mult Scler Relat Disord. 2021;48:102699.
192. Lucchinetti CF, Gavrilova RH, Metz I, Parisi JE, Scheithauer BW, Weigand S, et al. Clinical and radiographic spectrum of pathologically confirmed tumefactive multiple sclerosis. Brain. 2008;131(Pt 7):1759–75.
193. Abdoli M, Freedman MS. Neuro-oncology dilemma: tumour or tumefactive demyelinating lesion. Mult Scler Relat Disord. 2015;4(6):555–66.
194. Faissner S, Hoepner R, Lukas C, Chan A, Gold R, Ellrichmann G. Tumefactive multiple sclerosis lesions in two patients after cessation of fingolimod treatment. Ther Adv Neurol Disord. 2015;8(5):233–8.
195. Altintas A, Petek B, Isik N, Terzi M, Bolukbasi F, Tavsanli M, et al. Clinical and radiological characteristics of tumefactive demyelinating lesions: follow-up study. Mult Scler. 2012;18(10):1448–53.
196. Balloy G, Pelletier J, Suchet L, Lebrun C, Cohen M, Vermersch P, et al. Inaugural tumor-like multiple sclerosis: clinical presentation and medium-term outcome in 87 patients. J Neurol. 2018;265(10):2251–9.
197. Abou Zeid N, Pirko I, Erickson B, Weigand SD, Thomsen KM, Scheithauer B, et al. Diffusion-weighted imaging characteristics of biopsy-proven demyelinating brain lesions. Neurology. 2012;78(21):1655–62.
198. He J, Grossman RI, Ge Y, Mannon LJ. Enhancing patterns in multiple sclerosis: evolution and persistence. AJNR Am J Neuroradiol. 2001;22(4):664–9.
199. Perez Giraldo GS, Singer L, Cao T, Jamshidi P, Dixit K, Kontzialis M, et al. Differential diagnosis of tumor-like brain lesions. Neurol Clin Pract. 2023;13(5):e200182.
200. Hayashida Y, Hirai T, Morishita S, Kitajima M, Murakami R, Korogi Y, et al. Diffusion-weighted imaging of metastatic brain tumors: comparison with histologic type and tumor cellularity. AJNR Am J Neuroradiol. 2006;27(7):1419–25.
201. Hyland M, Bermel RA, Cohen JA. Restricted diffusion preceding gadolinium enhancement in large or tumefactive demyelinating lesions. Neurol Clin Pract. 2013;3(1):15–21.
202. Wingerchuk DM, Marignier R, Palace J, Paul F, Aktas O, Bennett JL, et al. IPND 2025: Revised consensus criteria, classification, and nomenclature for neuromyelitis optica spectrum disorders (poster P427). ECTRIMS 2025; Barcelona.

3 Autoimmune Non-demyelinating Diseases of Nervous System

3.1 Atopic Myelitis

3.1.1 Synonym

- Idiopathic eosinophilic myelitis; Atopic diathesis

3.1.2 Epidemiology

- A rare and likely underdiagnosed condition, with over 100 cases reported in the literature.

3.1.3 Etiology and Definition

- Occurs in patients with chronic atopic disorders, such as atopic dermatitis, asthma, or allergic rhinitis.
- It is characterized by localized, persistent inflammation of the spinal cord associated with an enhanced immunoglobulin E (IgE) response to environmental antigens, particularly house dust mite, less frequently to other antigens.
- Cross-reactivity between environmental allergens and central nervous system (CNS) antigens is suspected to be the underlying mechanism. It is hypothesized that peripherally produced IgE sensitizes mast cells located in the perivascular areas of the CNS (for example, extremely prevalent in the meninges), which then initiate blood-brain barrier disruption, vascular leakage, and inflammation through the release of vasoactive amines.

T. Uher, *Mimics and Red Flags of Multiple Sclerosis*,
https://doi.org/10.1007/978-3-031-98945-2_3

- It is speculated that a fraction of multiple sclerosis (MS) patients may initiate CNS inflammation because of increased IgE and atopic conditions.
- Inflammatory spinal cord lesions in atopic myelitis contain many eosinophils and T lymphocytes.

3.1.4 Clinical Features

- Spinal cord syndrome.
- The posterior columns are most affected, leading to sensory symptoms (which may include a positive Lhermitte's sign) and sphincter dysfunction being more frequent and severe compared to motor deficits.
- In rare cases where the anterior spinal cord is predominantly involved, motor deficits become more prominent.
- While most patients have a history of atopy, some cases occur without any such history.

3.1.5 Disease Course

- Although atopic disorders are common in children and typically diminish in adulthood, atopic myelitis can manifest at any age.
- Disease onset, progression, and improvement often align with seasonal fluctuations in environmental allergen concentrations in the air.
- The disease course can vary, presenting as acute, subacute, or chronically progressive with periods of fluctuation.

3.1.6 Brain Imaging

- Typically, normal, or age-related findings.

3.1.7 Spinal Cord Imaging

- Lesions distribution
  - The posterior or central portions of the cervical or thoracic spinal cord are most frequently affected.
  - The anterior portions of the spinal cord are rarely affected.
- Lesions morphology and signal
  - Typically, partial myelitis presents with short lesions (involving <3 spinal segments); longitudinally extensive transverse myelitis (LETM) is rare.
- Contrast enhancement
  - Frequently present mild/partial enhancement.

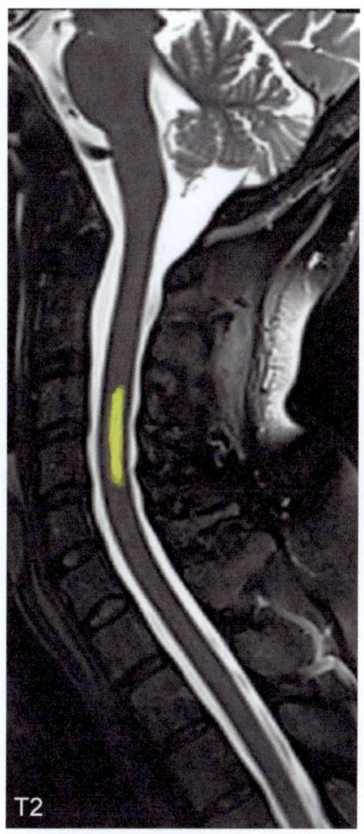

Fig. 3.1 Spinal cord lesion in atopic myelitis

- Perilesional changes
  - Local cord swelling.
- Evolution over time
  - Corticosteroid treatment can be associated with complete resolution of lesional pathology (Fig. 3.1).

3.1.8 Blood Work

- Typically, patients present with leukocytosis, eosinophilia, elevated IgE levels, and allergen-specific IgE antibodies to common environmental allergens, particularly house dust mites (Dermatophagoides pteronyssinus and Dermatophagoides farinae).
- Proportion of patients (12–66%) has normal IgE levels and eosinophil counts.
- Conversely, elevated IgE and mite-specific IgE antibodies can be found in patients without a history of atopy.
- Other routine blood tests usually return normal results.

3.1.9 Examination of CSF

- Frequently elevated concentration of protein.
- Cytology is usually normal, without eosinophils.
- Cerebrospinal fluid (CSF)-restricted oligoclonal bands (OCB) are negative.

3.1.10 Diagnosis

- Based on a history of atopy, spinal cord imaging, elevated IgE levels, and high eosinophil count in blood.

3.1.11 Differential Diagnosis

- Spinal cord tumors.
- In demyelinating diseases, eosinophil infiltration is typically absent on biopsy, except in some cases of patients with neuromyelitis optica spectrum disorders (NMOSD). However, patients with NMOSD often present with LETM, optic neuritis, positive anti-aquaporin 4 (AQP4) IgG antibodies, and a relapsing-remitting disease course.
- Parasitic infections, such as those caused by Toxocara canis, can lead to eosinophilic myelitis.
- Anterior spinal artery syndrome of ischemic etiology.
- Other conditions presenting with partial myelitis. Therefore, in atopic patients with neurological manifestations, this rare condition should also be considered.
- Hopkins syndrome (asthmatic amyotrophy).
  - Typically affects children with atopic asthma, but it can rarely occur in adults.
  - From days to a few weeks after an acute asthma attack, damage to the anterior horn cells may develop, resulting in the acute onset of flaccid paralysis in one or two limbs and severe muscle atrophy.
  - However, the site of pathology may not be limited to the anterior horns.
  - Some patients may also show additional involvement of the pyramidal and sensory spinal tracts, representing a transition between Hopkins syndrome and atopic myelitis.
  - The response to corticosteroids is poor, but relapses are rare.
  - It must be differentiated from Hirayama disease, a rare, nonfamilial form of monomelic benign juvenile brachial amyotrophy.

3.1.12 Treatment and Prognosis

- Corticosteroids are often effective in treatment.
- Most patients experience only mild neurological deficits and have a relatively benign disease course [1–5].

3.2 Autoimmune Encephalitis with Antibodies Against Neuronal Surface

3.2.1 Epidemiology

- The most frequent autoimmune encephalitis (AE) is the subtype with antibodies against NMDA receptors (NMDAR) andleucine-rich glioma-inactivated protein-1 (LGI1).
- Incidence of NMDAR 0.15/100.000/year.
- Incidence of LGI1 0.08/100.000/year [6, 7].

3.2.2 Etiology and Definition

- A heterogeneous group of immune-mediated conditions affecting the brain, but in some instances also the meninges, spinal cord, or peripheral nerves.
- Neuronal autoantibodies (NAAs) identified in AE target either
  - Intracellular antigens, which can be either intranuclear or intracytoplasmic. These are more likely to be associated with paraneoplastic conditions, or
  - Neuronal surface antigens, which are less likely to be associated with paraneoplastic conditions [8, 9].
- In some cases, AE may be preceded by viral infections (such as herpes simplex virus [HSV] encephalitis) or by the use of immune-modulating drugs (such as tumor necrosis factor (TNF)-alpha inhibitors and immune checkpoint inhibitors) [10].
- Currently, there are described more than 16 neuronal surface antibodies [10].
- Further information about AE associated with antibodies targeting intracellular antigens can be found in the chapter on "Paraneoplastic disorders." Details about other specific AE including glial fibrillary acidic protein (GFAP) astrocytopathy, NMOSD, myelin oligodendrocyte glycoprotein antibody-associated disease (MOGAD), or Hashimoto encephalopathy are provided in dedicated chapters.

3.2.3 Clinical Features

- The phenotypes are heterogeneous and may resemble other diseases.
- Often present with acute-onset psychiatric symptoms, cognitive decline, encephalopathy, seizures, or movement disorders [9, 11].
- Voltage-gated potassium channel VGKC-complex AE (Morvan syndrome) often presents with autonomic dysfunction, peripheral nerve hyperexcitability, and encephalopathy [12].
- Optic neuritis as an initial presentation of NMDAR-antibody AE has been reported in only a few cases [13, 14].
- Although some antibodies are linked to certain syndromes (such as oromandibular dyskinesia, cognitive/behavioral changes, and speech and autonomic dysfunction in NMDAR-antibody AE, or faciobrachial dystonic seizures in LGI1-antibody AE), there is marked clinical symptom overlap between the antibody subtypes (Table 3.1) [10, 11, 15].

Table 3.1 Anatomical-clinical syndromes and associated antibodies

Anatomical location	Clinical phenotype	Antibodies
Limbic encephalitis	Cognitive dysfunction, psychiatric symptoms, epilepsy	Hu, CRMP5/CV2, Ma2, NMDAR, AMPAR, LGI1, CASPR2, GAD65, GABA-B-R, DPPX, mGluR5, AK5, Neurexin-3α
Cortical/subcortical encephalitis	Cognitive dysfunction, epilepsy	PCA-2 (MAP1b), NMDAR, GABA A/B R, DPPX, MOG
Striatal encephalitis	Movement disorders	CRMP5/CV2, DRD2, NMDAR, LGI1, PD10A
Diencephalic encephalitis	Autonomic dysfunction and sleep disorders	Ma 1–2, IgLON5, DPPX, AQP4
Brainstem encephalitis	Cognitive dysfunction, movement disorders, bulbar signs, and symptoms	Ri, Ma 1–2, KLHL11, IgLON5, DPPX, AQP4, MOG, GQ1b
Cerebellitis or cerebellar degeneration	Cerebellar syndrome with ataxia	Hu, Ri, Yo, Tr, CASPR2, KLHL11, NIF, mGluR1, GAD65, VGCC
Meningo-encephalitis	Cognitive dysfunction, epilepsy, meningeal syndrome	GFAP or seronegative AE
Encephalomyelitis	Movement disorders including progressive encephalomyelitis with rigidity and myoclonus; stiff person syndrome; spinal cord syndromes, opticospinal manifestations	GAD65, Amphyphysin, Glycine receptor, PCA-2 (MAP1B), GABA A/B R, DPPX, CRMP5/CV2, AQP4, MOG
Neuropathy/neuronopathy	Sensory ataxia, sensori-motor neuropathy	Hu, PCA-2 (MAP1B), CRMP5, Amphiphysin, CASPR2, CASPR1, CONTACTIN1, NIF155
Autonomic neuropathy/ganglionopathy	Autonomic dysfunction	Hu, CRMP5, Anti-ganglionic AChR
Neuromuscular junction dysfunction	Myasthenic syndrome	VGCC, AchR
Myopathy	Motor weakness	Striational

Adapted from Abboud et al. [10]

3.2.4 Disease Course

- Acute or subacute onset (<3 months).
- Hyperacute or insidious onset is relatively rare.
- The most common course is monophasic.
- The relapsing-remitting course is rare. If clinical worsening occurs, it is usually explained by treatment failure or abrupt cessation of treatment.
- Although, a progressive course is more typical for some paraneoplastic syndromes, it might also occur in non-paraneoplastic AE (LGI1, CASPR2, DPPX, GAD65; see below for definitions of abbreviations) [9, 10, 15].

3.2.5 Brain and Spinal Cord Imaging

- NMDAR (N-Methyl D-Aspartate Receptor):
  - Mesiotemporal T2 hyperintensities and hypermetabolism on 18-fludeoxyglucose positron emission tomography (FDG-PET).
  - Later may develop hippocampal atrophy.
  - Discrete and nonspecific small lesions in deep white matter, thalamus, cerebellum, brainstem, or less frequently in basal ganglia (23–50%).
  - Transient or faint contrast enhancement of the cortex, meninges, and basal ganglia (25%).
- AMPAR (α-amino-3-hydroxy-5-methyl-4-isoxazolepropionic acid receptor)
  - Mesiotemporal T2 hyperintensities (90%), which might extend into anterior septal nuclei, insula, frontal, occipital, or cerebellar regions.
  - Might be mild, transient unilateral contrast enhancement of the hippocampus.
  - Later may develop hippocampal and amygdalar sclerosis.
- GABA-A-R (Gamma-Amino butyric acid-A Receptor)
  - All patients have extensive multifocal or diffuse cortical and subcortical T2 hyperintensities. Some patients exhibit rapid progression from focal mediotemporal and frontal T2 hyperintensities to brain atrophy and extensive bilateral lesions.
- GABA-B-R (Gamma-Amino butyric acid B Receptor)
  - The majority of patients exhibit uni- or bilateral T2 hyperintensities in the medial temporal lobe, including hippocampus and amygdala.
  - Sometime is present frontal and temporal leukencephalopathy, hippocampal laminar necrosis, brainstem encephalitis, cerebellar, basal ganglia lesions, or spinal cord lesions.
  - May be present contrast enhancement of the lesions.
  - Later may develop hippocampal or frontotemporal atrophy.
- LGI1 (Leucine-rich glioma-inactivated antibodies)
  - At the stage of faciobrachial dystonic seizures, magnetic resonance imaging (MRI) is usually normal.
  - At the stage of limbic encephalitis: uni- or bilateral T2 hyperintensities of mediotemporal lobes; sometime in basal ganglia; additionally can be mild, ill-defined contrast enhancement of T2 hyperintense regions.
  - Later frequently present hippocampal or whole brain atrophy, which might also develop in patients with previously normal MRI findings.
- CASPR2 (Contactin-associated protein-like 2; Morvan's syndrome)
  - Usually normal MRI.
  - Sometimes T2 hyperintensities in frontal, and mesiotemporal region or unspecific periventricular white matter lesions.
  - Later may develop hippocampal atrophy or sclerosis.
- DPPX (Dipeptidyl-peptidase-like protein 6)
  - Normal MRI in the majority of patients.
  - Unspecific patchy periventricular and subcortical white matter T2 lesions (30%).

- Glycine receptor
  - Normal brain MRI (70%) or T2 hyperintensities in temporal white matter.
  - Sometimes spinal cord lesions.
- DRD2 (Dopamine receptor 2)
  - T2 hyperintensities in caudate, putamen, globus pallidus, and substantia nigra (50%).
  - Later may develop basal ganglia atrophy and gliosis.
- GAD65 (Glutamic acid decarboxylase 65)
  - Although, antibodies against GAD65 target intracellular antigens, it is not considered a classical onconeruonal antibody and is associated with clinical features similar to antibodies against surface antigens. GAD65 receptors are located intracellularly but can transiently appear on the membrane of the synaptic cleft during neurotransmission.
  - Mediotemporal T2 hyperintensities.
  - Patients with ataxia have cerebellar atrophy.
  - Later may develop hippocampal sclerosis [16].
- Spinal cord is affected only rarely. AE associated with GABA-B-R or glycine receptor antibodies might be linked to LETM [16].
- Imaging red flags for diagnosis of AE
  - Normal imaging is considered as a red flag for the diagnosis of AE [11]. Although an MRI may be normal at the onset of symptoms, pathology may become apparent on follow-up imaging conducted days later [10, 16]. AE associated with LGI1, CASPR2, and immunoglobulin-like domain containing, cell adhesion molecule 5 (Ig-LON5) antibodies may exhibit only minimal pathology on MRI [11].
  - Progressive brain atrophy without lesional pathology or persistent lesion activity despite immunotherapy is atypical feature [11].
  - Although diffuse or patchy contrast enhancement of lesions may be seen in a few patients, intense enhancement is atypical.
  - Rarely may be extensive demyelination, meningeal enhancement, or cortical restricted diffusion [10, 16] (Fig. 3.2).

3.2.6 Blood Work

- Testing for NAAs should include analysis by two different techniques (brain immunohistochemistry and cell-based assay). However, in typical cases, an identification of the antibody with only one technique should suffice.
- Testing for NAAs in CSF and serum is essential. This is because CSF testing is more sensitive for certain antibodies, such as NMDAR and GFAP antibodies, whereas serum testing is more sensitive for others, including onconeuronal, LGI1, myelin oligodendrocyte glycoprotein (MOG), and aquaporin 4 (AQP4) antibodies [10, 15].
- Although the phenotype of the suspected AE may suggest a specific subtype, it is recommended to conduct a comprehensive panel examination. Furthermore, some patients may test positive for multiple NAAs (Table 3.1) [10].

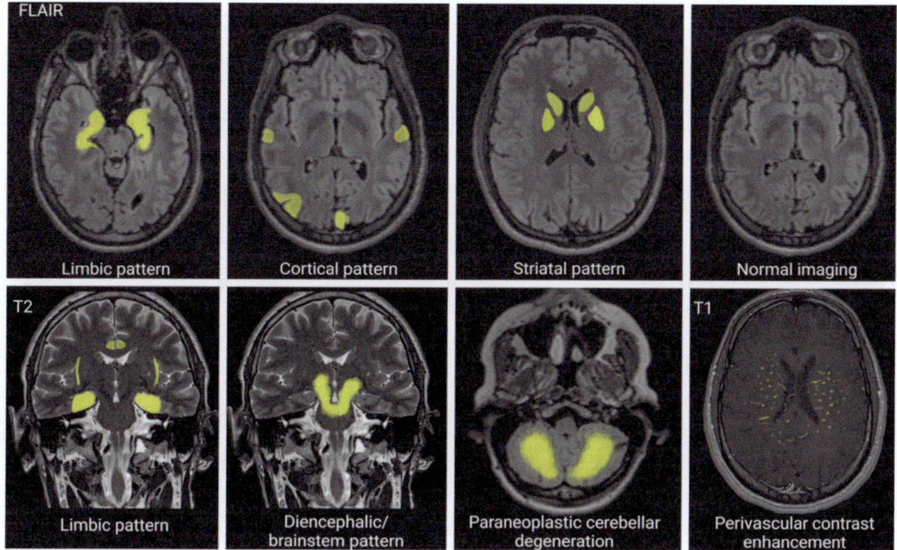

Fig. 3.2 MRI patterns in autoimmune and paraneoplastic encephalitis

- NNAs are detected in 0.23% of the general population when cell-based assays are used. However, the prevalence is higher (6%) when less specific, nonstandard methods such as enzyme-linked immunoassay (ELISA) are employed [17].
- Patients with various neurological diagnoses, including MS (15–20%) may have positive NAAs in their serum or CSF. MS patients with positive NAAs tend to be older but do not otherwise differ from those with negative NAAs [18]. The detection of NAAs in neurological patients should be interpreted with caution and should only be performed in suspected cases of AE [11, 18].

3.2.7 Examination of CSF

- Routine testing may yield normal findings, except for the presence of positive NAAs. However, some patients may show an inflammatory pattern without positive NAAs (seronegative AE).
- For example, in patients with NMDAR-antibody AE, completely normal CSF findings are very rare (5%). In contrast, the proportion of patients with LGI1-antibody AE who have normal CSF findings is much higher (54%).
- Majority of with AE have elevated concentration of protein and mild-to-moderate lymphocytic pleocytosis (usually 20–200 cells/mm3; up to <900 cells/mm^3).
- Often elevated IgG index and/or positive CSF-restricted OCB [10, 19, 20].
  - NMDAR, GABA-B-R, AMPAR, and DPPX-antibody AE frequently exhibit pleocytosis and positive CSF-restricted OCB.
  - In contrast, LGI1, IgLON5, CASPR2, and GlyR-antibody AE only rarely exhibit pleocytosis and positive CSF-restricted OCB.
  - CSF-restricted OCB positivity in AMPAR and NMDAR-antibody AE are almost always associated with pleocytosis.

  - Isolated CSF-restricted OCB positivity without pleocytosis may be present in patients with AE associated with LGI1, IgLON5, GlyR, and often with GAD65 antibodies [19, 20].

3.2.8 Biopsy

- Only rarely required in patients with atypical or mass-like lesions to exclude alternative diagnoses, because MRI findings are usually nonspecific [10, 21].

3.2.9 Diagnosis

- Patient with AE should meet the three criteria
  A. Subacute onset (<3 months) of typical clinical symptoms.
  B. At least one of the following (new focal CNS deficits, unexplained seizures, CSF pleocytosis, or MRI findings suggestive of encephalitis).
  C. Excluded alternative disorders.
- If these three criteria are fulfilled, patients should be assessed for distinct subtypes of AE [15].
- Bilateral limbic encephalitis as the only imaging finding may be sufficient to diagnose definite AE in suspected cases even in the absence of NAAs [9].

3.2.10 Differential Diagnosis

- A broad differential diagnosis should be considered to avoid misdiagnosis [11].
- Several conditions such as herpes simplex encephalitis, Wernicke encephalopathy due to thiamine deficiency, drug intoxications, prion diseases, Hashimoto encephalopathy, neoplasma or non-convulsive status epilepticus may resemble AE [8, 12].
- Hyperacute or insidious disease onset and absence of MRI or CSF pathology suggestive of AE should raise suspicion of a diagnosis other than AE [11].
- Documented rare cases of NMDAR-antibody AE in patients with MS. Therefore, newly occurring encephalopathy or epileptic seizures in patients with MS should raise suspicion of this condition.
- False-positive diagnosis of AE is often associated with overinterpretation of a nonspecific positive antibody result (50%), misinterpretation of nonspecific symptoms (18%), misinterpretation of nonspecific MRI findings (14%), unrecognized functional neurologic features (13%), or psychiatric diagnosis interpreted as AE.
- Most common disorders misdiagnosed as AE include (from most to less common): functional neurologic disorders; neurodegenerative dementia; psychiatric disease; non-specific cognitive syndrome (related to fibromyalgia, fatigue, sleep disorder, medication adverse reaction, or other comorbidities); neoplasm (glio-

blastoma, lymphoma); seizure disorder (nonimmune-mediated); infections (e.g., residual symptoms following previous viral encephalitis, human immunodeficiency virus [HIV] encephalopathy, Creutzfeldt-Jakob disease); mitochondrial disorders; adrenal insufficiency; Wernicke encephalopathy; small vessel vasculitis; Klein Levin syndrome (episodic hypersomnia with cognitive and behavioral changes) or MS [11].

3.2.11 Treatment and Prognosis

- In patients with an inflammatory CSF, antiviral and antibiotic treatment is usually indicated until a negative screening for infectious etiology is received.
- Early and aggressive immuno-modulatory treatment is associated with better prognosis of AE.
- Syndromes in which antibodies attack antigens on the surface of neurons are more likely to respond to immunotherapy than those involving intracellular antigens, which are often associated with cancer [9, 10, 12, 22].
- Cancer screening should be performed in most adults with AE.
- The most common neoplasms associated with AE are small cell lung cancer, thymic neoplasm, breast cancer, ovarian teratoma or carcinoma, testicular teratoma or seminoma, neuroblastoma, and lymphoma.
- NMDAR-antibody AE in young women is often associated with an ovarian teratoma (40%), in contrast LGI1-antibody AE is associated with cancer less frequently (10%) [23].

3.3 Bickerstaff's Brainstem Encephalitis

3.3.1 Epidemiology

- Anti-GQ1b antibody syndrome includes three disorders: Bickerstaff's brainstem encephalitis (BBE), Miller–Fischer syndrome (MFS), and more frequent Guillain–Barre syndrome (GBS):
  - BBE: Incidence <0.1/100.000/years.
  - MFS: incidence 0.01–0.18/100.000/year.
  - GBS: Incidence 1–2/100.000/year [24–27].

3.3.2 Etiology and Definition

- Although the pathophysiology of BBE is not clear, an immune-mediated process triggered by an infective agent such as Campylobacter jejuni, Mycoplasma pneumoniae, or Haemophilus influenzae was suggested [28].
- Discussed whether BBE is a distinct disease or a variant of MFS or GBS. There is considerable overlap of phenotypes among all three conditions [29].

- The GQ1b antigen is highly expressed in the paranodes and neuromuscular junctions of various cranial nerves (oculomotor, trochlear, and abducent), as well as in muscle spindles in the limbs, and the reticular formation in the brainstem. This explains clinical phenotype and positivity of anti-GQ1b IgG antibodies in BBE and MFS [28].
- The pathophysiology of ataxia in the GQ1b-antibody syndrome is still unclear. It has been proposed that ataxia in BBE and MFS might have a purely peripheral origin, involving abnormalities of the joint position sense and muscle spindle proprioception.

3.3.3 Clinical Features

- Clinical features of BBE are typically progressive and symmetric and include
  A. Progressive symmetrical external ophthalmoplegia with diplopia.
    - Palsy of voluntary extraocular muscles.
    - Initially 75%; later 100% of cases [29].
  B. Ataxia (truncal and limb).
    - Initially 58%; later 100% of cases.
    - Similarly to MFS, it is unclear whether the ataxia has a peripheral origin, characterized by abnormalities of joint position sense and muscle spindle proprioception, or a central origin, involving brainstem or cerebellar pathology [29, 30].
  C. Encephalopathy including disturbance of consciousness.
    - Initially 13%, later 74% of cases.
    - Hyperreflexia (34%); Babinski sign (40%); pupillary abnormalities; facial palsy (45%); internal ophthalmoplegia and bulbar palsy (34%); limbs weakness (initially 11%, later 60%); limbs sensory impairment (initially 19%, later 31%); pseudobulbar affect; decorticate-like posturing; nystagmus (27%); blepharoptosis and photophobia (initially 5%, later 29%) [29].
- Although 34% of patients may present with hyperreflexia, the majority exhibit absent or decreased tendon reflexes.
- Rarely may occur optic neuritis or area postrema syndrome.
- Sometime present an incomplete clinical triad. Patients may exhibit only ophthalmoplegia without ataxia or areflexia, and vice versa. In these cases, anti-GQ1b IgG positivity may assist in the diagnosis [25, 31].

3.3.4 Disease Course

- The median age of symptom onset is 39 years (range, 3–91 years) [29].
- The onset is subacute and symptoms nadir within 4 weeks.
- The disease course is monophasic and progressive [29, 32].
- BBE is typically preceded by an infection (92%).
  - Upper respiratory (66%), fever (14%), diarrhea (5%).

3.3.5 Brain Imaging

- The majority of cases show normal MRI.
- Only a minority of cases (11–30%) exhibit infra-tentorial (central mesencephalon, central pons, superior cerebellar peduncle, cerebellum) or supratentorial (thalamus, white matter, corpus callosum) T2 hyperintense lesions [29, 33] (Fig. 3.3).
- Might be contrast enhancement of brain lesions, leptomeninges, cranial nerves (mostly fourth, sixth, and second cranial nerves) or cauda equina [34, 35].
- Only 1% of patients with MFS have abnormal T2 lesions on MRI [33].

3.3.6 Spinal Cord Imaging

- Typically, normal [29].
- Documented case study with cord lesion in the dorsal cervical spinal cord [35].

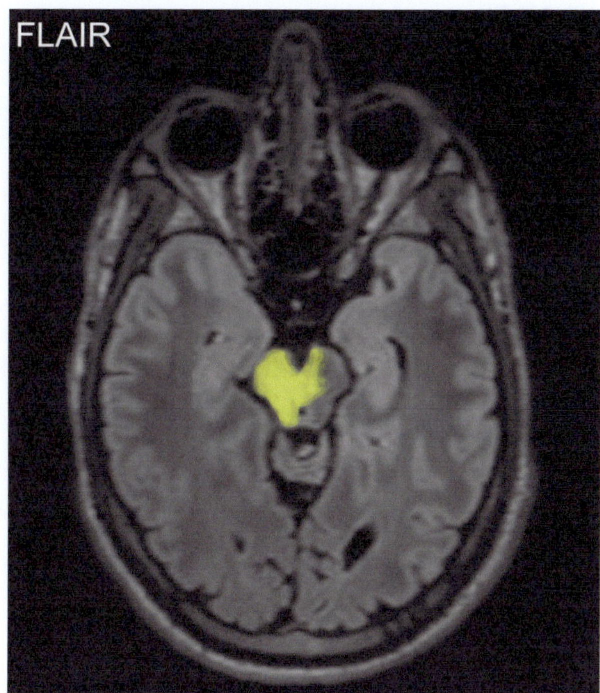

Fig. 3.3 A minority of patients with Bickerstaff's brainstem encephalitis exhibit infratentorial lesions

3.3.7 Blood Work

- Similarly to MFS, there is frequently an elevated concentration of anti-GQ1b IgG antibodies (60–70%) and anti-ganglioside GM1, anti-GD1a, or anti-GalNAc-GD1a IgG antibodies (20%) [28, 29, 32].
- Sometime may be detected serological evidence of recent Campylobacter jejuni infection (23%) [29].

3.3.8 Examination of CSF

- The concentration of protein is normal or elevated (59%).
- (range 0.10 to 6.78 g/l; elevation particularly in the second week of the disease).
- Cell count is normal or there is a mild pleocytosis (37%)
- (range 0–142 cells/mm^3; median 2 cells/mm^3).
- Might be proteino-cytological dissociation (35%)
- (19% in the first; 57% in the third-fourth week).
- CSF-restricted OCB are negative [28, 29].

3.3.9 Electrophysiology

- Abnormal motor nerve conduction studies (44%).
- Predominant axonal (38%) or demyelinating peripheral neuropathy (6%).
- Sometimes present denervation potentials [29].

3.3.10 Diagnosis

- The diagnosis is considered definite, if there is a typical clinical trial, alternative diagnoses are excluded, and patients test positive for anti-GQ1b antibodies.
- The diagnosis is considered probable in patients with a typical phenotype but negative (or unknown) anti-GQ1b antibodies [9].

3.3.11 Differential Diagnosis

- The similarities between BBE, MPS, and GBS may cause confusion.
  - BBE includes encephalopathy, altered consciousness (owing to involvement of the brainstem reticular activating system), and/or other CNS involvement, whereas MFS and GBS do not.
  - Patients fulfilling criteria for BBE (ophthalmoplegia, ataxia, encephalopathy) and simultaneous peripheral polyneuropathy may be diagnosed with combination of BBE and GBS [29].
  - Apart from BBE, imaging in MFS is almost always normal [28].

- Very rarely, BBE might be associated with optic neuritis, which must be distinguished from MS or NMOSD [34].
- MS is not associated with bilateral symmetrical ophthalmoplegia nor encephalopathy as observed in BBE. MS is also not associated with peripheral involvement as observed in GBS and MFS.
- Other mimics of BBE might include neoplasm or vascular disease of brainstem, Wernicke's encephalopathy, botulism, myasthenia gravis, pituitary apoplexy, acute disseminated encephalomyelitis (ADEM), Behçet's disease, CNS vasculitis, or CNS lymphoma [29].

3.3.12 Treatment and Prognosis

- Corticosteroids, plasmapheresis, and intravenous immunoglobulin [29].
- The majority of patients achieve complete recovery [28].

3.4 Chronic Lymphocytic Inflammation with Pontine Perivascular Enhancement Responsive to Steroids (CLIPPERS)

3.4.1 Epidemiology

- Prevalence <0.1/100.000
- Female/male ratio (2–4)/(6–8) [36, 37]

3.4.2 Etiology and Definition

- A chronic inflammatory disease characterized by perivascular histiolymphocytic infiltrates in the white matter of the CNS.
- The pathogenesis is poorly understood and is likely a heterogeneous condition with different pathways leading to similar clinical presentations. Approximately 20% of cases are associated with solid or hematological malignancies [37, 38].

3.4.3 Clinical Features

- Brainstem syndrome, most commonly involving ataxia (>90%), followed by cranial nerve involvement, central paresis, and dysarthria.
- Less common manifestations include altered facial sensation, nystagmus, diplopia, vertigo, cognitive deficit, bladder dysfunction, headache, or tremor.
- Uveitis, fewer, or encephalopathy is typically absent.
- Significant clinical and radiological improvement after corticosteroids (70–80%).

3.4.4 Disease Course

- Symptom onset is subacute and occurs around the age of 50 (range, 13–86).
- Course is usually relapsing remitting, less often monophasic. Malignancy-associated cases of CLIPPERS are associated with higher risk of relapsing course [36, 37].

3.4.5 Brain Imaging

- Lesions' location
  - Typically, bilateral lesions located at least in two of the following three locations including: pons, brachium pontis, and cerebellum.
  - However, lesions may be also present in cerebral cortex, basal ganglia, midbrain, medulla oblongata, or even corpus callosum with frequency decreasing with increasing distance from the pons.
- Lesions' appearance
  - Small punctate lesions may coalesce to form larger lesions.
  - Lesions are hyperintense on T2 images, but their signal is usually faint.
  - Markedly increased T2 signal of lesions is atypical.
  - Diffusion-weighted imaging (DWI) and angiography show normal findings.

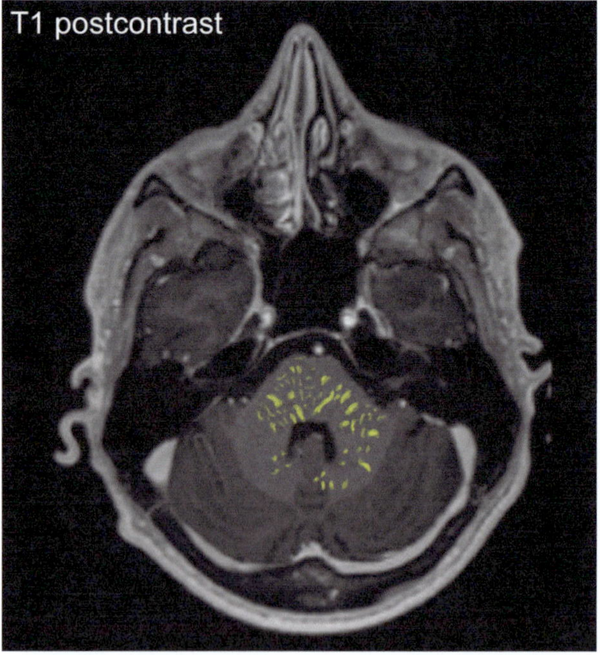

Fig. 3.4 Multiple punctate and curvilinear enhancement in chronic lymphocytic inflammation with pontine perivascular enhancement responsive to steroids (CLIPPERS)

- Contrast enhancement
  - Characteristic multiple punctate (dot-like, diameter <3 mm) and curvilinear gadolinium enhancement (PCGE) corresponds to the lumens of small vessels or perivascular areas of vessels. This MRI pattern resembles a 'salt-and-pepper' or 'peppering' of the pons (Fig. 3.4).
- Perilesional changes
  - No mass effect and minimal or no vasogenic edema.
  - Only rarely present perilesional mass effect during relapses.
- Evolution over time
  - Reduction of the number and volume of enhancing lesions is followed by corticosteroid treatment and correlates with improvement of clinical manifestations [39–41].
- Differential diagnosis of PCGE
  - A. intra-axial punctate hyperintense T1 lesions (non-post-contrast) can be seen also in some MS patients.
  - B. extra-axial punctate lesions related to the leptomeningeal enhancement (not typical for CLIPPERS).
  - C. exclusion of physiologic PCGE, which usually follow the anatomy of the deep medullary veins and do not show abnormal T2 signal.
  - D. pathologic PCGE not related to CLIPPERS
    1. collateral vessels in Moyamoya disease (T2 signal is normal).
    2. small vessels enlargement related to developmental or acquired venous drainage disturbances (T2 signal is normal).
    3. blood-brain barrier disruption of the small vessels (abnormal T2 signal): Endothelopaties (Susac's syndrome, posterior reversible encephalopathy syndrome [PRES], or post-radiotherapy changes); angiocentric infiltrates associated with infectious diseases complicated by secondary vasculitis; autoimmune diseases (connective tissue diseases, sarcoidosis, histiocytosis, vasculitis, and demyelinating diseases); prelymphoma states and lymphomas [39].

3.4.6 Spinal Cord Imaging

- Cord lesions may rarely occur [39].

3.4.7 Blood Work

- Routine blood tests are normal.

3.4.8 Examination of CSF

- Mildly elevated concentration of protein (50%).
- Mild mononuclear pleocytosis (40%).
- CSF-restricted OCB (25%) [38].

- Serological testing of CSF for Epstein-Barr virus (EBV) and varicella zoster virus (VZV) may be rarely positive. The role of these herpetic infections in the pathogenesis of malignancy-associated and non-malignancy-associated CLIPPERS is discussed. Therefore, serological testing is recommended [37, 42].

3.4.9 Diagnosis

- Based on clinical, MRI, and laboratory measures, sometimes on histopathology
- Often challenging and extensive investigations are mandatory to rule out alternative diagnoses because CLIPPERS is diagnosis of exclusion [37, 39, 40].

3.4.10 Differential Diagnosis

- Since most CLIPPERS mimickers require immunosuppressive therapies, it is necessary to exclude infectious diseases. Extensive investigations, including salivary gland biopsy, cerebral angiography, bone marrow biopsy, or whole-body FDG-PET scan, are often essential to reach the diagnosis. Brain biopsy should be performed when all investigations remain inconclusive and when CLIPPERS criteria are not met [39].
- All patients should undergo screening for associated malignancies, particularly hematological ones. Relapse between 2 and 12 months after initial corticosteroid treatment, high relapse rate, and highly elevated concentration of protein in CSF is associated with higher risk of associated lymphoma [43].
- Considering that hemophagocytic lympho-histiocytosis (HLH) is a treatable disease that may mimic CLIPPERS, the *HLH* gene should be examined in all patients with probable CLIPPERS [38].
- Brain biopsy should be reserved only for atypical cases to exclude alternative diagnoses such as CNS lymphoma, primary angiitis of CNS, lymphomatoid granulomatosis, autoimmune gliopathies (anti-myelin oligodendrocyte glycoprotein [MOG] or anti-glial fibrillary acidic protein [GFAP]), or low-grade glioma [39].
- Other mimics that should be considered in differential diagnosis include sarcoidosis, Sjögren's syndrome, neuro-Behçet's disease, MS, ADEM, NMOSD, Bickerstaff encephalitis, other autoimmune encephalitides, CNS infections, and paraneoplastic syndromes [40].
- Reported rare cases of patients with positive anti-MOG IgG presenting with a CLIPPERS-like brainstem syndrome and fulfilling the criteria for probable CLIPPERS. Although, these anti-MOG Ig positive (MOGAD) patients also respond well to corticosteroids, they are younger, exhibit leptomeningeal enhancement, large patchy brain T2 lesions, and differences in brain biopsy [44].

3.4.11 Treatment and Prognosis

- A longer duration of corticosteroid treatment during the acute phase is associated with a lower risk of future relapses. Indeed, relapses are often triggered by rapid corticosteroid tapering. Hence, it is recommended to administer high-dose intravenous corticosteroids for at least 10 days, followed by a very slow tapering regimen.
- Usually, lifelong immunosuppressive treatment is required to prevent relapses. It is often required combination of peroral corticosteroids (Prednison 20 mg/day or higher) with immunosuppressive treatment (methothexate 15 mg/week; azatioprine 150 mg/day; hydroxychloroquine 400 mg/day; or cyclophosphamide 1 g/month). Some patients may require anti-CD20, intravenous immunoglobulin or plasmapheresis. It is worth noting that all these treatment recommendations have not been systematically explored in clinical trials.
- Clinical follow-up and brain MRI are recommended every 3 months.
- Symptoms and MRI lesions can completely remit if effective treatment is provided within a certain time window. Delay in diagnosis and treatment is associated with poorer prognosis.
- Although the long-term prognosis is still not well defined, the mortality rate is estimated to be 10% in all patients, 30% in cases associated with malignancy, and 14–15% in patients with relapses [37].

3.5 Hashimoto Encephalopathy

- An immune-mediated disease characterized by subacute fluctuating encephalopathy, particularly affecting older patients.
- Clinical features may also include seizures, psychiatric symptoms, myoclonus, tremor, transient aphasia, lateralized motor or sensory deficits (resembling stroke-like episodes), sleep abnormalities, and gait difficulties.
- This often-misdiagnosed disease is associated with autoimmune Hashimoto thyroiditis.
- Most patients are euthyroid or subclinically hypothyroid (with increased serum thyroid-stimulating hormone (TSH) but have increased thyroid peroxidase (TPO) and positive thyroglobulin antibodies. However, the prevalence of thyroid antibodies is high in the general population (around 13% and rises with age), and their presence alone does not support a diagnosis in patients without objective clinical and paraclinical abnormalities typical for Hashimoto encephalopathy. Thyroid antibody testing is of limited value in the contemporary evaluation and diagnosis of autoimmune encephalopathies.
- Patients with Hashimoto encephalopathy does not have positive specific neural autoantibodies.
- Brain MRI is typically normal or may show nonspecific T2 hyperintensities in around 25% of patients.
- CSF usually shows an elevated concentration of protein. Mild pleocytosis may be observed in a small and elevated IgG index with CSF-restricted OCB in very small proportion of patients.

- Electroencephalography (EEG) commonly shows diffuse background slowing.
- The symptoms respond well to corticosteroids [45–47].

3.6 Myasthenia Gravis

3.6.1 Epidemiology

- Incidence 40–120/100.000/year
- The peak age of disease onset occurs between 20 and 40 years (a female predominance) and between 55 and 75 years (a male predominance) [48–50].

3.6.2 Etiology and Definition

- Myasthenia gravis (MG) is an autoimmune disease associated with antibodies directed against different postsynaptic membrane receptors at the neuromuscular junction resulting in muscle weakness [48, 49].

3.6.3 Clinical Features

- Fluctuations of muscle weakness over time, fatigue, worsening of symptoms after exercise, and a high variability in the distribution of muscle weakness, which may be asymmetric.
- There are no sensory and CNS signs or symptoms [48].
- Bulbar and ocular manifestations of MG can mimic MS and vice versa [51].

3.6.4 Brain and Spinal Cord Imaging

- Only age- and comorbidities-related findings.

3.6.5 Blood Work

- Commonly detected autoantibodies against
  - Acetylcholine receptor (AChR); highly specific for MG.
  - Muscle-specific kinase (MUSK).
  - Lipoprotein-related protein 4 (LRP4).
- Although, a few patients are seronegative, in many of these patients are present low-affinity or low concentrations of antibodies that are detectable only by more sensitive non-routine cell-based methods [48, 49].

3.6.6 Examination of CSF

- Normal.

3.6.7 Electrophysiology

- Repetitive nerve stimulation and single-fiber electromyography (EMG) show an increased jitter and decrement at repetitive stimulation. EMG is not required in patients with typical clinical features and positive autoantibodies but can be important for differential diagnosis in cases without detectable autoantibodies [48, 49].

3.6.8 Diagnosis

- Based on a combination of clinical, laboratory, neurophysiological data, and clinical response to cholinesterase inhibitors [48, 49].

3.6.9 Differential Diagnosis

- The comorbidity of MG and MS is more frequent than expected statistically. This association may be underdiagnosed because of the possible overlap of symptoms, particularly bulbar and ocular [51, 52].
- Paraneoplastic neuromuscular diseases include thymoma-associated MG and Lambert–Eaton myasthenic syndrome (LEMS), which is primarily associated with small cell lung cancer (SCLC). It is characterized by antibodies against presynaptic voltage-gated calcium channels and an incremental response during repetitive stimulation [48, 49].

3.6.10 Treatment and Prognosis

- Cholinesterase inhibitors, immunosuppressive and immuno-modulatory drugs, thymectomy, and supportive treatment. The prognosis is in general good, only 10–15% of patients have insufficient control of disease activity [48, 49, 53].

3.7 Primary Angiitis of the CNS (PACNS)

3.7.1 Synonyms

- Isolated CNS angiitis/vasculitis; granulomatous angiitis of the brain, primary vasculitis of the CNS [54, 55].

3.7.2 Epidemiology

- Incidence 0.24/100.000/years.
- Female/male ratio 1/1 [56, 57].

3.7.3 Etiology and Definition

- A non-infectious idiopathic transmural inflammation of the CNS vasculature of unknown etiology.
- Infectious (mainly VZV and Mycoplasma) or para-infectious factors are considered in pathophysiology [54, 55].
- Affects large, small, and medium-sized leptomeningeal and parenchymal arterial vessels of the brain or spinal cord.
- It involves the three subtypes
  - 58% granulomatous
  - 28% lymphocytics and
  - 14% necrotizing vasculitis [55]

3.7.4 Clinical Features

- Clinical manifestations are heterogeneous, nonspecific, and most frequently include
- Headache.
- Cognitive decline (50%).
- Focal deficits due to CNS infarctions with or without imaging correlate.
- Transitory ischemic attacks (TIA).
- Seizures, acute encephalopathy, spinal cord symptoms are less frequent.
- As compared to systemic vasculitis, constitutional symptoms such as fever, anorexia, malaise, or weight loss are uncommon [54, 55, 58].

3.7.5 Disease Course

- Symptom onset can be either acute, especially when larger vessels are affected, or more commonly, insidious.
- The clinical course can be relapsing remitting, especially when small vessels are affected, or it can be slowly progressive, sometimes aggressive [54, 55, 58].
- The median age of symptom onset is 50 years [56, 57].

3.7.6 Brain Imaging

- Lesions' location and appearance
  - Focal lesions are almost always present (>90%).
  - Multiple, bilateral T2 lesions (unilateral involvement is rare).
  - Mostly supratentorial: frontal > parietal > temporal > occipital.
  - Often cortical and subcortical distribution (65%) but also deep gray and white matter.
  - Less often in periventricular white matter mimicking findings in MS.

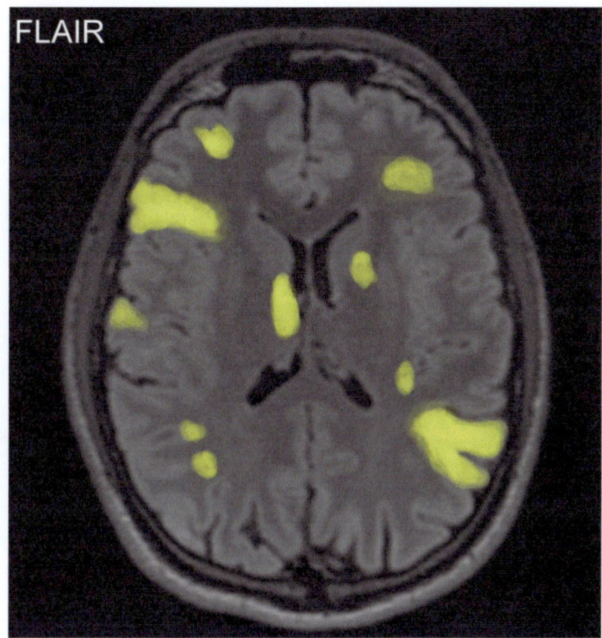

Fig. 3.5 MRI characteristics of primary angiitis of the CNS (PACNS)

- Rarely observed solitary tumor-like mass lesions (4%) (Fig. 3.5).
- Restricted diffusion observed in acute ischemic lesions ischemia.

- Contrast enhancement (<40%)
  - Usually parenchymal (89%), less commonly leptomeningeal (11%).
  - Lesions have variable ages (enhancing and non-enhancing lesions).
  - Sometimes observed PACNS-specific vessel wall thickening and intramural enhancement of large arteries [55, 56, 58, 59].
- Angiography
  - Alternating segments of stenosis with normal or dilated large or medium-sized vessels.
  - Arterial occlusions in many brain vessels are in the absence of advanced proximal vessel atherosclerosis or other pathology.
  - One abnormality in several arteries or several abnormalities in one artery is less consistent with primary CNS vasculitis.
  - Collateral blood flow may be seen.
  - Microaneurysms are rare.
  - Pathology is usually bilateral.
  - Frequently large arteries (such as the internal carotid and intracranial vertebral arteries, basilar artery, and their primary branches) and smaller arteries are simultaneously affected.
  - The sensitivity of angiography is 40–90%, but the specificity is only around 30%, because angiographic changes observed in vasculitis can be seen also in some non-vasculitic disorders (such as reversible cerebral vasoconstriction

  syndrome, CNS infections, cerebral arterial emboli, radiation vasculopathy, after subarachnoid hemorrhage or related to atherosclerosis) [55, 56, 58, 59].
  - Importantly, cerebral angiography might yield normal results because vascular pathology may affect very small arteries that are smaller than the resolution of angiography [60].
  - Magnetic resonance angiography (MRA) is less invasive than digital subtraction angiography (DSA), but it is less sensitive for small vessels pathology and vertebrobasilar circulation [56].
- Vessel wall MRI
  - Can help to distinguish PACNS from non-inflammatory vasculopathies such as atherosclerotic or in reversible cerebral vasoconstriction syndrome.
  - Circumferential type of the vessel wall enhancement is typical for infectious and or inflammatory vasculitis and affects mainly secondary and tertiary vessel segments. Eccentric type is typical for atherosclerosis and arterial hypertension and affects mainly primary and secondary vessel segments [54, 61].
- Other Features
  - Subarachnoid and parenchymal hemorrhages or microbleeds may sporadically occur [54, 55, 62].

3.7.7 Spinal Cord Imaging

- Pathological findings are rare (5%).
- Isolated spinal cord involvement may be rarely present in early disease stages, but over time almost all patients also have brain vasculitis.
- Thoracic cord is most often affected.
- Lesions usually show contrast enhancement.
- May be diffuse enhancement of conus, cauda equina, and nerve roots [55, 63].

3.7.8 Clinico-radiological Phenotypes of the PACNS

1. Negative angiography but biopsy-proven vasculitis
   - Markedly elevated concentration of protein in the CSF.
   - Meningeal or parenchymal enhancing lesions on MRI.
   - Favorably response to treatment.
   - Overall good prognosis [55].
2. A prominent leptomeningeal enhancement
   - Acute symptoms onset, often with cognitive impairment.
   - Angiography (MRA or DSA) is often negative.
   - Biopsy shows granulomatous vasculitis.
   - Most patients respond to corticosteroids and immunosuppression.
   - Overall good prognosis.

3. Biopsy-proven vasculitis with evidence of cerebral amyloid angiopathy
   - Biopsy shows a granulomatous vasculitis and vascular deposits of amyloid beta.
   - Usually a monophasic disease course.
   - Frequent cognitive dysfunction.
   - Enhancing meningeal lesions.
   - Good response to immunosuppressive treatment.
4. Rapidly progressive primary form
   - Many bilateral large cerebral vessel lesions on angiography.
   - Several bilateral cerebral infarctions.
   - Granulomatous or necrotizing vasculitis.
   - The response to immunosuppressive treatment is poor.
   - Often a fatal outcome.
5. Solitary tumor-like mass lesion (4%)
   - In 30% associated with cerebral amyloid angiopathy
   - Excision of the lesion or aggressive immunosuppressive therapy is often associated with a favorable outcome [55, 64, 65].
6. Intracerebral hemorrhage (11–12%)
   - Intraparenchymal or less often subarachnoidal hemorrhage.
   - Usually, present necrotizing vasculitis [55, 66].

3.7.9 Blood Work

- Routine testing is usually normal.
- The examination should include tests for erythrocyte sedimentation rate (ESR), C-reactive protein (CRP), anti-nuclear antibodies (ANA), antineutrophil cytoplasmic antibodies (ANCA), anti-phospholipid antibodies (APS), antibodies specific for different collagen vascular disorders, and serum angiotensin-converting enzyme (ACE) levels to exclude secondary vasculitis associated with systemic disease.

3.7.10 Examination of CSF

- Often abnormal findings (80–90%).
- Glucose level is usually normal.
- Elevated concentration of protein (sometimes markedly increased).
- Mild-to-moderate lymphomonocytic pleocytosis, sometimes with plasmatic cells.
- In case of marked pleocytosis (>250 cells/mm^3) should be considered alternative inflammatory or infectious disease.
- In contrast, mild pleocytosis can be present in non-vasculitic ischemic stroke or conditions such as Fabry disease or reversible cerebral vasoconstriction syndrome [54, 55, 59, 67].
- CSF-restricted OCB are present in around 20% [67].

3.7.11 OCT and Ophthalmological Assessment

- PACNS does not affect the eyes; therefore, ocular imaging including optical coherence tomography (OCT), may help identify its mimics, some of which may involve ocular pathology that remains asymptomatic.
- For example, branch retinal artery occlusions in the Susac's syndrome or embolic diseases, peripheral leakage on fluorescent angiogram in sarcoidosis, or subretinal pigment epithelium and vitreous opacity in CNS lymphoma [68].

3.7.12 Diagnosis

- Diagnosis is often delayed (75% diagnosed within 6 months) [55].
- Required presence of the following criteria:
  - Neurological deficit of unknown origin.
  - Brain angiography with typical features of vasculitis, or CNS biopsy showing histological features of vasculitis.
  - Findings cannot be explained by systemic vasculitis or any other disorder mimicking primary CNS vasculitis. PACNS is a diagnosis of exclusion [69].
- Diagnosis is definite in patients with
  - Biopsy-proven cerebral vasculitis showing transmural vascular inflammation of leptomeningeal or parenchymal vessels.
  - Sensitivity of biopsy is only 53–77%, because vasculitis affects arteries in a segmental way. Therefore, a negative biopsy may not exclude diagnosis of CNS vasculitis.
- Diagnosis is probable in patients with
  - Angiogram, MRI, and CSF findings are typical for vasculitis [54, 55, 62, 70]
- In addition, major (headache, stroke, cognitive impairment, focal neurological deficits) and minor (seizures, altered consciousness, psychiatric disorders) clinical features have been proposed, along with major (multiple parenchymal lesions, parenchymal/meningeal contrast enhancement, MRI angiography vessel abnormalities, vessel wall enhancement), and minor (parenchymal/subarachnoid hemorrhage, single parenchymal lesion) MRI features characteristic of PACNS, which could aid in diagnosis [71].

3.7.13 Differential Diagnosis

- Mimics of primary CNS vasculitis need to be always excluded because their treatment is often different. The most important mimics include
- Reversible cerebral vasoconstriction syndrome (RCVS)
  - The most common mimicker.
  - Heterogeneous group of disorders with brain vasoconstriction including Call-Fleming syndrome, post-partum angiopathy, drug-induced cerebral vasculopathy, migrainous vasospasm, and benign angiopathy.

- Clinically, there is recurrent sudden severe headache (thunderclap) and focal neurological deficits with or without seizures.
- Angiography shows multifocal segmental vasoconstrictions of brain arteries that resolves within 1–3 months.
- Complications include localized subarachnoid hemorrhage over the sulci, and less frequently, ischemic, or hemorrhagic strokes.
- Patient's history and normal CSF may help with diagnosis.
- Treated by oral nimodipine.

• Secondary CNS vasculitis (vasculitis caused by other systemic disorder)
  - Infections such as VZV, HIV, hepatitis C virus (HCV), parvovirus B19, cytomegalovirus (CMV), Mycoplasma pneumoniae, Borrelia burgdorferi, tuberculosis, Bartonella spp., Rickettsia spp., fungal infections, cysticercosis. The novel metagenomic next-generation sequencing may be used in patients with suspected vasculitis (especially those with chronic meningitis) to rule out an infectious process.
  - Systemic vasculitis in (ANCA)-associated vasculitis, Behçet's disease (5.3–14.3%), and less often polyarteritis nodosa, Henoch–Schönlein purpura, Kawasaki disease, giant-cell arteritis, Takayasu's arteritis, Wegener's granulomatosis (2%), or Churg–Strauss syndrome (4%).
  - Connective tissue diseases such as rheumatoid arthritis, Sjögren's syndrome, systemic lupus erythematosus (SLE), scleroderma, dermatomyositis, or other mixed connective tissue diseases.
  - Cerebral amyloid angiopathy (CAA) (three subtypes)
    - With deposition of amyloid beta without inflammation
      - Affects the older population with vascular risk factors. CSF does not show inflammatory pattern. Infarcts limited to one vascular territory and blood vessels calcifications favor underlying atherosclerotic process and not immune-mediated vasculitis.
    - With perivascular inflammation.
    - With granulomatous vasculitis (amyloid beta-related angiitis).
      - This subtype may mimic PACNS but occurs in older age, which is more often associated with cognitive impairment, seizures, intracerebral hemorrhages, and leptomeningeal enhancement but has lower frequency of infarctions.
  - Thrombotic vasculopathy rather than true inflammatory vasculitis can be observed in some patients with
    - Anti-phospholipid syndrome.
    - Sneddon's syndrome.
    - Ischemic cerebrovascular events.
    - Valvular emboli in bacterial endocarditis can result in occlusions of brain arteries mimicking a vasculitic pattern on angiography.
  - Hematologic malignancies such as Hodgkin's or less frequent non-Hodgkin lymphoma or intravascular lymphoma.
  - Other disorders with angiographic changes mimicking those found in PACNS are sarcoidosis (due to similar histological findings can be a differential diagnosis challenging), inflammatory bowel disease, graft-versus-host disease,

acute bacterial meningitis, cerebral autosomal dominant arteriopathy with subcortical infarcts and leukoencephalopathy (CADASIL), Sneddon's syndrome, or Susac's syndrome.
  - Drug-associated immune complex vasculitis [54, 55, 72].
- MS
  - In case that angiography does not show typical vasculitic pattern, the MRI findings in primary and secondary vasculitis can be undistinguishable from those seen in MS.
  - Patients with MS usually do not have marked elevation of protein in CSF, which is often present in vasculitis [57].
  - Central vein sign is present in the majority of MS lesions, whereas it is positive in only 14% of patients with PACNS [73].

3.7.14 Treatment and Prognosis

- Corticosteroids, cyclophosphamide, and other immunosuppressive agents such as TNF blockers or mycophenolate mofetil.
- The prognosis is variable and depends on phenotype, but overall, the long-term survival is reduced.
- MRI monitoring should include MR angiography 4–6 weeks after the treatment initiation and then every 3–4 months during the first year or when occur neurological worsening.
- In active patients may be required repeated CSF examination and repeated angiography [54, 55].
- Increased mortality is associated with occurrence of ischemic strokes [56].

References

1. Kira J, Yamasaki K, Kawano Y, Kobayashi T. Acute myelitis associated with hyperIgEemia and atopic dermatitis. J Neurol Sci. 1997;148(2):199–203.
2. Kira J, Isobe N, Kawano Y, Osoegawa M, Ohyagi Y, Mihara F, et al. Atopic myelitis with focal amyotrophy: a possible link to Hopkins syndrome. J Neurol Sci. 2008;269(1–2):143–51.
3. Matsuzono K, Suzuki M, Fujimoto S. A case report of atopic myelitis mimicking anterior spinal artery syndrome. Neurol Sci. 2020;41(4):969–71.
4. Gregoire SM, Mormont E, Laloux P, Godfraind C, Gilliard C. Atopic myelitis: a clinical, biological, radiological and histopathological diagnosis. J Neurol Sci. 2006;247(2):231–5.
5. Park CW, Choe WJ, Chun YI. Eosinophilic myelitis in the cervical cord mimicking intramedullary cord tumor. J Korean Neurosurg Soc. 2012;52(4):410–3.
6. Dubey D, Pittock SJ, Kelly CR, McKeon A, Lopez-Chiriboga AS, Lennon VA, et al. Autoimmune encephalitis epidemiology and a comparison to infectious encephalitis. Ann Neurol. 2018;83(1):166–77.
7. Zuliani L, Marangoni S, De Gaspari P, Rosellini I, Nosadini M, Fleming JM, et al. Epidemiology of neuronal surface antibody-mediated autoimmune encephalitis and antibody-based diagnostics. J Neuroimmunol. 2021;357:577598.
8. Rosenfeld MR, Dalmau JO. Paraneoplastic disorders of the CNS and autoimmune synaptic encephalitis. Continuum (Minneap Minn). 2012;18(2):366–83.

9. Graus F, Titulaer MJ, Balu R, Benseler S, Bien CG, Cellucci T, et al. A clinical approach to diagnosis of autoimmune encephalitis. Lancet Neurol. 2016;15(4):391–404.
10. Abboud H, Probasco JC, Irani S, Ances B, Benavides DR, Bradshaw M, et al. Autoimmune encephalitis: proposed best practice recommendations for diagnosis and acute management. J Neurol Neurosurg Psychiatry. 2021;92(7):757–68.
11. Flanagan EP, Geschwind MD, Lopez-Chiriboga AS, Blackburn KM, Turaga S, Binks S, et al. Autoimmune encephalitis misdiagnosis in adults. JAMA Neurol. 2023;80(1):30–9.
12. Jammoul A, Li Y, Rae-Grant A. Autoantibody-mediated encephalitis: not just paraneoplastic, not just limbic, and not untreatable. Cleve Clin J Med. 2016;83(1):43–53.
13. Yang HK, Kim JH, Park YH, Park KS, Kim JS, Hwang JM. Anti-NMDA-receptor optic neuritis in a patient with a history of encephalitis. Can J Ophthalmol. 2017;52(6):e216–e8.
14. Cheung SSL, Lau GKK, Chan KH, Wong IYH, Lai JSM, Tang WK, et al. Optic neuritis as the initial clinical presentation of limbic encephalitis: a case report. J Med Case Rep. 2018;12(1):357.
15. Dalmau J, Graus F. Diagnostic criteria for autoimmune encephalitis: utility and pitfalls for antibody-negative disease. Lancet Neurol. 2023;22(6):529–40.
16. Heine J, Prüss H, Bartsch T, Ploner CJ, Paul F, Finke C. Imaging of autoimmune encephalitis—relevance for clinical practice and hippocampal function. Neuroscience. 2015;309:68–83.
17. Lang K, Prüss H. Frequencies of neuronal autoantibodies in healthy controls: estimation of disease specificity. Neurol Neuroimmunol Neuroinflamm. 2017;4(5):e386.
18. Stevens-Jones O, Malmeström C, Constantinescu C, Dalla K, Nellgård B, Zelano J, et al. Presence of neural surface and onconeural autoantibodies in cerebrospinal fluid and serum in neurological diseases presents a potential risk for misdiagnosis. Eur J Neurol. 2023;30(9):2602–10.
19. Blinder T, Lewerenz J. Cerebrospinal fluid findings in patients with autoimmune encephalitis-a systematic analysis. Front Neurol. 2019;10:804.
20. Dürr M, Nissen G, Sühs KW, Schwenkenbecher P, Geis C, Ringelstein M, et al. CSF findings in acute NMDAR and LGI1 antibody-associated autoimmune encephalitis. Neurol Neuroimmunol Neuroinflamm. 2021;8(6)
21. Maat P, de Beukelaar JW, Jansen C, Schuur M, van Duijn CM, van Coevorden MH, et al. Pathologically confirmed autoimmune encephalitis in suspected Creutzfeldt-Jakob disease. Neurol Neuroimmunol Neuroinflamm. 2015;2(6):e178.
22. Titulaer MJ, McCracken L, Gabilondo I, Armangué T, Glaser C, Iizuka T, et al. Treatment and prognostic factors for long-term outcome in patients with anti-NMDA receptor encephalitis: an observational cohort study. Lancet Neurol. 2013;12(2):157–65.
23. Titulaer MJ, Soffietti R, Dalmau J, Gilhus NE, Giometto B, Graus F, et al. Screening for tumours in paraneoplastic syndromes: report of an EFNS task force. Eur J Neurol. 2011;18(1):19–e3.
24. Bogliun G, Beghi E, Italian GBSRSG. Incidence and clinical features of acute inflammatory polyradiculoneuropathy in Lombardy, Italy, 1996. Acta Neurol Scand. 2004;110(2):100–6.
25. Kuwabara S, Misawa S, Mori M. Bickerstaff brainstem encephalitis: more common than we think? J Neurol Neurosurg Psychiatry. 2013;84(11):1184.
26. Noioso CM, Bevilacqua L, Acerra GM, Della Valle P, Serio M, Vinciguerra C, et al. Miller Fisher syndrome: an updated narrative review. Front Neurol. 2023;14:1250774.
27. Sejvar JJ, Baughman AL, Wise M, Morgan OW. Population incidence of Guillain-Barre syndrome: a systematic review and meta-analysis. Neuroepidemiology. 2011;36(2):123–33.
28. Shahrizaila N, Yuki N. Bickerstaff brainstem encephalitis and Fisher syndrome: anti-GQ1b antibody syndrome. J Neurol Neurosurg Psychiatry. 2013;84(5):576–83.
29. Odaka M, Yuki N, Yamada M, Koga M, Takemi T, Hirata K, et al. Bickerstaff's brainstem encephalitis: clinical features of 62 cases and a subgroup associated with Guillain-Barre syndrome. Brain. 2003;126(Pt 10):2279–90.
30. Ropper AH, Shahani B. Proposed mechanism of ataxia in Fisher's syndrome. Arch Neurol. 1983;40(9):537–8.
31. Wakerley BR, Soon D, Chan YC, Yuki N. Atypical Bickerstaff brainstem encephalitis: ataxic hypersomnolence without ophthalmoplegia. J Neurol Neurosurg Psychiatry. 2013;84(11):1206–7.

32. Horton E, Krishnamoorthy S, Reynolds L. Bickerstaff's encephalitis. BMJ Case Rep. 2014;2014:bcr2014205336.
33. Ito M, Kuwabara S, Odaka M, Misawa S, Koga M, Hirata K, et al. Bickerstaff's brainstem encephalitis and Fisher syndrome form a continuous spectrum: clinical analysis of 581 cases. J Neurol. 2008;255(5):674–82.
34. Park JG, Bin CH, Park MS. Optic neuritis in a patient with Bickerstaff's brainstem encephalitis. J Clin Neurol. 2016;12(4):507–8.
35. Cuneo GL, Grazzini I, Guadagni M, Venturini E, Bianchi A. An atypical Bickerstaff's brainstem encephalitis with involvement of spinal cord. Neuroradiol J. 2016;29(5):396–9.
36. Taieb G, Mulero P, Psimaras D, van Oosten BW, Seebach JD, Marignier R, et al. CLIPPERS and its mimics: evaluation of new criteria for the diagnosis of CLIPPERS. J Neurol Neurosurg Psychiatry. 2019;90(9):1027–38.
37. Al-Chalabi M, DelCimmuto NR, Beran A, Devarasetty PP, Mhanna A, Mahfooz N, et al. Clinical characteristics, management, and outcomes of CLIPPERS: a comprehensive systematic review of 140 patients from 100 studies. Mult Scler Relat Disord. 2022;68:104112.
38. Taieb G, Kaphan E, Duflos C, Lebrun-Frenay C, Rigau V, Thouvenot E, et al. Hemophagocytic lymphohistiocytosis gene mutations in adult patients presenting with CLIPPERS-like syndrome. Neurol Neuroimmunol Neuroinflamm. 2021;8(3)
39. Taieb G, Duran-Pena A, de Chamfleur NM, Moulignier A, Thouvenot E, Allou T, et al. Punctate and curvilinear gadolinium enhancing lesions in the brain: a practical approach. Neuroradiology. 2016;58(3):221–35.
40. Dudesek A, Rimmele F, Tesar S, Kolbaske S, Rommer PS, Benecke R, et al. CLIPPERS: chronic lymphocytic inflammation with pontine perivascular enhancement responsive to steroids. Review of an increasingly recognized entity within the spectrum of inflammatory central nervous system disorders. Clin Exp Immunol. 2014;175(3):385–96.
41. Simon NG, Parratt JD, Barnett MH, Buckland ME, Gupta R, Hayes MW, et al. Expanding the clinical, radiological and neuropathological phenotype of chronic lymphocytic inflammation with pontine perivascular enhancement responsive to steroids (CLIPPERS). J Neurol Neurosurg Psychiatry. 2012;83(1):15–22.
42. Wang L, Holthaus EA, Jimenez XF, Tavee J, Li Y. MRI evolution of CLIPPERS syndrome following herpes zoster infection. J Neurol Sci. 2015;348(1–2):277–8.
43. Zhang L, Liu XH, Jin F, Liu MX, Zhang M, Zhang Y, et al. Chronic lymphocytic inflammation with pontine perivascular enhancement responsive to steroids (CLIPPERS) associated with or without lymphoma: comparison of clinical features and risk factors suggestive of underlying lymphomas. J Clin Neurosci. 2019;66:156–64.
44. Ferilli MAN, Papi C, Sabatelli M, Colosimo C, Iorio R. MOG autoimmunity mimicking CLIPPERS syndrome: case report and literature review. J Neuroimmunol. 2022;367:577875.
45. Valencia-Sanchez C, Pittock SJ, Mead-Harvey C, Dubey D, Flanagan EP, Lopez-Chiriboga S, et al. Brain dysfunction and thyroid antibodies: autoimmune diagnosis and misdiagnosis. Brain Commun. 2021;3(2):fcaa233.
46. Castillo P, Woodruff B, Caselli R, Vernino S, Lucchinetti C, Swanson J, et al. Steroid-responsive encephalopathy associated with autoimmune thyroiditis. Arch Neurol. 2006;63(2):197–202.
47. Laurent C, Capron J, Quillerou B, Thomas G, Alamowitch S, Fain O, et al. Steroid-responsive encephalopathy associated with autoimmune thyroiditis (SREAT): characteristics, treatment and outcome in 251 cases from the literature. Autoimmun Rev. 2016;15(12):1129–33.
48. Gilhus NE, Verschuuren JJ. Myasthenia gravis: subgroup classification and therapeutic strategies. Lancet Neurol. 2015;14(10):1023–36.
49. Punga AR, Maddison P, Heckmann JM, Guptill JT, Evoli A. Epidemiology, diagnostics, and biomarkers of autoimmune neuromuscular junction disorders. Lancet Neurol. 2022;21(2):176–88.
50. Pakzad Z, Aziz T, Oger J. Increasing incidence of myasthenia gravis among elderly in British Columbia, Canada. Neurology. 2011;76(17):1526–8.
51. Dehbashi S, Hamouda D, Shanina E. Co-occurrence of multiple sclerosis and myasthenia gravis: a case report and review of immunological theories. Mult Scler Relat Disord. 2019;34:135–6.

52. Bong JB, Lee MA, Kang HG. Newly diagnosed multiple sclerosis in a patient with ocular myasthenia gravis: a case report. Medicine (Baltimore). 2022;101(8):e28887.
53. Jacob S, Viegas S, Leite MI, Webster R, Cossins J, Kennett R, et al. Presence and pathogenic relevance of antibodies to clustered acetylcholine receptor in ocular and generalized myasthenia gravis. Arch Neurol. 2012;69(8):994–1001.
54. Paul SA, Roy D, Mondal GP, Bhattacharyya R, Ghosh KC, Das S, et al. Primary angiitis of central nervous system – a challenging diagnosis. J Neuroimmunol. 2022;366:577844.
55. Salvarani C, Brown RD Jr, Hunder GG. Adult primary central nervous system vasculitis. Lancet. 2012;380(9843):767–77.
56. Salvarani C, Brown RD Jr, Calamia KT, Christianson TJ, Weigand SD, Miller DV, et al. Primary central nervous system vasculitis: analysis of 101 patients. Ann Neurol. 2007;62(5):442–51.
57. Benseler SM, Silverman E, Aviv RI, Schneider R, Armstrong D, Tyrrell PN, et al. Primary central nervous system vasculitis in children. Arthritis Rheum. 2006;54(4):1291–7.
58. Kadkhodayan Y, Alreshaid A, Moran CJ, Cross DT 3rd, Powers WJ, Derdeyn CP. Primary angiitis of the central nervous system at conventional angiography. Radiology. 2004;233(3):878–82.
59. Kraemer M, Berlit P. Primary central nervous system vasculitis – an update on diagnosis, differential diagnosis and treatment. J Neurol Sci. 2021;424:117422.
60. Salvarani C, Brown RD Jr, Calamia KT, Christianson TJH, Huston J 3rd, Meschia JF, et al. Angiography-negative primary central nervous system vasculitis: a syndrome involving small cerebral vessels. Medicine (Baltimore). 2008;87(5):264–71.
61. Song JW, Shou H, Obusez EC, Raymond SB, Rafla SD, Kharal GA, et al. Spatial distribution of intracranial vessel wall enhancement in hypertension and primary angiitis of the CNS. Sci Rep. 2019;9(1):19270.
62. Birnbaum J, Hellmann DB. Primary angiitis of the central nervous system. Arch Neurol. 2009;66(6):704–9.
63. Salvarani C, Brown RD Jr, Calamia KT, Christianson TJ, Huston J 3rd, Meschia JF, et al. Primary CNS vasculitis with spinal cord involvement. Neurology. 2008;70(24 Pt 2):2394–400.
64. Molloy ES, Singhal AB, Calabrese LH. Tumour-like mass lesion: an under-recognised presentation of primary angiitis of the central nervous system. Ann Rheum Dis. 2008;67(12):1732–5.
65. Salvarani C, Brown RD Jr, Calamia KT, Christianson TJ, Huston J 3rd, Meschia JF, et al. Rapidly progressive primary central nervous system vasculitis. Rheumatology (Oxford). 2011;50(2):349–58.
66. Salvarani C, Brown RD Jr, Calamia KT, Christianson TJ, Huston J 3rd, Meschia JF, et al. Primary central nervous system vasculitis presenting with intracranial hemorrhage. Arthritis Rheum. 2011;63(11):3598–606.
67. Strunk D, Schulte-Mecklenbeck A, Golombeck KS, Meyer Zu Hörste G, Melzer N, Beuker C, et al. Immune cell profiling in the cerebrospinal fluid of patients with primary angiitis of the central nervous system reflects the heterogeneity of the disease. J Neuroimmunol. 2018;321:109–16.
68. Hajj-Ali RA, Calabrese LH. Central nervous system vasculitis: advances in diagnosis. Curr Opin Rheumatol. 2020;32(1):41–6.
69. Calabrese LH, Mallek JA. Primary angiitis of the central nervous system. Report of 8 new cases, review of the literature, and proposal for diagnostic criteria. Medicine (Baltimore). 1988;67(1):20–39.
70. Miller DV, Salvarani C, Hunder GG, Brown RD, Parisi JE, Christianson TJ, et al. Biopsy findings in primary angiitis of the central nervous system. Am J Surg Pathol. 2009;33(1):35–43.
71. Boulter DJ, Schaefer PW. Stroke and stroke mimics: a pattern-based approach. Semin Roentgenol. 2014;49(1):22–38.
72. Salvarani C, Hunder GG, Morris JM, Brown RD Jr, Christianson T, Giannini C. Aβ-related angiitis: comparison with CAA without inflammation and primary CNS vasculitis. Neurology. 2013;81(18):1596–603.
73. Maggi P, Absinta M, Grammatico M, Vuolo L, Emmi G, Carlucci G, et al. Central vein sign differentiates Multiple Sclerosis from central nervous system inflammatory vasculopathies. Ann Neurol. 2018;83(2):283–94.

Autoimmune and Inflammatory Multisystem Diseases

4

4.1 Anti-phospholipid Syndrome

4.1.1 Epidemiology

- Epidemiology is poorly understood.
- Incidence 2–5/100.000/year
- Prevalence 40–50/100.000
- Female/male ratio 3.5/1 [1]

4.1.2 Etiology and Definition

- Systemic autoimmune disorder associated with venous and/or arterial thrombosis, pregnancy morbidity, and other non-thrombotic manifestations in the presence of anti-phospholipid antibodies (aPL) directed against phospholipids and their cofactors.
- Proposed mechanisms of neuronal injury are
  - aPL interferes with endogenous anticoagulant mechanisms.
  - aPL binds directly to nervous tissue antigens.
  - aPL binds to endothelial cells and disrupt blood-brain barrier [2].

4.1.3 Subtypes

- Primary Anti-phospholipid syndrome (APS) (Hughes syndrome) (50%).
- Secondary APS (50%) [3].
  - Associated with other diseases, such as systemic lupus erythematosus (SLE) or malignancies [4, 5].

T. Uher, *Mimics and Red Flags of Multiple Sclerosis*,
https://doi.org/10.1007/978-3-031-98945-2_4

  - 10% of patients diagnosed with primary APS develop SLE within 10 years and re-diagnosed with secondary APS [6].
  - 30% of patients with SLE have aPL and among them around 10% will develop secondary APS [7].
- Catastrophic APS (Asherson's syndrome).
  - Rare, rapidly progressive variant [6].

4.1.4 Non-neurological Clinical Features

- The "20% rule" suggests that APS contributes to 20% of unprovoked deep vein thrombosis cases, 20–30% of strokes in adults under the age of 50, and 10–15% of recurrent fetal losses [21].
- Vascular thrombosis in any tissue, including pulmonary embolus.
- Pregnancy morbidity and fetal loss.
- Cardiac pathology (valve abnormalities, coronary artery disease, myocardial dysfunction, pulmonary hypertension, and intracardiac thrombi).
- Nephropathy (proteinuria, renal insufficiency, and arterial hypertension).
- Skin changes (livedo reticularis or racemosa, Raynaud phenomenon, oral ulcers, photosensitivity, and patchy hair loss).
- Arthralgias and other rheumatological symptoms.
- Hematological pathology (see below).

4.1.5 Neurological Clinical Features

- Stroke and transient ischemic attack (TIA)
  - Acute onset and rapid resolution of symptoms may indicate ischemic. Etiology rather than demyelinating event in multiple sclerosis (MS).
  - Strokes in young age (<50 years).
  - Atherosclerotic, cardioembolic, or vasculitis-like cause.
- Cerebral venous thrombosis.
- Acute ischemic encephalopathy.
- Reversible cerebral vasoconstriction syndrome
  - Rare condition with thunderclap headache and recurrent neurological deficit.
- Sneddon's syndrome
  - Slowly progressive thrombotic non-inflammatory vasculopathy.
  - Combination of stroke/TIA and livedo reticularis.
  - Sometimes also present headache, brain hemorrhage, seizures, or psychiatric symptoms.
  - Most common in young adult women.
  - Skin biopsy shows thrombosis of subcutaneous arterioles and capillary dilation with blood stagnation causing livedo reticularis.
  - Idiopathic (50%) or associated with autoimmune diseases (often APS) (50%). Almost half of the patients with this syndrome have positive aPL.

- Migraine (20%)
  - Often symptoms onset years before the diagnosis of APS.
  - 12% of migraine patients test positive for aPL, which is 2–6 times higher than the rate observed in the general population.
- Seizures (6–9%)
  - Might occur also in APS patients with normal magnetic resonance imaging (MRI) findings.
- Psychiatric symptoms (broad spectrum)
  - Cognitive dysfunction from mild to dementia (19–40%).
- Movement disorders (most often chorea 1.3–4.5%; others are rare).

4.1.6 Ocular Features

- Amaurosis fugax (5.4%)
  - Most common ocular pathology in APS.
  - Usually unilateral but can be also bilateral.
  - The rapid-onset of short (2–30 minutes) painless visual loss, followed by rapid and complete spontaneous recovery, distinguishes it from optic neuritis observed in MS.
- Anterior non-arteritic ischemic optic neuropathy (NAION)
  - Caused by ciliary blood vessel thrombosis.
  - Fundoscopy shows papillary edema with linear hemorrhages.
  - Might present with sudden complete or incomplete visual loss and impairment of color vision, resembling optic neuritis in MS.
  - Visual loss is not transient, unlike in the case of amaurosis fugax.
- Orbital ischemic syndrome (rare; occurs in catastrophic APS) [4, 5, 8].

4.1.7 Brain Imaging

- Lesions' location
  - Rarely normal MRI findings.
  - Lesions tend to be located in the deep or subcortical white matter rather than in the periventricular or juxtacortical white matter as observed in MS.
  - Involvement of the corpus callosum is less frequent, whereas involvement of the putamen is more common in APS compared to MS.
- Lesions' appearance
  - T2 hyperintense lesions in APS tend to be smaller in size compared to those seen in MS.
  - They typically do not exhibit the ovoid shape and perpendicular orientation to the lateral ventricles as lesions in MS.
  - Large territorial infarctions may occur in APS-associated ischemic strokes (Fig. 4.1).
  - T1 hypo-intense lesions ("black holes") may be present in APS as a result of ischemic events, leading to irreversible tissue damage.
  - Acute ischemic lesions show restricted diffusion.

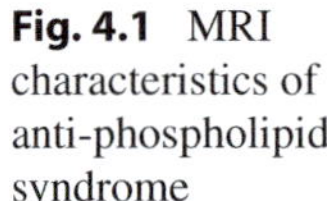

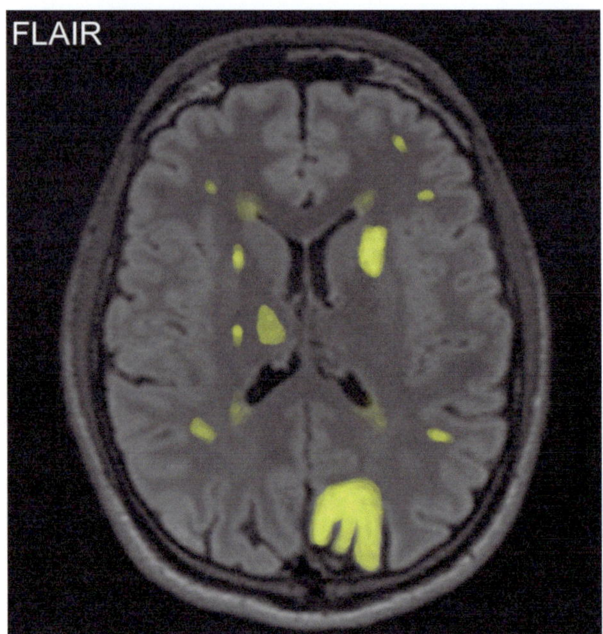

Fig. 4.1 MRI characteristics of anti-phospholipid syndrome

- Contrast enhancement
  - Usually absent, unless the MRI scan is performed during a subacute phase (>6 days from onset) of ischemic stroke showing gyriform enhancement in cortical gray matter.
- Evolution over time
  - Tend to remain static, maintaining shape and size over time.
  - In contrast, lesions in MS often show activity (new/enlarging lesions).
  - Partial resolution of lesions may occur following anticoagulation.
- Associated findings:
  - Lesions have an ischemic rather than inflammatory etiology.
  - The absence of the central vein sign (CVS) in APS may aid in the differential diagnosis from MS.
  - Other possible MRI findings include diffuse cortical atrophy, focal hemorrhage, cerebral microbleeds, or dural sinus thrombosis [4, 5, 9–11].

4.1.8 Spinal Cord Imaging

- Typically, normal findings, transverse myelitis is very rare (0.4–4%).
- Myelitis usually presents as longitudinally extensive transverse myelitis (LETM), most often in thoracic segments, and less frequently with short lesions mimicking MS.
- Often accompanied by swelling and spinal cord atrophy, which may resemble neuromyelitis optica spectrum disorders (NMOSD).
- Usually caused by vasculitis or thrombosis [4, 8, 10, 12].

4.1.9 Blood Work

- The frequency of aPL positivity in the serum of patients with APS is as follows
  - Anticardiolipin antibodies (70%).
  - Anti-beta 2 glycoprotein 1 (β2GP1) antibodies (10%).
  - Only lupus anticoagulant (15–20%).
  - Only ACA (25%) [1, 5].
- aPL positivity may occur in general population (2–5%), although typically in low titers and more frequently observed in older individuals [1, 13].
- aPL positivity is also detected in 2–88% of MS patients (a wide range), particularly during relapses, in older age, and in secondary progressive MS. However, the significance of aPL antibodies in MS remains unclear [2].
- Some patients with APS may exhibit mild thrombocytopenia, hemolytic anemia, prolonged activated partial thromboplastin time (aPTT) with a paradoxically prothrombotic state, and a history of false-positive serologic tests for syphilis (Venereal Disease Research Laboratory [VDRL] or rapid plasma reagin [RPR] tests).
- An acute thrombotic event might falsely normalize the aPTT; therefore, it is recommended to repeat this aPTT testing after recovery [14].

4.1.10 Examination of CSF

- Routine testing in primary APS typically yields normal results, without the presence of cerebrospinal fluid (CSF)-restricted oligoclonal bands (OCB).
- A minority of patients with rare APS-associated transverse myelitis may exhibit elevated concentration of protein and mild pleocytosis.
- Secondary APS is more frequently associated with mildly elevated concentration of protein and CSF-restricted OCB (15–65%) [9, 10].

4.1.11 Electrophysiology

- Although visual evoked potentials (VEP) in primary APS typically yield normal results, secondary APS may be associated with delayed latencies of the P100 wave [10, 15].
- Most patients exhibit normal nerve conduction studies or only signs of subclinical peripheral neuropathy [4].

4.1.12 Diagnosis

- The diagnosis of APS requires the presence of at least one clinical and one laboratory criterion, as per the 2006 Sydney revised APS classification criteria.
- Clinical criteria
  - Vascular venous or arterial thrombosis (superficial thrombophlebitis does not meet this criterion) and/or

  - Pregnancy morbidity (3 miscarriages <10 weeks, or 1 miscarriage ≥10 weeks, or premature birth before 34 weeks due to severe preeclampsia or placental insufficiency).
- Positive laboratory criteria
  - Anticardiolipin immunoglobulin G (IgG) and/or M (IgM), >40 IgG phospholipid units (GPL) or MPL (IgM phospholipid units), or >99th percentile.
  - Anti-beta-2-glycoprotein-I IgG and/or IgM, >99th percentile or >40 IU.
  - Lupus anticoagulant.
- aPL are not specific for APS. In the healthy population, they can be temporarily increased during infections or induced by drugs such as phenothiazines, procainamide, quinine, anti-tumor necrosis factor (TNF) agents, and others. Therefore, the positivity of aPL needs to be confirmed on two separate occasions, with tests performed at least 12 weeks apart. Additionally, aPL antibodies need to be present in sufficiently high titers, as mentioned above [13].
- The clinical significance of positive aPL titers <40 IU or isolated positivity of IgA isotypes remains unclear. The diagnostic role of IgA aPL remains controversial, and testing for IgA isotypes is reserved for patients with a strong clinical suspicion for APS but negative IgG and IgM aPL titers [16]. It is worth noting that IgA isotypes of anticardiolipin antibodiesa and anti-beta-2-glycoprotein-I are more commonly found in patients with SLE and are included in the diagnostic criteria for SLE [17].
- The diagnostic criteria may provide assistance, but they are not intended to solely diagnose APS. Diagnosis should always be established clinically because additional manifestations, known as "extra-criteria" or "non-criteria," may occur that cannot be exclusively explained by thrombotic phenomena. These manifestations may include neurological manifestations such as seizures, myelitis, chorea, migraine, or hematological and other manifestations.
- Cases of APS where patients do not meet the serological criteria with low titers or even an absence of aPL antibodies have been reported. These cases are referred to as "seronegative APS" [2].
- Whether MS patients with low-titer anticardiolipin antibodies positivity (5.6% of patients) represent a distinct subgroup of MS patients with atypical features such as absence of CSF-restricted OCB and milder disease course remains unclear [18].

4.1.13 Differential Diagnosis

- Patients with APS may develop transverse myelitis, retrobulbar neuritis, or any other neurological symptom typical for MS. Relapsing-remitting phenotype of APS, often termed "lupoid sclerosis," might also occur. Moreover, the age of symptom onset, typically between 20 and 50 years, overlaps with that of MS [1].
- Although MS patients might have positive aPL (2–44%) and ANA (2.5–25%, in low titers), they usually show negative anti-deoxyribonucleic acid (DNA) autoantibodies.
- Although APS patients have positive aPL in almost 100%, they have negative antinuclear antibodies (ANA) and anti-DNA autoantibodies.

- SLE patients have positive aPL in only 50–60% but frequently have positive ANA (98%) and anti-DNA (60%).
- Distinguishing between APS, MS-like APS syndrome, MS with aPL positivity, and coexistence of APS and MS can be challenging. Hence, it is suggested that a number of patients with APS may be misdiagnosed with MS [10].
- Screening for aPL in suspected MS patients should be reserved only for those presenting with atypical features, such as isolated myelitis, migraine, absence of OCB, high and persistent ANA titers, or history of vascular events and pregnancy morbidity [19], because aPL positivity is observed in some MS patients [2] and rarely in healthy individuals [1, 13].
- It is not advisable to test for aPL in patients at low risk of APS, such as older patients with thrombotic events or individuals with other risk factors for thromboembolism [20].
- aPL positivity is observed in 19–46% of NMOSD patients; however, APS patients do not typically test positive for aquaporin 4 (AQP4) IgG. Therefore, APS patients showing symptoms suggestive of NMOSD should undergo screening for anti-AQP4 IgG antibodies to rule out comorbid NMOSD [21].
- Other diseases mimicking APS include Behçet's disease, Sjögren's syndrome, migraine, cerebral small vessel disease (CSVD) or cerebral autosomal dominant arteriopathy with subcortical infarcts and leukoencephalopathy (CADASIL) [4, 5, 9–11].

4.1.14 Treatment and Prognosis

- Anticoagulation, although its use in patients with persistent aPL without a history of thrombosis, remains controversial [2].
- Some authors recommend a trial of oral anticoagulants for 6 months in patients with persistent aPL positivity and/or features suggesting APS [10].
- Corticosteroids, anti-CD20 therapy, intravenous immunoglobulin, or plasmapheresis may be considered in patients who exhibit disease activity despite anticoagulation or when severe non-thrombotic manifestations dominate.
- Hydroxychloroquine can be employed as an adjunctive drug in refractory cases [5].

4.2 Behçet's Disease

4.2.1 Epidemiology

- Highest prevalence (80–370/100.000) along the ancient Silk Road, stretching from eastern Asia to the Mediterranean, particularly in Turkey [22].
- Prevalence in USA 5.2/100.000 [23].
- Neuro-Behçet's disease (NBD) is present in approximately 10% (range 1.3–59%) of patients with Behçet's disease.
- Female/male ratio 1/2.8 [24, 25].

4.2.2 Etiology and Definition

- A multisystem inflammatory disorder of unknown origin causing perivasculitis, involving blood vessels of all sizes (small, medium, and large), types (arteries and veins), and tissues. However, this vaso-occlusive angiitis has venous predominance [24, 25].

4.2.3 Non-neurological Clinical Features

- Mucocutaneous
  - Painful round or oval oral aphthae/ulcers in almost all patients (97–99%)
  - However, recurrent aphthous stomatitis affects 10–20% of the general population; therefore, it should be interpreted cautiously when diagnosing Behçet's disease [45].
  - Genital aphthae/ulcers (scrotum or inguinal areas in males; vulva and inguina in females; or anorectal) can be painless and are present in vast majority of patients (85%).
  - Other skin changes may include pseudofolliculitis (acne-like lesions), erythema nodosum (50%), papulopustular lesions (85%), or pathergy reaction (60%) [25, 26].
  - Rarely patients never develop mucocutaneous manifestations [27].
- Ocular
  - Anterior, posterior, or combined uveitis (50%). Contrary to the Behçet's disease, uveitis in MS is rare and usually intermediate.
  - Retinal vasculitis.
  - Cells in vitreous on slit-lamp examination [25, 28].
- Rheumatological
  - Mono/oligo/polyarthritis or ankylosing spondylitis-like features (30–50%).
- Gastrointestinal
  - Esophageal ulceration, acute abdomen, proctorrhagia, chronic and recurrent diarrhea, or gastroduodenitis (1–30%).
- Vascular
  - Venous lesions with superficial phlebitis (25%), deep vein thrombosis (5%), vasculitic ulcers, or Budd–Chiari syndrome.
  - Arterial lesions resulting in thrombosis or aneurysm (4%).
- Epididymitis (5%) [24–26].

4.2.4 Neurological Clinical Features

A. Parenchymal (subacute meningo-encephalitis)
   - Brainstem
     - Sensori-motor deficit, cranial nerve palsy, cerebellar ataxia, Horner syndrome, sensorineural hearing loss (50%), and rarely internuclear ophthalmoplegia.

  - Can be combined with cerebral involvement ("brainstem plus").
- Cerebral
  - Headache (migraine or tension-type) (70%).
  - Patients with Behçet's disease who experience headaches but have normal MRI results are not diagnosed with NBD.
  - Movement disorders (dystonia, parkinsonism, chorea) are rare despite the frequent involvement of the basal ganglia.
  - Seizures are much less common in NBD compared to SLE due to milder cortical involvement (2.0–2.5%) [24–26].
- Spinal cord
  - Myelitis is rare but usually severe.
  - Cord involvement is almost always accompanied by simultaneous brain pathology. Isolated myelitis is extremely rare [25, 29].
- Asymptomatic ("silent") NDB
  - Patients show only abnormal MRI findings. Although clinical manifestations may develop in the future, they are usually less severe [30].

B. Non-parenchymal (20%)
- Cerebral venous thrombosis with intracranial hypertension (18%)
  - Caused by occlusion of venous channels due to dural venous thrombosis, cortical vein thrombosis, or deep cerebral vein thrombosis. All these conditions often occur together, and their clinical presentations are quite similar and nonspecific.
  - Often present with increased intracranial pressure including headache, papilledema, and elevated CSF pressure and focal neurological deficits.
  - Symptom onset is acute (30%), subacute, or chronic [24, 25].
- Intracranial aneurysm
  - Rare (0.2%) and probably not causatively associated with NBD.
- Extracranial aneurysm/dissection/stenosis
  - Vasculitis of the vasa vasorum might be the underlying pathology for aneurysm formation or arterial dissection [31].
  - May result in hemorrhagic or ischemic strokes, which are, however, uncommon in NBD (1.5%) [24, 32].

C. Peripheral (only 0.8%)
- Guillain–Barre syndrome, sensori-motor polyneuropathy, mononeuritis multiplex, autonomic neuropathy.
- Rarely neuromuscular junction disorders or myositis.

D. Other rare neurological manifestations
- Acute meningeal syndrome
  - Relatively common in case of aseptic meningitis, mixed pachymeningitis, or leptomeningitis.
- Tumor-like NBD
  - This form is rare and typically responds to corticosteroid, but to confirm the diagnosis, a brain biopsy is usually required.
- Neuropsychiatric symptoms
  - Delirium, confusion, severe cognitive impairment, affective and psychotic disorders.

- Optic neuropathy (not neuritis; rare; 0.4%)
  - Might be bilateral, recurrent, and simulate optic neuritis in MS.
  - Isolated or together with other manifestations of NBD [24, 25, 32].

4.2.5 Disease Course

- NBD typically presents a few years after the onset of systemic Behçet's disease. However, in around 6% of cases, it can precede systemic presentations by 3–6 years. Alternatively, NBD can also develop simultaneously with the onset of the first systemic symptoms of Behçet's disease.
- Symptoms onset is typically acute or subacute and occurs in young adults (20–40 years); disease onset in childhood is rare.
- Course is monophasic with a single relapse (1/3), relapsing-remitting (1/3), or chronic progressive (1/3). Relapsing course may convert to the chronic progressive course.
- Relapses in NBD are typically associated with systemic flare-ups, often accompanied by systemic symptoms such as fatigue, malaise, subfebrile fever, ulcers, or uveitis [24, 25, 32].

4.2.6 Brain Imaging

- MRI findings may be normal, but typically, they reveal lesions that can be challenging to differentiate from those observed in MS. At disease onset, 12% of patients meet the McDonald criteria for dissemination in space, but this proportion increases to 71% in later disease stages [33].
- Lesions' location
  - Follows the distribution of intra-axial veins in the central nervous system (CNS) [34].
  - Typical unilateral (rarely bilateral) mesodiancephalic (upper brainstem) lesion extending from basal ganglia and thalamus to midbrain along the long tracts and creating a "Cascade sign" (46%) [34].
  - Commonly lesions in pons and medulla oblongata (40%).
  - Less frequently in hypothalamus, cerebellar peduncles, and internal capsule (mainly posterior limb).
  - White matter lesions are not common. If present, located rather subcortically than periventriculary and often associated with brainstem lesions [24, 34, 35].
  - Contrary to MS, lesions in the corpus callosum, optic nerve, cortical gray matter, or U-fibers are rare [24].
  - Leukoencephalopathy-like pattern may manifest in advanced stages of the disease [36].
- Lesions' appearance and perilesional changes
  - Lesions are typically larger than in MS; tumefactive (mass-like) lesions may also occur [37].
  - Often with perifocal edema [24, 34, 35].

- In acute vasculitic lesions, diffusion-weighted imaging (DWI) typically demonstrates either unchanged or mildly increased signal, alongside increased signal on the apparent diffusion coefficient (ADC) maps, suggestive of vasogenic edema. Apart from the ischemic lesion (which can be also seen in NBD), there is no signal reduction on ADC maps, which typically indicates cytotoxic edema. These observations are similar to those seen in CNS vasculitis or SLE [38].
- Contrast enhancement
  - Often ring-like, dense, dotted, or leptomeningeal enhancement.
  - May occur perineural enhancement around the orbital optic nerve [24, 34, 35].
- Evolution over time
  - Although most patients typically present with a single lesion at disease onset, the lesion burden tends to accumulate over time, resembling the findings observed in MS.
  - Despite this, there is a trend for partial or even complete resolution of some lesions over time, a feature not typically observed in MS [24, 25, 34].
- Associated findings
  - Microbleeds (4–6%) (which are extremely rare in MS) [39].
  - Asymmetric brainstem and/or cerebellar atrophy without marked whole brain atrophy may occur in NBS but atypical for MS [24, 34].

4.2.7 Spinal Cord Imaging

- T2 hyperintense lesions and myelopathy are relatively rare (10%).
- Affects cervical or thoracic cord.
- Symmetrical or asymmetric involvement.
- Usually transverse myelitis, but anterior spinal artery syndrome or centrally located lesions can also occur.
- Longitudinally extensive transverse myelitis (LETM) is more often than short lesion and is associated with a worse prognosis.
- Often contrast enhancement and perifocal edema [24, 25, 32].
- Typical MRI patterns
  - "Bagel sign": lesion with hypo-intense center and hyperintense margin with or without contrast enhancement on axial T2 images.
  - "Motor neuron sign": symmetrical involvement of anterior horn cells [40] (Fig. 4.2).

4.2.8 Blood Work

- Might be elevated erythrocyte sedimentation rate and other serum inflammatory markers, which correlates with disease activity.
- Although examination of the human leukocyte antigen B51 (HLA-B51) allele (the most important genetic factor in Behçet's disease) could be conducted in suspected cases as supportive evidence, this examination is not useful in diagnosis because only a proportion of patients with NBD have a positive result for this haplotype [24, 25].

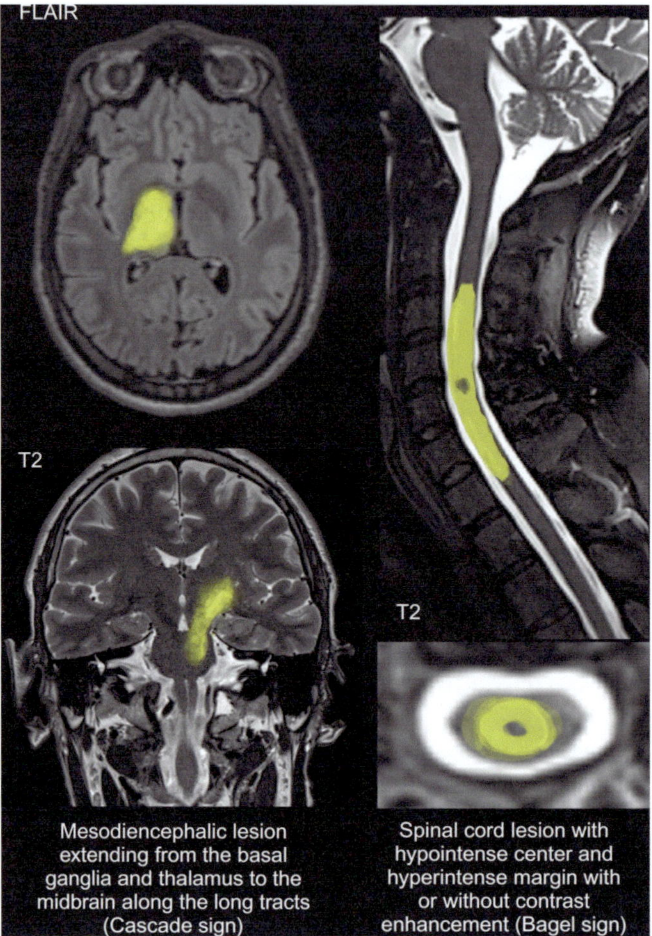

Fig. 4.2 MRI characteristics of neuro-Behçet's disease

4.2.9 Examination of CSF

- Elevated concentration of protein in most patients (only rarely normal).
- Glucose level is usually normal, which can aid in differentiation from infections or granulomatous processes.
- Increased concentration of interleukin 6 (IL-6).
- Initially may be neutrophil-dominant pleocytosis, which later evolves to lymphocyte-dominant pleocytosis or a mixed profile, typically with fewer than 200 cells/mm^3 (60–80%).
- CSF-restricted OCB might be sometimes present in parenchymal form of NBD (10.8%); thus, the presence of OCB cannot rule out NBD. OCB appear to be less stable compared with MS and may disappear after corticosteroid treatment [24, 25, 32, 41, 42].

4.2.10 OCT

- Optical coherence tomography (OCT) may show decreased retinal nerve fiber layer (RNFL) and macular thickness in patients with ocular involvement [43].

4.2.11 Electrophysiology

- Abnormal visual evoked potentials (VEP), including absent potentials, decreased amplitude with or without prolonged P100 latency, or only prolonged P100 latency, are present in 40% patients with NBD and 25% of patients with Behçet's disease without neurological involvement [44].

4.2.12 Diagnosis

- NBD is defined as a combination of neurologic manifestations in patients with Behçet's disease. Diagnosis may be straightforward in patients who fulfill the diagnostic criteria for Behçet's disease. In contrast, in some patients, diagnosis can be challenging because there is no specific diagnostic test, and NBD can precede systemic manifestations of Behçet's disease.
- Diagnosis of Behçet's disease requires:
  - Recurrent oral ulcerations (≥3 relapses over 12 months)plus two or more features from the following:
    1. Recurrent genital ulcerations.
    2. Eye lesions (anterior or posterior uveitis, cells in vitreous on slit-lamp examination, or retinal vasculitis).
    3. Skin manifestations (erythema nodosum, pseudo-foliculitis, papulopustular lesions or acneiform nodules in post-adolescent patients not on corticosteroids).
    4. Positive pathergy test (minor skin trauma or needle prick induces development of erythematous indurations, which may persist as papules or progress to pustules) [24, 25, 32].

4.2.13 Differential Diagnosis

- NBD should be considered in the differential diagnosis of stroke in young adults, MS, CNS vasculitis, movement disorders, intracranial hypertension, central venous thrombosis, or cerebral venous sinus thrombosis [24, 25].
- Chronic progressive NBD should be considered in patients with brainstem and cerebellar atrophy associated with leukoencephalopathy resembling MS [36].

4.2.14 Treatment and Prognosis

- Immunosuppressive drugs including corticosteroids (with slow tapering), oral cytostatics, TNF inhibitors (infliximab), anti-IL-6 (tocilizumab), or anti-CD20 therapies [24, 25].
- Most patients with acute relapse respond well to corticosteroids.
- Cyclosporin may worsen the disease.
- Neurological involvement is one of the most important causes of severe disability (65.4% after 17 years) and mortality (35.2% after 17 years) [25, 45].
- Predictors of poor outcome include young age at onset, male sex, brainstem or cerebellar symptoms, paresis, frequent relapses, primary progressive course, HLA-B51 allele, brainstem lesions and atrophy on MRI, high concentration of protein, and marked pleocytosis in CSF [24, 25].

4.3 Celiac Disease

4.3.1 Epidemiology

- Prevalence 700–1.400/100.000 [46].
- Estimated that >70% of cases remain undiagnosed [47].

4.3.2 Etiology and Definition

- Autoimmune T-cell-mediated enteropathy caused by the ingestion of gluten in genetically susceptible individuals.
- There is a strong genetic association with the HLA types DQ8 and DQ2 (DQA1 0501 and QQB1 0201 arranged either in cis or trans configuration). Approximately 70–100% of monozygotic twins and 10% of first-degree relatives are concordant for the disease [48].

4.3.3 Non-neurological Clinical Features

- The classical form of celiac disease (CD) presents with chronic diarrhea, anorexia, weight loss, abdominal distension, muscle wasting, and mood changes.
- Non-classical CD, the most common phenotype, typically presents with non-specific intestinal and extraintestinal manifestations including hematological (anemia due to iron deficiency), hepatic (mild elevation of transaminases), nutritional, musculoskeletal (arthralgia, arthritis, osteopenia/osteoporosis, sacroiliitis, short stature), dermatological (alopecia, chronic urticaria, dermatitis herpetiformis), stomatological (recurrent stomatitis, dental enamel defects), reproductive (unexplained fertility-related disorders), immunological (attenuated response to the hepatitis B virus vaccine, hyposplenism), fatigue, gastro-oesophageal reflux disease, and neurological symptoms (see below) [48].

4.3.4 Neurological Clinical Features

- Occurs in 4–60% of patients with CD.
- Heterogeneous manifestations can occur at any age, often leading to delayed diagnosis of CD and are often not associated with any gastrointestinal symptoms.
- Epilepsy is often associated with occipital calcifications and folate deficiency
- Cerebellar syndrome with gait ataxia, lower limb ataxia, dysarthria, or nystagmus is relatively common (29–43%). Gastrointestinal symptoms are present in only small proportion of these patients (<10%).
- Symptomatic or subclinical peripheral neuropathy (small-fiber sensory neuropathy, symmetric predominantly sensory neuropathy, mononeuritis multiplex, motor or sensori-motor polyneuropathy) is common (23–41%).
- Headaches (most often migraine or tension type) (42%).
- Cognitive deficit and affective disorders.
- Other rare complications may include acute generalized chorea, pseudotumor cerebri, cerebral vasculitis, stiff-man syndrome, myositis, neuromyotonia, myasthenic syndrome, or myelopathy [48–54].
- Epidemiological data on neurological complications are based on a limited number of studies with relatively small sample sizes and do not account for many undiagnosed patients. Therefore, the reported prevalence of patients with different neurological abnormalities might be highly overestimated.

4.3.5 Brain Imaging

- Small nonspecific T2 lesions in subcortical white matter (20–36%) (Fig. 4.3).
- Rarely diffuse white matter changes.
- A gluten-free diet does not lead to the resolution of white matter lesions, but it may halt the progression of white matter pathology.
- Accelerated brain atrophy, particularly in the cerebellum and cortical and deep gray matter structures, including the thalamus, may occur [51, 52, 54–56].
- The cause of white matter pathology is not clear, but an immune-mediated vasculitis is suggested as a potential cause [57].

4.3.6 Spinal Cord Imaging

- Even patients with rare CD-associated myelopathy typically exhibit normal findings on MRI [54].

4.3.7 Blood Work

- See "Diagnosis"

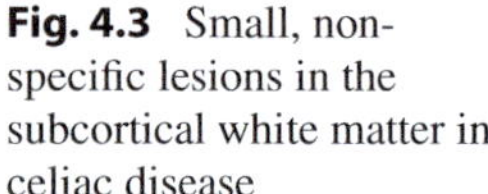

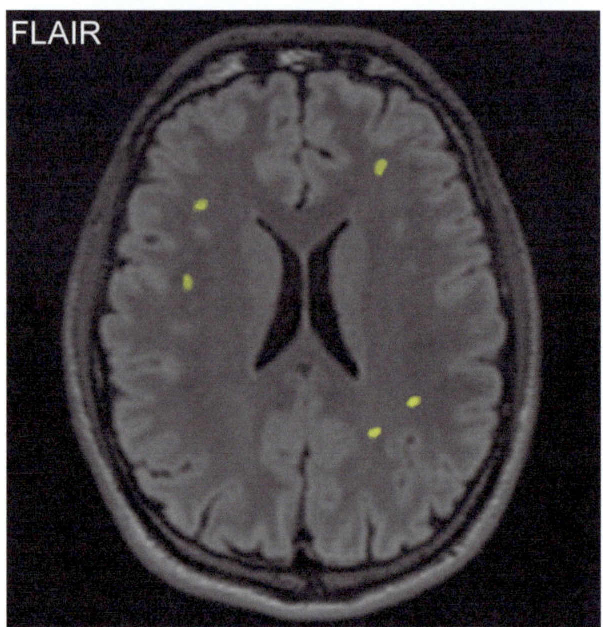

Fig. 4.3 Small, non-specific lesions in the subcortical white matter in celiac disease

4.3.8 Examination of CSF

- Routine CSF testing is expected to be normal, but a few case studies of patients with CD and elevated concentration of protein, pleocytosis, and positive CSF-restricted OCB, mimicking the findings seen in MS have been reported [58–60].
- Furthermore, a few cases of patients with immune-mediated rapid-onset gluten cerebellar ataxia due to gluten sensitivity associated with mild pleocytosis and CSF-restricted OCB exist [61].

4.3.9 Electrophysiology

- Occasionally present peripheral neuropathy [48, 54].

4.3.10 Diagnosis

- The diagnosis requires the detection of IgA anti-transglutaminase 2 (TG2) antibodies and characteristic histological changes on small intestinal biopsy (Marsh type 3a-c).
- Patients with positive IgA anti-TG2 and IgA anti-endomysial antibodies (EMA), but without duodenal villous atrophy (Marsh type 0 or 1), may still be considered as having a potential diagnosis of CD.

- Blood testing should be performed before initiation of gluten-free diet.
- Patients with IgA deficiency may only exhibit positive IgG antibodies [48, 54].

4.3.11 Differential Diagnosis

- A few case studies have described patients with CD and white matter lesions resembling those seen in MS. The absence of spinal cord lesions and OCB, along with the presence of peripheral involvement, may aid in distinguishing these patients from those with MS [62, 63].

4.3.12 Treatment and Prognosis

- Strict gluten-free diet.
- Intestinal and extraintestinal manifestations of CD may be irreversible if left untreated, but usually improve with gluten-free diet [48, 54].
- CD is associated with a slightly increased risk of non-Hodgkin lymphoma, especially in the gut [64].

4.4 Churg–Strauss Syndrome

4.4.1 Synonyms

- Eosinophilic granulomatosis with polyangiitis

4.4.2 Epidemiology

- Prevalence 1.1–1.4/100.000 (adults).
- Incidence 0.01–0.27/100.000/year [65–67].

4.4.3 Etiology and Definition

- Churg–Strauss syndrome (CSS) is caused by eosinophil-rich disseminated necrotizing vasculitis affecting small-to-medium blood vessels. It is associated with extravascular granulomas and occurs exclusively in patients with bronchial asthma and tissue eosinophilia. Vessel inflammation and eosinophilic proliferation contribute to organ damage.
- Neuronal damage is driven by vasculitis and/or eosinophil-mediated injury.
- CSS belongs to the group of antineutrophil cytoplasmic antibodies (ANCA)-associated vasculitidies, which includes three disorders:

  - CSS (stands between primary systemic vasculitis and hyper-eosinophilic disorders).
  - Granulomatosis with polyangiitis (GPA; Wegener granulomatosis).
  - Microscopic polyangiitis (MPA); (GPA, MPA, and other primary systemic vasculitidies are not associated with asthma and marked eosinophilia in the blood, and they exhibit different pathological findings compared to CSS [67, 68].

4.4.4 Clinical Features

- Clinical manifestations are variable, but typically there are three phases.
- Prodromal phase
  - Lasting from months to years; characterized by asthma bronchiale (96–100%) and rhinosinusitis with nasal polyps, allergic rhinitis, and recurrent or chronic sinusitis (47–93%). Some patients may also experience symptoms such as arthralgias, myalgias, malaise, fever, weight loss, otitis media, hearing loss, or facial nerve palsy.
  - The mean age of symptom onset is 40–60 years (range, 7–74) [65–67].
- Eosinophilic Phase
  - Characterized by peripheral eosinophilia and organ involvement (lungs: 60–70%; heart 30–50%; or gastrointestinal tract).
- Vasculitic Phase
  - Characterized by clinical manifestations of small vessel vasculitis.
  - Patients may have fever, fatigue, headache, and weight loss, renal (25%) or skin involvement (palpable purpura and nodules).
  - ANCA-positive patients have different phenotype (peripheral neuropathy, glomerulonephritis, purpura) as compared with ANCA-negative patients (myocardial involvement, lung infiltrates, gastrointestinal tract symptoms) [67].
  - Peripheral nervous system involvement is often:
    - Peripheral neuropathy due to vasculitis of the vasa nervorum includes mostly multiplex mononeuritis, less often sensory-motor polyneuropathy or cranial nerve neuropathy (55–75%).
    - Optic neuritis can be uni- or bilateral.
    - Neuronal compression resulting from granulomas, as seen in Wegener's granulomatosis, is typically absent.
  - CNS involvement is less often (5–39%) and include
    - Ischemic lesions/strokes (63% of patients with CNS pathology).
    - Posterior reversible encephalopathy syndrome (PRES) (37% of patients with CNS involvement).
    - Intracranial hemorrhages.
    - Oblongata or spinal cord involvement [69, 70].

4.4.5 Brain Imaging

- Multiple small punctate or large T2 hyperintensities in deep white matter of multiple vascular territories, often with restricted diffusion on DWI, indicating an ischemic origin.
- May occur typical ischemic lesions in cortical and subcortical regions.
- Other lesion locations include oblongata, cerebellum, or corpus callosum.
- Some patients may exhibit MS-like lesions (Fig. 4.4).
- Rarely manifests as hemorrhagic stroke, subarachnoid hemorrhage, or hypertrophic pachymeningitis.
- The frequency of focal lesions is similar to those seen in other ANCA-associated vasculitides, such as GPA or MPA [67, 70–73].

4.4.6 Spinal Cord Imaging

- The two case studies described patients with multifocal non-enhancing brain lesions and focal lesions in the cervical and thoracic spinal cord [70, 74].

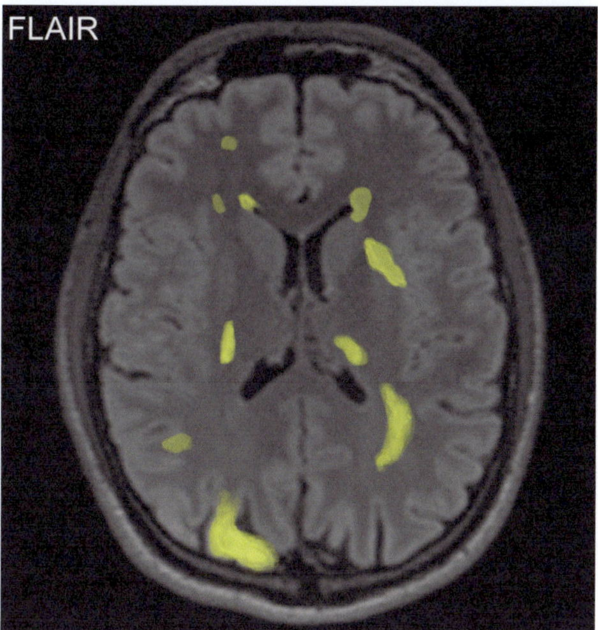

Fig. 4.4 Multiple sclerosis (MS)-like brain lesions in Churg–Strauss syndrome

4.4.7 Blood Work

- Positive ANCA need to be confirmed by the presence of myeloperoxidase (40%) [75].
- High total leukocyte counts with a very high proportion of eosinophils (>1500 cells/μL or >10%).
- Often high C-reactive protein (CRP), high erythrocyte sedimentation rate (ESR) and elevated IgE levels
- A high concentration (>80 pg/mL) of eotaxin-3, which is an eosinophil-attracting chemokine, has been found to have good sensitivity (87.5%) and specificity (98.6%) for the diagnosis of active CSS [76].

4.4.8 Examination of CSF

- Sporadically present low glucose (6–14%), mildly elevated protein (14–50%), mild pleocytosis (4–11%), eosinophils, and increased intracranial pressure [70].
- One case study described a patient with positive CSF-restricted OCB [74].

4.4.9 Diagnosis

- There are no widely accepted diagnostic criteria; however, one of the most used algorithms requires the presence of at least four of the six criteria
  - History of asthma.
  - Eosinophilia >10%.
  - Peripheral neuropathy.
  - Pulmonary infiltrates.
  - Paranasal sinus abnormality.
  - Extravascular eosinophils infiltrate on biopsy.
- Diagnosis is primarily based on clinical findings; therefore, organ biopsy is not always required. However, in "limited" forms of CSS affecting only single organs, biopsy is often necessary for accurate diagnosis [77].

4.4.10 Differential Diagnosis

- Idiopathic hyper-eosinophilic syndrome (HES) is also characterized by marked and persisting eosinophilia of unknown origin (>6 consecutive months) and organ dysfunction. However, unlike CSS, HES usually does not involve asthma, lacks vasculitis in biopsy specimens, and is ANCA negative [67].

4.4.11 Treatment and Prognosis

- Corticosteroids and cyclophosphamide can improve the outcome [67, 78].

- The prognosis is typically favorable, with around 90% of patients achieving remission. However, approximately 25% of patients may experience relapses, and around 10% may die due to systemic complications such as severe cardiac, gastrointestinal, or renal involvement.
- Untreated patients have a mortality rate of 50% at 3 months [79].

4.5 Cogan's Syndrome

4.5.1 Epidemiology

- Extremely rare disorder; only a few hundred cases have been reported [80].
- Females and males are affected equally [81–84].

4.5.2 Etiology and Definition

- The etiology of Cogan's syndrome (CS) remains unknown, but it is currently believed to be an autoimmune disorder. It often coexists with other autoimmune diseases, and histopathological examination of corneal tissue and cochlea reveals lymphocytic and plasma cell infiltration, suggesting a cell-mediated reaction. CS is associated with large and/or medium vessel vasculitis, although vessels of any size may be affected [81, 82].

4.5.3 Clinical Features

A. Eye symptoms (75%)
    - Typical CS: Non-syphilitic interstitial keratitis with granular and irregular corneal infiltrates of the cornea.
    - Atypical CS: Without non-syphilitic interstitial keratitis, but with glaucoma, conjunctivitis, uveitis, or episcleritis.
    - Rarely are ocular symptoms absent, and intestinal keratitis asymptomatic.
    - Other features include ocular redness (74%), photophobia (50%), ocular pain (50%), and decreased visual acuity (42%).

B. Audio-vestibular symptoms (75%)
    - Sudden onset of tinnitus, vestibular syndrome, and hearing loss.
    - In the early stages might be affected only one ear.
    - Typically, a progression of bilateral sensorineural hearing loss occurs over a span of 3–90 days, which may resemble Meniere's disease.
    - Time between onset of eye and audio-vestibular symptoms is usually <2 years. If the time exceeds 2 years, it is diagnosed as atypical CS.

C. Systemic vasculitis (15–30%)
    - More commonly seen in atypical CS and may affect any organ system.
    - Cardiovascular

    - Aortitis with aortic vasculitis (in 10% of patients) can lead to life-threating complications such as aortic aneurysm, dissection, or insufficiency.
- Neurological
    - In around 13% of patients and include stroke or TIA, myelopathy, seizures, meningitis, or encephalitis.
    - Peripheral or cranial neuropathy may rarely occur.
- Gastrointestinal
    - Diarrhea, anorexia, abdominal pain, mesenteric arteritis
- Other
    - Fever, headaches, polyarthralgia, arthritis, myalgia, splenomegaly, lymphadenopathy [81–85]

4.5.4 Disease Course

- The median age of symptom onset is 25 years (range, 5–63 years).
- The onset of the disease is typically preceded by a viral prodrome occurring a few weeks earlier [82–85].

4.5.5 Brain Imaging

- Often normal, but some patients may have ischemic strokes or multiple focal T2 hyperintensities in deep white matter compatible with cerebral vasculitis.
- Sometimes seen calcifications, narrowing, or soft tissue obliteration of the vestibular labyrinth and the cochlea [85–87].

4.5.6 Spinal Cord Imaging

- Reported case study of patient presenting with myelopathy [83].

4.5.7 Blood Work

- Blood tests typically reveal normal findings, although some patients may exhibit elevated concentrations of CRP, leukocyte count, and ESR.

4.5.8 Examination of CSF

- Routine testing typically yields normal results.
- Some patients may exhibit mildly elevated concentrations of protein and mild pleocytosis, or rarely present with a picture resembling aseptic meningitis [81, 82, 85, 87].

4.5.9 Diagnosis

- The diagnosis is often challenging, as it relies solely on the association between bilateral ocular and vestibulo-auditory symptoms, with no specific diagnostic tests available. Support for the diagnosis may be garnered from a positive response to corticosteroid treatment [81–84].
- Some patients may not present with interstitial keratitis at the onset of the disease; it may develop in later stages. Additionally, other patients may only exhibit sensorineural loss, without involvement of the eyes, with or without systemic vasculitis. These atypical phenotypes can further complicate the diagnosis of CS [87].

4.5.10 Differential Diagnosis

- Mainly Susac's syndrome (encephalopathy, typical brain MRI and eye involvement), Takayasu's arteritis (does not involve eyes and ears), polyarteritis nodosa, granulomatosis with polyangiitis (Wegener's granulomatosis), giant cell arteritis, rheumatoid arthritis, syphilis, and tuberculosis [82, 84].
- Compared to Meniere's disease, audio-vestibular involvement in CS is more severe, long-standing, without a period of complete remission, and often bilateral [87].
- Vogt–Koyanagi–Harada disease is a rare immune-mediated condition prevalent in Asia, characterized by chronic uveitis, alopecia, vitiligo, hearing loss, and potential systemic manifestations [88].

4.5.11 Treatment and Prognosis

- The recommendation is based on a limited number of case studies.
- Mild ocular involvement is treated using local corticosteroids.
- Inner ear pathology or systemic vasculitis is treated with corticosteroids, cyclophosphamide, azathioprine, methotrexate, cyclosporine, anti-CD20, anti-interleukin 6 (IL-6), or tumor necrosis factor (TNF)-alpha blockers. In some cases, patients may require cochlear implantation [81, 82].
- Patients without systemic vasculitis generally have a good prognosis without a reduction in life expectancy. However, patients with systemic involvement and severe vasculitis, such as aortitis, face a poor prognosis and an increased risk of premature death. Therefore, early diagnosis and anti-inflammatory treatment are crucial.
- More than 50% of patients have moderate to severe hearing loss despite therapy [81–83].

4.6 Cytotoxic T Lymphocyte Antigen 4 (CTLA-4) Haploinsufficiency

4.6.1 Epidemiology

- A rare genetic disorder with an unknown prevalence.

4.6.2 Etiology and Definition

- The CTLA-4 acts as a coinhibitory receptor on regulatory T cells. Its upregulation inhibits lymphocyte proliferation, whereas heterozygous mutations are associated with immune dysregulation and immunodeficiency. There is incomplete penetrance [89, 90].

4.6.3 Non-neurological Features

- The most frequent manifestations include autoimmune thrombopenia and hemolytic anemia, chronic diarrhea and inflammatory bowel disease, skin involvement (e.g., psoriasis), lymphoproliferation, or unusual and recurrent infections.
- The phenotype and age of symptom onset are highly variable, with some patients experiencing symptoms in late adulthood.
- Immune deficiency with recurrent infections.
- Hypogammaglobulinemia, diffuse lymphadenopathy, and hepatosplenomegaly.
- Autoimmune disorders (autoimmune hemolytic anemia or thrombocytopenia, skin diseases like psoriasis and others).
- Lymphoproliferation, granulomatous lymphocytic infiltration of various tissues, and malignancies (solid and hematological malignancies) [89–91].

4.6.4 Neurological Features

- They are highly variable and present in 11–32% of patients.
- Although immune and systemic manifestations typically precede neurological symptoms, in 5% of patients, the diagnosis of CTLA-4 haploinsufficiency is prompted by the presence of neurological manifestations.
- Commonly present headache, seizures (38%), or progressive focal neurological deficits (cerebellar ataxia, visual loss and optic atrophy, paraparesis) mimicking genetic neurodegenerative disorders or primary progressive MS (54%).
- Sometimes might be not clear whether neurological manifestations are caused by an autoimmune or by infiltrating lymphoproliferative process [89, 90, 92, 93].

4.6.5 Disease Course

- Median age of first autoimmune manifestations is 6 years (range 3–15), first infectious manifestations is 14 years (range 4–24), and first neurological manifestations is 18 years (range 15–45).
- Disease course is usually relapsing–remitting with subacute symptoms onset.
- May be present slowly progressive cognitive decline [93].

4.6.6 Brain Imaging

- T2 lesions are located mainly in the supratentorial peri- and para-ventricular white matter but may occur also in cortical and deep gray matter or infratentorial region.
- Periventricular lesions may be perpendicular to lateral ventricles and resemble Dawson fingers in MS.
- Lesions are often very large (tumefactive demyelination) and with contrast enhancement. The clinical symptoms are often disproportionally mild considering the size of the lesions.
- May be present diffuse bilateral leukoencephalopathy-like pattern.
- Commonly homogenous or ring-like contrast enhancement of lesions and/or leptomeninges.
- In general, CNS lesions exhibit a relapsing-remitting pattern (waxing and waning) and typically do not respond well to anti-inflammatory therapies, including corticosteroids [89, 90, 92, 93].

4.6.7 Spinal Cord Imaging

- Lesions are common, sometimes longitudinally extensive transverse myelitis (LETM).
- Frequently homogeneous contrast-enhancing [89, 90, 92, 93] (Fig. 4.5).

4.6.8 Blood Work

- Hypogammaglobulinemia across all Ig subclasses, including IgA, IgG, and IgM insufficiency, with low levels of IgG2 and IgG4 subclasses (80%).
- Lymphoproliferation.
- Low lymphocyte and natural killer (NK) cells count.
- Low levels of antimeasles and antimumps antibodies.

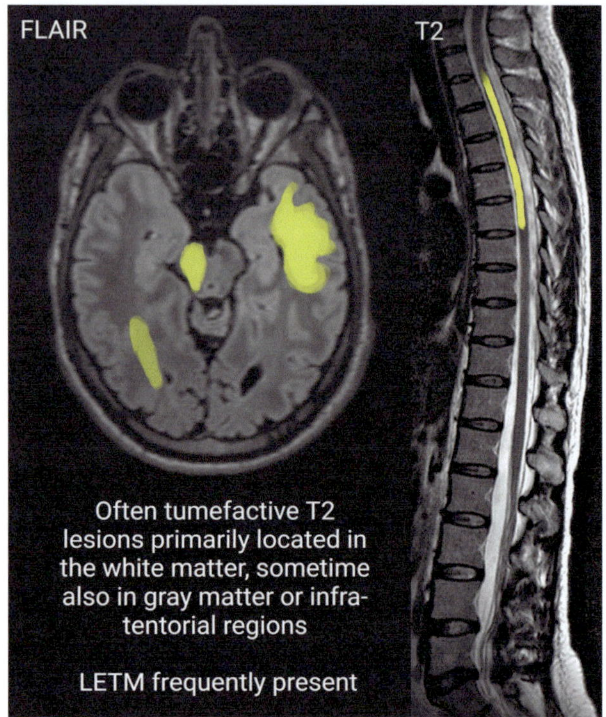

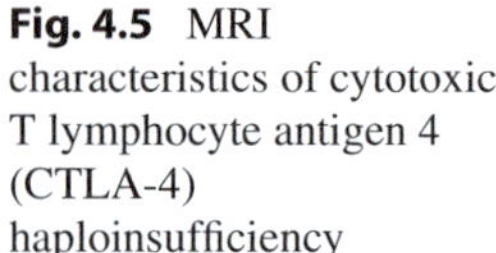
Fig. 4.5 MRI characteristics of cytotoxic T lymphocyte antigen 4 (CTLA-4) haploinsufficiency

4.6.9 Examination of CSF

- Mildly elevated concentration of protein.
- Mild to moderate pleocytosis (<50 cells/mm^3)
- Often elevated IgG index.
- CSF-restricted OCB in the majority of patients [89, 90, 92, 93].

4.6.10 Diagnosis

- Frequently delayed owing to the high variability of phenotypes and the rarity of the disorder. Early diagnosis through genetic molecular testing is crucial because treatment options are available [90, 93].

4.6.11 Treatment and Prognosis

- CTLA-4 fusion protein abatacept can stabilize the disease.
- Corticosteroids, sirolimus, and rituximab can be also used [89, 90, 93].

4.7 IgG4-Related Disease

4.7.1 Epidemiology

- Prevalence is unknown.
- Female/male ratio 1/3 [94, 95]

4.7.2 Etiology and Definition

- Immunoglobulin G4 (IgG4)-related disease (IgG4-RD) is a chronic inflammatory disease of unknown etiology, characterized by sclerosing inflammation and fibrosis resulting from the infiltration of IgG4-positive plasma cells and lymphocytes into single or multiple organs [94].

4.7.3 Non-neurological Features

- Diffuse infiltration may occur in various organs including the pancreas (most affected), bile ducts, gall bladder, lymph nodes, retroperitoneum, kidneys, breasts, prostate, lungs, bones, or skin.
- Some patients may develop inflammatory pseudotumors, which are mass lesions commonly found in the orbit, salivary glands, retroperitoneum, lymph nodes, lungs, kidneys, or other locations [94].

4.7.4 Neurological Features

- Neurological complications are rare (4–9%) and most commonly involve
- Hypophysitis.
  - Inflammation of the pituitary gland, often resulting in panhypopituitarism.
- Hypertrophic pachymeningitis.
  - Diffuse or focal thickening of the dura mater in the brain and/or spinal cord, which can result in cranial neuropathy, retro-orbital pain, visual loss, extra-ocular palsies, headache, seizures, or encephalopathy cognitive impairment.
- Perineural disease.
  - Migration of inflammatory cells along nerve tissue, particularly branches of the paravertebral, trigeminal, or optic nerves. This may cause compression and swelling of nerves (for example, optic nerve with visual loss).
  - Migration of inflammatory cells along nerve tissue, particularly branches of the paravertebral, trigeminal, or optic nerves, may cause nerve compression and swelling. This can lead to symptoms such as visual loss when the optic nerve is involved.
  - Peripheral neuropathy is extremely rare.

- Cerebral or spinal cord inflammatory pseudotumor.
  - This rare condition can occur in the meninges (resembling meningioma), ventricles, pituitary gland, cranial nerves, or parenchyma. The manifestations depend on the size and location of the lesion [96–100] (Fig. 4.6).

4.7.5 Disease Course

- Age of symptoms onset is usually >50 years (peak, 61–70 years) [94, 95], but teenagers and young adults can also be affected [100, 101].

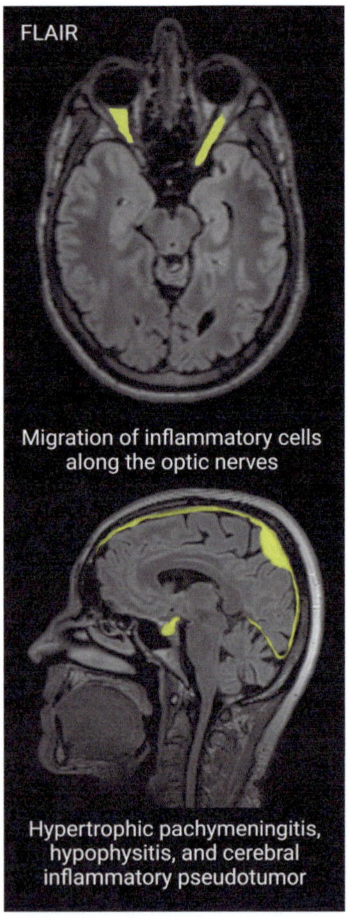

Fig. 4.6 MRI characteristics of IgG4–related disease

4.7.6 Brain and Spinal Cord Imaging

- Brain lesions are usually hypointense on T2 images owing to fibrosis and exhibit homogenous contrast enhancement [97].
- Presence of multiple unspecific brainstem, cortical, and subcortical lesions may mimic MS and other demyelinating diseases [101, 102].
- Involvement of the spinal cord is rare [100, 101].

4.7.7 Blood Work

- Routine blood tests are usually normal.
- Commonly normal also concentration of IgG4 (30%).
- Conversely, many other diseases such as parasitic infections, autoimmune diseases (such as Castleman's disease, rheumatoid arthritis, ANCA-associated vasculitis or even some patients with MS), allergic diseases, or pancreatic cancer may be associated with elevated levels of IgG4 (>135 mg/dL) [94, 103].

4.7.8 Examination of CSF

- IgG4-related pachymeningitis is typically associated with normal to mildly elevated concentrations of protein (median 0.72–0.99 g/L), variable mononuclear pleocytosis (median 14–24 cells/mm^3), elevated IgG index (75–100%), and positive CSF-restricted OCB (65–75%).
- Elevated concentrations of IgG4 in the CSF (>0.32 g/L) in almost all patients may aid in differential diagnosis (100%) [97, 102, 104].

4.7.9 Diagnosis

- The diagnosis is established through a combination of clinical, imaging, laboratory, and histopathological findings. The following criteria are necessary
  1. Diffuse or localized swelling or masses in one or more organs.
  2. Elevated serum IgG4 levels (>135 mg/dL).
  3. Dense lymphoplasmacytic infiltration, fibrosis, and/or obliterative phlebitis with IgG4-positive plasma cells on biopsy of the affected organs.
- The diagnosis is considered definite if all [94–96] criteria are fulfilled, probable if criteria 1 and 3 are fulfilled, and possible if criteria 1 and 2 are met [105].

4.7.10 Differential Diagnosis

- The diagnosis of IgG4-RD in the CNS is often delayed due to nonspecific imaging features that mimic findings observed in diseases such as neurosarcoidosis, rheumatoid arthritis, tuberculosis, other granulomatous diseases, vasculitic conditions (such as granulomatosis with polyangiitis, Behçet's disease, giant cell arteritis), or CNS lymphoma [106].

4.7.11 Treatment and Prognosis

- Treated IgG4-RD has favorable outcomes and excellent response to corticosteroids.
- The treatment response is better in early disease stages before extensive fibrosis develops. Therefore, early diagnosis is crucial to prevent extensive tissue involvement, which can lead to organ failure and often requires surgery.
- Corticosteroid withdrawal or tapering can sometimes trigger disease relapses, hence corticosteroid-sparing agents (azathioprine, mycophenolate mofetil, methotrexate), or anti-CD20 drugs may be required to control the disease [94].

4.8 Inflammatory Bowel Disease

4.8.1 Epidemiology

- Prevalence 1.300–2.000/100.000.
- Ulcerative colitis is slightly more prevalent than Crohn's disease [107, 108].
- The exact prevalence of neurological complications is unclear, with previous studies reporting a range between 0.25% and 47.5%. They are likely underreported [109–111].
- Prevalence of MS in patients with inflammatory bowel disease (IBD) is 0.2%, whereas the prevalence of IBD in patients with MS is around 0.6% [112].

4.8.2 Etiology and Definition

- Chronic idiopathic systemic disorders causing inflammation of the gastrointestinal tract, as well as extraintestinal complications. Their exact cause is unknown [107].
- Ulcerative colitis is a relapsing non-transmural inflammatory disease restricted to the colon.
- Crohn's disease is also a relapsing, but transmural inflammatory disease that may affect the entire gastrointestinal tract [107, 113].

4.8.3 Intestinal Features

- Commonly include bloody diarrhea, abdominal cramping, or weight loss [107].

4.8.4 Extraintestinal Non-neurological Features

- Can precede, accompany, or follow gastrointestinal symptoms.
- Common (25%; more frequent in Crohn's disease) and may include [107, 113]
  - Hematological (anemia, pro-coagulation state)
  - Ocular (iritis, uveitis)
  - Joint and bones (arthritis, osteoporosis)
  - Skin (erythema nodosum, pyoderma gangrenosum)
  - Hepatic and pancreatic (primary sclerosing cholangitis, pancreatitis)
  - Renal disorders
  - Cancer [107]

4.8.5 Neurological Features

- Caused by thromboembolic events, systemic and cerebral vasculitidies, malabsorption, or cerebral demyelination due to immune-related mechanisms. Usually include mainly
  - Peripheral neuropathy (radiculopathy, plexopathy, sensorimotor polyneuropathy) and myopathy are uncommon
  - Cerebrovascular disease (ischemic stroke or cerebral venous thrombosis) caused by thromboembolism, hypercoagulation state, vasculitis, or their combination
  - MS-like demyelinating conditions including myelopathy
  - Aseptic pachymeningitis
  - Encephalopathy, seizures and psychiatric symptoms [109, 110, 114, 115]

4.8.6 Brain Imaging

- Although some studies have noted a comparable rate of nonspecific T2 hyperintensities in the brain among patients with IBD and control groups [115, 116], other have observed a greater prevalence of nonspecific non-enhancing asymptomatic T2 hyperintensities in patients with IBD (42–75% in IBD compared to 16–45% in controls) [117–120].
- There are only rare case reports of IBD patients presenting with acute symptomatic brain lesions in
  - Periventricular white matter.

  - Subcortical white matter (inhomogeneous lesion with contrast enhancement extending into the midbrain, accompanied by mass effect, and mimicking glioblastoma).
  - Upper brainstem and medulla oblongata [121].
- Patients with IBD may exhibit accelerated gray matter atrophy [122].
- The origin of brain lesions is heterogeneous:
  - Ischemic mechanisms (atherosclerotic, thromboembolic).
  - Vasculitis (can result in stroke or migraine or be asymptomatic).
  - Demyelination (some lesions mimicking MS might not be associated with MS or radiologically isolated syndrome [RIS], but they may represent an MS-like syndrome linked to IBD).
  - Comorbidity with MS.
  - Opportunistic infection associated with immunosuppressive drugs.
  - Triggered by immuno-modulatory drugs such as TNF-alpha or very late antigen (VLA)-4 blocking agents.
  - Combined etiology of lesions [115–117, 121, 123, 124].

4.8.7 Spinal Cord Imaging

- Involvement of the spinal cord is rare but might mimic NMOSD or MS.
- Case studies reported patients with
  - Single or multiple contrast–enhancing short cord lesions.
  - Longitudinally extensive transverse myelitis (LETM) with a mass effect in cervical or thoracic segments [121, 125].

4.8.8 Examination of Blood and CSF

- Feacal calprotectin is a marker of neutrophil migration into the gastrointestinal tissue and is increased during the intestinal inflammation. It is used for monitoring and prediction of IBD, can differentiate IBD from irritable bowel syndrome but not between Crohn's disease and Ulcerative colitis [126].
- Routine CSF tests typically yield normal results. In patients with positive CSF-restricted OCB, comorbidity with MS should be ruled out [120].

4.8.9 Diagnosis

- There are no definitive diagnostic tests for Crohn's disease or ulcerative colitis, which are diagnosed clinically and confirmed by endoscopy, imaging, and biopsy. In IBD-unclassified patients, it is no possible to distinguish between ulcerative colitis and Crohn's disease (5–15%) [107, 127].

4.8.10 Differential Diagnosis

- The differential diagnosis of the CNS lesions on MRI in IBD patients with or without neurological symptoms can be challenging [121].
- Neurological manifestations typical of MS, characteristic lesions on MRI, involvement of the spinal cord, and the presence of CSF-restricted OCB may suggest the frequently observed coexistence of IBD with MS. The prevalence of MS in patients with Crohn's disease is five times higher than expected in the general population [112, 128, 129].

4.8.11 Treatment

- Immunosuppressive and immuno-modulatory drugs [107, 127].

4.9 Rheumatoid Arthritis

4.9.1 Epidemiology

- Prevalence 500–1.000/100.000 (adults)
- Prevalence rises with age and is highest in women older than 65 years [130]

4.9.2 Etiology and Definition

- A chronic autoimmune disease-causing inflammation of the synovium, the lining of the membranes that surround the joints (synovitis). Although the precise cause is unknown, around 50% of the risk for developing the rheumatoid arthritis (RA) is attributed to genetic factors.
- RA affects mostly small peripheral joints and distinguishes itself from spondyloarthritis (spondyloarthropathy), a group of conditions characterized by:
  - Inflammatory arthritis impacting the large joints in the spine, pelvis, or less frequently other large joints or
  - Inflammatory enthesitis (inflammation of the enthesis, the site where a tendon or ligament attaches to bone).
- The group of spondyloarthritides includes the following diagnoses
  - Ankylosing spondylitis (Morbus Bechterew)
  - Psoriatic arthritis
  - Reactive arthritis

- Enteropathic arthritis associated with inflammatory bowel disease (Crohn's disease or Ulcerative colitis)
- Juvenile spondyloarthritis
- Undifferentiated spondyloarthritis [131, 132]

4.9.3 Joint and Systemic Features

- RA affects small peripheral joints of the hands and feet and causes synovial tissue proliferation (pannus). Although it usually not affected the spine, subluxation of the atlantoaxial joint may occur.
- Pulmonary (pulmonary nodules, pleural effusion, and fibrosing alveolitis).
- Ocular (keratoconjunctivitis sicca, episcleritis, and scleritis).
- Vasculitis (nail fold and systemic).
- Cardiovascular (pericarditis, pericardial effusion, valvular heart disease, conduction defects, myocardial infarction, heart failure, peripheral vascular disease, and arterial hypertension).
- Cutaneous (palmar erythema, pyoderma gangrenosum, vasculitic rashes, and leg ulceration).
- Amyloidosis.
- Gastrointestinal symptoms.
- Osteoporosis.
- Renal disease.
- Or complications such as increased rate of infections and cancer.

4.9.4 Neurological and Imaging Features Related to RA

- Subluxation of the cervical vertebrae may result in spinal cord compression, myelopathy, and radiculopathy.
- Rheumatoid aseptic pachymeningitis can affect cranial nerves, including optic nerve. Rarely it may precede the occurrence of joints involvement. MRI may be associated with leptomeningeal thickening, contrast enhancement, and cortical lesions with restricted diffusion. Might be misdiagnosed with chronic subdural hematoma.
- Rheumatoid nodules (20% of individuals with RA) are typically found subcutaneously but rarely can also be found in other organs, such as the brain, often adjacent to the dura mater and/or choroid plexus. MRI shows hyperintensity on T1 and T2 images and occasionally contrast enhancement. They can manifest with symptoms or remain asymptomatic.
- CNS vasculitis.
- Unspecific T2 hyperintensities in subcortical or para-ventricular white matter (Fig. 4.7).
- Peripheral nerve entrapment, peripheral neuropathy, or mononeuritis multiplex.

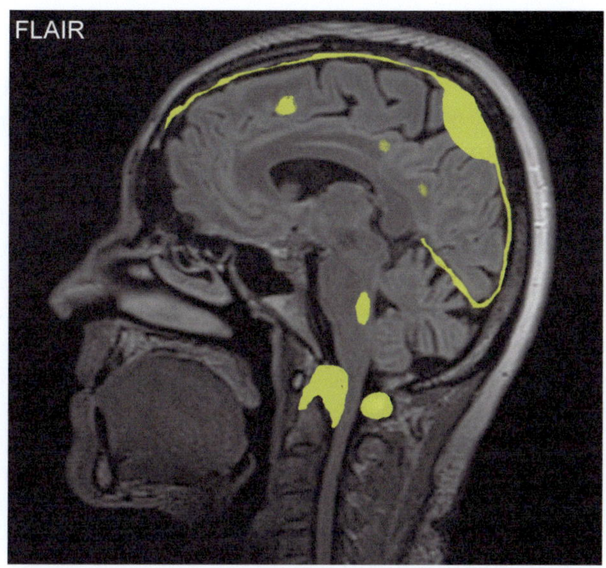

Fig. 4.7 Aseptic pachymeningitis, rheumatoid nodules, non-specific brain lesions, and pannus formation in the atlanto-axial joint in rheumatoid arthritis

4.9.5 Neurological and Imaging Features Unrelated to RA

- Cerebral hemorrhage or ischemic stroke (caused by serum hyper-viscosity from the elevated titers of circulating rheumatoid factor).
- Choroid plexus infiltration.
- Rheumatoid synovial infiltration of the spinal dura matter.
- Progressive multifocal leukoencephalopathy [131, 133–140].

4.9.6 Neurological and Imaging Features Related to Anti-TNF Drugs

- RA is probably not associated with higher risk of MS [141], but treatment of RA by TNF inhibitors increases risk of demyelinating diseases including MS and opportunistic infections of the CNS. The association between the use of anti-TNF drugs and the onset of demyelinating diseases is unclear and may be driven by altered immunological responses.
- Conversely, anti-TNF drugs reduce the likelihood of CNS vascular events and neurodegeneration, likely by regulating systemic inflammation [139, 142].
- There are case reports of patients with RA treated by anti-TNF drugs suffering from optic neuritis, MS, cranial and peripheral neuropathy [143]. In certain patients, demyelinating symptoms may resolve after discontinuing anti-TNF drugs and introducing systemic corticosteroids [144].

4.9.7 Blood Work

- Rheumatoid factor (IgM antibodies against the Fc fragment of IgG) is frequently positive (60–80%; in early RA only 40%), although it is not etiologically related to RA.
- However, low titers of rheumatoid factor are also found in about 1–5% of the general population, particularly among older individuals. The positivity is also more common in patients with various other inflammatory conditions (for example 52% of patients with primary and 98% patients with secondary Sjögren's syndrome), resulting in relatively low specificity for rheumatoid factor.
- The presence of rheumatoid factor of IgA and IgG isotypes in the absence of IgM is more common in mixed connective tissue disease than in RA.
- Anti-Citrullinated Protein Antibodies (ACPA) are more specific and sensitive for the diagnosis of RA and predict better more severe disease.
- Elevated levels of CRP and ESR rate are frequently present [131, 145, 146].

4.9.8 Examination of CSF

- Usually does not show specific abnormalities, but in patients with neurological complications such as aseptic pachymeningitis may be present inflammatory pattern with elevated protein and lymphocytic pleocytosis [133–135, 138].
- In these cases, CSF-restricted OCB can be absent, present, or can disappear following the treatment [137, 147].

4.9.9 Diagnosis

- Based on a combination of joint involvement; blood findings (Rheumatoid factor, ACPA, CRP, ESR) and duration of symptoms (ACR/EULAR 2010 criteria) [148].
- The presence of neurological involvement is confirmed through clinical assessment, imaging, and in some cases also histopathology [131, 133–139].

4.9.10 Treatment and Prognosis

- Disease-modifying antirheumatic drugs including anti-TNF-alpha drugs such as abatacept, rituximab, or tocilizumab [131].
- There is a possible association between anti-TNF medications and demyelination; therefore, non-anti-TNF drugs should not be used in the patients with preexisting demyelinating disorders of CNS [139].

- Untreated active RA results in joint damage, disability, and systemic complications.
- Higher rheumatoid factor titers predict a poorer prognosis and more severe disease [131].

4.10 Sarcoidosis

4.10.1 Epidemiology

- Incidence of systemic sarcoidosis
  - 3–10/100.000/year (Caucasians)
  - 35–80/100.000/year (African Americans)
- Among patients with systemic sarcoidosis
  - 5–10% of patients have clinical neurosarcoidosis (with or without systemic manifestations of sarcoidosis)
  - 10–25% of patients have asymptomatic neurosarcoidosis
  - Over long-term follow-up, 10–20% of patients present with isolated neurosarcoidosis, without manifestations of systemic sarcoidosis
- Risk factors include African American ethnicity and age 20–45 years (70%) and >50 years (30%) (two peaks of incidence).
- Female/male ratio 55/45 [149–154].
- Cigarette smokers have lower incidence compared to smokers (25 versus 75%) probably due to the immunosuppressive effect of tobacco exposure [155].

4.10.2 Etiology and Definition

- A multisystem disease characterized by a noncaseating granulomatous inflammatory exaggerated response to an unidentified antigen (possibly microbial), and there is ongoing debate about whether it is an autoimmune disease.
- A combination of environmental and genetic factors plays a role in pathogenesis of sarcoidosis [151, 156, 157]. Monozygotic twins have an 80-fold higher risk, whereas dizygotic twins have a seven-fold higher risk of developing sarcoidosis [158].

4.10.3 Non-neurological Clinical Features

- May be asymptomatic in many patients.
- The clinical manifestations result from the location of the granulomas.
- Sarcoidosis occurs mostly in the organs that are in closest with the external environment such as the lungs, skin, and eyes, and their draining lymph nodes.

- Most often affects the lungs and/or mediastinal lymph nodes (in 90% of cases), but it may involve any organ, ranging from a single lymph node or isolated organ to multi-organ involvement.
- Pulmonary (67–90%).
- Lymph nodes (10–20%).
- Hepatic (20–30%).
- Eye (10–50%) (see below)
  - Uveitis (20–50%): the most frequent ocular manifestation of systemic sarcoidosis presenting either as anterior uveitis (in young age) or panuveitis (in middle and older age).
- Skin (15–21%)
  - Often the first manifestation of disease (15–35%)
  - 20–40% of patients with cutaneous sarcoidosis lack systemic involvement
- Cardiovascular system
  - Arrhythmias, heart failure, pericardial disease, pulmonary hypertension, and sudden cardiac death
- Constitutional symptoms (20%)
  - Chills, weight loss, or fatigue [150–154, 156, 159]

4.10.4 Cranial Neuropathy

- 50–75% of patients with neurosarcoidosis.
- Caused by granulomatous invasion of the cranial nerve from meninges, infiltration of cranial nerve nuclei, fascicles, and nerves, basilar aseptic meningitis, or increased intracranial pressure.
- May affect multiple cranial nerves simultaneously or sequentially.
- Most common and typical manifestation of neurosarcoidosis occurs much more frequent than in MS. Multiple concurrent or serial cranial neuropathies should raise suspicion on neurosarcoidosis.
- Typically presents with a subacute onset and a progressive course.
- Around 80% of cases are associated with other neurological symptoms.
- MRI often reveals increased T2 signal within the nerve and nerve thickening with or without contrast enhancement and leptomeningeal contrast enhancement.
- Most often cranial neuropathies include
- Peripheral facial palsy (around 30%).
  - Most often cranial neuropathy in sarcoidosis
  - Often recurrent and bilateral (30–40%)
  - Simultaneous or sequential
  - Rarely Heerfordt syndrome (facial palsy, parotitis, anterior uveitis, fever)
  - >80% of patients exhibit some additional neurologic manifestation, which helps to distinguish it from Bell's palsy
- Optic neuritis, perineuritis or neuropathy (7–35%).
  - Usually subacute unilateral eye pain and vision loss
  - Slightly more often bilateral than unilateral (in MS in only 1%)

  - Affected optic nerve, but sometime also the optic chiasm, when chiasmal involvement may be associated with pituitary pathology
  - Although responds to corticosteroids, the visual recovery is often poor.
  - Less frequently may occur compressive optic neuropathy due to infiltration of the optic nerve or the presence of a mass-like lesion
- Vestibulocochlear neuropathy (3–17%)
  - Vestibular syndrome and hearing loss are frequently caused by selective vestibulocochlear nerve involvement or basilar leptomeningitis
- Other cranial neuropathies are less often.
- Need to be distinguished cranial neuropathies associated mainly with MS, NMOSD, Sjögren's syndrome, SLE, infections (such as Lyme disease, syphilis, human immunodeficiency virus [HIV], varicella-zoster virus [VZV], or herpes simplex virus [HSV]), brain neoplasms (such as glioma or meningioma), infiltrative malignancy (including lymphoma), histiocytosis, and Bell's palsy [151, 154, 159, 160].

4.10.5 Aseptic Meningitis

- 10–20% of patients with neurosarcoidosis.
- Most typical manifestation; in 40% of cases with sarcoidosis in CNS.
- Subacute onset; may become chronic.
- Clinical features include cranial neuropathy, hydrocephalus, headache, meningeal syndrome, or seizures, but no fewer.
- MRI shows thin leptomeningeal enhancement of pia matter and arachnoidea or rarely pachymeningitis with thick enhancement of dura matter.
- Often nodular component of contrast enhancement.
- MRI features often appear worse than clinical manifestations.
- Predilection at the base of the skull (basilar meningitis).
- May be complicated by hydro-cephalus (9%) due to involvement of arachnoid granulations (communicating) or compression of the aqueduct (obstructive).
- Meningitis may spread along the perivascular spaces into parenchyma or extend to spinal cord meninges.
- Not only leptomeningeal disease, but also dural inflammation (pachymeningitis) and a dural inflammatory mass mimicking a meningioma can occur.
- Needs to be distinguished mainly
  - In the case of leptomeningitis (inflammation of the pia mater and arachnoid mater), differential diagnosis include mainly fungal, tuberculous, and neoplastic meningitides (including lymphoma), brucellosis, Lyme disease, infiltrative histiocytosis, and glial fibrillary acidic protein (GFAP) antibody-associated syndromes.
  - In the case of pachymeningitis (inflammation of the dura mater), differential diagnosis include mainly IgG4-related disease, ANCA-associated vasculitis, infiltrative histiocytosis, meningioma, and intracranial hypotension.
  - MRI picture is often indistinguishable from these mimickers [151, 159, 160].

4.10.6 Hypothalamic/Pituitary Infiltration

- A part of parenchymal disease.
- 2–9% of patients with neurosarcoidosis.
- 10–25% of patients with brain parenchymal involvement.
- Frequently associated with hypopituitarism or syndrome of inappropriate antidiuretic hormone secretion (SIADH) (10–25%).
- Thickening and contrast enhancement of pituitary gland or stalk sometimes with extension into the hypothalamus.
- Needs to be distinguished IgG4-related disease, lymphocytic hypophysitis; granulomatous hypophysitis; xanthomatous hypophysitis, syphilis; tuberculosis, granulomatosis with polyangiitis, adenoma, germinoma, craniopharyngioma, Rathke cleft cyst, or infiltrative histiocytosis [151, 154, 159, 161, 162].

4.10.7 Brain Parenchymal Lesions

- 15–50% of patients with neurosarcoidosis.
- Caused by the spread of infiltration from the meninges (spread of leptomeningeal infiltration through perivascular spaces); brain tissue infiltration; focal vasculitis or venulitis; vascular compression from the infiltrate; or sinus thrombosis.
- Clinical manifestations usually include focal neurological deficit (5–10%), cognitive impairment, encephalopathy (5–10%), or seizures (14–15%).
- MRI features are nonspecific; most often MRI patterns include
- Small non-enhancing T2 lesions in periventricular and deep white matter
  - Most frequent type.
  - Usually iso-intense on T1-weighted images.
  - These lesions may be indistinguishable from lesions observed in MR or cerebral small vessel disease. They are prevalent even in older general population and patients with sarcoidosis but without clinical neurological complications, do not resolve with treatment, and do not correlate with neurological disability. Therefore, their link to neurosarcoidosis remains unclear.
- Enhancing mass lesions (6–37%)
  - Relatively common.
  - May abut dura matter and mimic meningioma (complication of the meningeal disease) or located in supra- or infratentorial white and gray matter (deep or cortical).
  - Frequently associated with nearby leptomeningeal involvement and are thought to represent the spread of leptomeningeal disease along the perivascular spaces.
  - May be large or diffuse and mistaken for neoplasms or tumefactive demyelination.
  - Although lesions are mostly hyperintense on T2, they may are also iso- or hypo-intense owing to high cellularity, similarly as seen in very cellular metastasis and CNS lymphoma.
  - T1 images usually show iso- or hypo-intense signal.

  - Sometime with persistent (>2 months), homogeneous, often punctate, or nodular contrast enhancement (6–37%)
  - Central necrosis, calcifications, or hemorrhages occur only rarely
  - Treatment may be sometimes associated with complete or near-complete resolution of the lesions
- Other potential brain/skull complications may include
  - Cystic or sclerotic skull (or other bones) involvement
  - Hydrocephalus due to leptomeningeal involvement (10%)
  - Rarely cavernous sinus or lacrimal gland involvement [151, 154, 159, 163]
- Needs to be distinguished mainly: ANCA-associated vasculitis, Behçet's disease, chronic lymphocytic inflammation with pontine perivascular enhancement responsive to steroids (CLIPPERS) (if affected the brainstem), CNS vasculitis, eosinophilic granulomatosis with polyangiitis, GFAP antibody-associated syndromes, granulomatosis with polyangiitis (GPA or Wegener's granulomatosis), histiocytosis, myelin oligodendrocyte glycoprotein antibody-associated disease (MOGAD), neoplasms (including CNS lymphoma), NMOSD, non-vasculitic vascular diseases, Sjögren's syndrome or tuberculosis [151, 152, 161].

4.10.8 Encephalopathy

- A part of parenchymal disease.
- Cognitive impairment; headache (32%); depression (60–66%) or other psychiatric manifestations including psychosis (20%) [151, 159, 164].

4.10.9 Vascular Disease

- A part of parenchymal disease.
- Ischemic and hemorrhagic stroke, cerebral small vessel disease (CSVD), embolism, atherosclerosisa, vasculitis and angioinvasive lymphoma are rare [151].

4.10.10 Myelopathy

- 19–26% of patients with neurosarcoidosis.
- Most often due to subpial intramedullary lesion.
- Typically, not an isolated or first manifestation of the neurosarcoidosis.
- Usually subacute onset; slowly progression.
- Frequently disabling.
- Mostly affects thoracic and less cervical spine, rarely conus or cauda equina.
- Typical nodular and linear leptomeningeal contrast enhancement (>50%) associated with intraparenchymal T2 hyperintensity, T1 hypo-intensity, and edema causing fusiform enlargements of the cord.
- Can be present bone marrow enhancement.
- Typically, dorsal column (subpial) ≥2 spinal segments and persistent (>2 months) enhancement despite of treatment.

- Often central canal contrast enhancement, which may together with the dorsal column enhancement resemble a trident on axial MRI (trident sign; 9%).
- Four main MRI patterns of neurosarcoidosis-associated myelitis:
  - Longitudinally extensive transverse myelitis (LETM) (45%)
  - Short tumefactive myelitis (23%)
  - Meningitis/meningoradiculitis (23%)
  - Anterior myelitis adjacent to disc degeneration (10%)
- Distinguished four stages of evolution of spinal cord lesions:
  - Phase 1: early inflammation with linear leptomeningeal enhancement along the spinal surface
  - Phase 2: centripetal spread of the leptomeningeal inflammatory process through the Virchow-Robin spaces into spinal cord parenchyma with faint enhancement and diffuse swelling
  - Phase 3: less prominent/absent swelling, focal or multiple enhancement
  - Phase 4: resolution of the inflammatory process and spinal cord atrophy
- Rarely occur calcifications, cyst formation, or extradural involvement.
- Extraspinal or extramedullary sarcoid granulomatous mass lesions are rare and cause compressive myelopathy.
- Difficult to diagnose, but spinal cord lesions with coexisting meningeal involvement with dural swelling and enhancement, may be a clue to neurosarcoidosis.
- Needs to be distinguished MS, NMOSD, GFAP antibody-associated syndromes, SLE, infectious diseases (such as tuberculosis, VZV, and HSV), non-inflammatory conditions (such as spondylotic myelopathy, metabolic diseases, or spinal dural AV fistulas) [151, 159, 165, 166] (Fig. 4.8).

4.10.11 Peripheral Involvement

- Peripheral neuropathy
  - Symptomatic neuropathy is rare (1–2% of patients with systemic disease).
  - Caused by direct granulomatous involvement of the nerve, by localized vasculitis or epineuriumand/or perineurinum involvement.
  - Polyneuropathy of large or small fibers, (poly)-radiculoneuropathy, mononeuritis multiplex, chronic inflammatory demyelinating polyradiculoneuropathy (CIDP), Guillain–Barre-like syndrome.
  - The most common type is symmetric axonal sensori-motor neuropathy.
  - Vast majority of patients (90%) have simultaneously subclinical muscle pathology. Hence, nerve and muscle biopsy should be performed together (for example, to distinguish from leprosy affecting only peripheral nerves but not muscles).
- Small-fiber neuropathy
  - Occurs often (30% of patients with systemic disease), normal conduction studies.

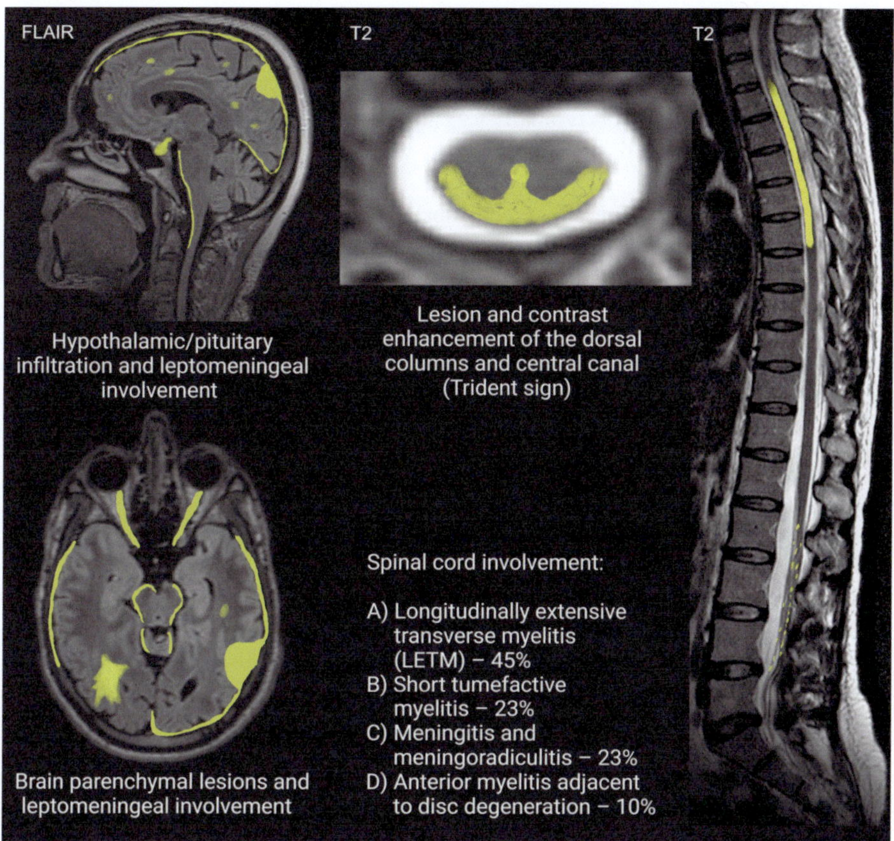

Fig. 4.8 MRI characteristics of neurosarcoidosis

  – Sensory loss, neuropathic pain, hyperhidrosis/hypohidrosis, cardiovascular dysautonomia, gastrointestinal dysmotility, sicca symptoms, and bladder and sexual dysfunction.
  – Probably only epiphenomenon (due to circulating inflammatory mediators) because there is no granulomatous involvement of the small fibers [151, 154, 159, 167].
- Myopathy
  – Asymptomatic (50–80%); symptomatic (only around 2%).
  – Acute, subacute, or chronic; relapsing or progressive disease course.
  – Needs to be distinguished mainly: inflammatory myositis (polymyositis/dermatomyositis, Sjögren's syndrome, rheumatoid arthritis, SLE, inclusion body myositis, and vasculitis), infectious myositis, and other myopathies (endocrine, toxic, metabolic, genetic) [151, 154, 159, 168].

4.10.12 Disease Course

- Relapsing-remitting or progressive.
- The onset of symptoms is typically less acute than in MS, NMOSD, or MOGAD.
- 75% of neurosarcoidosis cases manifest within 2 years following the onset of systemic sarcoidosis.
- 50–70% of patients experience the onset of neurosarcoidosis without exhibiting symptoms of systemic sarcoidosis.
- The mean age of symptoms onset is around 43 years [151, 159].

4.10.13 Blood Work

- There is no sensitive or specific test for sarcoidosis.
- May be elevated levels of acute-phase reactants.
- Sometime present increased concentration of vitamin D and calcium.
- Increase level of serum angiotensin-converting enzyme (ACE) present in only 60% of patients with pulmonary sarcoidosis and has low sensitivity (62%) and specificity (76%) for diagnosis of sarcoidosis [151].
- Serum chitotriosidase levels are elevated in patients with sarcoidosis, and they correlate with disease activity, severity, and multi-organ dissemination. Treatment with corticosteroids helps decrease its levels. Chitotriosidase is an enzyme produced by activated macrophages, and its levels can also be elevated in other conditions involving macrophage activation, such as Gaucher disease and certain infections. Therefore, although chitotriosidase levels can be helpful in supporting a diagnosis of sarcoidosis, they are not typically used as a standalone diagnostic test. Instead, they are often used in combination with other clinical and laboratory findings to aid in the diagnosis and monitoring of sarcoidosis. It is utilized in clinical practice to identify patients with active progression, detect relapses, and assess the effectiveness of treatment [169].
- Increased level of soluble interleukin 2 (IL-2) receptor has 88% sensitivity and 85% specificity for diagnosis [170].

4.10.14 Examination of CSF

- Frequently nonspecific abnormal findings (50–80%).
- CSF opening pressure may be elevated.
- Decreased glucose level is frequent, although it can also occur in bacterial, fungal, and mycobacterial infections, as well as malignancies.
- Elevated concentration of protein (sometime very high).
- Mild-to-moderate pleocytosis (usually <100 cells/mm^3); predominantly comprising lymphocytes; however, neutrophils may also be present during the acute phase; eosinophils are rare.
- Increased IgG index and/or CSF-restricted OCB (20–40%).

- CSF-restricted OCB (9–20%).
- Compared to MS, patients with neurosarcoidosis show more often increased albumin quotient (Qalb), elevated CSF lactate, and higher serum and CSF levels of soluble IL-2 receptor, but a lower frequency of intrathecal IgG synthesis and positive Measles-Rubella-Zoster (MRZ) reaction.
- ACE level in CSF has poor sensitivity and specificity for diagnosis.
- Increased CD4/CD8 ratio and IL-6 level [151, 153, 154, 166, 171, 172].

4.10.15 Diagnosis

- Diagnosing neurosarcoidosis might be challenging.
- If neurosarcoidosis is suspected, it is crucial to investigate for evidence of systemic sarcoidosis by conducting a physical examination, a dilated eye examination, a chest X-ray (abnormal in 50%), and laboratory tests [151].
- Additionally, whole-body contrast CT or 18-fludeoxyglucose positron emission tomography (FDG-PET) scans can be utilized to identify active lymph nodes and guide biopsy site. An active lesion on FDG-PET outside the CNS is detected in 22% of the patients with suspected neurosarcoidosis, thus providing potential biopsy site [173].
- Gallium scintigraphy may be used, if FDG-PET-CT is not available [154].
- Sarcoidosis is a pathologic diagnosis that primarily relies on biopsy due to the unspecific clinical and imaging presentation [151].
- However, biopsy is not always feasible in neurosarcoidosis because of the risk of permanent neurologic deficits induced by the procedure [154].
- Diagnostic criteria 2018 categorize patients into definite, probable, and possible neurosarcoidosis based on pathologic and clinical features [174].

4.10.16 Differential Diagnosis

- Because of variable phenotypes, neurosarcoidosis can mimic a number of neoplasms and infections and is called the great mimic [154].
- Biopsy, preferably of a lymph node, lesion, skin, or nerve, is recommended for definitive diagnosis and to differentiate from conditions such as granulomatous infections; sarcoid-like reactions to lymphomas or other malignancies or medications; tuberculosis; viral infections such as HIV; multisystem granulomatous syndromes (as seen in common variable immunodeficiency disease [CVID] or other immunodeficiency syndromes); and disease related to IgG4 [151].
- Patients with sarcoidosis presenting with neurological manifestations are typically diagnosed with neurosarcoidosis. However, when MRI reveals multiple "MS-typical lesions" without the presence of "neurosarcoidosis-typical lesions," the diagnosis of MS is favored. Although rare, the coexistence of systemic sarcoidosis and MS can occur. In such cases, close follow-up is essential to monitor disease progression and confirm the diagnosis of MS. The clinical and imaging presentations of neurosarcoidosis and MS often exhibit distinct characteristics.

In cases where the diagnosis is unclear, treatment options that are safe and effective for both conditions, such as corticosteroids, methotrexate, azathioprine, or cyclophosphamide, should be considered [175].

4.10.17 Treatment and Prognosis

- Corticosteroids, methotrexate, azathioprine, cyclophosphamide.
- TNF-alpha inhibitors (infliximab, adalimumab, etanercept); often combined with low-dose cytotoxic immunosuppressants such as methotrexate or azathioprine. Treatments for sarcoidosis such as TNF-alpha inhibitors may exacerbate MS.
- Anti-CD20 therapy, only case reports, probably not very effective.
- Anti-IL-6 therapy (tocilizumab) and Janus kinase (JAK) inhibitor (tofacitinib); only case reports.
- The absence of response to immunosuppressive treatment requires a reconsideration of the diagnosis.
- Important to recognize that clinical response might lag the MRI response, and treatment effect may become apparent only after several months of treatment.
- Neurologic involvement is associated with increased mortality [150, 153].
- Prognosis is highly variable with complete remission (27%), incomplete remission (32%), stable disease (24%), or deterioration (6%).
- Despite the increased utilization of new therapies, one-third of the patients experience stability, deterioration, or mortality (5%).
- Approximately 71% of patients have residual symptoms, and 29% functional impairment [152, 159, 171].

4.11 Sjogren's Syndrome

4.11.1 Synonyms

- Keratitis filamentosa

4.11.2 Epidemiology

- Prevalence 22–770/100.000.
- Incidence 3.5–3.9/100.000/years [176–179].
- In Europe is a prevalence 15 times higher than that in Asia.
- Female/male ratio 9–11/1.
- Highest incidence in middle-aged (50 years) post-menopausal females.
- Sjögren's syndrome (SjS) is frequently associated with other coexisting autoimmune diseases [176, 177].

4.11.3 Etiology and Definition

- Primary SjS is a systemic autoimmune disease characterized primary by chronic inflammation with periductal lymphocytic infiltrates of the exocrine glands, although SjS can affect any organ system.
- The precise etiology of SjS remains unknown, but one hypothesis suggests that the activation of mucosal epithelial cells, potentially triggered by viral stimulation (such as Epstein–Barr virus [EBV], human T-cell lymphotropic virus type I [HTVL-1], hepatitis C virus [HCV], or coxsackievirus), may initiate the activation of the innate and adaptive immune systems. This activation subsequently leads to the secretion of autoantibodies. These autoantibodies form immune complexes that perpetuate and intensify a cycle of immune system activation, ultimately resulting in tissue damage.
- Extra-glandular (extraepithelial) lymphocytic infiltration and complex deposition in organs, resulting from B-cell hyper-reactivity, can cause interstitial nephritis, primary biliary cholangitis, obstructive bronchiolitis, purpura, pneumonitis, cryoglobulinemia-associated glomerulonephritis, or peripheral neuropathy.
- Extra-glandular features of SjS are similar to those of SLE with the vasculitic features that are mediated by immune complexes and complement. However, in SjS, there is an increased frequency of lymphocytic infiltration into extra-glandular tissues, which is associated with a higher incidence of lymphoma compared to patients with SLE. There are similarities between primary SjS and SLE, suggesting that primary SjS may be a manifestation of SLE affecting the mucosal tissues [180, 181].

4.11.4 Subtypes

- Primary SjS
  - When it occurs alone or in association with organ-specific autoimmune disease, such as thyroiditis, primary biliary cirrhosis, or cholangitis [182].
- Secondary (or associated) SjS
  - When it occurs with other systemic autoimmune disease such as RA (26–31%), SLE (7–19%), systemic sclerosis (14–21%), scleroderma, dermatomyositis, and others [178, 182].

4.11.5 Glandular Features

- Dry eye/xerophthalmia (92.4%).
- Dry mouth/xerostomia (93.7%).
- Abnormal ocular tests (83%).
- Positive minor salivary gland biopsy (81.6%).
- Abnormal oral diagnostic tests (78%).
- Palpable parotid, submandibular, or lacrimal swelling (25%).

4.11.6 Extra-glandular Systemic Features

- Present in around 75% of patients.
- Arthralgias with morning stiffness or synovitis (41%).
- Raynaud syndrome (15%).
- Chronic bronchitis, bronchiolitis, interstitial lung disease, pleuritis, or pulmonary arterial hypertension (12–13%).
- Systemic symptoms such as fever, weight loss, or night sweats (10%).
- Renal manifestations such as interstitial nephritis or cryoglobulinemia-associated glomerulonephritis (5%).
- Benign lymphadenopathy or lymphoma (11%).
- Skin manifestations such as purpura, vasculitis, subacute cutaneous lupus, paniculitis, erythema nodosum, granuloma annulare, or amyloidosis (10–11%).
- Other rare (non-EULAR Sjögren's syndrome disease activity index [ESSDAI]) systemic features include acute pancreatitis (0.6%), dysphagia (2.7%), chronic gastritis (3.1%), pleuritis (1.6%), laryngitis (0.2%), sinusitis (0.5%), interstitial cystitis (0.7%), uveitis (0.9%), episcleritis (0.6%), orbital pseudotumor (0.2%), pericarditis (0.7%), heart valve disorders (0.5%), pulmonary hypertension, or myocarditis [180, 183].
- Three major features (dryness of the mouth and eyes, fatigue, and joint pain) are present vast majority of patients (>80%).
- Especially, fatigue is most disabling symptom [182].

4.11.7 Neurological Features

- Present in around 10–20% of patients.
- Usually occur together with other extra-glandular manifestations of SjS.
- Neurological complications manifest more frequently in patients who are already diagnosed with SjS (60–70%) [177, 184].
- However, in a considerable proportion of patients (30–40%), neurological complications precede the diagnosis of SjS by up to 2 years (mean 26; range 6–81 months) [184, 185]. This is particularly true for rare complications involving the CNS (2.6–3.6%), which commonly precede the diagnosis of SjS (52–80%).
- CNS involvement include wide range of presentations such as brain vasculitis, transverse myelitis, demyelinating lesions, rest-leg syndrome, hearing loss, meningitis, meningo-encephalitis, encephalitis, optic neuropathy, PRES, MS-like disease, stroke, seizures, movement disorders (chorea, dystonia, intention tremor, L-dopa-resistant parkinsonism, athetosis), internuclear ophthalmoplegia, nystagmus, spastic tetraparesis or cerebellar symptoms and reflect the localization of the focal CNS vasculitis (cryoglobulinaemia-related or not) [186–189].
- CNS focal/multifocal involvement
  - MS-like or NMOSD-like manifestations

    - Optic neuritis is rare, which may occur as the result of either demyelination or ischemic vasculitis. Can be bilateral, severe and in sometimes the first symptom of SjS.
    - Subacute transverse myelitis, most often longitudinally extensive transverse myelitis (LETM) is relatively rare [187].
    - Optic neuritis and myelitis may exhibit relapsing-remitting pattern; a high relapse rate; poor response to corticosteroids; and imaging features typical of NMOSD. Many of these patients meet diagnostic criteria for NMOSD and test positive for anti-aquaporin-4 (AQP4) IgG. These patients have likely a comorbid NMOSD rather than a neurological complication of SjS [190].
    - The prevalence of SjS is higher among individuals who test positive for anti-AQP4 IgG compared to those who test negative. Comorbid SjS and NMOSD are more common in females and are associated with a higher relapse rate, although not with a higher Expanded Disability Status Scale (EDSS) score [191].
    - Similarly, patients who meet the diagnostic criteria for MS can be diagnosed with MS and SjS. Distinguishing between MS-like complications and MS in some patients can pose a challenge, and the relationship between SjS and MS remains a subject of ongoing debate [189].
      - Stroke (rare)
      - Amyotrophic lateral sclerosis (ALS)-like symptoms (rare)
- CNS diffuse involvement
  - Cognitive dysfunction (from mild to dementia) (80%) [192]
  - Psychiatric symptoms
  - Aseptic meningo-encephalitis
    - Relatively common, associated with inflammation of meningeal vessels. Clinical manifestations include headache, meningeal signs, flu-like symptoms, focal neurological deficit, seizures, cranial neuropathy or cerebellar syndrome [186].
- Peripheral involvement
  - In 6.8–16.1% of patients (some studies reported prevalence of 59%).
  - Pure sensory axonal polyneuropathy (most often), sensori-motor neuropathy, neuronopathy, cranial nerve involvement, ataxic ganglionopathy, vasculitis (mononeuritis multiplex), poly-radiculo-neuropathy, CIDP, and small-fiber neuropathy.
  - Myositis with pain or weakness (2%).
  - Different mechanisms may be responsible for peripheral nervous system involvement including vasculitis of the vasa nervorum, lymphocytic infiltration of the dorsal ganglia, necrotizing vasculitis, or anti-neuronal antibodies [177, 183, 186, 193].
- Autonomic involvement
  - Rare (0.4%)
  - May include Adie's pupils, anhidrosis, arrhythmia, bowel/bladder, and GIT dysfunction or orthostatic hypotension [177, 183, 186, 193].

4.11.8 Disease Course of Neurological Manifestations

- Chronic progressive or relapsing-remitting.
- The symptoms' onset is insidious or acute (stroke-like) [187].

4.11.9 Brain Imaging

- Although some studies have reported an increased prevalence of nonspecific T2 hyperintense lesions in the white matter (usually asymptomatic) [194], other studies have not confirmed this finding [195].
- Brain lesions likely consist of a group of pathologies of heterogeneous origin and reflect either inflammatory demyelination or ischemic lesions due to vasculitis [194].
- Some patients with SjS exhibit MS-like lesions in the brain [186], and a considerable number of them meet the diagnostic criteria for MS [188].
- However, patients with SjS typically
  - Do not have lesions of corpus callosum.
  - Lesions are preferentialy located in cortical, juxtacortical, and deep white matter but not periventriculary [196].
  - Central vein sign (CVS) is infrequent compared to MS (11% versus 88%) [11].

4.11.10 Spinal Cord Imaging

- Cord lesions, when present, are often located in regions atypical for MS
  - Central (44.4%)—atypical for MS
  - Peripheral (37%)—typical for MS
  - LETM (31.3%)—atypical for MS
  - Dorsal (18.5%)—typical for MS [197]

4.11.11 Ultrasonography

- Ultrasonography of the major salivary glands, including the parotid and submandibular glands, can reveal hypoechoic or anechoic regions, aiding in diagnosis and ongoing monitoring. It has not been yet incorporated into diagnostic criteria [197].

4.11.12 Blood Work

- Patients with primary SjS often have positive various antibodies (listed below). In secondary SjS, their prevalence varies according to the underlying autoimmune condition.
- Anti-Sjögren's syndrome antigen B (SSB)/La (50–75%)
  - In MS, rarely positive (1–2%).

- Anti-Sjögren's syndrome antigen A (SSA)/Ro (73%)
  - In MS, rarely positive (3–13%).
  - Anti-SSB/Ro and Anti-SSB/La are typically positive together [183, 198, 199].
  - Positive testing may occur years prior to symptoms onset; therefore, close follow-up is necessary for the positive asymptomatic patients [200].
  - Some NMOSD patients test positive for anti-SSA or anti-SSB antibodies (7.7–12%), among whom a proportion have comorbid SjS [201, 202].
- Rheumatoid factor (50%)
  - In MS, rarely positive (1–2%).
  - Although rheumatoid factor and anti-SSB antibodies are not included in the classification criteria, they are considered as key markers of the disease.
- Anti-double stranded deoxyribonucleic acid (dsDNA) antibodies are important in the diagnosis of SLE, but they are typically absent in SjS.
- Anti-ANA are more frequently positive (80%) than in MS (18–33%).
- Occasionally, present decreased levels of C3 (13.4%) and C4 (14.6%) complement components, which are normal or slightly increased in MS.
- High levels of cryoglobulins (7%) [180, 183, 199, 203].
- Elevated erythrocyte sedimentation rate (60%), which is not seen in MS [189].
- Anti-phospholipid antibodies (<13%)
  - Diagnostic criteria for antiphospholipid syndrome are fulfilled only rarely (1.4%).
  - May be positive also in MS (6–21%) and healthy controls (1–9%) [199, 204].

4.11.13 Examination of CSF

- Only some patients exhibit an inflammatory pattern in CSF, and its presence and extent are independent of whether the peripheral or central nervous system is affected.
- Mildly elevated concentration of protein and albumin quotient (30%)
- Cytology is normal or presents mild pleocytosis (8–107 cells/μL) (14%)
- OCB
  - Absent (42%) (pattern I)
  - CSF-restricted OCB (17%) (pattern II)
  - Combination of CSF-restricted and corresponding OCB (8%) (pattern III)
  - Corresponding serum and CSF OCB IgG in 33% (pattern IV)
- Patients with secondary SjS associated with other systemic autoimmune diseases have a higher rate of inflammatory changes in CSF and a more prevalent presence of CSF-restricted OCB (71%) [205].

4.11.14 OCT

- Abnormally reduced retinal nerve fiber layer (RNFL) and macular ganglion cell inner plexiform layer (GCIPL) thicknesses are common, associated with visual loss, and may indicate the severity of xerophthalmia. They also correlate with levels of anti-SSB antibodies [206].

4.11.15 Electrophysiology

- Abnormal findings on VEP are frequent (83%) in patients with primary SjS and CNS involvement who meet the criteria for MS [207].

4.11.16 Diagnosis

- Established in patients with a score of 4 or more (maximum score is 9) according to the 2017 American Congress of Rheumatology/European League Against Rheumatism (ACR-EULAR) Classification Criteria for Primary SjS.
- The criteria can be applied only to patients who have at least one symptom of ocular or oral dryness or the systemic manifestations suggestive of primary SjS.
- However, these criteria cannot be applied in patients with active HCV infection, after radiotherapy of the cervical spine, sarcoidosis, graft-versus-host disease, receipt of anticholinergic drugs, and disease associated with IgG4 [208].
  A. Focus score of ≥1 in biopsy (three points)
    - At least one mononuclear-cell infiltrate containing ≥50 inflammatory cells per 4 mm^2 of minor labial salivary gland.
    - A biopsy of minor salivary glands is usually performed in patients suspected of having SjS, but with absent anti-SSA antibodies, which are negative in 25% of SjS patients.

  B. Presence of anti-SSB and anti-SSA antibodies in serum (3 points):
    - Isolated positivity of only anti-SSB in the absence of anti-SSA antibodies is unspecific and is not considered to be a criterion for the diagnosis.
    - In the case of anti-SSA/Ro, only anti-Ro60 should be considered because anti-Ro52 is unspecific for SjS.
    - Although anti-SSA/Ro antibodies are unspecific for SjS, anti-SSB/La antibodies seem to be more specific.

  C. Sjögren's International Collaborative Clinical Alliance (SICCA) ocular staining score of ≥5 (one point)
    - An ophthalmologist performs examination with fluorescein and lissamine green staining. Score ranges from 0 to 12.

  D. Schirmer test of ≤5 mm per 5 min (one point)
    - A measurement of tear production by inserting filter paper on the conjunctiva in the lower eyelid and assessing the amount of moisture.

  E. Unstimulated whole salivary flow of ≤0.1 mL per minute (1 point)
    - A measurement of the rate of salivary flow by collecting saliva in a tube for at least 5 min after the patient has swallowed.
- The EULAR SjS Disease Activity Index (ESSDAI) assesses systemic complications in 12 domains and is used only in clinical trials [209].
- Younger patients have a lower frequency of sicca syndrome and positive salivary gland biopsy, but a higher frequency of activity in the constitutional, cutaneous, and laboratory features of SjS [203].
- SjS patients with neurological manifestations have less frequent signs of glandular disease and are more often seropositive for anti-SSA/Ro antibodies compared to patients without neurological involvement [188].

4.11.17 Differential Diagnosis

- General
  - Since symptoms such as dry mouth or eyes, limb pain, and fatigue are very common and nonspecific, early diagnosis of SjS can be challenging. The presence of systemic complications may prompt clinicians to consider SjS in the differential diagnosis [208].
  - ANA are the most encountered autoantibodies in primary SjS. A positive ANA result in a patient presenting with sicca features should raise suspicion for SjS and prompt further evaluation to confirm or exclude the diagnosis [203].
  - Sometimes a clear distinction between MS, primary SjS, and SLE patients can be difficult because clinical and laboratory features and MRI lesions may be indistinguishable.
  - For differential diagnosis, it is important to note that despite sicca symptoms are often rare at the beginning, almost all patients with SjS and CNS involvement have serological and histological evidence of an inflammatory affection of salivary glands typical of SjS [188].
  - Patients diagnosed with SjS should undergo regular screening for neurological status [188].
- MS
  - SjS similarly to other rheumatological diseases are often challenging in the differential diagnosis of demyelinating disorders of CNS, especially in patients with first symptoms of SjS being demyelinating event. In these patients, the diagnosis of SjS was delayed by 2–5 years [187, 188]. Many of these patients were initially diagnoses with MS. However, older age, progressive phenotype, systemic symptoms, a positive Schirmer's test, and elevated levels of ANA or anti-SSB/A antibodies resulted in further examination and diagnosis of SjS 188).
  - In a study involving 440 MS patients, the investigation for SjS diagnosis yielded positive results in 0.91% of the patients [210]; however, another study of 439 MS patients reported comorbid SjS in a much higher proportion of patients (10.9%) [276].
  - Other review study suggested that the overall prevalence of primary SjS among MS patients is generally low, ranging from 0% to 3.3%, a prevalence comparable to that observed in the general population [189].
  - It is worth noting that a significant number of MS patients exhibit symptoms of sicca syndrome, yet they do not meet the criteria for a diagnosis of SjS. These symptoms may be often attributed to medication side effects, comorbidities, or autonomic dysfunction [210, 211].
  - In contrast, some authors recommend performing a Schirmer's test in patients with a phenotype compatible with SjS and MS, primary progressive phenotype, or suspected diagnosis of MS refractory to treatment, testing for serum anti-SSA/B antibodies, and salivary gland biopsy, because there is no other separating biomarker. This should be considered especially in patients who develop sicca symptoms or signs of systemic disease [188, 189].

  - Rheumatologic autoantibodies (ANA, SSA/B, rheumatoid factor, anticardiolipin antibodies, or lupus anticoagulant) are frequently found in MS patients and are not associated with disease severity or systemic rheumatologic diseases. Therefore, these tests should be performed only in suspected cases [199].
- NMOSD
  - The prevalence of SjS in anti-aquaporin-4 (AQP4) IgG-positive NMOSD is relatively high (2–20%). This prevalence is notably higher compared to anti-AQP4 IgG-negative NMOSD patients.
  - Anti-AQP4 positive patients with comorbid SjS are more frequently females, have more often positive OCB, and a greater relapse rate compared to AQP4-positive patients without comorbid SjS [191].
  - Among cases of coexisting NMOSD and SjS, the diagnosis of NMOSD preceded that of primary SjS in 50% of cases, with a median interval of 3.5 years. Notably, only 50–60% of patients with both conditions exhibited sicca syndrome, which is less frequent compared to SjS patients without neurological involvement [212].
  - In some patients, it may be unclear whether they suffer from coexisting SjS and MS or NMOSD, or if they have neurological complications of SjS [188].

4.11.18 Treatment

- Muscarinic agonists for the treatment of oral and to lesser extent ocular dryness.
- Hydroxychloroquine may be used for arthralgia.
- The heterogeneity of the disease phenotypes and treatment responses suggests that a more individualized approach to therapy is required to improve better outcomes in patients with SjS.
- Corticosteroids and immunosuppressants used in accordance with guidelines for SLE and other connective tissue diseases [180, 213].
- Extra-glandular manifestations of SjS, including those in CNS, are treated usually with cyclophosphamide or rituximab in combination with corticosteroids.
- The majority of disease-modifying drugs used in MS are ineffective in patients with SjS and CNS involvement [188].
- The disease progression in SjS patients presenting with myelopathy, whether meeting the criteria for NMOSD or not appears comparable. Hence, individuals with SjS-associated myelopathy warrant aggressive treatment akin to that employed for NMOSD patients [190].

4.11.19 Prognosis

- In general, primary SjS is not associated with an increase mortality, but a small proportion of patients may have a severe extra-glandular involvement such as vasculitis, hypocomplementaemia, or cryoglobulinaemia and be at increased risk of mortality [214].

- Cryoglobulinaemia, low complement fractions, higher number of inflammatory infiltrates in the salivary gland biopsy, and male sex predict neurological involvement and more severe disease course [180, 215].
- Patients with primary SjS have an increased risk of B-cell lymphoma (by a factor of 15 to 44), as compared with the general population [178, 180].

4.12 Susac's Syndrome

4.12.1 Synonyms

- Retinocochleocerebral vasculopathy; small infarctions of cochlear, retinal, and encephalic tissue (SICRET) syndrome [216].

4.12.2 Epidemiology

- Prevalence 0.14/100.000 (Europe); probably underestimated.
- Female/male ratio 3.5/1 [217–219].

4.12.3 Etiology and Definition

- Susac's syndrome (SuS) is considered as an autoimmune inflammation affecting small arterial vessels with occlusive microangiopathy and endotheliopathy. The vasculitis in the SuS affects the brain, inner ear, and retina. The etiology and mechanism remain unknown [220].
- Brain biopsy shows microinfarcts; thickened hyalinized vessel walls; collagen deposition; CD8+ infiltrates; perivascular lymphocytic cuffing in the leptomeninges; enlarged and reactive endothelial cells leading to near occlusion of the vessels [221].

4.12.4 Clinical Features

- Typical triad includes encephalopathy with headache, sensorineural hearing loss, and multiple recurrent branch retinal arterial occlusions (BRAO).
- SuS can be easily distinguished from MS when all typical features of the syndrome are present. However, the clinical triad is often incomplete (only 13–15% at disease onset and >85% after months). On average, the completion of the triad typically takes around 5 months. However, in some patients, it may extend over years, resulting in delays in diagnosis [216, 217, 222].
- Encephalopathy (70–75%).
  - The most common manifestation [217]

  - If not present within the 2 years from disease onset, it is unlikely to develop in the future.
  - Develop acutely (stroke-like) or subacutely.
  - Vertigo, ataxia, gait disorder, sensory symptoms (25%)
  - Upper motor neuron syndrome (20%)
  - Affective disorders, behavioral changes, psychosis, apathy, somnolence, or coma may prevent patients from reporting hearing and visual symptoms.
  - Other rare symptoms include sphincter symptoms, dysarthria, nausea and vomiting, seizures, or diplopia.
  - Progressive cognitive decline may result in dementia [217, 220, 223, 224]
- Headache (60–80%)
  - May be severe, associated with nausea and vomiting, and undistinguishable from migraine or tension headache.
  - Usually responds to analgesics.
  - All patients with new-onset migraine with visual symptoms and the corpus callosum lesions should have an ophthalmological review and audiometry to exclude SuS [217, 223–225].
- Vestibulocochlear symptoms (60–80% at disease onset).
  - Caused by arteriolar microinfarctions of the cochlear apex and vestibular labyrinth.
  - Roaring tinnitus and vertigo with nystagmus are frequently associated with hearing loss or may precede it.
  - Hearing loss is acute or subacute, unilateral, or bilateral, simultaneous, or sequential, steady or fluctuating. Usually sensorineural, low, or mid-tone frequencies and pantonal. Over time may include also high frequencies, may become severe, and require cochlear implantation.
  - Hearing loss and tinnitus are atypical symptoms of MS, which can aid in the differential diagnosis from SuS. Audiometry may appear normal when the cause is cortical pathology associated with MS. Conversely, brainstem auditory evoked potentials (BAEP) are often abnormal in MS but normal in SuS. Once hearing loss and tinnitus occur, they often become permanent [216, 217, 220, 225].
- Eye symptoms (40–50% at disease onset)
  - They can be sole symptoms of SuS.
  - Occasionally, retinal occlusions may be asymptomatic, and ophthalmological examination is necessary to confirm ocular involvement.
  - Patients complain about photopsias, scintillating scotomas, visual field defects, decreased visual acuity, or any other visual deficits.
  - BRAO is rarely observed in other diseases and can aid in distinguishing SuS from other diagnoses. Fluorescein angiogram may show multiple BRAO with non-filling of retinal vessels and typical hyperfluorescence of the arterial vessel walls. These findings may be absent in the very early stages but can develop later, making repeat imaging necessary. Conversely, they often resolve in more chronic stages of the disease.
  - The presence of arteriolar wall hyperfluorescence indicates compromised integrity of the retinal vessel wall. It serves as a marker of disease activity. It

is typically not observed in other retinal vasculitides and requires differentiation from fluorescein leakage. In more chronic stages, arteriolar wall hyperfluorescence often resolves and may no longer be detectable [223, 226, 227].
  - The eye involvement in SuS is well recognized in uveitis referral centers but is often missed by general ophthalmologists [227].
  - In suspected cases, fluorescein angiography should be performed, even in patients without visual symptoms or when fundoscopy yields normal results [224].
- Systemic manifestations
  - Skin involvement such as livedo reticularis or livedo racemosa (5%).
  - Arthralgias and symptomatic or asymptomatic myopathy [217, 223].

4.12.5 Disease Course

- Age of symptoms onset is between 20 and 40 years (range, 2.5–72) [217]
- There are three subtypes of disease course
  - Monophasic (54%): typically presenting with encephalopathy; often limited to 1–2 years; has relatively good prognosis, if treated early.
  - Polyphasic (42%): recurrent BRAO and hearing loss relapses without encephalopathy but with brain MRI changes. The time between relapses can be even many years.
  - Chronic progressive (4%): fluctuating progression of disease without remissions; most severe and potentially fatal phenotype [217, 228].

4.12.6 Brain Imaging

- Lesions' location and appearance
  - T2 lesions "snowball lesions," in the corpus callosum (78%).
  - Involvement of central fibers of callosal body (between the ventricular surface and superior aspect of the corpus callosum) and splenium with sparing of periphery (e.g., lateral portions of corpus callosum) is pathognomonic for SuS.
  - Radial "icicle" or "spoke" lesions arising from the roof of the callosum, and "string of pearls" appearance of punctate microinfarcts in the internal capsule may be present.
  - Lesions in the corpus callosum may exhibit a hypo-intense correlate on T1-weighted images in chronic stages, described as "punched out holes."
  - On the contrary, involvement of the callososeptal interface is characteristic of MS or, to a lesser extent, ischemia, and it can aid in the differential diagnosis from SuS. Involvement of corpus callosum may help to distinguish SuS from cerebral vasculitis, which does not typically affect corpus callosum.
  - Additionally, often present multi-focal, rounded, small (3–7 mm) T2 hyperintense lesions in perivetricular and subcortical white matter, deep gray metter, cerebellum, or pons (70–100%) (Fig. 4.9).
  - May be present restricted diffusion of lesions.

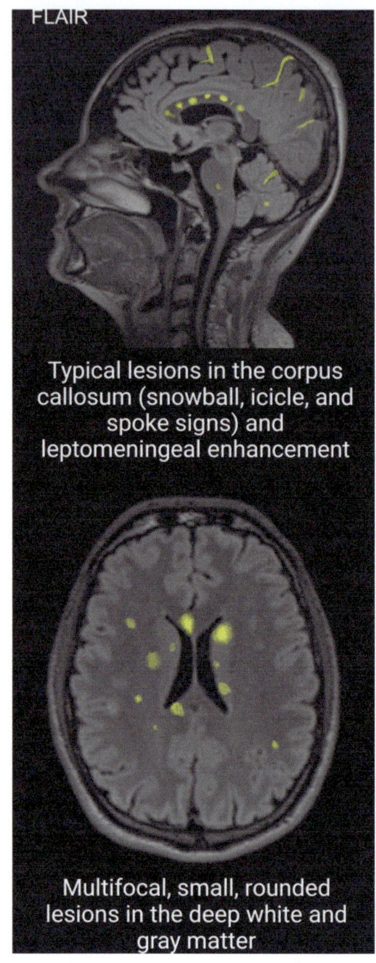

Fig. 4.9 MRI characteristics of Susac's syndrome

- Contrast enhancement
  - Frequently present during acute relapses (50%).
  - Leptomeningeal enhancement (20–40%) is usually not observed in MS or acute disseminated encephalomyelitis (ADEM) and may support the diagnosis of SuS.
- Evolution over time
  - The punctate lesions can fully resolve [216, 217, 225, 228, 229].

4.12.7 Spinal Cord Imaging

- The case study reported a patient with SuS exhibiting spinal cord lesions located paracentrally and laterally [230].

4.12.8 Blood Work

- Normal

4.12.9 Examination of CSF

- Often disrupted blood-brain barrier with markedly elevated concentration of protein (mean 1.6–1.8 g/L).
- Mild pleocytosis (median cell count of 12 cells/μL) (45%).
- CSF-restricted OCB (4–15%).
- CSF analysis primarily focuses on excluding alternative diagnoses [216, 217, 222, 225].

4.12.10 OCT

- 68% of eyes show reduced retinal nerve fiber layer (RNFL) thickness.
- Detects retinal involvement, which is important especially in later disease stages, when BRAO and arteriolar wall hyperfluorescence might not be detectable [231].

4.12.11 Histology

- Brain, muscle, and skin biopsies are unspecific and rather help to exclude other diseases. The diagnosis can be established with less-invasive techniques, and biopsy findings might not be helpful, thus leading to false-negative results [216].

4.12.12 Diagnosis

- Diagnostic criteria were proposed in 2016 [216]
- For definite diagnosis of SuS each of the following criterions (1; 2; 3) with subcriteria (a; b) must be met.

1. Brain involvement
   A. Clinical: New cognitive impairment, behavioral changes, focal neurological symptoms, or headache (headache must be a new symptom, must precede the other symptoms by less than 6 months, and must be described as migrainous or oppressive, not as a trigemino-autonomous headache).
   B. Brain MRI: hyperintense, multifocal, round small T2 lesions, ≥1 of them in the corpus callosum ("snowball")
   – To fulfil point 1, a patient must have ≥1 clinical feature and typical MRI.
2. Retinal involvement

- Clinical signs and symptoms are not required (retinal involvement can be asymptomatic).
- Ophthalmological examination shows
  A. ≥1 BRAO in fluorescein angiography or fundoscopy.
  B. Arterial wall hyperfluorescence with focal segmental staining of the arterial wall near the site of obstruction, or
  C. Characteristic signs of retinal branch ischemia in fundoscopy, or
  D. OCT with sectorial damage of the inner retinal layers from the RNFL through to the outer plexiform layer.
     – To fulfil point 2, at least ≥1 ophthalmological feature (from 4) needs to be present.
     – Visual field deficits or scintillating scotoma may support the diagnosis and help with differential diagnosis but are not sufficient to fulfil the diagnostic criteria for retinal involvement.

- Vestibulocochlear involvement, particularly at disease onset, may be asymptomatic, or the symptoms may be subtle or intermittent, which can complicate the diagnosis.
  A. Clinical: new tinnitus, hearing loss, or peripheral vertigo.
  B. Examination of inner ear function shows hearing loss confirmed by an audiogram (pure-tone or speech audiogram, favorably for low or mid-tone frequencies), or vestibular vertigo confirmed by objective examinations such (caloric testing of the vestibular organ, nystagmography, and/or vestibular evoked myogenic responses).
     – To fulfil point 3, at least ≥1 of the objective clinical findings needs to be present.
  - Probable SuS is diagnosed in patients with incomplete triad, when only 2 of the three (1–3) criteria are fulfilled (for example, patient with headache, typical MRI, objective hearing loss, but without ophthalmological involvement). These patients should be closely monitored.
  - Possible SuS is diagnosed in patients showing some clinical or paraclinical findings typical of SuS.
  - Clinical features without typical MRI pathology or vice versa, typical MR features without clinical manifestations are not sufficient for the diagnosis of SuS.
  - The application of diagnostic criteria assists making the decision whether to treat the patient aggressively or to rather wait and monitor [216].

4.12.13 Differential Diagnosis

- In patients with typical triad and MRI features, diagnosis of SuS is not difficult to establish. However, at early disease stages, the triad is only sometimes complete [217], making an early diagnosis challenging. Therefore, misdiagnosis or delayed diagnosis occurs often. Median diagnostic delay is 3–7 months, but in some patients, it reaches many years [217, 225].

- Patients with visual and vestibulocochlear symptoms have greater diagnostic delay [225]. Delay in treatment initiation may be associated with relapses, disease progression, and irreversible organs damage [216, 232].
- MS, migraine, cerebrovascular diseases such as cerebral vasculitis, and stroke are the most common misdiagnoses of Susac's syndrome [219, 225].
- In contrast to MS, Uhthoff and Lhermitte's phenomena are absent, and neurological symptoms are less likely to spontaneously remit [224].
- Other SuS mimics represent ADEM, Meniere's disease, CNS vasculitis, retinal vasculitis with or without systemic disease, adult-onset leukoencephalopathy with axonal spheroids and pigmented glia (ALSP), microembolic stroke, histoplasmosis, viral encephalitis, Hashimoto's encephalitis, or CNS lymphoma [224, 225].

4.12.14 Treatment and Prognosis

- Owing to its rarity and often delayed diagnosis, treatment trials for Susac's syndrome do not exist. Therefore, treatment is typically empirical.
- The treatment must be aggressive, needs to be initiated early, and maintained long enough to prevent permanent visual loss, deafness, and dementia.
- Corticosteroids, methotrexate, azathioprine, mycophenolate mofetil, cyclosporine, cyclophosphamide, intravenous immunoglobulins, anti-CD20, TNF-alpha inhibitors (infliximab), or plasmapheresis are used [216, 223, 227, 232].
- Immune treatment for MS, such as interferon-beta, may cause exacerbation of the disease; however, TNF inhibitors can be beneficial [224, 233].
- Chronic marihuana use may increase disease activity of SuS [234]
- Roughly half of the patients experience remission without significant disability, while the other half may develop dementia. In some cases, severe brain atrophy is observed, though a fulminant fatal course is rare [219, 235].

4.13 Systemic Lupus Erythematosus (SLE)

4.13.1 Epidemiology

- Prevalence 30–50/100.000 [236].
- Neuropsychiatric complications of systemic lupus erythematosus (NPSLE) affect 20–90% of patients with SLE. The wide range is attributed to the lack of a clear definition of NPSLE [237–239].
- Demyelinating NPSLE affects only 1.3% of patients with SLE [240].
- Black, Hispanic, and Asian patients have higher prevalence and disease activity of SLE.
- Female/male ratio 7–15/1 [241].

4.13.2 Etiology and Definition

- The SLE is chronic systemic autoimmune disease with alterations in immune system activity that result in autoimmunity targeting nucleic acids and their associated proteins and tissue-damaging inflammation. Although, the etiology of SLE is unknown multiple genetic, epigenetic, and environmental risk factors probably play a role [242].
- The pathogenesis of NPSLE is multifactorial, involving inflammatory processes, multiple autoimmune antibodies, blood–brain barrier dysfunction, complement activation, and immune complexes, which result in vasculopathy, cytotoxicity, and autoantibody-mediated neuronal damage.
- In patients, it may often be unclear whether the nature of the NPSLE presentations can be attributed to vascular or inflammatory mechanisms [239, 243].
- NPSLE include a heterogeneous group of neurologic (central, peripheral, and autonomous) and psychiatric manifestations diagnosed in patients with SLE in which other causes are excluded [244].

4.13.3 Non-neurological Systemic Features

- SLE is one of the most heterogeneous diseases regarding phenotype and treatment response. For more details, see the section "Diagnosis" [241].

4.13.4 Neurological Features

- Headache (migraine, benign intracranial hypertension, etc.) (12.2–28.3%) [245].
- Cerebrovascular disease including stroke (8–15%).
- Movement disorder (0.9%).
- Aseptic pachymeningitis (0.3–7.0%) [244].
- Myelopathy/myelitis (relatively rare; 1–2%).
  - May be the first presentation of NPSLE.
  - Often dominating motor and bowel/blader involvement, contrary to MS in which is more often dominating sensory manifestations [245].
  - Onset is chronic progressive with ascending neurological symptoms, subacute progressive, or a hyperacute-catastrophic.
  - Disease course can be relapsing-remitting or progressive [245–247].
  - It is debated whether it constitutes a separate demyelinating condition or rather a complication of SLE [248].
- Psychiatric manifestations
  - Cognitive dysfunction (23–60%), affective disorders (7.4–65%), acute confusional state (0.9–7.0%), psychosis [238, 244].
- Ocular manifestations (1%)
  - Optic neuritis/neuropathy
    - Uni-or bilateral, severe, often painless (but can be painful).

    - The acute/subacute onset is frequently followed by progressive visual loss over weeks [249, 250], which is considered atypical for optic neuritis in MS, where progression longer than 14 days is atypical [251].
    - Considered as a part of SLE demyelinating syndrome (see below).
    - Worse prognosis compared to that in optic neuritis in MS.
  - Ischemic neuropathy.
  - Retrochiasmal lesions.
  - All ocular complications require early and aggressive treatment to avoid irreversible visual loss [249, 250].
- Seizures (7–20%)
  - More frequent compared to MS, where it occurs in only 2–3% [244, 245].
- Demyelinating syndrome (also called "lupoid sclerosis") (0.9–2.7%).
  - Rare [244, 252] but in approximately 40% of patients, it represents the first manifestation of SLE [240, 253].
  - Characterized by demyelination with relative preservation of axons.
  - Presents as an acute or relapsing encephalomyelitis with discrete CNS lesions disseminated in space and time, potentially mimicking MS [240].
  - Myelitis and optic neuritis are the most common presentations.
  - There are five subtypes of demyelinating NPSLE (2017 criteria) [240, 254]:
  - Lupoid sclerosis sharing common features with NMO.
    - 13.5% of patients satisfy the 2006 criteria for NMO [240].
    - This subtype of has highest disease activity [240, 254].
  - Lupoid sclerosis sharing common features with NMOSD
    - 50% of patients satisfy the 2007 criteria for NMOSD [240].
    - Optic neuritis associated with transverse myelitis (not longitudinally extensive transverse myelitis [LETM]) is present in 28.6% and isolated optic neuritis (can be bilateral) in 14.3% of patients with this demyelinating NPSLE subtype [240, 254].
    - Current diagnostic criteria of NMOSD unify traditional NMO and modern NMOSD definition into one group [255].
    - Currently, patients with SLE fulfilling diagnostic criteria for NMOSD are considered to have coexistence of the two diseases (NMOSD and SLE) [248, 255, 256] and not demyelinating NMO subtype of demyelinating NPSLE [240].
  - Lupoid sclerosis affecting brain or brainstem (11–12%)
    - Clinical manifestations are heterogeneous and depend on location and extent of demyelination.
    - Common cognitive dysfunction, acute confusional state, coma, psychosis, headache, seizures, or aseptic meningitis [240, 254].
    - May be dominant brainstem or cerebellar involvement (7.0%).
    - Some patients satisfied the McDonald 2010 criteria for MS (1%) [257]. These patients are considered to have coexistence of the SLE and MS [248] and not the demyelinating subtype of NPSLE [240]. This rare coexistence is usually not associated with a more severe phenotype for either entity [257, 258].

    - However, a great proportion of patients with demyelination may not fulfill criteria for either MS or SLE. These patients exhibit lupus-like autoimmune features (like arthritis or skin changes) and are not formally diagnosed with SLE, but with "demyelination with autoimmune features (DAF)," which describes patients in this "gray zone" [248].
  - Clinically isolated syndrome (CIS) (30%)
    - Refers to first clinical demyelinating event NPSLE [240, 254].
- Autonomic nervous system involvement (0.08–1.3%)
- Peripheral involvement
  - Acute inflammatory demyelinating polyradiculoneuropathy (Guillain–Barré syndrome) (0.08–1.2%), mononeuropathy single/multiplex (0.9–6.9%), myasthenia gravis (0.2%), cranial neuropathy (1%), plexopathy, and polyneuropathy (1.5–5.4%) [244].

4.13.5 Disease Course

- The age of symptoms onset is between 15 and 45 years.
- Disease course of NPSLE is usually relapsing remitting, persistently active, only serologically active, or with prolonged remission.
- Less frequently non-relapsing progressive course [241].

4.13.6 Brain Imaging

- Patients with NPSLE commonly show nonspecific abnormalities on MRI.
- Brain MRI is normal (50%) or shows small cortical and subcortical T2 hyperintense white matter lesions secondary to small vessel vasculopathy (e.g., small ischemic lesions) (50%).
- Brain abnormalities on MRI are most frequently seen in patients with NPSLE demyelinating syndrome ("lupoid sclerosis").
- Demyelinating syndrome sharing common features with NMO/NMOSD:
  - Not associated only with spinal cord lesions, but frequently also with brain T2 hyperintensities (57.1%) located mainly in hypothalamus, periventricular region, corpus callosum, and the brainstem.
- Demyelinating syndrome prominently involving the brain/or brainstem
  - Associated with T2 hyperintense lesions localized periventriculary, in deep white matter region, cortico-subcortical region, corpus callosum or in the brainstem (mostly pons, mesencephalon, and cerebellar peduncles).
  - Often atypical, large, and confluent.
  - Rarely, focal lesions may completely resolve following treatment.
  - Contrast enhancement is rare, but occasionally is present in parenchyma, optic nerves, or leptomeninges [240, 254, 259].
  - Brain microbleeds are common (>50%) [260].
  - May occur brain atrophy and basal ganglia calcifications (Fahr's disease) because of chronic inflammation in brain [254].

4.13.7 Spinal Cord Imaging

- Although, spinal cord lesions are less frequent in NPSLE, they are observed in around 70% of patients with demyelinating subtypes of NPSLE [254].
- Single short lesion or LETM with mild leptomeningeal enhancement.
- Demyelinating syndrome sharing common features with NMO/NMOSD is associated with
  - LETM is common (in 78.6% of the NMO/NPSLE and 57.1% of the NMOSD/NPSLE patients).
  - Spinal cord lesions are in cervical and less thoracic segments.
  - May be present mild contrast enhancement of lesions (30%).
  - Two distinct subtypes of the cord involvement:
    A. Pathology involving mainly white matter, which is associated with a relapsing disease course, central paraparesis with hyperreflexia, fulfill criteria for NMO, and often has lupus anticoagulant positivity.
    B. Pathology involving mainly gray matter, which is often associated with prodromes including fever, urinary retention, and flaccidity with hyporeflexia causing diagnostic delay in some patients. This subtype is associated with higher risk of irreversible paraplegia despite a monophasic course [249, 261].
- In general, brain and spinal cord MRI features have limited utility in distinguishing between demyelinating syndrome of NPSLE and MS, even if spinal cord involvement in SLE has often characteristics of LETM [10, 245, 262] (Fig. 4.10).

4.13.8 Blood Work

- Proportion of patients with MS (2.5–25%) has ANA positivity in low titers (its clinical significance is unclear) and anti-phospholipid antibodies (5–33%), but anti-DNA antibodies are very rare in MS. This may help differentiate MS from SLE, where anti-DNA antibodies are positive in 60% of patients and ANA are positive in 98% [10, 241, 245].
- Type 1 interferon pathway activation is low in MS but high in SLE and NMOSD. The evaluation of this signature is, however, often not available [241, 245].

4.13.9 Examination of CSF

- Mildly elevated concentration of protein with disruption of blood–brain barrier, and less frequently increased opening pressure of CSF.
- Often mild pleocytosis (<100 cells/mm^3), which tends to be more pronounced than in MS.
- CSF-restricted OCB are not frequently present (10–20%) and may disappear after successful immunotherapy [245, 254, 263]

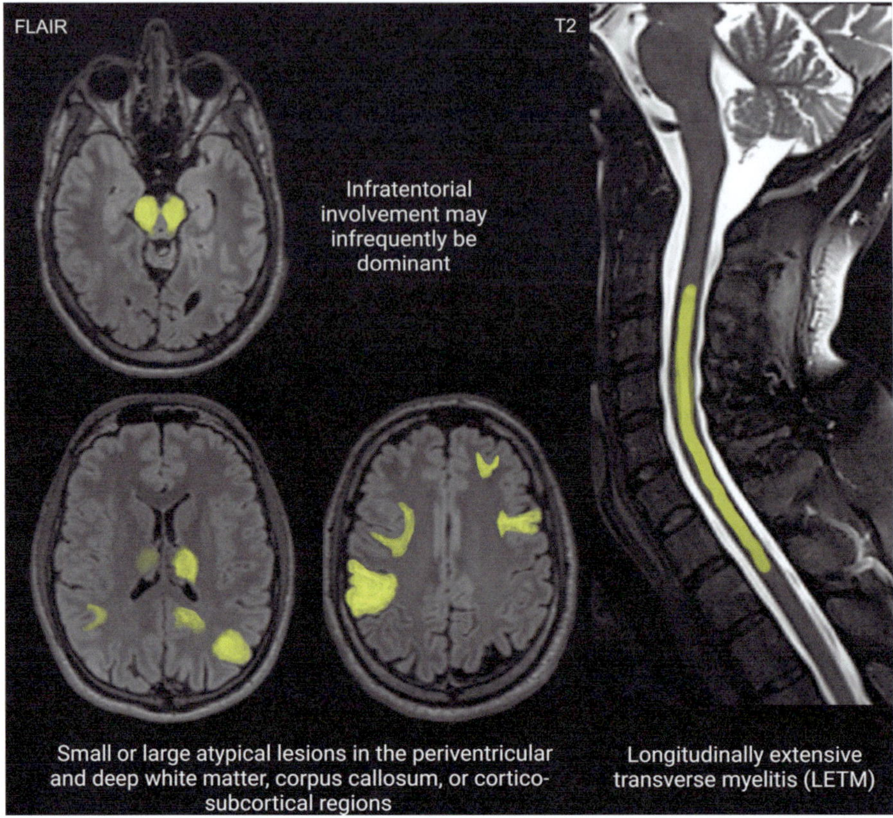

Fig. 4.10 MRI characteristics in systemic lupus erythematosus (SLE)

4.13.10 Examination of Blood and CSF in Different Subtypes of Demyelinative NPSLE

- Sharing common features with NMO
  - Anti-AQP4 IgG positivity (62.5%)
  - Hyperproteinorrachia and pleocytosis in the CSF
  - CSF-restricted OCB (22.2%)
- Sharing common features with NMOSD
  - Anti-AQP4 IgG positivity (10%)
  - Hyperproteinorrachia and pleocytosis in the CSF
  - CSF-restricted OCB (<10%)
- Demyelinating syndrome prominently involving the brain
  - Hyperproteinorrachia and pleocytosis in the CSF, but negative OCB
- Demyelinating syndrome prominently involving the brainstem and CIS
  - CSF is usually normal [240, 254]

4.13.11 Diagnosis of SLE

- The new European League Against Rheumatism (EULAR) and American College of Rheumatology (ACR) revised classification of SLE was published in 2019 [264].

A. Presence of ANA in titer >1:80.
   - ANA can also occur in other autoimmune diseases or in patients taking certain drugs, such as anticonvulsants, TNF inhibitors, or some antidepressants. Additionally, some MS patients may have ANA in low titers (<1:320). ANA negativity is rare in SLE patients. Although ANA-negative patients may not fulfill classification criteria for SLE (required for entering a clinical trial), in some cases, clinical diagnosis of SLE is possible.

B. In addition to a positive ANA, patients need to achieve a total score of 10 or more on the ACR/EULAR classification criteria. This score is based on 22 criteria with distinct weights.
   - Constitutional: Fever (weight = 2)
   - Cutaneous: Non-scaring alopecia (2); Oral ulcers (2); Subacute cutaneous or discoid lupus (4); Acute cutaneous lupus (6)
   - Arthritis: Synovitis with swelling or effusion in two joints or tenderness in two joints plus 30 min of morning stiffness (6)
   - Neurological: Delirium (2); Psychosis (3); Seizure (5)
   - Serositis: Pleural or pericardial effusion (5); Acute pericarditis (6)
   - Hematological: Leucopenia (3); Thrombocytopenia (4); Autoimmune hemolysis (5)
   - Renal: Proteinuria >0.5 g/24 h (because of reserve of kidneys, most patients with nephritis have normal renal functions, therefore creatinine level is not useful marker here) (4); Renal biopsy class II or V lupus nephritis (8); Renal biopsy class III or IV lupus nephritis (10)
   - Anti-phospholipid antibodies: Anti-cardiolipin or anti-beta 2 glycoprotein 1 antibodies or lupus anticoagulant (2)
   - Complement proteins: Low C3 or low C4 (3); Low C3 and low C4 (4); Highly specific antibodies: Anti-dsDNA antibody (6); and anti-Smith antibody (anti-Sm) (6).

4.13.12 Diagnosis of NPSLE

- There is no gold standard for diagnosis.
- According to the 1999 criteria patient can be diagnosed with NPSLE if meet the case definition for neuropsychiatric lupus (19 items) and in addition meet 3 or more of the ACR (non-NPSLE) criteria for SLE.
- If a patient meets the definition for a neuropsychiatric syndrome but meets an insufficient number of ACR criteria for SLE, the patient may be classified as having possible NPSLE [237].

- The 1999 ACR nomenclature failed to identify CIS as a demyelinating syndrome secondary to SLE suggesting the need for updated criteria [240].
- Isolated optic neuritis is not considered CIS because it is classified as cranial neuropathy according to the 1999 nomenclature [237].
- A major limitation of all classifications of NPSLE is the lack of definitions for individual manifestations, lack of standardization, and absence of validation studies [265]. Limited knowledge of the clinical, laboratory, and imaging features, as well as the limitations associated with diagnosing NPSLE, delays its diagnosis and treatment [240].

4.13.13 Differential Diagnosis

- General
  - Demyelinating syndrome secondary to SLE (demyelinating NPSLE) is rare condition but may represent a diagnostic challenge as it can mimic MS and other demyelinating and infectious diseases, neoplastic and paraneoplastic syndromes. Therefore, diagnosis needs to be made only after a careful and comprehensive examination [254].
- MS
  - Central demyelinating syndrome mimicking MS can be the first clinical manifestation of SLE patients. Therefore, screening for specific serological markers (anti-dsDNA, ANA, anti-phospholipid antibodies) is recommended in the suspected patients with CIS [240, 254].
  - Anti-phospholipid antibodies are suggestive of SLE or primary anti-phospholipid syndrome rather than MS. The absence of CSF-restricted OCB and LETM in NPSLE can also be a distinguishing feature between SLE and MS.
  - In a patient with demyelinating event suggestive of MS red flags should be assessed, including renal involvement, rash, arthritis, arthralgias, myalgias, headache, meningismus, cerebrovascular disease, cerebral venous sinus thrombosis, livedo reticularis, recurrent spontaneous abortion, thrombotic events, seizures, photosensitivity, Raynaud's phenomenon, sicca syndrome, psychiatric symptoms or peripheral neuropathy. If present, the diagnosis of NPSLE should be considered in differential diagnosis. These manifestations can also suggest primary or secondary anti-phospholipid syndrome associated with SLE [245, 253, 266, 267].
  - Specific tests to differentiate between MS and SLE do not exist and in many patients, the diagnosis can only be made after a long-term follow-up [245].
  - The coexistence of demyelinating syndrome in a patient with SLE represents a major challenge. It is not clear whether such a patient has a neurologic manifestation of the SLE or the patient has two different diseases. The resolving of this question has high clinical relevance, because treatment for SLE and MS differ significantly [248].

- NMOSD
  - The presence of anti-AQP4 IgG may aid in differentiating NPSLE from NMOSD.
- PML
  - PML needs to be ruled out in patients with NPSLE presenting with isolated brain MRI lesions without spinal cord and optic nerve involvement [240].

4.13.14 Treatment

- Neuropsychiatric manifestations in SLE patients should be first evaluated and treated as in those without SLE, and secondarily attributed to SLE and treated accordingly [265].
- For the treatment of SLE and NPSLE are used hydroxychloroquine, corticosteroids (at lowest possible dose), oral immunosuppressants (mycophenolate mofetil, azathioprine, methotrexate, ciclosporin, leflunomide), or anti-B cell activating factor (BAFF) and anti-CD20 treatments in severe cases [241, 252, 254].

4.13.15 Prognosis

- 15-year survival is about 90% [268].
- Early treatment is associated with better outcomes.
- The prognosis is heterogenous: complete or partial remission (50%); stable course despite treatment (25%); disease progression or death (25%).
- The NMO subtype of demyelination is associated with the worst prognosis, a high frequency of relapses, clinical worsening, and death in 50% of cases.
- The NMOSD subtype of demyelination with optic neuritis associated with transverse myelitis (not LETM) or isolated optic neuritis has better prognosis compared to patients with NMO subtype with LETM.
- Patients presenting with CIS has the best prognosis with clinical improvement in >90% of cases [240, 254].

4.14 Other Autoimmune Multisystem Diseases

4.14.1 Ankylosing Spondylitis

- Chronic and progressive autoimmune spondyloarthritis primarily affecting the spine and sacroiliac joints, but it also presents with various extra-articular manifestations such as uveitis, aortitis, or inflammatory bowel disease.
- Although neurological complications are rare, they may include MS-like symptoms characterized by brain lesions fulfilling the dissemination in space criteria and the presence of spinal cord lesions.

- In patients with infra-tentorial and spinal cord lesions, distinguishing whether neurological manifestations are a complication of ankylosing spondylitis or comorbid with MS can be challenging or nearly impossible, especially when lesion activity (contrast enhancement and the occurrence of new T2 lesions) is observed.
- Case studies have reported cases of patients with CSF-restricted OCB.
- HLA-B27 positivity is observed in 85% of White patients with ankylosing spondylitis, compared to only 8% of controls [269–271].

4.14.2 Relapsing Polychondritis

- Autoimmune systemic disease characterized by painful relapses of inflammation primarily affecting cartilaginous and proteoglycan-rich tissues.
- These include the cartilage of the ear and nose, which present a typical manifestation often absent in early disease stages, as well as the joints, tracheobronchial tree, skin, and kidneys. The inflammatory process leads to deformation and functional impairment of the affected tissues.
- During relapses, levels of CRP and ESR are frequently elevated.
- Approximately 3% of patients experience neurological complications due to vasculitis affecting the peripheral or central nervous system. These complications may manifest as cranial neuropathy, headache, aseptic pachymeningitis, limbic encephalitis, rhombencephalitis, cerebral infarction, ataxia, seizures, confusion, psychosis, or cognitive symptoms.
- Diagnosis primarily relies on clinical presentation since there are no specific paraclinical tests or histological patterns. There is no characteristic brain MRI pattern. However, CSF analysis may reveal elevated concentration of protein and pleocytosis.
- Treatment typically involves the use of immunosuppressive drugs [272, 273].

4.14.3 Sneddon's Syndrome

- Autoimmune disorder with endothelial dysfunction, particularly affecting medium and small-sized vessels.
- Disorder is characterized by the combination of livedo racemosa (a net-like pattern of vessels in the skin) or livedo reticularis and ischemic strokes.
- Often associated with anti-phospholipid antibody syndrome (50–80% of cases have positive anti-phospholipid antibodies), systemic lupus erythematosus, and valvulopathies.
- Angiography reveals vasculopathy in 75% of cases [274].

4.14.4 Systemic Sclerosis and Localized Scleroderma

- Autoimmune disorder characterized by inflammation, vascular injury, and fibrosis, spanning a spectrum of phenotypes from localized scleroderma to systemic sclerosis.
- Neurological complications are relatively common and encompass brain white matter lesions and calcifications, brain atrophy, brain vasculitis, transverse myelitis, peripheral and cranial neuropathy, dysautonomia, or myopathy.
- CNS involvement may manifest as seizures, headache, focal neurological deficits, or cognitive impairment.
- Some patients may exhibit an inflammatory pattern in CSF, including the presence of CSF-restricted OCB.
- Diagnosis is typically confirmed using biopsy of the lesions [275].

References

1. Dabit JY, Valenzuela-Almada MO, Vallejo-Ramos S, Duarte-Garcia A. Epidemiology of antiphospholipid syndrome in the general population. Curr Rheumatol Rep. 2022;23(12):85.
2. D'Angelo C, Franch O, Fernandez-Paredes L, Oreja-Guevara C, Nunez-Beltran M, Comins-Boo A, et al. Antiphospholipid antibodies overlapping in isolated neurological syndrome and multiple sclerosis: neurobiological insights and diagnostic challenges. Front Cell Neurosci. 2019;13:107.
3. Hughes GR. Migraine, memory loss, and "multiple sclerosis". Neurological features of the antiphospholipid (Hughes') syndrome. Postgrad Med J. 2003;79(928):81–3.
4. Leal Rato M, Bandeira M, Romao VC, Aguiar de Sousa D. Neurologic manifestations of the antiphospholipid syndrome – an update. Curr Neurol Neurosci Rep. 2021;21(8):41.
5. Ricarte IF, Dutra LA, Abrantes FF, Toso FF, Barsottini OGP, Silva GS, et al. Neurologic manifestations of antiphospholipid syndrome. Lupus. 2018;27(9):1404–14.
6. Levine JS, Branch DW, Rauch J. The antiphospholipid syndrome. N Engl J Med. 2002;346(10):752–63.
7. Unlu O, Zuily S, Erkan D. The clinical significance of antiphospholipid antibodies in systemic lupus erythematosus. Eur J Rheumatol. 2016;3(2):75–84.
8. Kim JH, Lee SI, Park SI, Yoo WH. Recurrent transverse myelitis in primary antiphospholipid syndrome—case report and literature review. Rheumatol Int. 2004;24(4):244–6.
9. Cuadrado MJ, Khamashta MA, Ballesteros A, Godfrey T, Simon MJ, Hughes GR. Can neurologic manifestations of Hughes (antiphospholipid) syndrome be distinguished from multiple sclerosis? Analysis of 27 patients and review of the literature. Medicine (Baltimore). 2000;79(1):57–68.
10. Ferreira S, D'Cruz DP, Hughes GR. Multiple sclerosis, neuropsychiatric lupus and antiphospholipid syndrome: where do we stand? Rheumatology (Oxford). 2005;44(4):434–42.
11. Maggi P, Absinta M, Grammatico M, Vuolo L, Emmi G, Carlucci G, et al. Central vein sign differentiates Multiple Sclerosis from central nervous system inflammatory vasculopathies. Ann Neurol. 2018;83(2):283–94.
12. Criteria for diagnosis of Behcet's disease. International Study Group for Behcet's Disease. Lancet. 1990;335(8697):1078–80.

13. Miyakis S, Lockshin MD, Atsumi T, Branch DW, Brey RL, Cervera R, et al. International consensus statement on an update of the classification criteria for definite antiphospholipid syndrome (APS). J Thromb Haemost. 2006;4(2):295–306.
14. Koike T, Sueishi M, Funaki H, Tomioka H, Yoshida S. Anti-phospholipid antibodies and biological false positive serological test for syphilis in patients with systemic lupus erythematosus. Clin Exp Immunol. 1984;56(1):193–9.
15. Paran D, Chapman J, Korczyn AD, Elkayam O, Hilkevich O, Groozman GB, et al. Evoked potential studies in the antiphospholipid syndrome: differential diagnosis from multiple sclerosis. Ann Rheum Dis. 2006;65(4):525–8.
16. Sebastiani GD, Galeazzi M, Tincani A, Piette JC, Font J, Allegri F, et al. Anticardiolipin and anti-beta2GPI antibodies in a large series of European patients with systemic lupus erythematosus. Prevalence and clinical associations. European Concerted Action on the Immunogenetics of SLE. Scand J Rheumatol. 1999;28(6):344–51.
17. Petri M, Orbai AM, Alarcon GS, Gordon C, Merrill JT, Fortin PR, et al. Derivation and validation of the Systemic Lupus International Collaborating Clinics classification criteria for systemic lupus erythematosus. Arthritis Rheum. 2012;64(8):2677–86.
18. Vilisaar J, Wilson M, Niepel G, Blumhardt LD, Constantinescu CS. A comparative audit of anticardiolipin antibodies in oligoclonal band negative and positive multiple sclerosis. Mult Scler. 2005;11(4):378–80.
19. IJdo JW, Conti-Kelly AM, Greco P, Abedi M, Amos M, Provenzale JM, et al. Anti-phospholipid antibodies in patients with multiple sclerosis and MS-like illnesses: MS or APS? Lupus. 1999;8(2):109–15.
20. Pengo V, Tripodi A, Reber G, Rand JH, Ortel TL, Galli M, et al. Update of the guidelines for lupus anticoagulant detection. Subcommittee on Lupus Anticoagulant/Antiphospholipid Antibody of the Scientific and Standardisation Committee of the International Society on Thrombosis and Haemostasis. J Thromb Haemost. 2009;7(10):1737–40.
21. Lee EJ, Lim YM, Kim SY, Lee J, Kim H, Jin JY, et al. The clinical and prognostic value of antinuclear antibodies in NMO-IgG seropositive neuromyelitis optica spectrum disorder. J Neuroimmunol. 2019;328:1–4.
22. Yurdakul S, Hamuryudan V, Yazici H. Behcet syndrome. Curr Opin Rheumatol. 2004;16(1):38–42.
23. Calamia KT, Wilson FC, Icen M, Crowson CS, Gabriel SE, Kremers HM. Epidemiology and clinical characteristics of Behcet's disease in the US: a population-based study. Arthritis Rheum. 2009;61(5):600–4.
24. Borhani-Haghighi A, Kardeh B, Banerjee S, Yadollahikhales G, Safari A, Sahraian MA, et al. Neuro-Behcet's disease: an update on diagnosis, differential diagnoses, and treatment. Mult Scler Relat Disord. 2020;39:101906.
25. Al-Araji A, Kidd DP. Neuro-Behcet's disease: epidemiology, clinical characteristics, and management. Lancet Neurol. 2009;8(2):192–204.
26. Yazici H, Fresko I, Yurdakul S. Behcet's syndrome: disease manifestations, management, and advances in treatment. Nat Clin Pract Rheumatol. 2007;3(3):148–55.
27. Lueck CJ, Pires M, McCartney AC, Graham EM. Ocular and neurological Behcet's disease without orogenital ulceration? J Neurol Neurosurg Psychiatry. 1993;56(5):505–8.
28. Casselman P, Cassiman C, Casteels I, Schauwvlieghe PP. Insights into multiple sclerosis-associated uveitis: a scoping review. Acta Ophthalmol. 2021;99(6):592–603.
29. Leker RR, Steiner I. Isolated intracranial hypertension as the only sign of cerebral venous thrombosis. Neurology. 2000;54(10):2030.
30. Yesilot N, Shehu M, Oktem-Tanor O, Serdaroglu P, Akman-Demir G. Silent neurological involvement in Behcet's disease. Clin Exp Rheumatol. 2006;24(5 Suppl 42):S65–70.
31. Pannone A, Lucchetti G, Stazi G, Corvi F, Ferguson TL, Massucci M, et al. Internal carotid artery dissection in a patient with Behcet's syndrome. Ann Vasc Surg. 1998;12(5):463–7.
32. Kalra S, Silman A, Akman-Demir G, Bohlega S, Borhani-Haghighi A, Constantinescu CS, et al. Diagnosis and management of Neuro-Behcet's disease: international consensus recommendations. J Neurol. 2014;261(9):1662–76.

33. Borhani Haghighi A, Sarhadi S, Farahangiz S. MRI findings of neuro-Behcet's disease. Clin Rheumatol. 2011;30(6):765–70.
34. Kocer N, Islak C, Siva A, Saip S, Akman C, Kantarci O, et al. CNS involvement in neuro-Behcet syndrome: an MR study. AJNR Am J Neuroradiol. 1999;20(6):1015–24.
35. Kurtuncu M, Tuzun E, Akman-Demir G. Behcet's disease and nervous system involvement. Curr Treat Options Neurol. 2016;18(5):19.
36. Kanoto M, Hosoya T, Toyoguchi Y, Oda A. Brain stem and cerebellar atrophy in chronic progressive neuro-Behcet's disease. Eur J Radiol. 2013;82(1):146–50.
37. Jade J, Chung K, Arendse M, Hussain Z, White D. Neuro-Behcet's disease presenting with tumour-like lesions and responding to rituximab. J Clin Neurosci. 2016;32:139–41.
38. Hiwatashi A, Garber T, Moritani T, Kinoshita T, Westesson PL. Diffusion-weighted MR imaging of neuro-Behcet's disease: a case report. Neuroradiology. 2003;45(7):468–71.
39. Albayram S, Saip S, Hasiloglu ZI, Teke M, Ceyhan E, Tutuncu M, et al. Evaluation of parenchymal neuro-behcet disease by using susceptibility-weighted imaging. AJNR Am J Neuroradiol. 2011;32(6):1050–5.
40. Uygunoglu U, Siva A. Behcet's syndrome and nervous system involvement. Curr Neurol Neurosci Rep. 2018;18(7):35.
41. Al-Araji A, Sharquie K, Al-Rawi Z. Prevalence and patterns of neurological involvement in Behcet's disease: a prospective study from Iraq. J Neurol Neurosurg Psychiatry. 2003;74(5):608–13.
42. Saruhan-Direskeneli G, Yentür SP, Mutlu M, Shugaiv E, Yesilot N, Kürtüncü M, et al. Intrathecal oligoclonal IgG bands are infrequently found in neuro-Behçet's disease. Clin Exp Rheumatol. 2013;31(3 Suppl 77):25–7.
43. Atas M, Yuvaci I, Demircan S, Guler E, Altunel O, Pangal E, et al. Evaluation of the macular, peripapillary nerve fiber layer and choroid thickness changes in Behcet's disease with spectral-domain OCT. J Ophthalmol. 2014;2014:865394.
44. Stigsby B, Bohlega S, al-Kawi MZ, al-Dalaan A, el-Ramahi K. Evoked potential findings in Behcet's disease. Brain-stem auditory, visual, and somatosensory evoked potentials in 44 patients. Electroencephalogr Clin Neurophysiol. 1994;92(4):273–81.
45. Hirohata S, Kikuchi H, Sawada T, Nagafuchi H, Kuwana M, Takeno M, et al. Retrospective analysis of long-term outcome of chronic progressive neurological manifestations in Behcet's disease. J Neurol Sci. 2015;349(1–2):143–8.
46. Singh P, Arora A, Strand TA, Leffler DA, Catassi C, Green PH, et al. Global prevalence of celiac disease: systematic review and meta-analysis. Clin Gastroenterol Hepatol. 2018;16(6):823–36 e2.
47. Gatti S, Lionetti E, Balanzoni L, Verma AK, Galeazzi T, Gesuita R, et al. Increased prevalence of celiac disease in school-age children in Italy. Clin Gastroenterol Hepatol. 2020;18(3):596–603.
48. Catassi C, Verdu EF, Bai JC, Lionetti E. Coeliac disease. Lancet. 2022;399(10344):2413–26.
49. Gobbi G, Bouquet F, Greco L, Lambertini A, Tassinari CA, Ventura A, et al. Coeliac disease, epilepsy, and cerebral calcifications. The Italian Working Group on Coeliac Disease and Epilepsy. Lancet. 1992;340(8817):439–43.
50. Croall ID, Sanders DS, Hadjivassiliou M, Hoggard N. Cognitive deficit and white matter changes in persons with celiac disease: a population-based study. Gastroenterology. 2020;158(8):2112–22.
51. Hadjivassiliou M, Croall ID, Grunewald RA, Trott N, Sanders DS, Hoggard N. Neurological evaluation of patients with newly diagnosed coeliac disease presenting to gastroenterologists: a 7-year follow-up study. Nutrients. 2021;13(6)
52. Hadjivassiliou M, Croall ID, Zis P, Sarrigiannis PG, Sanders DS, Aeschlimann P, et al. Neurologic deficits in patients with newly diagnosed celiac disease are frequent and linked with autoimmunity to transglutaminase 6. Clin Gastroenterol Hepatol. 2019;17(13):2678–86 e2.
53. Luostarinen L, Himanen SL, Luostarinen M, Collin P, Pirttila T. Neuromuscular and sensory disturbances in patients with well treated coeliac disease. J Neurol Neurosurg Psychiatry. 2003;74(4):490–4.

54. Hadjivassiliou M, Sanders DS, Grunewald RA, Woodroofe N, Boscolo S, Aeschlimann D. Gluten sensitivity: from gut to brain. Lancet Neurol. 2010;9(3):318–30.
55. Currie S, Hadjivassiliou M, Clark MJ, Sanders DS, Wilkinson ID, Griffiths PD, et al. Should we be 'nervous' about coeliac disease? Brain abnormalities in patients with coeliac disease referred for neurological opinion. J Neurol Neurosurg Psychiatry. 2012;83(12):1216–21.
56. Kieslich M, Errazuriz G, Posselt HG, Moeller-Hartmann W, Zanella F, Boehles H. Brain white-matter lesions in celiac disease: a prospective study of 75 diet-treated patients. Pediatrics. 2001;108(2):E21.
57. Pratesi R, Gandolfi L, Friedman H, Farage L, de Castro CA, Catassi C. Serum IgA antibodies from patients with coeliac disease react strongly with human brain blood-vessel structures. Scand J Gastroenterol. 1998;33(8):817–21.
58. Habek M, Hojsak I, Barun B, Brinar VV. Downbeat nystagmus, ataxia and spastic tetraparesis due to coeliac disease. Neurol Sci. 2011;32(5):911–4.
59. Dietrich W, Erbguth F. Neurological complications of inflammatory intestinal diseases. Fortschr Neurol Psychiatr. 2003;71(8):406–14.
60. Finsterer J, Leutmezer F. Celiac disease with cerebral and peripheral nerve involvement mimicking multiple sclerosis. J Med Life. 2014;7(3):440–4.
61. Newrick L, Hoggard N, Hadjivassiliou M. Recognition and management of rapid-onset gluten ataxias: case series. Cerebellum Ataxias. 2021;8(1):16.
62. Pengiran Tengah CD, Lock RJ, Unsworth DJ, Wills AJ. Multiple sclerosis and occult gluten sensitivity. Neurology. 2004;62(12):2326–7.
63. Hadjivassiliou M, Sanders DS, Grunewald RA. Multiple sclerosis and occult gluten sensitivity. Neurology. 2005;64(5):933–4. author reply -4
64. Catassi C, Bearzi I, Holmes GK. Association of celiac disease and intestinal lymphomas and other cancers. Gastroenterology. 2005;128(4 Suppl 1):S79–86.
65. Watts RA, Lane SE, Bentham G, Scott DG. Epidemiology of systemic vasculitis: a ten-year study in the United Kingdom. Arthritis Rheum. 2000;43(2):414–9.
66. Kahn JE, Bletry O, Guillevin L. Hypereosinophilic syndromes. Best Pract Res Clin Rheumatol. 2008;22(5):863–82.
67. Greco A, Rizzo MI, De Virgilio A, Gallo A, Fusconi M, Ruoppolo G, et al. Churg-Strauss syndrome. Autoimmun Rev. 2015;14(4):341–8.
68. Jennette JC, Falk RJ, Bacon PA, Basu N, Cid MC, Ferrario F, et al. 2012 revised International Chapel Hill Consensus Conference Nomenclature of Vasculitides. Arthritis Rheum. 2013;65(1):1–11.
69. Wolf J, Bergner R, Mutallib S, Buggle F, Grau AJ. Neurologic complications of Churg-Strauss syndrome—a prospective monocentric study. Eur J Neurol. 2010;17(4):582–8.
70. Liu S, Guo L, Fan X, Zhang Z, Zhou J, Tian X, et al. Clinical features of central nervous system involvement in patients with eosinophilic granulomatosis with polyangiitis: a retrospective cohort study in China. Orphanet J Rare Dis. 2021;16(1):152.
71. Hemmett J, Qirjazi E, Weir MA, Moussa M, Landry YD, Gunaratnam L. Cardiac, renal, and central nervous system dysfunction with eosinophilia: eosinophilic granulomatosis with polyangiitis. Lancet. 2015;385(9966):480.
72. Xu D, Xu H, Wang F, Wang G, Wei Q, Lei S, et al. Multiple distinctive demyelinating lesions caused by eosinophilic granulomatosis with polyangiitis: case report and literature. Review. 2019:10.
73. Andre R, Cottin V, Saraux JL, Blaison G, Bienvenu B, Cathebras P, et al. Central nervous system involvement in eosinophilic granulomatosis with polyangiitis (Churg-Strauss): report of 26 patients and review of the literature. Autoimmun Rev. 2017;16(9):963–9.
74. Mittal S, Acsadi A, Cruz L, Aglio T, Ek K, Lakshminarayanan S, et al. A rare case of Churg Strauss syndrome associated with cervical spine and brain involvement (P4.037). Neurology. 2014;82(10 Suppl):P4.037.
75. Radice A, Bianchi L, Sinico RA. Anti-neutrophil cytoplasmic autoantibodies: methodological aspects and clinical significance in systemic vasculitis. Autoimmun Rev. 2013;12(4):487–95.

76. Zwerina J, Bach C, Martorana D, Jatzwauk M, Hegasy G, Moosig F, et al. Eotaxin-3 in Churg-Strauss syndrome: a clinical and immunogenetic study. Rheumatology (Oxford). 2011;50(10):1823–7.
77. Masi AT, Hunder GG, Lie JT, Michel BA, Bloch DA, Arend WP, et al. The American College of Rheumatology 1990 criteria for the classification of Churg-Strauss syndrome (allergic granulomatosis and angiitis). Arthritis Rheum. 1990;33(8):1094–100.
78. Cohen P, Pagnoux C, Mahr A, Arene JP, Mouthon L, Le Guern V, et al. Churg-Strauss syndrome with poor-prognosis factors: a prospective multicenter trial comparing glucocorticoids and six or twelve cyclophosphamide pulses in forty-eight patients. Arthritis Rheum. 2007;57(4):686–93.
79. Guillevin L, Cohen P, Gayraud M, Lhote F, Jarrousse B, Casassus P. Churg-Strauss syndrome. Clinical study and long-term follow-up of 96 patients. Medicine (Baltimore). 1999;78(1):26–37.
80. Cogan D. Syndrome of nonsyphilitic interstitial keratitis and vestibuloauditory symptoms. Arch Ophthalmol. 1945;33:144–9.
81. Greco A, Gallo A, Fusconi M, Magliulo G, Turchetta R, Marinelli C, et al. Cogan's syndrome: an autoimmune inner ear disease. Autoimmun Rev. 2013;12(3):396–400.
82. Shamriz O, Tal Y, Gross M. Autoimmune inner ear disease: immune biomarkers, audiovestibular aspects, and therapeutic modalities of Cogan's syndrome. J Immunol Res. 2018;2018:1498640.
83. Vollertsen RS, McDonald TJ, Younge BR, Banks PM, Stanson AW, Ilstrup DM. Cogan's syndrome: 18 cases and a review of the literature. Mayo Clin Proc. 1986;61(5):344–61.
84. Tayer-Shifman OE, Ilan O, Tovi H, Tal Y. Cogan's syndrome—clinical guidelines and novel therapeutic approaches. Clin Rev Allergy Immunol. 2014;47(1):65–72.
85. Grasland A, Pouchot J, Hachulla E, Bletry O, Papo T, Vinceneux P, et al. Typical and atypical Cogan's syndrome: 32 cases and review of the literature. Rheumatology (Oxford). 2004;43(8):1007–15.
86. Casselman JW, Majoor MH, Albers FW. MR of the inner ear in patients with Cogan syndrome. AJNR Am J Neuroradiol. 1994;15(1):131–8.
87. Migliori G, Battisti E, Pari M, Vitelli N, Cingolani C. A shifty diagnosis: Cogan's syndrome. A case report and review of the literature. Acta Otorhinolaryngol Ital. 2009;29(2):108–13.
88. Standardization of Uveitis Nomenclature (SUN) Working Group. Classification criteria for Vogt-Koyanagi-Harada disease. Am J Ophthalmol. 2021;228:205–11.
89. Ayrignac X, Goulabchand R, Jeziorski E, Rullier P, Carra-Dallière C, Lozano C, et al. Two neurologic facets of CTLA4-related haploinsufficiency. Neurol Neuroimmunol Neuroinflamm. 2020;7(4)
90. Ayrignac X, Carra-Dallière C, Marelli C, Taïeb G, Labauge P. Adult-onset genetic central nervous system disorders masquerading as acquired neuroinflammatory disorders: a review. JAMA Neurol. 2022;79(10):1069–78.
91. Schubert D, Bode C, Kenefeck R, Hou TZ, Wing JB, Kennedy A, et al. Autosomal dominant immune dysregulation syndrome in humans with CTLA4 mutations. Nat Med. 2014;20(12):1410–6.
92. Rovshanov S, Göçmen R, Barişta İ, Çağdaş D, Üner A, Çilingir V, et al. A rare central nervous system involvement due to CTLA-4 gene defect. Noro Psikiyatr Ars. 2022;59(3):248–52.
93. Coustal C, Goulabchand R, Labauge P, Guilpain P, Carra-Dallière C, Januel E, et al. Clinical, radiologic, and immunologic features of patients with CTLA4 deficiency with neurologic involvement. Neurology. 2023;101(15):e1560–e6.
94. Stone JH, Zen Y, Deshpande V. IgG4-related disease. N Engl J Med. 2012;366(6):539–51.
95. Uchida K, Masamune A, Shimosegawa T, Okazaki K. Prevalence of IgG4-related disease in Japan based on nationwide survey in 2009. Int J Rheumatol. 2012;2012:358371.
96. Goulam-Houssein S, Grenville JL, Mastrocostas K, Munoz DG, Lin A, Bharatha A, et al. IgG4-related intracranial disease. Neuroradiol J. 2019;32(1):29–35.
97. Baptista B, Casian A, Gunawardena H, D'Cruz D, Rice CM. Neurological manifestations of IgG4-related disease. Curr Treat Options Neurol. 2017;19(4):14.

98. Joshi D, Jager R, Hurel S, Pereira SP, Johnson GJ, Chapman M, et al. Cerebral involvement in IgG4-related disease. Clin Med (Lond). 2015;15(2):130–4.
99. Lu LX, Della-Torre E, Stone JH, Clark SW. IgG4-related hypertrophic pachymeningitis: clinical features, diagnostic criteria, and treatment. JAMA Neurol. 2014;71(6):785–93.
100. Qi Z, Liu J, Li G, Zhang Y. Immunoglobulin G4-related spinal intramedullary inflammatory pseudotumor: a case report and literature review. Front Neurol. 2022;13:878414.
101. Qing P, Lu C, Yan B, Liu C, Fox DA, Zhao Y, et al. Case report: IgG4-related intracranial lesions mimicking multiple sclerosis in a 14-year-old girl. Front Neurol. 2022;13:1007153.
102. Regev K, Nussbaum T, Cagnano E, Giladi N, Karni A. Central nervous system manifestation of IgG4-related disease. JAMA Neurol. 2014;71(6):767–70.
103. Ebbo M, Grados A, Bernit E, Vely F, Boucraut J, Harle JR, et al. Pathologies associated with serum IgG4 elevation. Int J Rheumatol. 2012;2012:602809.
104. Levraut M, Cohen M, Bresch S, Giordana C, Burel-Vandenbos F, Mondot L, et al. Immunoglobulin G4-related hypertrophic pachymeningitis: a case-oriented review. Neurol Neuroimmunol Neuroinflamm. 2019;6(4):e568.
105. Umehara H, Okazaki K, Masaki Y, Kawano M, Yamamoto M, Saeki T, et al. Comprehensive diagnostic criteria for IgG4-related disease (IgG4-RD), 2011. Mod Rheumatol. 2012;22(1):21–30.
106. Fenderson J, Berenberg J, Tom L, Gress F. IgG4-related disease: imitating a great imitator. Hawaii J Med Public Health. 2015;74(9 Suppl 2):22–6.
107. Baumgart DC, Sandborn WJ. Inflammatory bowel disease: clinical aspects and established and evolving therapies. Lancet. 2007;369(9573):1641–57.
108. Dahlhamer JM, Zammitti EP, Ward BW, Wheaton AG, Croft JB. Prevalence of inflammatory bowel disease among adults aged ≥18 years—United States, 2015. MMWR Morb Mortal Wkly Rep. 2016;65(42):1166–9.
109. Lossos A, River Y, Eliakim A, Steiner I. Neurologic aspects of inflammatory bowel disease. Neurology. 1995;45(3 Pt 1):416–21.
110. Oliveira GR, Teles BC, Brasil EF, Souza MH, Furtado LE, de Castro-Costa CM, et al. Peripheral neuropathy and neurological disorders in an unselected Brazilian population-based cohort of IBD patients. Inflamm Bowel Dis. 2008;14(3):389–95.
111. Ferro JM, Oliveira SM. Neurology of inflammatory bowel disease. J Neurol Sci. 2021;424:117426.
112. Wang X, Wan J, Wang M, Zhang Y, Wu K, Yang F. Multiple sclerosis and inflammatory bowel disease: a systematic review and meta-analysis. Ann Clin Transl Neurol. 2022;9(2):132–40.
113. Rothfuss KS, Stange EF, Herrlinger KR. Extraintestinal manifestations and complications in inflammatory bowel diseases. World J Gastroenterol. 2006;12(30):4819–31.
114. Benavente L, Moris G. Neurologic disorders associated with inflammatory bowel disease. Eur J Neurol. 2011;18(1):138–43.
115. Dolapcioglu C, Guleryuzlu Y, Uygur-Bayramicli O, Ahishali E, Dabak R. Asymptomatic brain lesions on cranial magnetic resonance imaging in inflammatory bowel disease. Gut Liver. 2013;7(2):169–74.
116. Hart PE, Gould SR, MacSweeney JE, Clifton A, Schon F. Brain white-matter lesions in inflammatory bowel disease. Lancet. 1998;351(9115):1558.
117. Geissler A, Andus T, Roth M, Kullmann F, Caesar I, Held P, et al. Focal white-matter lesions in brain of patients with inflammatory bowel disease. Lancet. 1995;345(8954):897–8.
118. Chen M, Lee G, Kwong LN, Lamont S, Chaves C. Cerebral white matter lesions in patients with Crohn's disease. J Neuroimaging. 2012;22(1):38–41.
119. Zikou AK, Kosmidou M, Astrakas LG, Tzarouchi LC, Tsianos E, Argyropoulou MI. Brain involvement in patients with inflammatory bowel disease: a voxel-based morphometry and diffusion tensor imaging study. Eur Radiol. 2014;24(10):2499–506.
120. Stovicek J, Liskova P, Lisy J, Hlava S, Keil R. Crohn's disease: is there a place for neurological screening? Scand J Gastroenterol. 2014;49(2):173–6.
121. de Lau LM, de Vries JM, van der Woude CJ, Kuipers EJ, Siepman DA, Sillevis Smitt PA, et al. Acute CNS white matter lesions in patients with inflammatory bowel disease. Inflamm Bowel Dis. 2009;15(4):576–80.

122. Agostini A, Benuzzi F, Filippini N, Bertani A, Scarcelli A, Farinelli V, et al. New insights into the brain involvement in patients with Crohn's disease: a voxel-based morphometry study. Neurogastroent Motil. 2013;25(2):147.
123. Agranoff D, Schon F. Are focal white matter lesions in patients with inflammatory bowel disease linked to multiple sclerosis? Lancet. 1995;346(8968):190–1.
124. Dolapcioglu C, Dolapcioglu H. Structural brain lesions in inflammatory bowel disease. World J Gastrointest Pathophysiol. 2015;6(4):124–30.
125. Yang Y, Zhang Y. Acute transverse myelitis in an adult-patient with underlying ulcerative colitis: a case report. BMC Gastroenterol. 2022;22(1):161.
126. WGW P, Chubb SP, Gillett MJ, Vasikaran SD. Faecal calprotectin. Clin Biochem Rev. 2018;39(3):77–90.
127. Lamb CA, Kennedy NA, Raine T, Hendy PA, Smith PJ, Limdi JK, et al. British Society of Gastroenterology consensus guidelines on the management of inflammatory bowel disease in adults. Gut. 2019;68(Suppl 3):s1–s106.
128. Kitchin LI, Knobler RL, Friedman LS. Crohn's disease in a patient with multiple sclerosis. J Clin Gastroenterol. 1991;13(3):331–4.
129. Gupta G, Gelfand JM, Lewis JD. Increased risk for demyelinating diseases in patients with inflammatory bowel disease. Gastroenterology. 2005;129(3):819–26.
130. Symmons D, Turner G, Webb R, Asten P, Barrett E, Lunt M, et al. The prevalence of rheumatoid arthritis in the United Kingdom: new estimates for a new century. Rheumatology (Oxford). 2002;41(7):793–800.
131. Scott DL, Wolfe F, Huizinga TW. Rheumatoid arthritis. Lancet. 2010;376(9746):1094–108.
132. Sieper J, Poddubnyy D. Axial spondyloarthritis. Lancet. 2017;390(10089):73–84.
133. Cianfoni A, Falcone C, Faustini F, Lauriola L, Imbesi S, Della Marca G, et al. Rheumatoid leptomeningitis: magnetic resonance imaging and pathologic findings—a case report. J Neuroimaging. 2010;20(2):192–4.
134. Bathon JM, Moreland LW, DiBartolomeo AG. Inflammatory central nervous system involvement in rheumatoid arthritis. Semin Arthritis Rheum. 1989;18(4):258–66.
135. Lee Ching C, Kenyon L, Berk M, Park C. Rheumatoid meningitis sine arthritis. J Neuroimmunol. 2019;328:73–5.
136. Takahashi M, Yamamoto J, Idei M, Nakano Y, Soejima Y, Saito T, et al. Multiple intracranial nodules associated with rheumatoid arthritis: case report. Neurol Med Chir. 2014;54(4):317–20.
137. Defty H, Sames E, Doherty T, Hughes R. Case report of transverse myelitis in a patient receiving etanercept for rheumatoid arthritis. Case Rep Rheumatol. 2013;2013:728371.
138. Miyaue N, Yabe H, Yamanishi Y, Tada S, Ando R, Nagai M. Three cases of rheumatoid meningitis with elevated CSF neopterin levels. J Neuroimmunol. 2020;348:577396.
139. Atzeni F, Talotta R, Masala IF, Gerardi MC, Casale R, Sarzi-Puttini P. Central nervous system involvement in rheumatoid arthritis patients and the potential implications of using biological agents. Best Pract Res Clin Rheumatol. 2018;32(4):500–10.
140. Yagita K, Shinde A, Suenaga T. Rheumatoid meningitis can present MRI findings that mimic chronic subdural haematoma. BMJ Case Rep. 2019;12(8)
141. Letarouilly JG, Vermersch P, Flipo RM. Therapeutic consequences in patients with both inflammatory rheumatic diseases and multiple sclerosis. Rheumatology (Oxford). 2023;62(7):2352–9.
142. Bernatsky S, Renoux C, Suissa S. Demyelinating events in rheumatoid arthritis after drug exposures. Ann Rheum Dis. 2010;69(9):1691–3.
143. Bosch X, Saiz A, Ramos-Casals M. Monoclonal antibody therapy-associated neurological disorders. Nat Rev Neurol. 2011;7(3):165–72.
144. Sicotte NL, Voskuhl RR. Onset of multiple sclerosis associated with anti-TNF therapy. Neurology. 2001;57(10):1885–8.
145. Westwood OM, Nelson PN, Hay FC. Rheumatoid factors: what's new? Rheumatology (Oxford). 2006;45(4):379–85.

146. Mendez-Rayo T, Ochoa-Zárate L, Posso-Osorio I, Ortiz E, Naranjo-Escobar J, Tobón GJ. Interpretation of autoantibodies in rheumatological diseases. Rev Colomb Reumatol (Eng Ed). 2018;25(2):112–25.
147. Nissen MS, Nilsson AC, Forsberg J, Milthers J, Wirenfeldt M, Bonde C, et al. Use of cerebrospinal fluid biomarkers in diagnosis and nonitoring of rheumatoid meningitis. Front Neurol. 2019;10:666.
148. Kay J, Upchurch KS. ACR/EULAR 2010 rheumatoid artvhritis classification criteria. Rheumatology (Oxford). 2012;51 Suppl 6:vi5–9.
149. Joubert B, Chapelon-Abric C, Biard L, Saadoun D, Demeret S, Dormont D, et al. Association of prognostic factors and immunosuppressive treatment with long-term outcomes in neurosarcoidosis. JAMA Neurol. 2017;74(11):1336–44.
150. Ungprasert P, Carmona EM, Utz JP, Ryu JH, Crowson CS, Matteson EL. Epidemiology of sarcoidosis 1946–2013: a population-based study. Mayo Clin Proc. 2016;91(2):183–8.
151. Bradshaw MJ, Pawate S, Koth LL, Cho TA, Gelfand JM. Neurosarcoidosis: pathophysiology, diagnosis, and treatment. Neurol Neuroimmunol Neuroinflamm. 2021;8(6)
152. Fritz D, Voortman M, van de Beek D, Drent M, Brouwer MC. Many faces of neurosarcoidosis: from chronic meningitis to myelopathy. Curr Opin Pulm Med. 2017;23(5):439–46.
153. Iannuzzi MC, Rybicki BA, Teirstein AS. Sarcoidosis. N Engl J Med. 2007;357(21):2153–65.
154. Pawate S. Sarcoidosis and the nervous system. Continuum (Minneap Minn). 2020;26(3):695–715.
155. Ungprasert P, Crowson CS, Matteson EL. Smoking, obesity and risk of sarcoidosis: a population-based nested case-control study. Respir Med. 2016;120:87–90.
156. Valeyre D, Prasse A, Nunes H, Uzunhan Y, Brillet PY, Müller-Quernheim J. Sarcoidosis. Lancet. 2014;383(9923):1155–67.
157. Rose NR, Bona C. Defining criteria for autoimmune diseases (Witebsky's postulates revisited). Immunol Today. 1993;14(9):426–30.
158. Fingerlin TE, Hamzeh N, Maier LA. Genetics of sarcoidosis. Clin Chest Med. 2015;36(4):569–84.
159. Fritz D, van de Beek D, Brouwer MC. Clinical features, treatment and outcome in neurosarcoidosis: systematic review and meta-analysis. BMC Neurol. 2016;16(1):220.
160. Carlson ML, White JR Jr, Espahbodi M, Haynes DS, Driscoll CL, Aksamit AJ, et al. Cranial base manifestations of neurosarcoidosis: a review of 305 patients. Otol Neurotol. 2015;36(1):156–66.
161. Smith JK, Matheus MG, Castillo M. Imaging manifestations of neurosarcoidosis. AJR Am J Roentgenol. 2004;182(2):289–95.
162. Langrand C, Bihan H, Raverot G, Varron L, Androdias G, Borson-Chazot F, et al. Hypothalamo-pituitary sarcoidosis: a multicenter study of 24 patients. QJM. 2012;105(10):981–95.
163. Bathla G, Watal P, Gupta S, Nagpal P, Mohan S, Moritani T. Cerebrovascular manifestations of neurosarcoidosis: an underrecognized aspect of the imaging spectrum. AJNR Am J Neuroradiol. 2018;39(7):1194–200.
164. Krumholz A, Stern BJ. Neurologic manifestations of sarcoidosis. Handb Clin Neurol. 2014;119:305–33.
165. Murphy OC, Salazar-Camelo A, Jimenez JA, Barreras P, Reyes MI, Garcia MA, et al. Clinical and MRI phenotypes of sarcoidosis-associated myelopathy. Neurol Neuroimmunol Neuroinflamm. 2020;7(4)
166. Pawate S, Moses H, Sriram S. Presentations and outcomes of neurosarcoidosis: a study of 54 cases. QJM. 2009;102(7):449–60.
167. Vital A, Vital C. Clinical Neuropathology practice guide 3–2014: combined nerve and muscle biopsy in the diagnostic workup of neuropathy—the Bordeaux experience. Clin Neuropathol. 2014;33(3):172–8.
168. Cohen Aubart F, Abbara S, Maisonobe T, Cottin V, Papo T, Haroche J, et al. Symptomatic muscular sarcoidosis: lessons from a nationwide multicenter study. Neurol Neuroimmunol Neuroinflamm. 2018;5(3):e452.

169. Bennett D, Cameli P, Lanzarone N, Carobene L, Bianchi N, Fui A, et al. Chitotriosidase: a biomarker of activity and severity in patients with sarcoidosis. Respir Res. 2020;21(1):6.
170. Eurelings LEM, Miedema JR, Dalm V, van Daele PLA, van Hagen PM, van Laar JAM, et al. Sensitivity and specificity of serum soluble interleukin-2 receptor for diagnosing sarcoidosis in a population of patients suspected of sarcoidosis. PLoS One. 2019;14(10):e0223897.
171. Leonhard SE, Fritz D, Eftimov F, van der Kooi AJ, van de Beek D, Brouwer MC. Neurosarcoidosis in a tertiary referral center: a cross-sectional cohort study. Medicine (Baltimore). 2016;95(14):e3277.
172. Vlad B, Neidhart S, Hilty M, Ziegler M, Jelcic I. Differentiating neurosarcoidosis from multiple sclerosis using combined analysis of basic CSF parameters and MRZ reaction. Front Neurol. 2023;14:1135392.
173. Fritz D, van de Beek D, Brouwer MC, Booij J. Whole-body 18F-FDG PET-CT in the diagnosis of neurosarcoidosis. Mayo Clin Proc. 2020;95(5):1082–4.
174. Stern BJ, Royal W 3rd, Gelfand JM, Clifford DB, Tavee J, Pawate S, et al. Definition and consensus diagnostic criteria for neurosarcoidosis: from the Neurosarcoidosis Consortium Consensus Group. JAMA Neurol. 2018;75(12):1546–53.
175. Tyshkov C, Pawate S, Bradshaw MJ, Kimbrough DJ, Chitnis T, Gelfand JM, et al. Multiple sclerosis and sarcoidosis: a case for coexistence. Neurol Clin Pract. 2019;9(3):218–27.
176. Qin B, Wang J, Yang Z, Yang M, Ma N, Huang F, et al. Epidemiology of primary Sjogren's syndrome: a systematic review and meta-analysis. Ann Rheum Dis. 2015;74(11):1983–9.
177. Carvajal Alegria G, Guellec D, Mariette X, Gottenberg JE, Dernis E, Dubost JJ, et al. Epidemiology of neurological manifestations in Sjogren's syndrome: data from the French ASSESS Cohort. RMD Open. 2016;2(1):e000179.
178. Patel R, Shahane A. The epidemiology of Sjogren's syndrome. Clin Epidemiol. 2014;6:247–55.
179. Thurtle E, Grosjean A, Steenackers M, Strege K, Barcelos G, Goswami P. Epidemiology of Sjögren's: a systematic literature review. Rheumat Ther. 2024;11(1):1–17.
180. Mariette X, Criswell LA. Primary Sjogren's syndrome. N Engl J Med. 2018;379(1):97.
181. Nocturne G, Mariette X. Advances in understanding the pathogenesis of primary Sjogren's syndrome. Nat Rev Rheumatol. 2013;9(9):544–56.
182. Meijer JM, Meiners PM, Huddleston Slater JJ, Spijkervet FK, Kallenberg CG, Vissink A, et al. Health-related quality of life, employment and disability in patients with Sjogren's syndrome. Rheumatology (Oxford). 2009;48(9):1077–82.
183. Retamozo S, Acar-Denizli N, Rasmussen A, Horvath IF, Baldini C, Priori R, et al. Systemic manifestations of primary Sjogren's syndrome out of the ESSDAI classification: prevalence and clinical relevance in a large international, multi-ethnic cohort of patients. Clin Exp Rheumatol. 2019;37 Suppl 118(3):97–106.
184. Jamilloux Y, Magy L, Hurtevent JF, Gondran G, de Seze J, Launay D, et al. Immunological profiles determine neurological involvement in Sjogren's syndrome. Eur J Intern Med. 2014;25(2):177–81.
185. Lafitte C, Amoura Z, Cacoub P, Pradat-Diehl P, Picq C, Salachas F, et al. Neurological complications of primary Sjogren's syndrome. J Neurol. 2001;248(7):577–84.
186. Alunno A, Carubbi F, Bartoloni E, Cipriani P, Giacomelli R, Gerli R. The kaleidoscope of neurological manifestations in primary Sjogren's syndrome. Clin Exp Rheumatol. 2019;37 Suppl 118(3):192–8.
187. Delalande S, de Seze J, Fauchais AL, Hachulla E, Stojkovic T, Ferriby D, et al. Neurologic manifestations in primary Sjogren syndrome: a study of 82 patients. Medicine (Baltimore). 2004;83(5):280–91.
188. Afzali AM, Moog P, Kalluri SR, Hofauer B, Knopf A, Kirschke JS, et al. CNS demyelinating events in primary Sjogren's syndrome: a single-center case series on the clinical phenotype. Front Neurol. 2023;14:1128315.
189. Masi G, Annunziata P. Sjogren's syndrome and multiple sclerosis: two sides of the same coin? Autoimmun Rev. 2016;15(5):457–61.
190. Kim SM, Waters P, Vincent A, Kim SY, Kim HJ, Hong YH, et al. Sjogren's syndrome myelopathy: spinal cord involvement in Sjogren's syndrome might be a manifestation of neuromyelitis optica. Mult Scler. 2009;15(9):1062–8.

191. Akaishi T, Takahashi T, Fujihara K, Misu T, Fujimori J, Takai Y, et al. Impact of comorbid Sjogren syndrome in anti-aquaporin-4 antibody-positive neuromyelitis optica spectrum disorders. J Neurol. 2021;268(5):1938–44.
192. Tezcan ME, Kocer EB, Haznedaroglu S, Sonmez C, Mercan R, Yucel AA, et al. Primary Sjogren's syndrome is associated with significant cognitive dysfunction. Int J Rheum Dis. 2016;19(10):981–8.
193. Ramos-Casals M, Brito-Zeron P, Solans R, Camps MT, Casanovas A, Sopena B, et al. Systemic involvement in primary Sjogren's syndrome evaluated by the EULAR-SS disease activity index: analysis of 921 Spanish patients (GEAS-SS Registry). Rheumatology (Oxford). 2014;53(2):321–31.
194. Morgen K, McFarland HF, Pillemer SR. Central nervous system disease in primary Sjogrens syndrome: the role of magnetic resonance imaging. Semin Arthritis Rheum. 2004;34(3):623–30.
195. Harboe E, Beyer MK, Greve OJ, Goransson LG, Tjensvoll AB, Kvaloy JT, et al. Cerebral white matter hyperintensities are not increased in patients with primary Sjogren's syndrome. Eur J Neurol. 2009;16(5):576–81.
196. Karathanasis DK, Rapti A, Nezos A, Skarlis C, Kilidireas C, Mavragani CP, et al. Differentiating central nervous system demyelinating disorders: the role of clinical, laboratory, imaging characteristics and peripheral blood type I interferon activity. Front Pharmacol. 2022;13:898049.
197. Hammenfors DS, Brun JG, Jonsson R, Jonsson MV. Diagnostic utility of major salivary gland ultrasonography in primary Sjogren's syndrome. Clin Exp Rheumatol. 2015;33(1):56–62.
198. de Andres C, Guillem A, Rodriguez-Mahou M, Lopez Longo FJ. Frequency and significance of anti-Ro (SS-A) antibodies in multiple sclerosis patients. Acta Neurol Scand. 2001;104(2):83–7.
199. Solomon AJ, Hills W, Chen Z, Rosenbaum J, Bourdette D, Whitham R. Autoantibodies and Sjogren's syndrome in multiple sclerosis, a reappraisal. PLoS One. 2013;8(6):e65385.
200. Arbuckle MR, McClain MT, Rubertone MV, Scofield RH, Dennis GJ, James JA, et al. Development of autoantibodies before the clinical onset of systemic lupus erythematosus. N Engl J Med. 2003;349(16):1526–33.
201. Pittock SJ, Lennon VA, de Seze J, Vermersch P, Homburger HA, Wingerchuk DM, et al. Neuromyelitis optica and non organ-specific autoimmunity. Arch Neurol. 2008;65(1):78–83.
202. Birnbaum J, Atri NM, Baer AN, Cimbro R, Montagne J, Casciola-Rosen L. Relationship between neuromyelitis optica spectrum disorder and Sjogren's syndrome: central nervous system extraglandular disease or unrelated, co-occurring autoimmunity? Arthritis Care Res (Hoboken). 2017;69(7):1069–75.
203. Brito-Zeron P, Acar-Denizli N, Ng WF, Zeher M, Rasmussen A, Mandl T, et al. How immunological profile drives clinical phenotype of primary Sjogren's syndrome at diagnosis: analysis of 10,500 patients (Sjogren Big Data Project). Clin Exp Rheumatol. 2018;36 Suppl 112(3):102–12.
204. Ramos-Casals M, Brito-Zeron P, Font J. The overlap of Sjogren's syndrome with other systemic autoimmune diseases. Semin Arthritis Rheum. 2007;36(4):246–55.
205. Pars K, Pul R, Schwenkenbecher P, Suhs KW, Wurster U, Witte T, et al. Cerebrospinal fluid findings in neurological diseases associated with Sjogren's syndrome. Eur Neurol. 2017;77(1–2):91–102.
206. Yang JM, Sung MS, Ji YS, Heo H, Park SW. Analysis of clinical factors associated with retinal morphological changes in patients with primary Sjogren's syndrome. PLoS One. 2016;11(6):e0157995.
207. Alexander EL, Malinow K, Lejewski JE, Jerdan MS, Provost TT, Alexander GE. Primary Sjogren's syndrome with central nervous system disease mimicking multiple sclerosis. Ann Intern Med. 1986;104(3):323–30.
208. Shiboski CH, Shiboski SC, Seror R, Criswell LA, Labetoulle M, Lietman TM, et al. 2016 American College of Rheumatology/European League Against Rheumatism classification

criteria for primary Sjogren's syndrome: a consensus and data-driven methodology involving three international patient cohorts. Ann Rheum Dis. 2017;76(1):9–16.
209. Seror R, Ravaud P, Mariette X, Bootsma H, Theander E, Hansen A, et al. EULAR Sjogren's Syndrome Patient Reported Index (ESSPRI): development of a consensus patient index for primary Sjogren's syndrome. Ann Rheum Dis. 2011;70(6):968–72.
210. Annunziata P, De Santi L, Di Rezze S, Millefiorini E, Capello E, Mancardi G, et al. Clinical features of Sjogren's syndrome in patients with multiple sclerosis. Acta Neurol Scand. 2011;124(2):109–14.
211. Flachenecker P, Reiners K, Krauser M, Wolf A, Toyka KV. Autonomic dysfunction in multiple sclerosis is related to disease activity and progression of disability. Mult Scler. 2001;7(5):327–34.
212. Prasad CB, Kopp CR, Naidu G, Sharma V, Misra DP, Agarwal V, et al. Overlap syndrome of anti-aquaporin 4 positive neuromyelitis optica spectrum disorder and primary Sjogren's syndrome: a systematic review of individual patient data. Rheumatol Int. 2023;44:2807.
213. Ramos-Casals M, Brito-Zeron P, Bombardieri S, Bootsma H, De Vita S, Dorner T, et al. EULAR recommendations for the management of Sjogren's syndrome with topical and systemic therapies. Ann Rheum Dis. 2020;79(1):3–18.
214. Singh AG, Singh S, Matteson EL. Rate, risk factors and causes of mortality in patients with Sjogren's syndrome: a systematic review and meta-analysis of cohort studies. Rheumatology (Oxford). 2016;55(3):450–60.
215. Carubbi F, Alunno A, Cipriani P, Bartoloni E, Baldini C, Quartuccio L, et al. A retrospective, multicenter study evaluating the prognostic value of minor salivary gland histology in a large cohort of patients with primary Sjogren's syndrome. Lupus. 2015;24(3):315–20.
216. Kleffner I, Dorr J, Ringelstein M, Gross CC, Bockenfeld Y, Schwindt W, et al. Diagnostic criteria for Susac syndrome. J Neurol Neurosurg Psychiatry. 2016;87(12):1287–95.
217. Dorr J, Krautwald S, Wildemann B, Jarius S, Ringelstein M, Duning T, et al. Characteristics of Susac syndrome: a review of all reported cases. Nat Rev Neurol. 2013;9(6):307–16.
218. Seifert-Held T, Langner-Wegscheider BJ, Komposch M, Simschitz P, Franta C, Teuchner B, et al. Susac's syndrome: clinical course and epidemiology in a Central European population. Int J Neurosci. 2017;127(9):776–80.
219. Susac JO. Susac's syndrome: the triad of microangiopathy of the brain and retina with hearing loss in young women. Neurology. 1994;44(4):591–3.
220. Susac JO, Hardman JM, Selhorst JB. Microangiopathy of the brain and retina. Neurology. 1979;29(3):313–6.
221. Hardy TA, O'Brien B, Gerbis N, Barnett MH, Reddel SW, Brewer J, et al. Brain histopathology in three cases of Susac's syndrome: implications for lesion pathogenesis and treatment. J Neurol Neurosurg Psychiatry. 2015;86(5):582–4.
222. Kleffner I, Duning T, Lohmann H, Deppe M, Basel T, Promesberger J, et al. A brief review of Susac syndrome. J Neurol Sci. 2012;322(1–2):35–40.
223. Sauma J, Rivera D, Wu A, Donate-Lopez J, Gallego-Pinazo R, Chilov M, et al. Susac's syndrome: an update. Br J Ophthalmol. 2020;104(9):1190–5.
224. Buzzard KA, Reddel SW, Yiannikas C, Sean Riminton D, Barnett MH, Hardy TA. Distinguishing Susac's syndrome from multiple sclerosis. J Neurol. 2015;262(7):1613–21.
225. Triplett JD, Qiu J, O'Brien B, Gopinath S, Trewin B, Spring PJ, et al. Diagnosis, differential diagnosis and misdiagnosis of Susac syndrome. Eur J Neurol. 2022;29(6):1771–81.
226. Egan RA, Hills WL, Susac JO. Gass plaques and fluorescein leakage in Susac syndrome. J Neurol Sci. 2010;299(1–2):97–100.
227. Papasavvas I, Teuchner B, Herbort CP Jr. Susac syndrome (Retino-cochleo-cerebral vasculitis), the ophthalmologist in the role of the whistleblower. J Ophthalmic Inflamm Infect. 2020;10(1):27.
228. Rennebohm R, Susac JO, Egan RA, Daroff RB. Susac's syndrome—update. J Neurol Sci. 2010;299(1–2):86–91.
229. Susac JO, Murtagh FR, Egan RA, Berger JR, Bakshi R, Lincoff N, et al. MRI findings in Susac's syndrome. Neurology. 2003;61(12):1783–7.

230. Hua le H, Donlon SL, Okuda DT. A case of Susac syndrome with cervical spinal cord involvement on MRI. J Neurol Sci. 2014;337(1–2):228–31.
231. Ringelstein M, Albrecht P, Kleffner I, Buhn B, Harmel J, Muller AK, et al. Retinal pathology in Susac syndrome detected by spectral-domain optical coherence tomography. Neurology. 2015;85(7):610–8.
232. Rennebohm RM, Susac JO. Treatment of Susac's syndrome. J Neurol Sci. 2007;257(1–2):215–20.
233. Laird PW, Newman NJ, Yeh S. Exacerbation of Susac syndrome retinopathy by interferon Beta-1a. Arch Ophthalmol. 2012;130(6):804–6.
234. Shields RA, Kleinman RA, Smith SJ, Sanislo SR, Nguyen QD. A fatal case of Susac syndrome: the importance of ophthalmic examination in confirming the diagnosis. Am J Ophthalmol Case Rep. 2018;12:18–20.
235. Andour H, Rostoum S, Regragui Y, Fikri M, Jiddane M, Touarsa F. Fulminant Susac syndrome-a rare cause of coma: the history of the fatal course in a young man. SAGE Open Med Case Rep. 2023;11:2050313x221149826.
236. Lim SS, Drenkard C, McCune WJ, Helmick CG, Gordon C, Deguire P, et al. Population-based lupus registries: advancing our epidemiologic understanding. Arthritis Rheum. 2009;61(10):1462–6.
237. The American College of Rheumatology nomenclature and case definitions for neuropsychiatric lupus syndromes. Arthritis Rheum. 1999;42(4):599–608.
238. Vivaldo JF, de Amorim JC, Julio PR, de Oliveira RJ, Appenzeller S. Definition of NPSLE: does the ACR nomenclature still hold? Front Med (Lausanne). 2018;5:138.
239. Hanly JG. Avoiding diagnostic pitfalls in neuropsychiatric lupus: the importance of attribution. Lupus. 2017;26(5):497–503.
240. Piga M, Chessa E, Peltz MT, Floris A, Mathieu A, Cauli A. Demyelinating syndrome in SLE encompasses different subtypes: do we need new classification criteria? Pooled results from systematic literature review and monocentric cohort analysis. Autoimmun Rev. 2017;16(3):244–52.
241. Dorner T, Furie R. Novel paradigms in systemic lupus erythematosus. Lancet. 2019;393(10188):2344–58.
242. Crow MK. Pathogenesis of systemic lupus erythematosus: risks, mechanisms and therapeutic targets. Ann Rheum Dis. 2023;82(8):999–1014.
243. Popescu A, Kao AH. Neuropsychiatric systemic lupus erythematosus. Curr Neuropharmacol. 2011;9(3):449–57.
244. Sarwar S, Mohamed AS, Rogers S, Sarmast ST, Kataria S, Mohamed KH, et al. Neuropsychiatric systemic lupus erythematosus: a 2021 update on diagnosis, management, and current challenges. Cureus. 2021;13(9):e17969.
245. Magro Checa C, Cohen D, Bollen EL, van Buchem MA, Huizinga TW, Steup-Beekman GM. Demyelinating disease in SLE: is it multiple sclerosis or lupus? Best Pract Res Clin Rheumatol. 2013;27(3):405–24.
246. Ropper AH, Poskanzer DC. The prognosis of acute and subacute transverse myelopathy based on early signs and symptoms. Ann Neurol. 1978;4(1):51–9.
247. Li XY, Xiao HB, Pai P. Myelitis in systemic lupus erythematosus. J Clin Neurosci. 2017;44:18–22.
248. Nikolopoulos D, Kitsos D, Papathanasiou M, Kapsala N, Garantziotis P, Pieta A, et al. Demyelinating syndromes in systemic lupus erythematosus: data from the "Attikon" lupus cohort. Front Neurol. 2022;13:889613.
249. de Andrade FA, Guimaraes Moreira Balbi G, Bortoloti de Azevedo LG, Provenzano Sa G, de Moraes V, Junior H, Mendes Klumb E, et al. Neuro-ophthalmologic manifestations in systemic lupus erythematosus. Lupus. 2017;26(5):522–8.
250. Siatkowski RM, Scott IU, Verm AM, Warn AA, Farris BK, Strominger MB, et al. Optic neuropathy and chiasmopathy in the diagnosis of systemic lupus erythematosus. J Neuroophthalmol. 2001;21(3):193–8.

251. Solomon AJ, Arrambide G, Brownlee WJ, Flanagan EP, Amato MP, Amezcua L, et al. Differential diagnosis of suspected multiple sclerosis: an updated consensus approach. Lancet Neurol. 2023;22(8):750–68.
252. Bertsias G, Ioannidis JP, Boletis J, Bombardieri S, Cervera R, Dostal C, et al. EULAR recommendations for the management of systemic lupus erythematosus. Report of a Task Force of the EULAR Standing Committee for International Clinical Studies Including Therapeutics. Ann Rheum Dis. 2008;67(2):195–205.
253. Theodoridou A, Settas L. Demyelination in rheumatic diseases. J Neurol Neurosurg Psychiatry. 2006;77(3):290–5.
254. Chessa E, Piga M, Floris A, Mathieu A, Cauli A. Demyelinating syndrome in SLE: review of different disease subtypes and report of a case series. Reumatismo. 2017;69(4):175–83.
255. Wingerchuk DM, Banwell B, Bennett JL, Cabre P, Carroll W, Chitnis T, et al. International consensus diagnostic criteria for neuromyelitis optica spectrum disorders. Neurology. 2015;85(2):177–89.
256. Wingerchuk DM, Lennon VA, Pittock SJ, Lucchinetti CF, Weinshenker BG. Revised diagnostic criteria for neuromyelitis optica. Neurology. 2006;66(10):1485–9.
257. Fanouriakis A, Mastorodemos V, Pamfil C, Papadaki E, Sidiropoulos P, Plaitakis A, et al. Coexistence of systemic lupus erythematosus and multiple sclerosis: prevalence, clinical characteristics, and natural history. Semin Arthritis Rheum. 2014;43(6):751–8.
258. Jacome Sanchez EC, Garcia Castillo MA, Gonzalez VP, Guillen Lopez F, Correa Diaz EP. Coexistence of systemic lupus erythematosus and multiple sclerosis. A case report and literature review. Mult Scler J Exp Transl Clin. 2018;4(2):2055217318768330.
259. Aisen A, Gabrielsen T, McCune W. MR imaging of systemic lupus erythematosus involving the brain. AJR Am J Roentgenol. 1985;144(5):1027–31.
260. Yeoh H, Lee JY, Lee YJ, Park DW, Kim TY, Ahn GY, et al. Relationship between cerebral microbleeds and white matter MR hyperintensities in systemic lupus erythematosus: a retrospective observational study. Neuroradiology. 2019;61(3):265–74.
261. Birnbaum J, Petri M, Thompson R, Izbudak I, Kerr D. Distinct subtypes of myelitis in systemic lupus erythematosus. Arthritis Rheum. 2009;60(11):3378–87.
262. Kim SS, Richman DP, Johnson WO, Hald JK, Agius MA. Limited utility of current MRI criteria for distinguishing multiple sclerosis from common mimickers: primary and secondary CNS vasculitis, lupus and Sjogren's syndrome. Mult Scler. 2014;20(1):57–63.
263. McLean BN, Miller D, Thompson EJ. Oligoclonal banding of IgG in CSF, blood-brain barrier function, and MRI findings in patients with sarcoidosis, systemic lupus erythematosus, and Behcet's disease involving the nervous system. J Neurol Neurosurg Psychiatry. 1995;58(5):548–54.
264. Aringer M. EULAR/ACR classification criteria for SLE. Semin Arthritis Rheum. 2019;49(3S):S14–S7.
265. Bertsias GK, Ioannidis JP, Aringer M, Bollen E, Bombardieri S, Bruce IN, et al. EULAR recommendations for the management of systemic lupus erythematosus with neuropsychiatric manifestations: report of a task force of the EULAR standing committee for clinical affairs. Ann Rheum Dis. 2010;69(12):2074–82.
266. Miller DH, Weinshenker BG, Filippi M, Banwell BL, Cohen JA, Freedman MS, et al. Differential diagnosis of suspected multiple sclerosis: a consensus approach. Mult Scler. 2008;14(9):1157–74.
267. Miller TM. Differential diagnosis of myotonic disorders. Muscle Nerve. 2008;37(3):293–9.
268. Tektonidou MG, Lewandowski LB, Hu J, Dasgupta A, Ward MM. Survival in adults and children with systemic lupus erythematosus: a systematic review and Bayesian meta-analysis of studies from 1950 to 2016. Ann Rheum Dis. 2017;76(12):2009–16.
269. Mignarri A, Dotti MT, Battisti C, Vallone I, Federico A. Occurrence of ankylosing spondylitis and multiple sclerosis-like syndrome in a HLA-B27 positive patient. Neurol Sci. 2009;30(4):329–32.

270. Cellerini M, Gabbrielli S, Bongi SM. Cerebral magnetic resonance imaging in a patient with ankylosing spondylitis and multiple sclerosis-like syndrome. Neuroradiology. 2001;43(12):1067–9.
271. Tan FU, Tellioğlu S, Aydin G, Erdemoğlu AK, Keleş I. Ankylosing spondylitis and multiple sclerosis in an HLA-B27 negative patient. Acta Neurol Belg. 2004;104(4):169–72.
272. Jeon CH. Relapsing polychondritis with central nervous system involvement: experience of three different cases in a single center. J Korean Med Sci. 2016;31(11):1846–50.
273. Borgia F, Giuffrida R, Guarneri F, Cannavo SP. Relapsing polychondritis: an updated review. Biomedicines. 2018;6:3.
274. Wu S, Xu Z, Liang H. Sneddon's syndrome: a comprehensive review of the literature. Orphanet J Rare Dis. 2014;9:215.
275. Amaral TN, Peres FA, Lapa AT, Marques-Neto JF, Appenzeller S. Neurologic involvement in scleroderma: a systematic review. Semin Arthritis Rheum. 2013;43(3):335–47.
276. Bucak E, Konen FF, Seeliger T, Jendretzky KF, Nay S, Grote-Levi L, et al. Comorbid Sjögren's disease in Multiple Sclerosis (Poster P615). ECTRIMS 2025; Barcelona.

5 Infectious Diseases

5.1 Brain Abscess

5.1.1 Epidemiology

- Incidence 0.4–0.9/100.000/year [1].

5.1.2 Etiology and Definition

- Caused by bacteria, mycobacteria, fungi, or parasites.
- Most common in patients with immunosuppression; disruption of the natural protective barriers surrounding the brain (surgery, trauma, mastoiditis, sinusitis, or dental infection); a systemic source of infection, especially in patients with underlying cardiac or pulmonary disease (e.g., arteriovenous fistulas).
- For example, fungi are responsible for 90% of brain abscess cases among solid-organ transplant recipients [2, 3].
- Bacteria may enter the brain through:
  - 50% contiguous spread
  - 30% hematogenous dissemination
  - 20% unknown mechanisms [3]
- At the beginning occurs early cerebritis (focal infection without a capsule or pus formation) with an inflammatory response, including edema. It resolves or progresses into the formation of a capsule (around 10 days after infection), characterized by the accumulation of fibroblasts and vascularization [4].

T. Uher, *Mimics and Red Flags of Multiple Sclerosis*,
https://doi.org/10.1007/978-3-031-98945-2_5

5.1.3 Clinical Features

- Typically include headache, fever, focal neurological deficits, psychiatric symptoms, or seizures. Consciousness is often not altered.
- The abscess may progress rapidly and unexpectedly, irrespective of the initial level of disease severity [3, 4].

5.1.4 Brain Imaging

- Lesions' location:
  - Variable
- Lesions' appearance:
  - Fluid-attenuated inversion recovery (FLAIR) and T2-weighted magnetic resonance images (MRI):
    Hyperintense necrotic center with pus.
    Hyperintense zone of (vasogenic) edema surrounding the abscess.
    Relatively hypo-intense rim (capsule of the abscesses). The rim is usually smooth and complete (in glioblastoma is usually irregular and incomplete).
  - T1-weighted MRI:
    Hypo-intense necrotic center with pus and a hypo-intense zone of edema surrounding the abscess.
    The capsule is relatively hyperintense [4–7].
  - Diffusion-weighted imaging (DWI):
    Offer valuable assistance in differential diagnosis [5].
    Centrally restricted diffusion with a markedly decreased signal on apparent diffusion coefficient (ADC) maps [4].
    Necrotic or cystic brain tumors typically exhibit a converse pattern with a hypo-intense signal on DWI [8]. Nevertheless, necrotic metastases may occasionally demonstrate restricted diffusion as well [9]. Smoother inner wall, satellite lesions, and occurrence of low-intensity capsule may favor abscess before brain tumor [10].
    Some immunocompromised patients with abscesses may occasionally not exhibit restricted diffusion [11].
  - Susceptibility-weighted imaging (SWI):
    "Dual rim" consists of two concentric rims around the abscess: hyperintense inner layer and hypo-intense outer layer surrounding the central cavity (75%), which may help in distinguishing an abscess from a glioblastoma.
    Also visible on T2 images [6, 7]
- Contrast enhancement:
  - Diffuse enhancement at the stage of cerebritis
  - Later (>10 days) thin (open or closed) ring-shaped enhancement of the abscess wall (continuous component on the ventricular side), but no central enhancement [4, 6, 7].
- Perilesional changes:
  - Edema and mass effect [4–7] (Fig. 5.1).

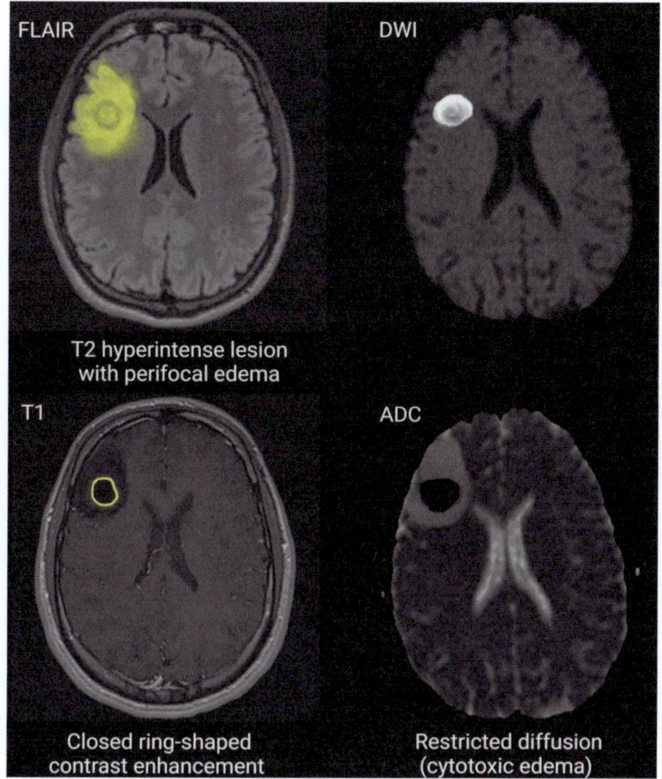

Fig. 5.1 MRI characteristics of a brain abscess

5.1.5 Blood Work

- Unspecific elevation of inflammatory markers may be present [12].

5.1.6 Examination of CSF

- Elevated concentration of protein and pleocytosis (>90%).
- Inflammatory patterns and positive cultures are notably prevalent, especially in individuals with coexisting meningitis (6–22%) [13].
- Data about cerebrospinal fluid (CSF)-restricted oligoclonal bands (OCB) are not available.
- Lumbar puncture should only be performed if meningitis is suspectted or if there is a concern about abscess rupture into the ventricular system. Spinal tap can be performed only in patients who do not have contraindications for this procedure [4].

5.1.7 Diagnosis

- Based on neurological manifestations and imaging.
- Almost any brain abscess with a diameter of at least 1 cm is amenable to stereotactic aspiration, regardless of location in the brain. The aspiration can be needed for the identification of the causative pathogen [4].

5.1.8 Differential Diagnosis

- The differential diagnosis includes primary and secondary metastatic brain tumors, demyelination, bacterial meningitis, epidural abscess, and subdural empyema, or central nervous system (CNS) lymphoma [4].

5.1.9 Treatment and Prognosis

- Antimicrobial therapy should be started already when there is a suspicion of a brain abscess because a treatment delay is associated with worse outcomes.
- Corticosteroids should be reserved only for patients with massive brain edema (utilized in 50% of cases) since they may impede the transport of antimicrobial agents across the blood–brain barrier.
- Anticonvulsants are usually not indicated if patients do not have epilepsy.
- Abscess rupture into the ventricular system results in ventriculitis, often leading to a subsequent hydrocephalus, and is associated with high mortality (27–85%).
- Most patients experience a favorable outcome, with either no or minimal sequelae (70%), but approximately 15% of patients die [3, 4].

5.2 Brucellosis

5.2.1 Synonyms

- Undulant fever; Mediterranean fever; Malta fever [14].

5.2.2 Epidemiology

- Incidence 500.000/worldwide/year [15, 16].
- Occurs globally, but is most common in the Mediterranean basin (Portugal, Spain, Southern France, Italy, Greece, Turkey, and North Africa), Arabian Peninsula, India, and central and southern America [17].

5.2.3 Etiology and Definition

- Zoonotic infection caused by the aerobic bacteria genus Brucella.
- Usually transmitted by eating or drinking unpasteurized or raw dairy products (where Brucella can survive up to 3 months); by eating undercooked meat; contamination via wounds through contact with infected animals; inhalation, or rarely by direct person-to-person spread (via sexual contact, tissue transplantation, or blood transfusion).
- Suggested pathophysiological mechanisms of neurobrucellosis include direct neuropathic effect of bacteria; deleterious cytokine or endotoxin release; and an immunopathologic host reaction to Brucella within organ systems [14, 16, 18].

5.2.4 Disease Course

- Distinguished two phases of brucellosis:
  - The acute phase, which begins 2–4 weeks after incubation period and presents with unspecific symptoms such as fever, fatigue, weight loss, sweats malaise, anorexia, headaches, muscle aches, and arthralgia.
  - Chronic phase includes neurological and other systemic manifestations, which may occur months to years after infection onset.
- Distinguished three phases of neurobrucellosis:
  - Acute meningitis or meningo-encephalitis
  - Chronic peripheral form (radiculopathy)
  - Chronic CNS infection (meningo-encephalitis, myelitis, cerebellar involvement, cranial nerve palsies) [16, 19, 20].

5.2.5 Systemic Clinical Features

- Multisystem disease involving organ systems such as musculoskeletal, nervous, hematologic, cardiopulmonary, or genitourinary [14, 17].

5.2.6 Neurological Features

- Neurobrucellosis occurs in 4–7% of patients with brucellosis; can be the only manifestation of brucellosis; and may present without any systemic features.
- Meningitis/meningo-encephalitis (37%).
  - Most often, complication
  - Acute, chronic, or recurrent
  - May be associated with intracranial hypertension, encephalopathy, headache, altered consciousness, meningism

- Cranial neuropathies
  - Vestibulocochlear nerve pathology is the most frequent and commonly associated with sensorineural hearing loss
  - Sixth and seventh cranial nerves are less frequent
  - Optic neuropathy or optic disc edema simulating optic neuritis in MS
- Vascular complications including sinus thrombosis, aneurysms, ischemic strokes, or subarachnoid hemorrhages.
- Seizures
- Cognitive decline and behavioral changes
- Progressive myelitis
- PNS involvement (7% of cases with neurological complications).
  - Acute, subacute, or chronic polyradiculoneuropathies (often proximally dominant); may mimic Guillain–Barré syndrome
  - Peripheral neuropathy [18, 19, 21, 22].

5.2.7 Brain Imaging

- Normal (55%) or pathological findings (45%), including:
- Leptomeningeal enhancement
- Non-specific periventricular and subcortical white matter
  - Sometimes diffuse, leukoencephalopathy-like lesions
  - Rarely brainstem lesions
  - May mimic findings observed in multiple sclerosis (MS)
- Cranial nerve involvement
- Brain abscesses and granulomas [16, 19, 23–26].

5.2.8 Spinal Cord Imaging

- Focal myelitis or longitudinally extensive transverse myelitis (LETM) with or without contrast enhancement.
- Nerve root enhancement
- Typical vertebral endplates and sacroiliac joints involvement (spondylitis).
- Intramedullary or paravertebral abscesses [23, 24].

5.2.9 Blood Work

- Routine tests are normal or show mildly elevated C-reactive protein (CRP) and/or erythrocyte sedimentation rate (ESR) [19].

5.2.10 Examination of CSF

- Low glucose and elevated concentration of protein (median 0.83 g/L). However, severe hyperproteinorrhachia and severe hypoglycorrhachia are rare and may indicate rather tuberculosis.
- Lymphocytic pleocytosis (median 75 cells/mm^3)
- Typically, corresponding OCB in serum and CSF (pattern IV) [19, 20, 27].

5.2.11 Diagnosis

- Bacterial isolation is the gold standard, but the sensitivity is low (10–30%).
- In the absence of a positive culture, the diagnosis relies on:
  - Serum agglutination testing:
    Detects antibodies to Brucella species
    Cross-reactivity with Yersinia, vibrio cholera, and E. coli
    Positive in patients with previous brucellosis infection, thus positive results cannot distinguish from active infection
  - Enzyme-linked immunosorbent assay (ELISA) (Brucellacapt) in serum and CSF
  - Polymerase chain reaction (PCR) or CSF metagenomic next-generation sequencing (mNGS)
- Diagnosis requires the presence of all four criteria:
  - Symptoms and signs suggestive of neurobrucellosis not explained by other neurological diseases
  - Positive CSF culture for Brucella or positive Brucella immunoglobulin G (IgG) agglutination titer in the blood
  - Lymphocytic pleocytosis and elevated concertation of protein in CSF
  - An effect of antibiotics [19].

5.2.12 Differential Diagnosis

- Can mimic any systemic disease; therefore is often misdiagnosed or diagnosed with significant delay (2–12 months after symptom onset) [19].
- Frequent mimickers of neurobrucellosis include:
  - MS [25, 26, 28, 29].
  - Chronic meningitis in tuberculosis or neurocryptococcosis
  - Processes with a skull base predominance (tuberculosis or sarcoidosis) [19].

5.2.13 Treatment and Prognosis

- There is no consensus on the choice of antibiotic, dose, and duration of antimicrobial treatment. Usually used combination of three different antibiotics over 3 to 6 months. Patients must be followed up regularly due to the risk of relapse, which occurs in 5–15% of patients.

- Corticosteroids may have a positive effect.
- Mortality rate in the post-antibiotic era is low (0–5.5%).
- Permanent deafness is the most common residual deficit (20–30%) [16, 19, 30].

5.3 COVID-19

5.3.1 Etiology and Definition

- Highly contagious infection caused by the severe acute respiratory syndrome coronavirus 2 (SARS-CoV-2).
- The SARS-CoV-2 virus is primarily transmitted through inhalation of aerosols containing infectious particles.
- Neurological complications are relatively common (30%). Such complications may result from the direct effects of the virus on the nervous system, para-infectious or post-infectious immune-mediated responses, or the systemic effects of coronavirus disease 19 (COVID-19).
- COVID-19 also induces a prothrombotic state.

5.3.2 Respiratory Disease

- Acute upper and/or lower respiratory tract infection accompanied by constitutional symptoms.
- Chest X-rays or computed tomography (CT) scans may show ground-glass opacities and consolidations with a bilateral and peripheral distribution.
- Laboratory findings often include lymphopenia and mild elevations in inflammatory markers in the blood.

5.3.3 Neurological Involvement

- The most often complications include olfactory deficits, muscle weakness, and muscle damage.
- Long-COVID-19
  - Associated with fatigue, muscle weakness, headache, cognitive impairment, and brain fog.
- Encephalitis
  - Rare conditions that develop over hours to days.
  - Neurological manifestations may include headache, fever, seizures, meningism, encephalopathy, decreased consciousness, and focal deficits.
  - Brain MRI findings are either normal or show nonspecific changes, such as parenchymal lesions, leptomeningeal enhancement, micro-hemorrhages, edema, or acute necrotizing encephalopathy.
  - Brain lesions can extend into the spinal cord.
  - Electroencephalography (EEG) findings are often abnormal.

  - CSF analysis may be normal or show pleocytosis. Protein concentration may be elevated, and matched OCB may be detected. The presence of SARS-CoV-2 in CSF without accompanying clinical and/or radiological manifestations is insufficient to diagnose COVID-19-associated encephalitis.
  - Antiviral therapy and, in some cases, corticosteroids may be beneficial.
- Acute disseminated encephalomyelitis (ADEM)
  - Typically occurs weeks after an infection and is considered a post-infectious disease.
  - Clinical manifestations are similar to encephalitis.
  - Imaging shows confluent white matter lesions in the brain and sometimes also in the spinal cord (but isolated myelitis is extremely rare).
  - CSF findings are similar to those in encephalitis, with normal cytology or, less frequently, pleocytosis.
  - Treatment includes corticosteroids, intravenous immunoglobulin, and plasmapheresis.
  - If the virus is detected in the CSF, immunosuppressive treatment must be administered with caution, and antiviral therapy should be considered.
- Cerebrovascular disease
  - Symptoms typically begin around 10 days after the respiratory illness.
  - More common in patients with pre-existing risk factors for cerebrovascular disease.
  - COVID-19 is associated with a prothrombotic state.
- Neurodegenerative and autoimmune CNS diseases
  - Some studies suggest an association between COVID-19 infection and an increased risk of developing Parkinson's disease and Alzheimer's disease.
- Guillain-Barré syndrome (and Miller Fisher variant or other neuropathies)
  - Symptoms usually onset 7–24 days after the respiratory illness.
  - CSF shows normal cytology with elevated concentration of protein.
  - Electromyography (EMG) and nerve conduction studies show acute inflammatory demyelinating polyneuropathy (AIDP).
  - Brain MRI is normal; however, spinal cord imaging may reveal contrast enhancement of the caudal nerve roots.
- Muscular damage

5.3.4 Diagnosis

- PCR, which confirms the presence of SARS-CoV-2 ribonucleic acid (RNA).

5.3.5 Differential Diagnosis:

- A history of recent COVID-19 infection in patients with ADEM or myelitis should raise suspicion of a link to the infection.
- In patients with MS, COVID-19 infection may be associated with accelerated brain atrophy.

5.3.6 Treatment and Prevention

- Antiviral drugs, symptomatic treatment, monoclonal antibodies, and vaccination [31–37].

5.4 Epstein–Barr Virus (EBV)

5.4.1 Etiology

- A relatively benign, long-term, latent infection in the resting memory B cells.
- Over 90% of the population in adulthood has been infected.
- The EBV infection increases risk for certain cancers and autoimmune disorders, including MS, through mechanisms that are incompletely understood.
- EBV-associated neurological symptomatic complications are almost always the result reactivation of latent virus in the setting of severe immunosuppression (often after solid-organ transplantation and hematopoietic stem cell transplantation), and only rarely occur in immunocompetent individuals.

5.4.2 Non-neurological Features of Acute Infection

- Fever, malaise, lymphadenopathy, pharyngitis, upper respiratory symptoms, headache, or diarrhea.

5.4.3 Neurological Clinical, Imaging, and Laboratory Features

- Rare (0.5–7.5%), but their spectrum is wide.
- Symptoms onset is typically 1–3 weeks after the onset of respiratory symptoms, but occasionally much later.
- Most often are EBV-associated meningitis and encephalitis.
- Aseptic meningitis
  - In immunocompetent patients probably frequent, but almost always self-limiting condition with headache, stiff neck, and fewer. In immunosuppressed patients, the course is often progressive.
- Encephalitis
  - Focal neurological deficit, seizures, encephalopathy.
  - Resembles herpes simplex virus (HSV)-associated encephalitis and may occur even in the absence of systemic manifestations of EBV infection.
  - Brain MRI often normal or with symmetric T2 hyperintensities in deep gray matter (basal ganglia, thalamus), brainstem, cerebellum, corpus callosum, limbic cortex, optic nerves, or spinal cord.
  - MRI lesions may occasionally show contrast enhancement, edema, and restricted diffusion.

  - Antiviral treatment is typically associated with a complete resolution of imaging abnormalities.
  - CSF shows pleocytosis, mildly elevated protein, atypical lymphocytes, CSF-restricted OCB, and antibodies to EBV viral capsid antigen (VCA)
  - Often difficult to diagnose, therefore often underdiagnosed.
  - Together with human herpesvirus 6 (HHV-6), might be involved in the pathogenesis of Rasmussen's encephalitis.
- Psychiatric syndromes
  - Alice in Wonderland syndrome with distortions in the orientation, shape, and size of objects (dysmetropsia), body image disturbance (aschematia), and the tendency for linear objects to appear curvy (metamorphosia). Usually, self-limiting condition with a good prognosis and duration ranging from days to 3 months.
  - Acute psychosis
- ADEM
  - Associated with infectious mononucleosis or EBV reactivation.
- Acute cerebellitis with ataxia
- Brain hemorrhage
- Cranial neuropathy
- Myelitis
  - Rare
  - May present as longitudinally extensive transverse myelitis (LETM)
  - CSF shows lymphocytic pleocytosis and elevated protein
  - High-dose corticosteroids are effective
- Peripheral neuropathy
  - Mononeuritis multiplex, brachial plexopathy, or Guillain–Barré syndrome

5.4.4 Diagnosis

- Acute EBV infection:
  - A positive serum EBV-specific IgM and IgG to the viral capsid antigen (VCA IgG, IgM) and a positive IgG to the early antigen (EA IgG), but a negative IgG to the nuclear antigen (EBNA IgG).
  - A rise in IgG level, the disappearance of VCA-IgM and EA IgG, and the appearance of EBNA IgG at the follow-up support a diagnosis of acute infection.
- No established diagnostic criteria of EBV-associated CNS infections.
- Although, diagnosis may be supported by positive serology in CSF and PCR for EBV DNA in CSF, there are some challenges.
  - EBV DNA might be sometime detected also in healthy people.
  - Positive PCR for EBV DNA may be caused by co-infection, when EBV may be reactivated secondary to inflammatory responses from other pathogens.
  - The presence of EBV may be caused by contamination from EBV-infected lymphocytes.
- Although, direct isolation of the virus in brain biopsy or culture may also support the diagnosis, it is usually not used.

5.4.5 Treatment

- There are no guidelines, only case reports of using ganciclovir and acyclovir with or without corticosteroids.
- Prognosis is good, usually without residual deficit (85%) [38–43].

5.5 Hepatitis C (HCV)

5.5.1 Epidemiology

- Prevalence 2800/100.000 (globally) [44].

5.5.2 Etiology

- Caused by hepatitis C virus; RNA virus.
- The mechanisms underlying the association between HCV infection and extrahepatic manifestations are not yet fully understood and include:
  A. Neuroinvasion and direct damage: Peripheral blood mononuclear cells can mediate the entry of HCV into the CNS through the blood-brain barrier and infect the brain microvascular endothelial cells.
  B. Glial activation and macrophage infiltration: Some complications are driven by the proliferation of B lymphocytes with monoclonal and polyclonal production of antibodies, with the activity of the rheumatoid factor or cryoglobulins. Cryoglobulins are immunoglobulins able to clump together at temperatures below 37 °C and cause organ damage through either vascular sludging (Hyperviscosity syndrome, associated) or immune-mediated (Vasculitis). HCV infection causes an increase in cryoglobulin production by B lymphocytes clones followed by the precipitation of immune complexes and HCV-associated cryoglobulinemic vasculitis affecting medium and small blood vessels with transmural fibrinoid necrosis, thrombotic lumen occlusion, and infiltration of polymorphonuclear cells. The vasculitis is associated with ischemic tissue damage. Cryoglobulinemia may be caused also by other infections, autoimmune disorders, or malignancies [45, 46].
- The presence of HCV in an extrahepatic and immune-privileged site could be a potential source of late relapse after antiviral therapy. Therefore, inactive and treated HCV infection may be associated with HCV-associated inflammatory complications [47].

5.5.3 Hepatic Clinical Features

- Severe acute and chronic hepatitis.
- If left untreated, it leads to chronic active hepatitis (80%), cirrhosis, and hepatocellular carcinoma.

5.5.4 Extrahepatic Non-neurological Clinical Features

- HCV is considered as a systemic disease associated with a wide range of extrahepatic complications (>30 types). They may include insulin resistance and type 2 diabetes, ophthalmological, renal, gastrointestinal, thyroid, cardiovascular, joint, and skin manifestations.
- May prevail over hepatic symptoms or aggravate them.
- Cryoglobulinemia is frequent (30% of patients) and might be asymptomatic (20%) or symptomatic (10%), sometimes associated with severe systemic vasculitis.

5.5.5 Neurological Clinical Features and Imaging

- Wide range of complication affecting major proportion of infected patients without cirrhosis (50%).
- Do not correlate with severity of liver disease or viral replication rate.
- Acute or subacute encephalopathy.
  - Often due to ischemic damage associated with vasculitis.
- Cerebrovascular events
  - Ischemic stroke, lacunar syndrome, and rarely hemorrhages
  - Rarely represent the initial clinical manifestation of HCV infection
- Leukoencephalitis, encephalomyelitis, and ADEM
  - Immune-mediated mechanism, rather than direct CNS damage
  - Perivascular infiltrates of T lymphocytes and microglia nodules corresponding with CNS vasculitis
  - Encephalopathy, focal neurological deficit, seizures
- Cognitive and psychiatric manifestations.
  - Present in 50% of patients with chronic infection
  - Anxiety, depression, and fatigue
  - Cognitive impairments frequently occur before the development of cirrhosis and are independent of liver function or viral load.
  - Hepatic encephalopathy in patients with liver cirrhosis of different etiologies is caused by severe hepatocellular damage or porto-systemic shunts [45, 47, 48].
- Optic neuritis.
- Partial or transverse myelitis.
  - Not frequent, but probably underreported complication
  - Hypothesized antibody-mediated autoimmune demyelination, rather than direct CNS damage, which is supported by the presence of anti-HCV antibodies in CSF, but not always also the viral RNA. However, a combination of both mechanisms is possible.
  - Short lesions or longitudinally extensive transverse myelitis (LETM) with or without contrast enhancement. Sometime only the cases of partial myelitis often involving dorsal and lateral parts of the cord.
  - Frequently corticosteroids-responsive relapsing-remitting pattern of myelitis mimicking MS or neuromyelitis optica spectrum disorders (NMOSD).

  - Case studies of anti-aquaporin-4 (AQP4) IgG and HCV positive patients with LETM
  - Patients with myelitis may have normal brain MRI.
  - Hepatitis viruses should be considered in differential diagnosis of myelitis of unknown etiology [45, 49–57] (Fig. 5.2).
- Peripheral neuropathy (40–75%)
  - Sensory predominant symmetrical polyneuropathy, mononeuritis multiplex, or asymmetrical sensory neuropathy (with affected large or small fibers).
  - Less demyelinating polyneuropathy or poly-radiculonephropathy.
  - Pure motor neuropathies and autonomic neuropathies are rare.
  - In general, peripheral involvement is more frequent and severe in patients with cryoglobulinemia, affecting periphery in more than 60%, whereas CNS involvement occurs in only 6%.
  - Pathogenesis is indirect (inflammatory) because the virus itself does not invade the nerves and muscles.
  - Rarely HCV-associated monoclonal gammopathy of undetermined significance (MGUS)-associated anti-myelin associated glycoprotein (MAG) neuropathy [45, 48].

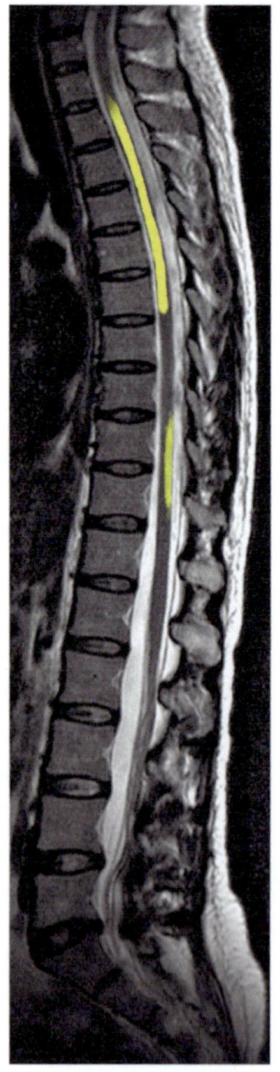

Fig. 5.2 Myelitis in hepatitis C (HCV)

5.5.6 Blood Work

- In addition to cryoglobulin, chronic HCV infection is frequently associated with positivity for antinuclear antibodies (ANA), anti-Sjogren's syndrome A (SSA)/anti-Sjogren's syndrome B (SSB) antibodies, and antineutrophil cytoplasmic antibodies (ANCA), reflecting an activation and proliferation of B lymphocytes. In these scenarios, it is required to distinguish between HCV-associated extrahepatic manifestations or a coexisting autoimmune disorder.

5.5.7 Examination of CSF

- Patients with CNS involvement have:
- Normal or mildly elevated concentration of protein and mild pleocytosis or normal cytology.
- Typically, anti-HCV antibodies are present in the CSF, but positive PCR results documenting the presence of viral RNA are rare.
- CSF-restricted OCB is usually absent [45, 47, 49, 55].

5.5.8 Diagnosis

- Confirmed through laboratory testing (ELISA and PCR).

5.5.9 Treatment and Prognosis

- Antiviral drug treatment (direct-acting antivirals) reaches sustained virological response in >95% of cases.
- Extrahepatic complications often respond to corticosteroids.
- Significant mortality and morbidity is associated with mixed cryoglobulinemia, which is treated using antiviral therapy to eliminate the viral trigger and immunosuppressive therapy (corticosteroids and anti-CD20 therapies) to inhibiting B-cell proliferation [45].

5.6 Herpes Simplex Virus (HSV) Infections

5.6.1 Epidemiology

- Infected two-thirds of the population.
- 10–20% of all viral encephalitides.
- Incidence 0.2–0.4/100.000/year.
- There is no age, sex, or seasonal predilection, but more common in immunocompromised patients [42, 58, 59].

5.6.2 Cause and Definition

- Double-stranded DNA HSV type 1 (HSV-1) and type 2 (HSV-2) transmitted through human-to-human close oral or genital contact.
- Viruses enter the CNS either by direct spread through the olfactory or trigeminal nerves or, less frequently, by hematogenous spread.
- Neurologic complications are caused by primary infection (often in young age) or by reactivation of latent disease (more frequent in older age), [42, 60]

5.6.3 Clinical Features

- Non-neurological clinical features:
  - HSV-1 mainly causes herpes labialis and HSV-2 causes genital herpes.
- HSV encephalitis
  - The most common neurologic complication of HSV-1 (<10% HSV-2)
  - More often in children and older patients
  - Seizures (32%) or refractory status epilepticus
  - Abnormal behavior (23%), confusion and/or disorientation (13%)
  - Altered consciousness (13%)
  - Fever, autonomic dysfunction, dysphagia, headache, meningeal signs
- HSV aseptic meningitis
  - Usually caused by HSV-2 infection (40% of cases have a history of genital lesions)
  - Associated with diffuse leptomeningeal enhancement or thickening
  - 20% recurrent meningitis
- HSV cranial and peripheral neuropathy
  - Rare; MRI may show nerve contrast enhancement [42, 60, 61]
- HSV myelitis and myeloradiculitis
  - Rare; occurs more frequently in immunocompromised patients
  - Usually caused by HSV-2 infection
  - Often longitudinally extensive transverse myelitis (LETM), sometimes with a corresponding dermatomal rash
  - Probably more frequent in the thoracolumbar than cervical region [61, 62].

5.6.4 Brain Imaging in HSV Encephalitis

- Lesions' location:
  - 5% of cases have a normal MRI, but majority of cases exhibit typical in pathology the medial temporal lobes (95%).
  - 55% of cases also have extratemporal involvement in the insula, cingulate, inferolateral frontal, posterior occipital, frontal, or parietal cortex.
  - 15% of cases have a pure extratemporal involvement.
  - Pathology is often bilateral, but asymmetric.
  - Brainstem and basal ganglia are typically spared, but can be also affected.

- Lesions' appearance:
  - T2 hyperintense and T1 iso- of hypo-intense lesions.
  - Often hemorrhage, necrosis, and cortical gray matter edema (Fig. 5.3)
  - Early frequently present restricted diffusion indicating cytotoxic edema (60–70%) associated with worse prognosis
- Contrast enhancement (50%)
  - Variable patterns of enhancement, including cortical gyral, leptomeningeal, diffuse, or ring-like [61, 63].

5.6.5 Spinal Cord Imaging

- Can occur lower thoracic and/or lumbosacral myelitis with cauda equina syndrome during reactivation of herpes simplex virus 2 (HSV-2) (Elsberg syndrome) with contrast enhancement and hemorrhagic necrosis on MRI [64].

5.6.6 Blood Work

- Normal

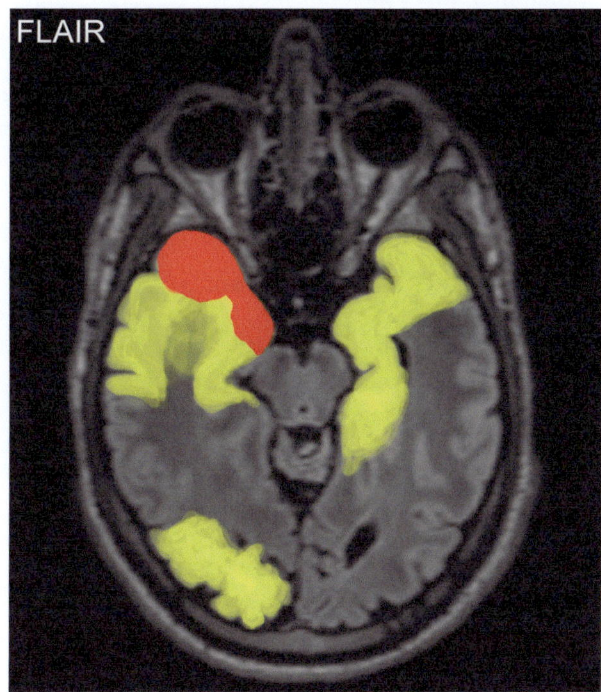

Fig. 5.3 Herpes simplex virus (HSV) encephalitis with hemorrhage, necrosis, and cortical gray matter edema

5.6.7 Examination of CSF

- Commonly elevated concentration of protein and lymphocytic pleocytosis.
- Pleocytosis in CSF may be absent in up to 26% of cases, in immunocompromised patients and healthy individuals.
- Anti-HSV antibodies typically appear later, so they cannot be used for early diagnosis [65, 66].

5.6.8 Diagnosis

- Detecting HSV-1/HSV-2 DNA through PCR (sensitivity of 96%; specificity 99%).
- The heterogeneous clinical presentations can make diagnosis challenging. Additionally, very early phases of encephalitis and immunocompromised patients may lack pleocytosis and show a false-negative PCR. Therefore, in suspected cases should be repeated CSF examination after 3–7 days [42, 60, 65].

5.6.9 Differential Diagnosis

- Asymmetric temporal lobe involvement on MRI may resemble findings seen in the infiltrative tumoral process, cerebral infarction, paraneoplastic limbic encephalopathy, systemic lupus erythematosus (SLE), Hurst hemorrhagic leukoencephalitis, Japanese encephalitis, or meningovascular syphilis. However, isolated temporal lobe involvement is rarely seen in these mimickers. They do not respond to antiviral treatments, and chronic atrophic changes (can be with calcifications) are more prominent in HSV encephalitis than in other mimicking conditions [61].

5.6.10 Treatment and Prognosis

- Intravenous acyclovir (10 mg/kg every 8 hours for 14 to 21 days).
- Acyclovir resistance should be considered in progressing patients despite antiviral treatment (occurs in 28% patients with HSV-1 infections who have undergone transplantation). In these cases, alternative antivirotics (foscarnet, brincidofovir) are recommended.
- Corticosteroids are usually not used.
- The mortality rate is high (untreated patients 70%; treated patients 5.5–11.9%).
- More than 62–87% of treated patients have residual deficit.
- Delay in diagnosis and treatment is associated with worse prognosis.
- Approximately 20% of patients develop after 2–6 weeks autoimmune N-methyl-D-aspartate receptor (NMDAR) encephalitis, which may mimic HSV encephalitis relapse [42, 60].

5.7 Human Immunodeficiency Virus (HIV)

5.7.1 Epidemiology

- People living with HIV: 39 million (worldwide).
- People acquiring HIV: 1.3 million/year.
- People dying from HIV-related causes: 613.000/year [67].
- Subtle neurological involvement (such as minor cognitive or motor disorders) is observed in approximately 20% of HIV patients, even in those treated with antiretroviral therapy [68]. However, the incidence of moderate-to-severe dementia is only 1% in 2000 [69].

5.7.2 Etiology and Definition

- HIV-1, a retrovirus, induces significant cluster of differentiation 4 (CD4) lymphocytes depletion leading to progressive immunodeficiency. Although the CD4 receptor serves as the primary target for HIV-1, the virus can also infect CD4-negative cells, such as astrocytes.
- Preferentially, HIV-1 replicates in T lymphocytes and macrophages. Following HIV infection and integration into the host-cell genome, the virus can remain latent, exerting no immediate influence on cell functions, for years [70, 71].
- HIV enters the nervous system shortly after infection, although productive CNS infection typically occurs after the onset of systemic immunosuppression. The brain may serve as a reservoir for HIV replication due to the potential hindrance posed by the blood-brain barrier against the penetration of antiretrovirals and because HIV might be sequestered within the macrophages located within the CNS [70].
- Chronic immune activation leads to the dysregulation of macrophages, causing an overproduction of pro-inflammatory cytokines and chemokines within the central and peripheral nervous system resulting in HIV-related neurological complications [70, 72].
- In summary, HIV-related neurological involvement may stem from the direct effects of HIV on the nervous system, HIV-related immune dysfunction leading to CD4 cell depletion, as well as from associated opportunistic infections and neoplasms [70, 73].

5.7.3 Clinical Features

- Cognitive dysfunction, vacuolar myelopathy, and sensory neuropathy are the most common neurological complications associated with HIV.
- Other acquired immunodeficiency syndrome (AIDS) related complications typically precede the presentation of neurological manifestations.
- Although combined antiretroviral therapy (cART) has led to a decreased incidence of neurological complications, HIV-associated neurological issues continue to contribute significantly to morbidity [70, 73].

- HIV-associated neurocognitive disorder (HAND)
  - Wide range of HIV-related cognitive dysfunctions, spanning from asymptomatic cognitive impairment to dementia.
  - Phenotype includes not only cognitive deficits (subcortical profile), but also gait disturbance, tremor, impairment of fine manual dexterity, or rapid eye movement abnormalities.
  - Particularly manifest in later stages of the disease. Despite the availability of cART, it remains relatively prevalent (40–45%).
  - Develops slowly over the course of weeks-months.
  - There is no specific marker; diagnosis is established through neuropsychological testing [74, 75].
- Vacuolar myelopathy
  - Spinal cord biopsy (autopsy) reveals vacuolar changes in the ascending and descending tracts, along with intralamellar vacuolation in the white matter of the spinal cord [70] in nearly half of clinically asymptomatic patients [76].
  - Often occurs simultaneously with severe forms of HAND in patients with advanced immunosuppression. However, there are also cases of patients with relatively preserved CD4 cell levels [77].
  - Slowly progressive, painless, spastic paraparesis, with sensory ataxia and neurogenic bladder [70] (Fig. 5.4).
- Sensory neuropathy:
  - In the early stages, it occurs in only 3% of patients, but subclinical neuropathy is present in 36% of patients with AIDS [78, 79].
  - Encompasses mainly distal sensory polyneuropathy and antiretroviral toxic neuropathy. In both conditions, negative and positive sensory symptoms predominate, whereas motor weakness is rare and typically confined to the distal muscles of the foot.
  - Peripheral involvement may also include polymyositis, cranial neuropathy, motor neuron disease, or inflammatory demyelinating polyneuropathy [70].
- Other neurological manifestations:
  - HIV-related demyelinating leukoencephalopathy can develop in patients who fail cART. This condition is characterized by CNS infiltration of HIV-infected monocytes and macrophages, leading to extensive destruction of white matter. Acute encephalopathy and immune reconstitution inflammatory syndrome (IRIS) may be associated with this complication [70].
  - Infective endocarditis with emboli into CNS (may occur not only in HIV but also in cytomegalovirus [CMV], tuberculosis, or varicella-zoster virus [VZV]).
  - Cognitive disorders may also be caused by infections such as syphilis, CMV, or John Cunningham virus (JCV). In cases of CMV encephalitis, seizures, delirium, and brainstem syndromes are more commonly observed, the progression of symptoms tends to be faster (occurring over days to weeks), and brain MRI scans often appear normal or show signs of periventriculitis. PCR testing for CMV is usually positive (90%) [70].
  - Encephalitis (acute HIV, CMV, HSV, West Nile virus infection, etc.).
  - Meningitis (Cryptococcus, HIV, tuberculosis, syphilis, etc.).

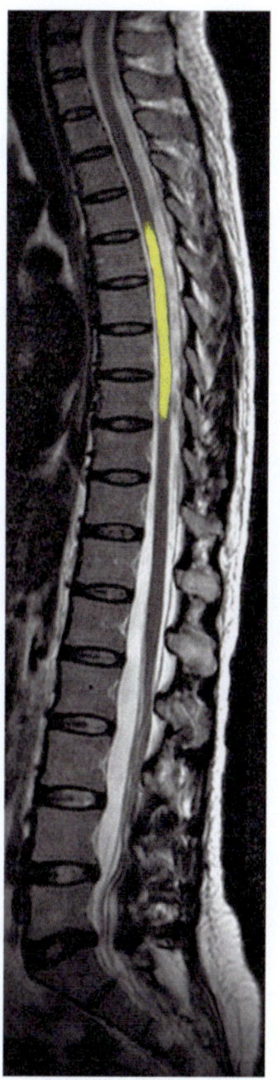

Fig. 5.4 Human immunodeficiency virus (HIV)-associated vacuolar myelopathy

- Mass lesion in brain (toxoplasmosis, JCV, lymphoma, abscess, etc.).
- Myelopathy/radiculopathy (CMV, HIV, VZV, borreliosis) [73].
- Neuro-ophthalmological manifestations are prevalent among symptomatic and asymptomatic HIV patients (60%) and encompass a variety of complications such as eye movement disorders (51%), visual field defects (39%), optic neuropathy (31%), papilloedema (27%), and ocular motor nerve palsies (26%) [80].

5.7.4 Brain Imaging

- MRI frequently appear normal during the early disease stages.
- If brain pathology is present, it tends to be non-specific and can be attributed to various factors, including the direct effects of HIV, antiretroviral treatment, opportunistic infections, neoplasms, vascular diseases, or metabolic disorders.
- HIV encephalopathy typically exhibits diffuse, confluent, and bilateral T2 hyperintensities and global brain atrophy.

- HIV-related focal lesions typically occur in the deep white matter, although they may occasionally appear in the cortico-subcortical region or brainstem. These hyperintensities are indicative of increased interstitial water content rather than demyelination. Importantly, these lesions can often be reversible with cART, which can help differentiate them from age-related and ischemic changes.
- HIV-related complications such as progressive multifocal leukoencephalopathy (PML), lymphoma, and toxoplasmosis present with focal lesions on MRI.
- Cryptococcosis often does not show changes on MRI, whereas tuberculosis may display findings suggestive of meningitis.
- IRIS can occur after commencement of cART [70, 81].

5.7.5 Spinal Cord Imaging

- MRI findings in HIV-associated vacuolar myelopathy include either a normal scan or non-specific T2 hyperintensities predominantly in the white matter of the lateral and posterior columns of the thoracic segments, often forming a longitudinally extensive transverse myelitis (LETM)-like pattern.
- HIV-associated myelitis is less common than vacuolar myelopathy and can present as LETM, edema, and contrast enhancement [70].

5.7.6 Blood Work

- Apart from decreased CD4 cell count and HIV viral load present normal results.
- CD4 count:
  - >500 (cell/mm^3) usually not associated with complications.
  - 200–500 can be associated with HAND.
  - <200 frequently associated with toxoplasmosis, HIV encephalopathy, cryptococcosis, PML, or lymphoma [81, 82].

5.7.7 Examination of CSF

- There is no specific CSF pattern.
- Concentrations of glucose and protein are frequently normal.
- Pleocytosis is present in around 40% of patients with untreated acute or chronic HIV infection (almost all patients have detectable HIV-1 RNA in the CSF) [70, 83].
- CSF-restricted OCB (pattern II or III) are often positive (51%) [84–86].
- HIV-1 could be isolated in CSF (80%) and detected using PCR (90%) in asymptomatic patients receiving cART [87].
- In certain patients, particularly those with HIV-associated dementia, viral load in the CSF may surpass plasma levels (30%). The administration of cART is effective in reducing viral load in the CSF [88].

5.7.8 Electrophysiological Studies

- Delayed latencies in visual evoked potentials (VEP) are observed in 57% of patients with neurological manifestations and in 42% of patients without neurological complications [80].
- Somatosensory evoked potentials (SSEP) frequently exhibit delayed latencies of central potentials, typically localized to the thoracolumbar spinal cord [89].

5.7.9 Diagnosis

- Through a combination of laboratory tests (decreased CD4 cell count; antigen/antibody testing; PCR) [90].

5.7.10 Differential Diagnosis

- HIV significantly decreases the risk of developing MS, and comorbid HIV and MS is extremely rare. Positive effects of cART on disease activity in MS activity was reported in few studies but further studies are needed to confirm and clarify the immunological mechanisms of treatment effect [91].
- In addition, absence of typical MRI features of MS in HIV-positive patients and response to cART should usually not lead to major diagnostic problems [85].
- The differential diagnosis of HIV-associated myelopathy/myelitis mainly includes vitamin B12 deficiency; syphilitic myelitis, VZV myelitis, tuberculous myelitis, and CMV myeloradiculitis [70].

5.7.11 Treatment and Prognosis

- Although cART significantly reduces the occurrence of HIV-associated dementia and other neurological complications, mild neurological disorders are still commonly reported [75].
- cART stands as the sole treatment option to prevent or slow the progression of HAND. However, it proves effective in only a proportion of patients [74]. HAND may significantly impact survival, quality of life, and everyday functioning [92].
- There is currently no effective treatment for HIV-associated myelopathy. Only a few case reports have suggested some potential benefit of cART [93].
- With adequate treatment, HIV is associated with no reduction in lifespan and a rare occurrence of opportunistic infections [94].
- Conversely, chronic, untreated HIV infection results in progressive immunodeficiency, culminating in AIDS within a median period of 10–11 years following primary infection [75].

5.8 Human T-Lymphotropic Virus Type I (HTLV-1) Myelopathy

5.8.1 Synonyms

- Tropical spastic paraparesis

5.8.2 Epidemiology

- Out of an estimated 5 to 10 million individuals who are infected with a life-long infection, approximately 2–4% develop myelopathy, and 2–5% develop adult T-cell leukemia-lymphoma.
- Female/male ratio 2–4/1 [95–98].
- The infection is predominantly prevalent in Japan, West and Sub-Saharan Africa, Latin America-Caribbean, Melanesia, the Middle East, and central Australia. The reason for its geographical distribution remains unknown.
- HTLV-1 may occur in clusters of high endemicity in regions where the virus is otherwise of low prevalence or absent, such as Europe or North America [95].

5.8.3 Etiology and Definition

- The HTLV-1 virus (RNA retrovirus) primarily infects CD4+ lymphocytes and, to a lesser extent, other types of leukocytes. These infected cells can traverse the blood-brain barrier and enter the CNS. HTLV-1 induces functional abnormalities in the infected cells and triggers an inflammatory response. Excessive cytotoxic and autoimmune reactions to HTLV-1-infected cells lead to damage in the spinal cord. Therefore, the disease manifests as progressive demyelination and neuronal loss within the CNS. The anterior and lateral columns of the thoracic spinal cord are particularly susceptible to damage [96, 97].
- The risk factors for developing myelopathy are not clear, but may include a high load of virus [96].
- The transmission routes encompass sexual contact, blood transfusion, organ transplantation, vertical transmission (transplacental), and breastfeeding [95, 98].

5.8.4 Clinical Features

- Symmetric (less frequent asymmetric) spastic paraparesis, with more pronounced symptoms proximally.
- Other commonly observed manifestations include:
  - Lumbar pain with or without radicular irritation
  - Minor sensory changes on lower limbs
  - Bowel, bladder, sexual dysfunction, and dysautonomia

- Less frequently or rarely observed manifestations include:
  - Encephalopathy with mild to severe cognitive deficit,
  - Involvement of upper limbs
  - Optic atrophy or neuritis
  - Other cranial nerve deficits, deafness, nystagmus, cerebellar signs, exaggerated jaw jerk, hyperreflexia, hand tremor, convulsions, muscular atrophy and fasciculation, peripheral neuropathy, sensory level, polyradiculopathy, and meningitis.
- Rarely are other organ systems manifestations associated with immune hypersensitivity conditions:
  - Uveitis; dermatitis; myositis; arthritis; vasculitis; pulmonary alveolitis with abnormal findings on chest X-ray; secondary Sjögren's syndrome; ichthyoses; cryoglobulinemia; monoclonal gammopathy; or adult T-cell leukemia/lymphoma [97, 99–103].

5.8.5 Disease Course

- The mean age of symptom onset is 40–50 years [101, 104–106].
- The median time between infection and symptom onset is 3.3 years (range, 0.3–30) [104].
- The clinical course varies widely, with 80–90% of cases exhibiting slow progression, whereas 10–20% may experience acute onset and rapid progression of spastic paraparesis.
- Older age is correlated with a faster rate of progression [97, 99–102].

5.8.6 Brain Imaging

- Usually, nonspecific T2 hyperintensities in the subcortical and periventricular white matter (50–70%).
- Lesions can occur in the brainstem (cortispinal tract, medial lemniscus, or middle cerebral peduncle) [99, 107, 108].

5.8.7 Spinal Cord Imaging

- Normal findings, or only focal atrophy (25%).
- Spinal cord lesions and atrophy (75%).
  - Initially affected the middle to lower thoracic spinal cord, but over time pathology progress to cervical segments.
  - Longitudinally extensive lesions may mimic NMOSD.
  - The lesions are predominantly situated in the white matter of the lateral columns but may also affect adjacent gray matter and anterior nerve roots .
  - In acute stage rarely focal edema and contrast enhancement [103, 108–111] (Fig. 5.5).

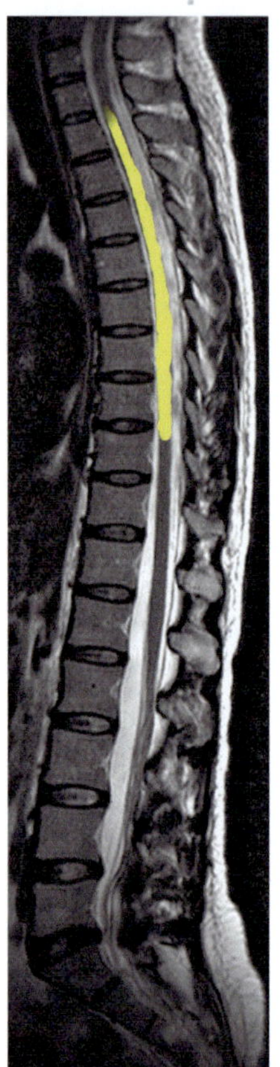

Fig. 5.5 Human T-lymphotropic virus type I (HTLV-1)–myelopathy

5.8.8 Examination of Blood and CSF

- May be present lobulated lymphocytes in blood and CSF.
- Mildly elevated concentration of protein and mild pleocytosis (30%).
- CSF-restricted OCB is present in majority of patients (64%) (pattern II: 14%; pattern III: 50%; and pattern IV: 32%) [108, 112, 113].

5.8.9 Electrophysiology

- Signs of peripheral neuropathy (30%) [114].

5.8.10 Diagnosis

- Established through serologic testing.

  1. Step: blood ELISA or agglutination screening test (sensitivity 100%, sensitivity >90%).

  2. Step: confirmatory Western blot to exclude false positivity and differentiate between HTLV-1 and HTLV-2 (sensitivity and specificity >97%).

- Although confirmatory PCR can detect provirus DNA in blood mononuclear cells, it is seldom utilized due to its high cost and low sensitivity.
- Anti-HTLV-1 antibodies can be detected in the CSF with a high CSF/serum ratio.
- HTLV-1 provirus can be cultured from CSF lymphocytes [95, 97, 115–117].

5.8.11 Differential Diagnosis

- Given that the clinical phenotype of HTLV-1 infection may resemble the spinal forms of primary progressive MS, it is advisable to consider HTLV-1 infection in patients with MS who reside or have resided in endemic areas [95].
- HTLV-1 infection may mimic NMOSD attacks including their response to corticosteroids. HTLV-1 serology should be performed in double (aquaporin-4 [AQP4]/myelin oligodendrocyte glycoprotein [MOG])-seronegative patients from high-risk areas [103].
- There are four known types of HTLV: HTLV-1, HTLV-2, HTLV-3, and HTLV-4. HTLV-2 is typically nonpathogenic but may lead to mild neurological disease resembling HTLV-1 infection, as well as chronic lung infection [95].

5.8.12 Treatment and Prognosis

- There is no curative treatment. Evidence suggests the efficacy of high-dose corticosteroids for induction and low-dose corticosteroids for maintenance therapy. The use of antiretroviral therapy, danazol, pentoxifylline, or interferon-alpha lacks supportive data [118].
- Approximately half of patients become dependent on wheelchairs within 20 years [119].

5.9 Lyme Neuroborreliosis

5.9.1 Etiology and Definition

- An infection by spirochetes (Borrelia) transmitted from vertebrate animals to humans through ticks of the genus Ixodes (zoonosis).
- In North America is caused primarily by Borrelia burgdorferi sensu stricto, but in Europe primarily by Borrelia afzelii and Borrelia garinii and less commonly by Borrelia burgdorferi sensu stricto [120, 121].

5.9.2 Epidemiology

- Affects the nervous system in 10–15% of infected individuals [120].
- Incidence 10–110/100.000/year [122, 123].

5.9.3 Stage 1 (Early Localized Lyme disease; After 1–4 Weeks from Infection)

- Erythema migrans:
  - Occurs days after the bite, and can persist for weeks
  - Asymptomatic (usually without, but sometimes with itching) cutaneous lesion at the site of inoculation
  - Expands day by day as the spirochetes migrate centrifugally and results in a usually large erythroderm (>5 cm in diameter)
  - Central area can return to its normal, causing a target-like appearance (80% in Europe; 20% in the USA)
  - Some patients have no erythema (20%) [120, 121, 124].

5.9.4 Stage 2 (Early Disseminated Lyme Disease; After Weeks to 4 Months from Infection)

- Non-specific flu-like signs and symptoms:
  - Might occur already during the first days-weeks after infection
  - Subfebrile state (high fever is uncommon)
  - Fatigue (54%)
  - Subjective fever and/or chills (39%), or objective fever (16%)
  - Anorexia (26%)
  - Headache (42%)
  - Neck stiffness (35%)
  - Myalgias (44%)
  - Arthralgias (44%)
  - Regional lymphadenopathy (23%) [125].
- Skin involvement
  - Multiple erythema migrans lesions (25% of patients in USA; rare in Europe) occurring week/s after infection
  - Borrelial lymphocytoma (single bluish-red swelling with a dense lymphocytic infiltration of the cutis and subcutis, located most on the earlobe in children and near the nipple in adults).
- Lyme carditis
  - Rare (only 1% of Lyme disease cases)
  - Does not occur if the early Lyme disease is appropriately treated.
  - May be complicated with fluctuating degrees of atrioventricular block; atrial fibrillation; sick sinus syndrome; diffuse myocardial involvement; acute myocarditis; valvular heart disease; sudden cardiac arrest or chronic cardiomyopathy.
  - Even without therapy may be self-limited condition. Treated carditis has usually excellent prognosis [126–128].

- Ocular involvement
  - Reported during all stages of Lyme disease
  - Most often a non-specific self-limited follicular conjunctivitis (10% of early Lyme disease cases).
  - Other rare ocular abnormalities include keratitis; iridocyclitis; retinal vasculitis; choroiditis; uveitis; optic neuropathy; retrobulbar optic neuritis; papillitis; neuroretinitis; non-arteritic ischemic optic neuropathy; or papilledema secondary to raised intracranial pressure [129–131].
  - Optic neuritis (diagnosis of exclusion) may be bilateral and be associated with optic nerve edema [132].
- Early Lyme neuroborreliosis
  - Cranial neuropathy (43–67%)
    Facial nerve palsy is the most common (75% of all Lyme neuroborreliosis-associated cranial neuropathies)
  - Isolated lymphocytic meningitis (6–10%)
    Inflammation in the subarachnoid space (meningitis; in children may cause raised intracranial pressure and a pseudo-tumor-like manifestations)
    The meningeal syndrome often presents as mild, characterized by a low-grade headache, without fever, and meningismus
    Untreated patients may have alternating episodes of meningitis and remissions
  - Painful radiculopathy/radiculitis/radiculoneuritis (30–66%)
    Often misdiagnosed
    Unlike mechanical radiculopathies, often a few adjacent dermatomes are involved
    Sensory deficits may be subtle, motor deficit may be severe.
    Rarely plexopathy, mononeuropathy, or mononeuropathy multiplex.
    Cauda equina may be also affected
  - Meningo-radiculo-neuritis (Bannwarth syndrome; 3%)
    With or without cranial neuritis
    Often with uni-lateral (70%) or bilateral (30%) facial palsy
    Severe, migrating radicular pain and sensitive symptoms; motor deficit occurs usually later
    Can be combined by peripheral nerve palsies
    Often initially misdiagnosed with discopathic radicular syndrome
    Meningeal or encephalitic features are not common, but sometimes may occur a confusional state or minor neurological signs.
    Typically resolves spontaneously in 5–6 months without antibiotic treatment [120, 121, 133–136].
  - Ischemic stroke
    Rare and controversial association with Lyme neuroborreliosis. Likely secondary to infection-induced cerebral endarteritis, similar as in other infections such as syphilis or TB [128, 137].

5.9.5 Stage 3 (Late disseminated Lyme Disease; After >4 Months from Infection)

- Only a minority of untreated patients develop all three clinical stages of the disease.
- Acrodermatitis chronica atrophicans
  - A mild bluish-red skin discoloration with swelling typically appears on the extensor surfaces of the hands and feet [121, 128].
- Arthritis
  - 30% of patients with Lyme disease in the USA, but only <10% in Europe
  - The incubation period ranges from days to years. Borrelia frequently spreads to joints, tendons, or bursae in the early stages of infection. This initial phase is often asymptomatic or marked by transient or migratory arthralgias. In the majority of patients, Lyme arthritis manifests as a late-stage complication, typically occurring 3–6 months after infection.
  - Mono- or oligo-articular large joint arthritis
  - Intermittent episodes or persistent arthritis with joint swelling, large effusions, and relatively little pain, especially the knee [138, 139].
- Late Lyme neuroborreliosis (extremely rare)
  - Encephalomyelitis (parenchymal CNS disease)

    Might occur in early and late disseminated stages.

    Spinal or brain involvement with spastic paraparesis; ataxia; cranial nerve palsies; deafness; bladder dysfunction; and cognitive impairment.

    Diagnosis requires an inflammatory pattern of CSF with intrathecal synthesis of antibodies against Borrelia.

    Usually responsive to antibiotics.

    May mimic MS [121, 128, 134, 140].
  - Axonal polyneuropathy

    Predominantly sensory; nerve biopsy shows similar changes to those in meningoradiculitis; CSF can be normal.

    In some patients occurs mononeuropathy multiplex [121, 128, 134, 140].
  - Encephalopathy

    Confusional state, mild dementia, or psychiatric symptoms
  - Reported also rare cases of patients with serologic evidence suggesting exposure to Borrelia infection and motor neuron disease, movement disorders (e.g., parkinsonism), myelitis, myoclonus, and opsoclonus [120, 134].
- Post-Treatment Lyme Disease Syndrome (3–10%)
  - Might occur in treated and untreated patients
  - Condition accepted by a consensus of clinicians
  - Presence of cognitive dysfunction, fatigue, fibromyalgia-like pain, depression, and poor quality of life persisting for months to years
  - Most commonly develop in patients with Lyme neuroborreliosis
  - There is no CSF pleocytosis and intrathecal antibody production
  - No consensus about its cause and treatment, but long-term antibiotic therapy does not provide benefit indicating that this syndrome is not caused by a residual, treatable infection. Therefore, it should not be referred to as "chronic Lyme disease."

- Whether this syndrome represents a real entity, a post-illness phenomenon, or are influenced by anchoring bias, is yet to be determined [121, 134, 141].

5.9.6 Brain Imaging

- Lyme neuroborreliosis may be associated with normal imaging findings (40–64%)
- Lesions' location
  - Unspecific T2 hyperintense lesions in periventricular and subcortical white matter; sometime in brainstem or basal ganglia.
  - Owing to the frequent involvement of the corpus callosum, there is speculation about its secondary autoimmune mechanism.
  - Number of lesions is variable (range from the recent study, 1–27).
  - Lesions may be confluent.
- Lesions' appearance
  - Lesions size is usually between 2 and 3 mm in diameter.
  - May be present MS-like appearance or perilesional edema.
- Contrast enhancement
  - Cranial nerve enhancement
  - Leptomeningeal enhancement
  - Enhancement of white matter lesions may show ring-like pattern
- Evolution over time
  - T2 lesions frequently persist even after successful treatment [142–149]

5.9.7 Spinal Cord Imaging

- Spinal cord involvement is very rare.
- Usually diffuse or small multi-focal T2 hyperintensities.
- Can occur longitudinally extensive transverse myelitis (LETM) with hyperintense signal in the gray matter ("H-sign").
- Sometime present contrast enhancement of nerve roots [148] (Fig. 5.6).

5.9.8 Blood Work

- Routine testing typically yields normal results
- For other details see "Diagnosis"

5.9.9 Examination of CSF

- Normal or slightly decreased glucose level.

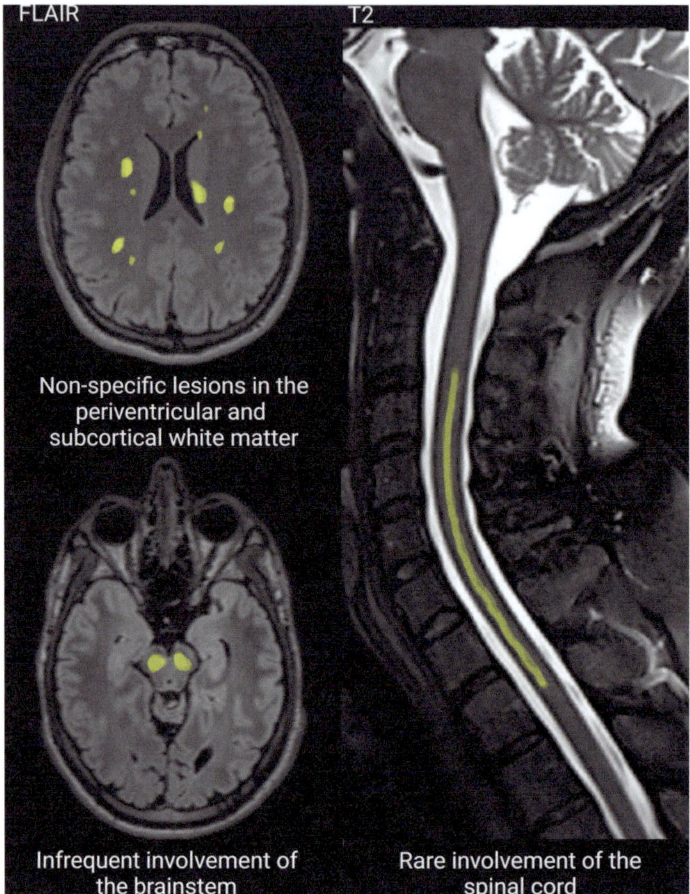

Fig. 5.6 MRI characteristics of lyme neuroboreliosis

- Modest elevation of concentration of protein (<2 g/L).
- Lymphocyte and monocyte pleocytosis (<150 cells/mm^3).
- Intrathecal production of Borrelia-specific antibodies in the CNS should be associated with a CSF:serum ratio of antibodies (antibody index) >1.5 [120, 121].
- Elevated IgG and IgM index and CSF-restricted OCB are typically present after 4 weeks from infection (90%) and may persist for many years after successful therapy. In chronic stages, the detection of intrathecal antibody production is less frequent (50%). Therefore, the elevation of IgG antibodies in the CSF may indicate not only an acute infection but also a past infection [150, 151].
- Elevated levels of chemokine (C-X-C motif) ligand 13 (CXCL13), a B-cell attracting chemokine, are often observed in conditions involving B-cell proliferation (including lymphoma, NMDAR-antibody encephalitis or MS) and spirochetal infections (Lyme disease, syphilis, leptospirosis). In clinical practice, elevated level of CXCL13 can offer supplementary diagnostic support, assess

active infection, and evaluate treatment response in cases of Lyme disease. Elevated CXCL13 is often present before the positivity of IgM and IgG antibodies and may, therefore, assist in the differential diagnosis in the very early stages of the disease [120, 152].
- The follow-up examination of CSF is typically recommended after 2 months, but usually only in cases that are unresponsive to antibiotics.

5.9.10 Electrophysiology

- Nerve conduction studies frequently reveal axonal neuropathy in patients with peripheral neuropathy [134].

5.9.11 Diagnosis

- Direct evidence of Borrelia through cultivation or PCR testing exhibits low sensitivity and is only feasible during the early stages of the disease (typically at the onset of erythema migrans).
- Sensitivity of PCR in the acute infection:
  - Synovial fluid 78%
  - Skin biopsy 69–76%
  - CSF 40%
  - Blood 20%
- The sensitivity of electron microscopy is low (13–15%).
- The serologic testing yields negative results during the erythema migrans stage. Therefore, diagnosis primarily depends on demonstrating the host's immune response to the infection, typically occurring 2–6 weeks after infection.
- Serologic testing involves a two-step approach:
  - Screening with an ELISA or immunofluorescent assay, followed by
  - Validation of positive/borderline test with a Western blot
- In the case of negative ELISA for IgG, but positive Western blot (which should be done if ELISA is negative), it is advised to repeat the serology after time.
- After the first 4–6 weeks of infection occur IgM antibodies occur, which tend to decrease after 3 months and may remain positive for several months. However, some patients may not develop IgM.
- Infections of longer duration have a dominant IgG response. IgG antibodies usually develop 2–4 weeks after the appearance of IgM.
- Isolated IgM positivity may occur only within a relatively short time window during the very early stages of the disease before IgG antibodies develop. In this case, it is recommended to perform follow-up testing of IgM and IgG after 6–8 weeks. If IgM positivity persists, it is likely not associated with Lyme disease but with antigen cross-reactivity, which is often seen in patients with conditions such as SLE, other rheumatological diseases, MS, or B19 parvovirus infection, indicating non-specific immune activation.

- Patients with sole peripheral nervous system involvement may exhibit normal findings in CSF; therefore, a negative result cannot definitively exclude peripheral involvement.
- The antibody response in the CNS reflects the past or current presence of Borrelia in the CNS. The positive antibodies in the CSF may persist at elevated levels for years following successful treatment. Therefore, normal CSF cytology without pleocytosis but with positive antibodies response can rule out an active CNS infection.
- May be present serologic cross-reactivity with syphilis [120, 121, 134, 153, 154].
- Lyme disease does not cause false-positive syphilis screens. However, syphilis might cause false-positive testing for Lyme disease [155].
- There is ongoing debate regarding whether immunosuppression, such as that seen in AIDS, might exacerbate the natural progression of spirochetal diseases like Lyme disease. Case study has reported MS patient undergoing natalizumab treatment concurrently with Lyme neuroborreliosis. Immunological responses in this case were found to be normal. Despite the patient experiencing highly active MS, there was no observed clinical or MRI deterioration of MS. As a result, it was concluded that discontinuation of natalizumab might not be necessary in such cases [156].

5.9.12 Differential Diagnosis

- Lyme neuroborreliosis can be easily misdiagnosed as MS due to similarities in their clinical manifestations, hyperintense T2 lesions in brain white matter, and the presence of CSF-restricted OCB [157].
- Cross-reactivity, also known as molecular mimicry, has been demonstrated between myelin basic protein (MBP) and borelia outer surface protein 39 (OSP-39), as well as other neural antigens. This phenomenon can lead to an immune response against Borrelia that inadvertently initiates an autoimmune attack against CNS antigens, resembling MS. [158, 159].
- Moreover, MS patients often exhibit chronic isolated IgM positivity against Borrelia, which is not indicative of Lyme disease but rather nonspecific immune activation. This serologic response can mimic Lyme neuroborreliosis.
- Has been speculated that Lyme neuroborreliosis may trigger the onset of MS or exacerbate disease activity in MS.
- Although rare, coexistence of MS and Lyme neuroborreliosis has been documented. In some patients, it remains unclear whether they have Lyme disease, MS, or both conditions [157].

5.9.13 Treatment and Prognosis

- Lyme neuroborreliosis is often treated by parenteral antibiotics, including intravenous penicillin, ceftriaxone (1 g twice daily is usually sufficient), or cefotaxime [134]. However, number of studies have found that oral doxycycline is comparably effective [160]. Amoxicillin or cefuroxime axetil demonstrates comparable efficacy to doxycycline [161].

- Several studies have endorsed the use of oral doxycycline in adults with meningitis, cranial neuritis, and radiculitis, reserving parenteral antibiotics solely for cases involving parenchymal CNS involvement, severe neurological symptoms, or when oral regimens fail.
- There is insufficient evidence to support prolonged antibiotic treatment for reducing the risk of post-Lyme syndrome. Recommended 10–14 days of antibiotic therapy; or up to 21–28 days in patients with CNS involvement or in chronic stages is usually sufficient.
- Combination of different antibiotics is not recommended.
- Doxycycline should be avoided in women who are pregnant or breastfeeding, and in children younger than 8 years [134, 154, 162].
- Appropriately treated patients have a long-term favorable outcome, but several patients have decreased cognitive performance.
- Even without therapy, Lyme disease is often self-limited condition [128, 134].

5.10 Progressive Multifocal Leukoencephalopathy (PML)

5.10.1 Epidemiology

- More than half of the adult population has been exposed to John Cunningham virus (JCV) (15% within the second; 80% within the seventh and eighth decades of life) [163].
- Natalizumab (NTZ) accounts for around 5% and HIV for 50–80% of all PML cases [164].
- Up to date, there have been reported around 800 PML cases of MS patients treated with NTZ, and only a few cases on other treatments for MS such as fingolimod, dimethyl fumarate, or anti-CD20 therapy [164–167].
- Patients on NTZ treatment with a higher risk of PML are those, who have:
  - High JCV seropositivity (JCV-index >1.5)
  - History of previous treatment with immunosuppressants and
  - Longer NTZ treatment (>24 months)
  - The risk of PML in patients with all of these risk factors is <1% [166, 167].

5.10.2 Etiology and Definition

- Pathophysiology:
  - PML is CNS lytic infection of white and gray matter cells by a JCV, which is human polyomavirus type 2.
  - PML affects only immunocompromised patients, especially those with alterations of cell-mediated immune responses [168] associated with conditions such as HIV, lymphoproliferative diseases, sarcoidosis, rheumatological dis-

orders, after organ transplants, inborn errors of immunity, immuno-modulatory treatments or high-age [166, 169, 170].
  - Granule cell neuronopathy is a distinct disease entity of JCV-associated disease affecting granule cells of the cerebellum [171]. In 5% of cases occurs simultaneously with PML [172].
- Infection:
  - Asymptomatic JCV infection typically occurs during childhood or in early adulthood through ingestion.
  - Following a period of asymptomatic viremia, JCV establishes latent persistent infection in the kidney, lymphoid organs, bone marrow, possibly also brain without any pathological effect on target tissues.
  - In immunosuppressed patients, JCV can reactivate (bone marrow is proposed as a reservoir), undergo viral genetic changes, and become a pathogenic neurotropic virus causing lytic multiplication of the virus in oligodendrocytes, astrocytes, and, less frequently, in cerebellar granular cell layer and cortical neurons.
- Disease stages:
  - Disease onset of PML is dated at the time entering of JCV into the brain and infection of oligodendrocytes [166, 167].
  - The initial stage of PML is clinically asymptomatic, with MRI lesions (representing inflamed perivascular spaces) typically manifesting 3–6 months after the onset of the infection.
  - The following symptomatic stage has two variants:
    A. Without immune reconstitution "classic PML," which is seen in immunosuppressed patients such as untreated HIV patients. The prognosis of this variant of PML is worse because patients lack an effective immune response to JCV infection.
    B. With immune reconstitution, which is typical for patients on immunomodulatory treatment such as NTZ. This variant has better prognosis because patients may reconsitute an effective immune response to JCV infection after discontinuation of immuno-modulatory treatment [164, 166, 167, 173].

5.10.3 Clinical Features

- Neurological manifestations are variable and depend on the location and extent of brain damage.
- The disease onset is subacute, and the course is progressive.
- Often present speech abnormalities, cognitive and behavioral changes, motor weakness, visual or brainstem symptoms.
- Distinguishing between PML and MS relapse can be challenging or almost impossible, but PML usually does not affect optic nerve and spinal cord [166, 167].

- NTZ-associated PML has more asymptomatic cases as compared with HIV-associated PML [167].
- Granule cell neuronopathy causes cerebellar syndrome [171].
- The sudden clinical and MRI worsening during the PML is often attributed to the rapid PML associated immune reconstitution inflammatory syndrome "PML-IRIS."
  - Observed in 20% of HIV-associated PML cases, particulary after initiation of combined antiretroviral therapy (cART) [174].
  - It is frequent in NTZ-associated PML, particularly after discontinuation of treatment or removal of drug by plasme exchange [175].
  - Caused by a regenerated cellular immune response against JCV-infected brain cells. This is associated with overshooting inflammation and pronounced lymphoid infiltrates in PML lesions and the surrounding white matter. The IRIS may result in brain damage and clinical worsening.
  - The term PML-IRIS should be used only in patients with the extreme and clinically relevant CNS inflammatory response because a continuum of inflammation is noted in PML, and there is no consensus on the definition of PML-IRIS based on MRI or other features [167].

5.10.4 Brain Imaging

- Although there are no pathognomonic MRI characteristics of PML, there are some frequently observed features:
- Lesions' location:
  - T2 hyperintensities dominantly in subcortical/juxtacortical white matter, often involving of U-fibers.
  - May be present leukocortical lesions, which do not respect the borders between the white matter and cortical gray matter.
  - Dominantly located in the frontal > occipital > and parietal lobes.
  - Asymmetric.
  - As disease progresses, lesions may progress into deeper white matter.
  - Although cortical and deep gray matter can be affected, there is dominant involvement of white matter.
  - Rarely affected corpus callosum, brainstem (10% of patients) and the cerebellum.
- Lesions' appearance:
  - T2-weighted images:

    Mono- or multi-focal lesions

    Can be microcystic and confluent

    Sharp borders towards the cortical gray matter, but often poorly demarcated towards white matter

    Small lesions can be difficult to differentiate from MS lesions

    Milky way appearance ("punctuate pattern")

    - Primary T2 hyperintense lesions may be surrounded by multiple small punctate T2 hyperintensities.
    - They suggest an inflammatory response in the lesion, therefore may not be seen in severely immune-suppressed patients.
    - Often show contrast enhancement and may have hypo-intense correlate on T1 images (Fig. 5.7).
  - T1-weighted images:

    Lesions typically appear iso-intense on T1 images during the early stages of the disease but become hypo-intense in advanced stages due to irreversible demyelination and the absence of remyelination.
  - DWI:

    Restricted diffusion, particulary at the borders of lesion and in lesions with active viral replication and swollen infected oligodendrocytes. ADC values are low (cytotoxic edema), normal or high (vasogenic edema).
- Contrast enhancement (30–40%)
- Perilesional changes:
  - Without mass effect
- Evolution over time:
  - PML lesions are detectable on MRI typically 3–6 months before clinical symptoms. The duration of this subclinical phase depends on the lesion size and location.
  - MRI pathology progresses over time due to the progression of JCV-induced disease and/or inflammatory response controlling the infection. Therefore, stable lesions are usually not associated with the PML.

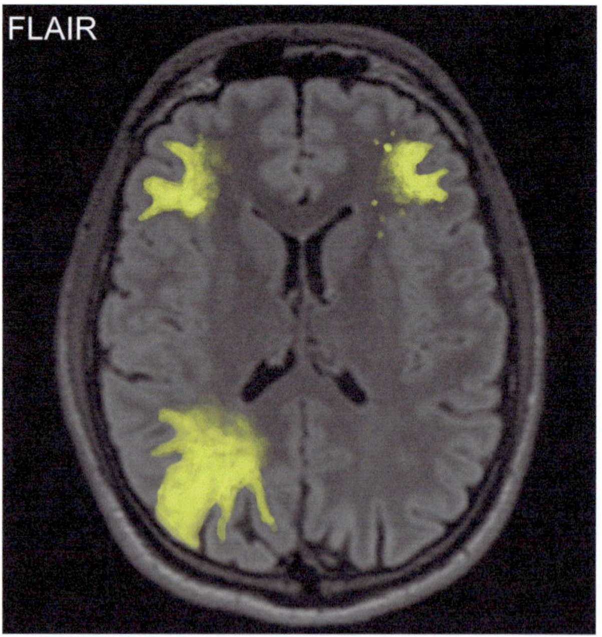

Fig. 5.7 MRI characteristics of progressive multifocal leukoencephalopathy (PML)

- PML-IRIS is suspected in cases of marked inflammation with new or increasing linear, punctate, or rim-like contrast–enhancing lesions; edema; and mass effect.
- Granule cell neuronopathy is associated with cerebellar atrophy.

5.10.5 PML Subtypes According to Brain MRI

A. Classical PML
  - Observed in immunosuppressed patients with minimal JCV-directed immune response (for example, untreated HIV patients or patients with hematologic malignancies).
  - No mass effect.
  - Contrast enhancement is usually absent.

B. Inflammatory PML
  - Observed in patients with functional immune system such as patients on NTZ, or HIV patients treated with cART.
  - Often "milky way appearance" pattern.
  - May be vasogenic perilesional edema and mass effect.
  - Often contrast enhancement, mainly at lesion borders.
  - Periphery of active lesions shows restricted diffusion.
  - Contrast enhancement and perilesional edema may be present already at the early disease stages and reflect the amount of inflammatory or antiviral immune activity [164, 166, 167, 171, 176–180].

5.10.6 Spinal Cord Imaging

- WM of the spinal cord is only rarely affected [181].

5.10.7 Blood Work

- Routine blood testing is normal.
- In JVC-infected patients are detectable anti-JCV IgG (JCV seropositivity) against different regions of the primary capsid protein of the JCV [166, 167].
- The seroconversion rate in either direction is 3–13% per year [182, 183].
- JCV seronegative patients on NTZ should be tested for JCV-index in serum at least every 6 months [184].
- The level of JCV-index in serum may be influenced by previous immunomodulatory treatment affecting levels of immunoglobulins, such as anti-CD20 therapies. Therefore, caution should be made, when interpreting JCV antibody indices to assess the risk of PML for patients on current or recent anti-CD20 therapy [185].

5.10.8 Examination of CSF

- Routine testing is usually normal or can show slightly elevated concentration of protein or mild pleocytosis [167, 186].
- CSF-restricted OCB are positive in around 50% of patients with HIV-associated PML [186].
- The detection of JCV-DNA through PCR exhibits high specificity (100%) but lower sensitivity (60–80%) for identifying JCV infection.
- In general, patients with NTZ-associated PML have a lower number of JCV-DNA copies (<200 copies/mL) as compared with HIV-associated PML [167].
- Patients in the early stages of PML with small lesion volumes are more likely to exhibit very low CSF viral loads (a small number of JCV copies) or even undetectable JCV-DNA in CSF. This can initially lead to uncertainty regarding the diagnosis. Hence, in these cases, repeated CSF sampling may be necessary [187].
- Nevertheless, the typical MRI pattern of PML and the rise in JCV antibody titers in suspected cases, even in the absence of detectable viral JCV-DNA in the CSF, should offer significant support for diagnosing PML [166].
- In rare cases, some patients may exhibit false-positive JCV-DNA in the CSF, which could be due to contamination or limitations of the PCR method. In such instances, repeated testing may be necessary [188].

5.10.9 Diagnosis

- Presence of brain lesions on MRI is required for the diagnosis of PML.
- Diagnosis is based on typical MRI features, clinical presentation, and direct detection of JCV-DNA in CSF by quantitative PCR or histologically [189].
- MRI is highly sensitive in detecting PML, even in asymptomatic patients.
- Lesion activity in patients on NTZ treatment should always rise a suspicion of PML [166, 167].

5.10.10 Differential Diagnosis

- HIV encephalopathy exhibit bilateral symmetrical periventricular white matter lesions, which are poorly demarcated. In contrast, PML exhibit usually asymmetric distribution of well-demarcated (at least partially) lesions located particularly in juxtacortical white matter.
- CNS lymphomas typically exhibit greater edema and homogeneous contrast enhancement of lesions compared to PML.
- MS lesions are mainly localized in periventricular white matter, infra-tentorial region and spinal cord region; show a central vein sign; and do not show a punctate or milky-way-like pattern.
- Other diagnoses mimicking PML may include posterior reversible encephalopathy syndrome (PRES), white matter injury from chemoradiation, ADEM, or diffuse low-grade glioma [166, 190].

5.10.11 Treatment and Prognosis

- Extended interval dosing (5–6 weeks) of NTZ reduces the risk of PML in patients with MS [191].
- Monitoring of JCV-index in serum improve early detection of PML.
- In the ideal scenario, the PML is diagnosed in subclinical patients based on MRI findings and detection of anti-JCV IgG, because early detection of PML in asymptomatic patients is associated with better outcomes.
- Restoring JCV-specific immunity is the most important step for treating of PML. This can be achieved by for example, by initiation of cART in HIV-infected patients or discontinuation of immunosuppressive or immuno-modulating therapy that caused PML.
- Early discontinuation of these immuno-modulatory treatments is associated with better outcomes [164, 166, 167].
- The positive effect of plasmapheresis or immunoadsorption to enhance drug clearance in NTZ-associated PML cases is not confirmed and needs to be weighed with the potential risk of triggering PML-IRIS [192].
- There are no established treatments to prevent PML progression. Several studies are testing the effect of various antiviral drugs, immunoglobulins, cytotoxic T lymphocytes, mefloquine, mirtazapine, pembrolizumab, or immune checkpoint inhibitors with promising results [167, 193].
- PML-IRIS is treated with high-dose corticosteroids to minimize the brain damage associated with an excessive immune response to JCV infection. In contrast, high and prolonged doses of corticosteroids might reduce effective viral clearance and lead to worse outcomes.
- An effect of maraviroc remains controversial [167].
- NTZ-associated PML causes death in 15–20% of symptomatic and 4% of asymptomatic patients. Furthermore, it causes a severe disability in a considerable proportion of patients [194, 195].
- The mortality rate is higher in patients with HIV [195].
- In general, immuno-modulatory treatment-associated PML has a better prognosis compared to PML in patients with lymphoproliferative diseases or HIV, because an immune competence in patients on immuno-modulatory treatment can be restored more easily by drug discontinuation [167, 195].

5.11 Syphilis

5.11.1 Epidemiology

- The incidence of primary and secondary syphilis in Western countries is 2–10/100.000/year, but in some geographical regions, it is much higher [196, 197].
- Currently, documented around 18 million cases of syphilis worldwide (2012) [198].

- Epidemiological data on neurosyphilis are scarce, but the estimated prevalence is 0.8–2.5% of patients with syphilis [197].
- The rate of neurosyphilis is two-fold higher in patients with HIV [199].

5.11.2 Etiology and Definition

- Early in infection, the spirochaete bacterium Treponema pallidum (T. pallidum) disseminates throughout the body, including in the CNS.

5.11.3 Disease Course

- Primary Stage:
  - Within 3 weeks of exposure (range, 10–90 days), individuals develop sores known as chancres at the site where the bacteria entered the body. During this stage, patients are contagious.
- Secondary Stage:
  - Approximately 2–12 weeks after the development of chancres, a rash may appear. Patients experience systemic symptoms such as fever, fatigue, weight loss, hair loss, swelling of the lymph nodes, and headaches. This stage is also contagious.
- Latent (Hidden) Stage:
  - Patients progress to this stage if left untreated. This stage may occur between the primary and secondary stages. It can persist for years, and some patients may experience a relapse of the infection.
- Tertiary (Late) Stage:
  - Typically occurs years-decades after the primary infection, although not all individuals with syphilis progress to this stage. Symptoms may include vasculitis, cardiac abnormalities, psychiatric and neurological syndromes, and blindness.
- Although, neurosyphilis may occur at any stage of syphilis, most often is seen in the secondary stage [197, 200, 201].

5.11.4 Asymptomatic Neurosyphilis

- Asymptomatic presence of T. pallidum in CSF or only the headache.
- Neuroinvasion may resolve spontaneously or may progress to persistent inflammation, especially in immunosuppressed patients [200].

5.11.5 Clinical Features of Early Neurosyphilis

- Syphilitic meningitis

  - Occurs <2 years from infection.
  - Meningeal syndrome.
  - Cranial neuropathies (most often II, VII, or VIII nerve) associated with visual (optic neuropathy) or hearing loss.
- Meningovascular disease
  - 5–10 years from infection but may also occur in later stages of disease.
  - Vasculitis affecting all types of arteries and leading to brain or rarely spinal cord a/symptomatic infarcts or strokes [197].
  - Thrombosis of the spinal vessels due to vasculitis can cause a rare syphilitic myelitis with acute or subacute motor deficit [202].

5.11.6 Clinical Features of Late Neurosyphilis

- Tabes dorsalis
  - Frequent in the pre-penicillin era, but currently rare.
  - Caused by demyelination of the posterior columns, dorsal roots, and dorsal root ganglia in the spinal cord.
  - Associated with a sensory gait ataxia with profoundly impaired proprioception, diminished reflexes, bowel and bladder dysfunction, and lancinating pains in the abdomen and extremities [197, 203].
- Syphilitic dementia (dementia paralytica)
  - Insidious onset, personality, and behavioral changes.
  - Progresses to quadriparesis; incontinence; aphasia; tremor; myoclonus; ataxia; and Argyll Robertson pupils, which react poorly to light but briskly to accommodation [197].
- Syphilitic gumma (granulomatous lesions)
  - May develop in any body tissue.
  - Symptoms are related to their size and location.
  - Typically, a symptom of tertiary syphilis, but it can also occur during the early stages of the disease [197, 204].

5.11.7 Brain Imaging

- Early stages
  - Syphilitic meningitis

    Can be present leptomeningeal or cranial nerves enhancement
  - Meningovascular disease

    Angiography may reveal segmental narrowing, irregularity, or occlusions of vessels, but may be also normal

    Sometime vessels wall thickening and contrast enhancement

    The middle cerebral artery is often affected [197, 205].
- Late stages:
  - Syphilitic dementia and encephalitis

Sometime normal MRI findings [206] or
Bilateral non-specific subcortical T2 hyperintensities, occasionally with a leukoencephalopathy-like pattern.
Brain atrophy (particularly frontal and mesiotemporal lobe) [197, 205].
Occasionally, cortical hypointensities on SWI due to iron deposition in activated microglial rod cells resembling PML [207].
  - Syphilitic gumma
    T1-hypo-intense and T2-hyperintense nodular mass usually arising from the pia mater (is meningeal-based) comprising adjacent cerebral cortex.
    Present contrast enhancement and perilesional edema
    Usually without restricted diffusion
    Can increase uptake on 18-fludeoxyglucose positron emission tomography (FDG-PET)
    May be misdiagnosed as neoplasm [197, 204, 205].

5.11.8 Spinal Cord Imaging

- Early stages:
  - Syphilitic (meningo) myelitis.
    No specific imaging patterns.
    Although, some patients may have even normal spinal cord imaging, many patients have longitudinally extensive transverse myelitis (LETM) mimicking NMOSD.
    Lesions usually centrally or ventrally located, often in the thoracic cord segments.
    Sometimes present "owl-eyes sign" with bilaterally symmetric ovoid T2 hyperintensities in the anterior horn cells.
    Some patients have superficial "strip-like" contrast enhancement of the cord, meningeal thickening, small-medium vessel endarteritis, and lymphoplasmacytic infiltrates or show a "flip-flop sign" (T2 hypo-intense and T1 hyperintense lesions).
    Contrast enhancement might be present in spinal lesions, in the cauda equina and/or in the spinal nerve roots, which needs to be distinguished, for example, from spreading of malignancy, lymphoma, sarcoidosis, or Lyme disease [202, 205, 208].
- Late stages:
  - Tabes dorsalis
    LETM affecting particularly dorsal columns of the spinal cord.
    With or without contrast enhancement and the spinal atrophy.
    The pattern may resemble vitamin B12, copper deficiency or paraneoplastic myelitis.
  - Myelopathy
    Can be associated with compression of the spinal cord by gumma or osteitis [197, 205] (Fig. 5.8).

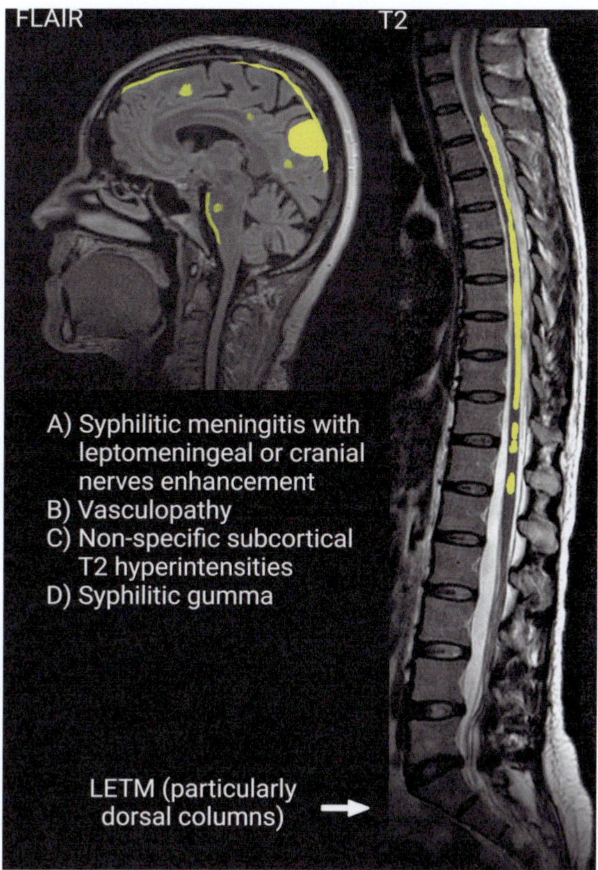

Fig. 5.8 MRI characteristics of neurosyphilis

5.11.9 Blood Work

- Treponemal and nontreponemal tests are required to make a diagnosis of syphilis. Nontreponemal test is used as the initial screen, which is followed in positive cases by a confirmatory treponemal test.
- This algorithm may miss patients with primary or latent syphilis, in whom the nontreponemal tests have lower sensitivity.
- Nontreponemal tests
  - Measure non-specific antibodies made in response to a synthetic cardiolipin, cholesterol, and lecithin antigen complex.
  - May show false-negative results (particularly in late syphilis or in HIV)
  - May show false-positive tests (particularly in HIV, autoimmune disorders, pregnancy, injection drug abuse and in low titers)
  - Titers correlate with disease activity
  - They include:

    Rapid Plasma Reagin (RPR) test

    Venereal Disease Research Laboratory (VDRL) test

- Treponemal tests
  - Measure antibodies to T. pallidum organisms.
  - More sensitive (>95%) than nontreponemal tests but are less specific for active syphilis. Additionally, test positivity remains for life, even after treatment.
  - They include:
    T. pallidum particle agglutination assay (TPPA)
    Fluorescent treponemal antibody absorption (FTA-ABS)
    Automated enzyme and chemiluminescent immunoassays measuring antibodies to recombinant T. pallidum proteins.

5.11.10 Examination of CSF

- Usually elevated concentration of protein (75%).
- Protein level might be normal in the late neurosyphilis (25%).
- Mild to moderate pleocytosis (predominantly lymphocytic, rarely also eosinophils).
- Pleocytosis tends to be more prominent in early neurosyphilis stages than in late-stage manifestations and may be absent in up to half of late-stage cases.
- CSF-restricted OCB is present in half of the patients with neurosyphilis [197, 209, 210].
- Normal CSF findings might be seen in patients with ocular or otologic forms of infection or sometime in patients with "burned-out" tabes dorsalis.
- The CSF VDRL test is recommended for diagnosing neurosyphilis. However, although it has high specificity, false positives can occur in patients with CNS malignancies or significant CSF blood contamination [197]. However, its sensitivity is low (30–88%), presenting a significant limitation [211, 212].
- If the CSF VDRL yields a negative result, the next step is a CSF treponemal assay. Although this test is more sensitive, it is less specific compared to the CSF VDRL. A negative CSF treponemal test provides strong reassurance against neurosyphilis.
- Similarly, as in the case of blood testing, negative result does not differentiate between previously treated and untreated neurosyphilis [197].
- Routine CSF analysis is not recommended for individuals with primary or secondary syphilis unless they exhibit clinical signs of neurosyphilis, ocular syphilis, or otosyphilis. This recommendation applies equally to patients with HIV co-infection and syphilis [199].
- Antibiotic treatment typically leads to improvement of pleocytosis within 6 months and normalization within 2 years. However, an increase in protein levels may persist permanently [213].

5.11.11 Diagnosis

- Owing to the difficulty in directly detecting bacteria in the tissue or CSF, diagnosis primarily relies on serologic testing of antibodies. However, there is no single test with high sensitivity and specificity to definitively confirm or exclude the diagnosis of syphilis. Even serologic testing from CSF cannot definitively confirm or exclude the diagnosis of syphilis.
- CSF VDRL is highly specific, but has low sensitivity; therefore negative result cannot rule out syphilis.
- CSF treponemal test has lower specificity than the VDRL and also cannot distinguish between previously treated syphilis and active infection [197].

5.11.12 Differential Diagnosis

- Syphilis is often referred to as the "great imitator" because it can mimic the symptoms of other conditions. This similarity can lead to misdiagnosis, particularly in the early stages. If left untreated, it can cause irreversible changes and may not respond well to treatment. Therefore, it is recommended to have a low threshold for testing for syphilis [197, 214].
- Owing to the potential risk of meningovascular neurosyphilis leading to CNS infarctions, testing for syphilis is advised for all stroke patients, particularly in regions with high syphilis prevalence, patients with a history of meningitis or encephalitis, young and sexually active individuals without typical cerebrovascular risk factors, or those experiencing recurrent and unexplained strokes [197].
- Syphilis testing is also recommended for patients presenting with new-onset psychiatric symptoms of unclear etiology, particularly in regions with a high prevalence of syphilis. Many patients with syphilitic dementia are misdiagnosed [209].
- The presentation of neurosyphilis may rarely manifest in atypical forms such as syphilitic amyotrophy, pure cerebellar ataxia, limbic encephalitis, or Parkinson's syndrome [197, 214].
- Has been hypothesized that neurosyphilis could trigger or coexist with conditions such as myelin oligodendrocyte glycoprotein antibody-associated disease (MOGAD) or NMOSD, underscoring the importance of testing for these diseases in patients with suspected neurosyphilis [215].

5.11.13 Treatment and Prognosis

- High-dose intravenous penicillin, or ceftriaxone as an alternative.
- Otherwise, there is no established alternative treatment; therefore for patients who have a penicillin allergy, skin testing and desensitization is recommended.
- Antibiotics should lead to improvement of symptoms. An effect of treatment is better in patients with early disease stages than in those with later disease stages, in whom clinical deficit may be irreversible [197].

5.12 Tuberculosis

5.12.1 Epidemiology

- Has been diagnosed in 10 milion people worldwide (2018).
- 2/3 of cases are diagnosed in India (most often), China, Indonesia, Philippines, Pakistan, Nigeria, Bangladesh, and South Africa [216].

5.12.2 Etiology and Definition

- Mycobacteria tuberculosis spread from the lungs via bloodstream to CNS.
- The clinical manifestations primarily result from the host immune response to mycobacteria [217].

5.12.3 Tuberculosis Subtypes

- Pulmonary
- Extra-pulmonary (except of CNS involvement)
- Neurotuberculosis represents the most severe form of extra-pulmonary form of tuberculosis and affects 5–10% of patients with the disease.

5.12.4 Tuberculous Meningitis

- The most common and most severe form of neurotuberculosis (70–80% of neurotuberculosis cases and 1–4% of all tuberculosis cases) often affecting children and adolescents.
- The onset is insidious (in children acute) with non-specific symptoms such as somnolence, apathy, irritability, anorexia, nausea, signs of raised intracranial pressure or higher temperature for 1–3 weeks which is followed by meningeal syndrome (but some patients might not develop it).
- Often present cranial neuropathy (29–38%).
- Imaging:
  - Normal or shows diffuse basal leptomeningeal enhancement with enhancing exudates.
  - A similar pattern of leptomeningeal enhancement may also be seen in, rheumatoid arthritis, sarcoidosis, carcinomatous meningitis, or other types of infectious meningitis.
  - Typically coexists with the spinal meningitis (arachnoiditis).
  - Can be complicated by hydrocephalus, vasculitis, ischemic stroke (from vascular compression or arteritis), cerebral venous thrombosis or optochiasmatic arachnoiditis (usually without visual loss) [216, 218–221].

5.12.5 Brain Parenchymal Tuberculosis

- Isolated or combined with meningitis (28–65%)
- There are different forms:
- Cerebritis
  - Angiitis may cause brain infarctions and strokes.
  - Present in 30–45% of patients with tuberculous meningitis.
  - May be complicated with brain edema and encephalopathy.
- Cerebral abscess (like any other bacterial abscess).
- Miliary Tuberculosis
  - Often present in severely immunocompromised patients.
  - MRI reveals small T2 hypo-intense lesions (2–3 mm in diameter), which may not be visible on non-contrast MRI sequences.
- Tuberculous mycotic aneurysm
- Tuberculomas (tuberculous granulomas) (3–39%)
  - Clinical manifestations depend on the size and location of these solitary or multiple mass lesions located in the brain parenchyma, meninges or in the ventricular system.
  - Well-circumscribed granulomas typically appear hypointense on T1 and T2-weighted images and exhibit ring or patchy homogeneous contrast enhancement. Caseating granulomas with liquefaction may have a hyperintense core and hypo-intense rim on T2 images and show restricted diffusion [216, 218–220].

5.12.6 Spinal Cord Tuberculosis

- Spinal cord tuberculous meningitis (arachnoiditis):
  - Rare, slowly (weeks to months) progressive, chronic form of tuberculosis, which occurs alone or in combination with brain involvement.
  - MRI shows thick, linear intradural enhancement, which may fill out the entire subarachnoid space.
  - May progress to syringomyelia (spinal cord cavitation).
- Tuberculous myelitis
  - Majority of patients have had coexisting meningeal or pulmonary tuberculosis.
  - Rapidly or slowly progressive transverse myelitis or radiculo-myelopathy, often leading to severe motor deficit.
  - In endemic regions, responsible for 19% of all longitudinally extensive transverse myelitis (LETM) cases.
  - Cervico-dorsal cord is the most affected. Pathology affects a single or multiple spinal cord levels.
  - Often present spinal meningeal enhancement.
  - Etiology is related to the immune-mediated mechanisms and respond to corticosteroids.

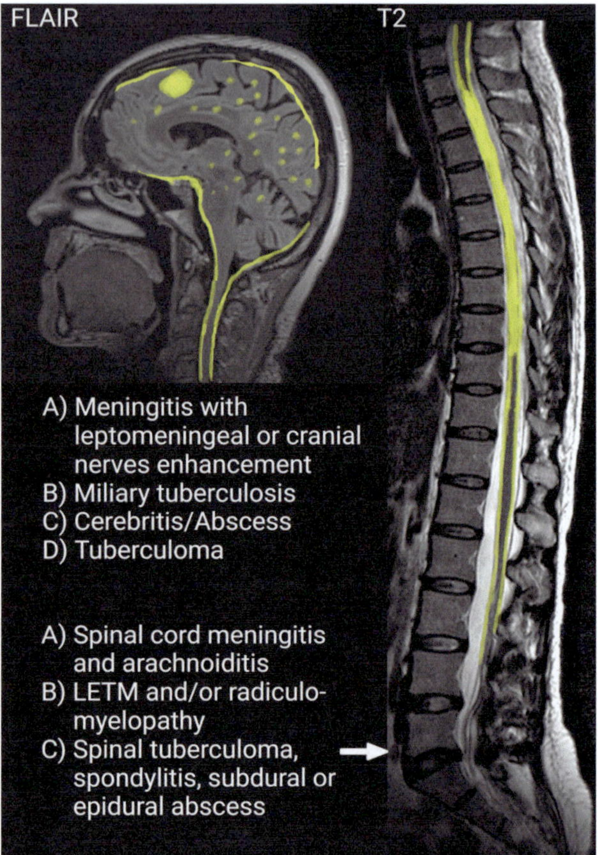

Fig. 5.9 MRI characteristics of neurotuberculosis

- Spinal tuberculoma
- Tuberculous spondylitis
- Subdural/epidural tuberculous abscess [216, 218–222] (Fig. 5.9).

5.12.7 Blood Work

- A positive Mantoux tuberculin skin test has low sensitivity and, furthermore, cannot distinguish between active disease and latent infection.
- Similarly, positive QuantiFERON-TB Gold testing helps to diagnose latent and active tuberculosis, but it cannot distinguish between latent and active disease. False positivity may occur in infections with non-tuberculous mycobacteria. However, a false-negative result (25% of active tuberculosis cases) does not rule out active infection [223].
- Negative QuantiFERON-TB results should be interpreted with caution in patients treated with any corticosteroids (risk of false negativity or indeterminate results) [224].

- Culturing CSF for mycobacteria takes weeks.
- Ziehl–Neelsen smear microscopy of CSF for acid-fast bacilli is often insensitive unless performed by experienced personal [217].
- Due to often comorbidity, all patients with tuberculosis should be tested for HIV [225].

5.12.8 Examination of CSF

- Markedly increased concentration of protein (often >2.5 g/L)
- Glucose is low <40 mg/dL (50–85%)
- Pleocytosis usually >100/mm^3 (range 20–1000/mm^3). During the initial days, polymorphonuclear leukocytes predominate, later followed by a shift towards lymphocytic predominance.
- Detecting bacteria directly within the CNS poses a challenge due to the low concentration of bacilli in the CSF. Although the PCR test is a highly specific diagnostic tool for tuberculosis, false-negative results are not uncommon [217, 218]. Therefore, a negative PCR test does not definitively rule out neuro-TB, and treatment should be initiated in suspected cases based on clinical and other paraclinical findings [226].
- CSF-restricted OCB (20%) [227].

5.12.9 Diagnosis

- Non-specific symptoms are often associated with delayed diagnosis and treatment. Moreover, diagnostic methods exhibit shortcomings in terms of sensitivity and speed, necessitating procedures such as lumbar puncture or biopsy [225].
- Neurotuberculosis may mimic MS at least at the onset of infection, and differential diagnosis may require extensive workup [228].
- In suspected patients, chest X-ray and QuantiFERON or tuberculin skin tests are required. Chest X-ray may show active or past tuberculosis infections in 40–52% of patients with neurotuberculosis [229, 230].

5.12.10 Treatment and Prognosis

- Antituberculous medications and corticosteroids [218].
- Patients with tuberculosis on antituberculous medication may develop new tuberculous granulomas and experience worsening of the disease due to a delayed-type immune response to mycobacteria. This paradoxical reaction is treated by corticosteroids [231].
- The prognosis is often poor, with the mortality around 16% [216].
- The mortality in patients with tuberculous meningitis is 20–50% [217, 218].

5.13 Varicella Zoster Virus (VZV) Infection

5.13.1 Epidemiology

- One in 4.000 chickenpox infections exhibits with VZV-associated CNS complications, most often VZV cerebellitis.
- VZV-associated CNS complications are very rare in immunocompetent, but relatively common in older individuals and immunocompromised people.
- By the age of 85, 50% of the general population will develop herpes zoster.
- The mean incidence of herpes zoster is around 320/100.000/year [42, 232–234].

5.13.2 Cause

- Double-stranded DNA virus is transmitted through human-to-human close oral or genital contact.
- After primary infection with chickenpox, VZV travels from the skin through sensory nerves or via hematogenous spread and persists in the cranial (usually trigeminal or geniculate) or the dorsal root (usually thoracic) nerve ganglia.
- VZV enters the CNS either by direct spread through the olfactory or trigeminal nerves or, less frequently, by hematogenous spread.
- Neurologic complications are caused by primary infection or by reactivation of latent disease.
- In case of VZV reactivation, viremia is usually absent, because viral particles are transported via the nerves. However, in immunosuppressed patients may occur also viremia and VZV may spread into the lungs, liver or CNS and cause meningitis, encephalitis, or myelitis.
- The cause of VZV-associated complications are either infectious or immune-mediated [42, 61, 234–236].

5.13.3 Clinical Features and Imaging

- VZV can affect every location of the neuraxis, including the retina, cranial nerves, brain, spinal cord, peripheral nerves, and skin.
- Herpes Zoster:
  - The virus reactivates and travels along a sensory nerve into the skin, where infects epithelial cells and cause vesicular rash (synonyms: shingles, herpes zoster, or acute herpetic neuralgia).
  - Some cases may have dermatomal zoster-like neuropathic pain without the rash responding to antiviral therapy (Zoster Sine Herpete).
- Herpes zoster ophthalmicus
  - Periorbital vesicular rash involving the tip of the nose (Hutchinson sign).
  - May be complicated by cranial neuropathies (III, IV, or VI); retinal necrosis; retinal detachment; keratitis; uveitis; iritis; or scleritis/episcleritis.

- Zoster oticus (Rumsay Hunt syndrome)
  - Caused by reactivation of VZV in the geniculate ganglion of the facial nerve.
  - Vesicular rash involving the external ear, ipsilateral tongue, or palate; a peripheral facial nerve (palsy and loss of taste) and vestibulocochlear neuropathy (hearing loss and vestibular syndrome).
- C2 or C3 herpes zoster
  - May be complicated with cranial nerve palsies.
- Other cervical, thoracic, or lumbosacral herpes zosters
  - May be complicated with radiculitis and peripheral nerve palsies.
- VZV meningo-encephalitis, meningoradiculitis and cerebellitis
  - Caused by virus reactivation and productive virus infection during immunosuppression.
  - Can occur in the absence of rash.
  - Diagnosis is confirmed either by detecting VZV DNA through PCR or by identifying anti-VZV antibodies in the CSF.
  - VZV encephalitis and meningitis

    Focal neurological deficit, seizures, delirium or meningismus.

    Usually self-limiting and not serious, but in immunosuppressed patients may be severe or progress into chronic encephalitis.
  - VZV cerebellitis

    One of the most common complications of VZV infection with ataxia, nystagmus, vomiting, headache, and sometimes also lethargy, meningismus, and fever.

    Neurologic manifestations of VZV infection may precede skin rash by several weeks.
- VZV-associated vasculopathy and stroke
  - Caused by productive virus infection of cerebral arteries, resulting in pathological vascular remodeling.
  - Should be suspected in patients with a recent history of herpes zoster or varicella infection presenting with neurological manifestations.
  - In around 30% of patients is absent skin rash preceding vasculopathy
  - At least 12 months following the VZV infections, there is an increased risk of ischemic (more frequently) and hemorrhagic stroke (less frequently), CNS vasculitis, myocardial infarction, spinal cord infarction, subarachnoid hemorrhage, cerebral aneurysm, arterial dissection, ectasia, or vessel wall enhancement.
  - This risk is even higher in patients after herpes zoster ophthalmicus.
  - VZV is responsible for 30–40% cases of childhood ischemic strokes and transient cerebral arteriopathies.
  - MRI is abnormal in almost all patients. Ischemic or hemorrhagic lesions are typically located in gray-white matter junction, but also may occur in cortical and deep gray matter or white matter.
  - Angiography shows segmental constrictions (63–70%), often with poststenotic dilatation. There are affected only large (13%), only small (37%), or both types of arteries (50%). Therefore, normal angiogram (30–37%), which

is not able to image small arteries, does not exclude the small vessel vasculopathy.
  - This treatable cause of stroke remains often undiagnosed because 30% of patients has no history of zoster rash; 30% have normal CSF; VZV DNA is often absent in CSF; and an average time between herpes zoster and stroke is 4.2 months [42, 232, 234, 237, 238].
- Giant cell arteritis (temporal arteritis)
- Ocular involvement
  - Occur particularly in severely immunocompromised patients
  - Acute or progressive retinal necrosis (caused also by CMV or HSV)
  - Retrobulbar optic neuritis
  - Central retinal artery occlusion
  - Might be associated with T2 hyperintensities and contrast enhancement in one or both optic nerves, optic tracts and lateral geniculate bodies, the post-synaptic optic radiations or optic cortex [234, 239].
- VZV myelopathy
  - Rare
  - Caused by three different mechanisms:
    A. Post-infectious type typically presents as a self-limiting, monophasic spastic paraparesis occurring in immunocompetent patients days to weeks after acute varicella or zoster. Skins rash of often missing.
    B. Direct VZV infection occurring mostly in immunocompromised patients might be associated with subacute or insidious, progressive, and sometimes fatal severe myelitis. MRI frequently shows longitudinally extensive transverse myelitis (LETM) with serpiginous lesions, mild edema and a variable pattern of contrast enhancement, which may appear irregular, linear, nodular, heterogeneous, patchy, or meningeal. The spinal cord lesions are often located at a level of the dermatomal skin rash (if present). Diagnosis is supported by the presence of PCR VZV DNA and/or anti-VZV IgG antibodies in CSF.
    C. Spinal ischemic stroke due to vasculopathy with restricted diffusion on MRI and positive serology.
- VZV myeloradiculitis and plexitis/radiculitis
  - Rare and painfull
  - Often associated with enhancement or thickening of nerve roots [61, 234, 236, 240, 241] (Fig. 5.10).
- VZV-associated Guillain-Barre syndrome (extremely rare) [242].

5.13.4 Blood Work

- Routine testing typically yields normal results.

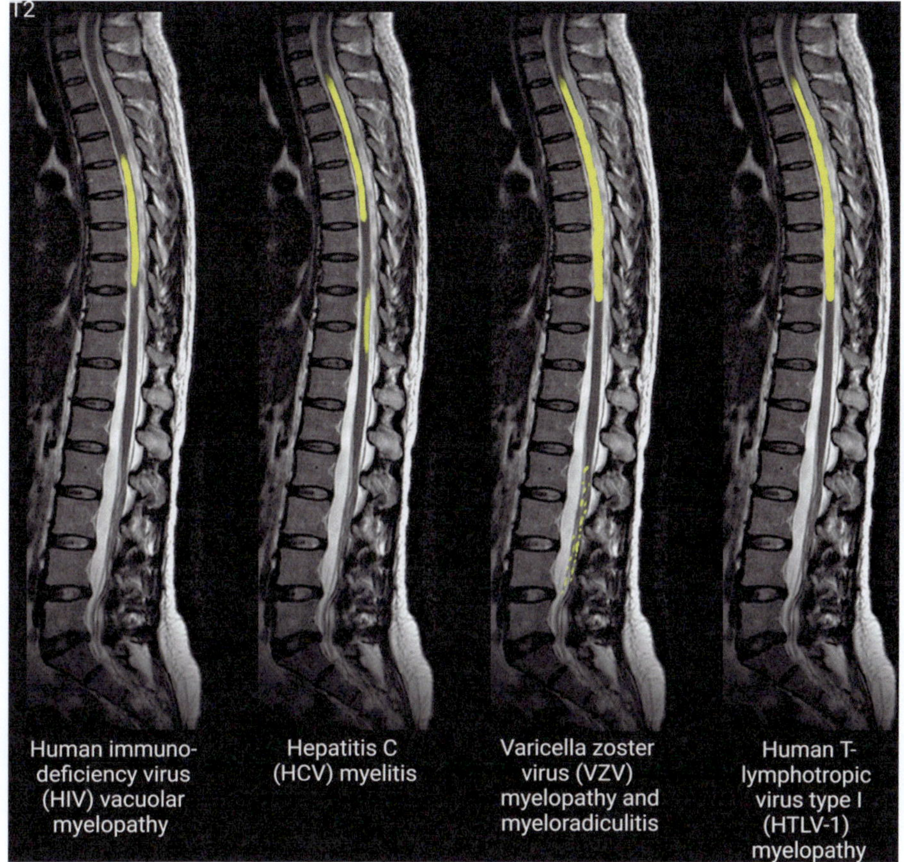

Fig. 5.10 MRI characteristics of infectious myelopathies

5.13.5 Examination of CSF

- Patients with CNS involvement have commonly:
- Normal glucose but elevated concentration of protein
- Mild lymphocytic pleocytosis <100 cells/mm^3 (60–70%)
- Red blood cells and CSF-restricted OCB directed against VZV [237].

5.13.6 Diagnosis

- In acute infection should be based on clinical symptoms (vesicular rash) and PCR detecting VZV DNA, whereas later stages rely on detecting the VZV IgG in CSF.
- Intrathecal synthesis of VZV-specific IgG can be supported by elevated CSF VZV antibody index to 1.5 or higher [42, 237].

5.13.7 Treatment and Prognosis

- Usually, self-limited infection in healthy children without any treatment.
- In selected cases (for example immunosuppressed patients, or herpes zoster ophthalmicus or oticus) may be used antiviral drugs, which may shorten the duration of rash.
- Oral corticosteroids (for example Prednisone 1 mg/kg) may be used in patients with zoster oticus, herpes zoster ophthalmicus, or VZV vasculopathy.
- Vaccination prevents 90% of infections; the rest of 10% infections are mild [42, 234].

5.14 Whipple Disease

5.14.1 Epidemiology

- Incidence 0.1/100.000/year.
- Caucasians are more frequently affected, suggesting a possible genetic predisposition [243, 244].

5.14.2 Etiology and Definition

- Chronic, multi-systemic, granulomatous bacterial infection caused by the bacterium, Tropheryma whipplei (T. whipplei). This bacterium is found in wastewaters and is transmitted in feces and saliva [243, 244].

5.14.3 Systemic Clinical Features

- The clinical phenotype is variable and may include:
  A. asymptomatic seroconversion
  B. self-limited primary infection (e.g., pneumonia, gastroenteritis)
  C. chronic asymptomatic carriage or
  D. chronic symptomatic infection occurring in predisposed individuals, especially those with immunodeficiency
- Classic Whipple disease (WD) includes gastrointestinal and systemic manifestations such as fever, chronic migratory arthralgias, and weight loss [244].

5.14.4 Neurological Clinical Features

- Nervous system is affected in 10–40% of patients with WD. Some of these patients might have isolated neurological involvement without histologic evidence of intestinal involvement.

- Neurological involvement typically includes the triad of:
  - Supranuclear ophthalmoplegia (32%)
  - Fluctuating cognitive impairment or rapidly progressing dementia (28%)
  - Oculo-masticatory myorhythmia or oculo-facial-skeletal myorhythmia, which are pathognomonic of WD (16%). In some patients occur only in later disease stages. They are defined as smooth, continuous, slow (1–3 Hz), convergent-divergent nystagmus, concurrent contractions of the masticatory muscles, supranuclear vertical gaze palsy, and occasionally, rhythmic movements of the limbs.
- Other neurological manifestations include:
  - Encephalopathy with decreased consciousness, apathy, confusion, or psychiatric symptoms (27%)
  - Seizures (14%)
  - Upper motor neuron syndrome (14%)
  - Nystagmus (14%)
  - Hypothalamic involvement with hypersomnia, polyuria, polydipsia, hyperphagia, central hypothermia, and change in libido (11%)
  - Cerebellar ataxia (10%)
  - Headache (10%)
  - Extrapyramidal movement disorder (7%)
  - Cranial neuropathy (7%)
  - Peripheral neuropathy mainly attributed to nutritional deficiencies caused by malabsorption (6%)
  - Other rare features include myelopathy; recurrent strokes secondary to WD endocarditis; Wernicke's encephalopathy; aseptic pachymeningitis; and myopathy [244–248].

5.14.5 Disease Course

- The mean age of symptom onset is around 50–60 years [243, 244].
- Disease course is progressive or relapsing-remitting [244].

5.14.6 Brain Imaging

- MRI may appear normal.
- Otherwise, there is brain atrophy or non-specific T2 hyperintensities, particularly in the subcortical white matter, brainstem, hypothalamus, or mesial temporal lobes.
- Lesions may have mass effect and contrast enhancement (ring or nodular, rarely leptomeningeal) [249–252].

5.14.7 Spinal Cord Imaging

- Rare case studies have demonstrated myelopathy with T2 hyperintense longitudinally extensive transverse myelitis (LETM)-like lesions with discrete peripheral enhancement.
- The volume of the lesion and contrast enhancement significantly decrease after corticosteroid treatment [251, 252].

5.14.8 Examination of CSF

- Routine tests typically yield normal results, without OCB positivity. However, a few case studies have described patients with elevated concentrations of protein, pleocytosis, and rarely, also the presence of CSF-restricted OCB [248, 250].

5.14.9 Diagnosis

- The diagnosis of WD may be very challenging, especially in absence of systemic manifestations of disease [252].
- Diagnosis requires clinical manifestations of WD and two out of three positive results in the following tests:
  1. Periodic acid schiff (PAS) staining shows foamy macrophages in tissue (small bowel, synovia, brain) or CSF.
  2. Detection of T. whipplei or detection of the specific 16S rRNA of the bacterium from cerebral or CSF material by PCR.
  3. Immunohistochemical staining with T. whipplei antibodies from the intestinum or other affected organs.
- Testing for WD in the CNS is essential even if the patient presents no neurological symptoms. If histological or PCR analysis yields positive results in CNS tissue or CSF samples, the patient may not necessarily exhibit neurological manifestations [253].

5.14.10 Differential Diagnosis

- Includes neurodegenerative diseases with dementia, including multiple system atrophy, progressive supranuclear palsy, and systemic infectious/inflammatory diseases such as sarcoidosis, vasculitis, Behçet's disease, and paraneoplastic syndromes [245].

5.14.11 Treatment and Prognosis

- There are no randomized controlled trials, and a consensus regarding the type and duration of antibiotic treatment is lacking.

- Corticosteroids may exhibit a positive effect on clinical and imaging features, leading to a response that mimics autoimmune disorders [251, 252].
- Brain involvement often represents the most severe complication.
- Treated patients typically do not exhibit permanent neurological deficits. However, some individuals with relapsing disease, severe CNS manifestations, or immune reconstitution inflammatory syndrome (IRIS) may have a poor prognosis despite antibiotic therapy, with potentially fatal complications [244, 245].

5.15 Other Bacterial, Parasitic, and Fungal Infections

5.15.1 Cat Scratch Disease

- Epidemiology:
  - Incidence 22.000 cases/year in USA.
- Etiology:
  - Caused by Bartonella henselae.
  - Half of cats are asymptomatic carriers of this bacteria.
  - Transmitted through scratches or bites from infected cats, tics or fleas.
  - More often affects children and immunosuppressed patients, but rarely also immunocompetent adults.
- Non-neurological clinical features:
  - Primary skin lesion at the inoculation site (vesicle); may be unnoticed.
  - Tender regional uni-lateral lymphadenopathy after 1–2 weeks, which can persist months (80–95%).
  - Malaise and anorexia (75%).
  - Low-grade (sometime prolonged) fever (9%).
  - Myalgia, arthralgia, or arthritis (10%).
  - Rarely hepatosplenomegaly, endocarditis, glomerulonephritis.
  - Parinaud oculoglandular syndrome with granulomatous conjunctivitis and ipsilateral periauricular lymphadenopathy.
  - Bacillary angiomatosis with neovascular proliferation in the skin or the internal organs (peliosis) is rare.
- Neurological clinical features (11%)
  - Neuroretinitis with acute uni-lateral visual field loss (2%).
  - Encephalopathy/encephalitis

    Headache, confusion, and seizures 1–6 weeks after the onset of lymphadenopathy.
  - Multiple cranial neuropathies (rare)

    Sometime affecting the optic nerve with progressive, bilateral or uni-lateral, painless or painful vision loss.
  - Cerebral arteritis
  - Transverse myelitis
  - Radiculitis, polyneuritis, neuralgic amyotrophy, Guillan-Barré syndrome

- Imaging features:
  - May be present non-specific subcortical T2 hyperintensities in brain
  - Rarely brain abscess
  - Myelitis is a associated with unspecific spinal cord T2 hyperintensities
- Examination of CSF:
  - CSF may show mild lymphocytic pleocytosis and CSF-restricted OCB
- Diagnosis:
  - Confirmed by serology and PCR. Serologic tests are also positive in patients with previous (often asymptomatic) exposure. However, high titers strongly indicate active or recent infection. PCR has higher specificity, but lower sensitivity compared to serology.
- Differential diagnosis:
  - Rarely comorbid with Lyme disease (share the same tick vector)
  - Needs to be distinguished from Lyme neuroborreliosis
  - Rarely may mimic MS
- Treatment:
  - Lymph node biopsy is usually not indicated, and infection is treated with antibiotics [254–261].

5.15.2 Chagas Disease (American Trypanosomiasis)

- Endemic (Central and South America) infection caused by the protozoan Trypanosoma cruzi. Worldwide infected around ten million people.
- Transmitted to humans by the infected feces of blood-sucking triatomine bugs.
- The asymptomatic phase (latent period), which may last three or more decades, is followed by digestive, cardiac, or neurologic symptoms in a third of patients.
- The acute phase of the infection is usually asymptomatic or associated with non-specific symptoms (fever, eyelid, and face edema, conjunctivitis, lymphadenopathy, hepatosplenomegaly, or anasarca).
- Severe acute cases with tumor-like granulomas, meningo-encephalitis or myocarditis are rare and occur in immunosuppressed patients or infants.
- Autonomic dysfunction occurs from the early phase of disease due to sympathetic and parasympathetic cells destruction. Patients exhibit cardiomyopathy, arrhythmias, megacolon, or sphincter dysfunction.
- In the chronic phase, the involvement of CNS is rare and occurs only in immunosuppressed patients. It is called acute Chagas disease reactivation, which is very similar to the severe acute phase including meningo-encephalitis, myocarditis, and cerebral granulomas.
- Often causes of cryptogenic and cardioembolic strokes in endemic regions.
- Diagnosis through the direct detection of the protozoan in the blood or CSF.
- Treatment (trypanocidal drugs) is underused due to frequently delayed diagnosis [262, 263].

5.15.3 Cryptococcal Meningitis

- Epidemiology:
  - Incidence 223.100/year (globally)
- Etiology:
  - Opportunistic infection caused by Cryptococcus species (encapsulated fungus) occurring mostly in immunosuppressed patients.
- Clinical features:
  - Cryptococcus may cause isolated pulmonary infections; Isolated cutaneous infections; Isolated eye infection (ocular palsies, papilledema, retinal disease with or without vitritis, or optic nerve infiltration); Isolated prostate infection; Life-threatening meningo-encephalitis; or Disseminated infections.
  - There are rare cases of Cryptococcal meningitis in MS patients on immunomodulatory treatments such as fingolimod (most cases), natalizumab, or dimethyl fumarate.
  - Clinical features of meningo-encephalitis include headache, encephalopathy, fever, nausea or vomiting, somnolence, malaise, meningeal signs, focal neurological deficit, seizures, or photophobia. Sometimes they can mimic relapse of MS.
  - Symptoms onset is usually subacute or insidious over several weeks, less often acutely.
  - Some patients may have parenchymal brain involvement, high intracranial pressure, and cranial neuropathies.
  - Restoration of pathogen-specific immunity particularly in patients with CNS infections may result in the immune reconstitution inflammatory syndrome (IRIS), which is associated with high morbidity and mortality.
- Imaging features
  - Gelatinous pseudocysts in basal ganglia or less frequent in subcortical white matter (typical feature).
  - Parenchymal nodules/cryptococcomas often seen in basal ganglia with or without nodular contrast enhancement (typical feature).
  - Patients may exhibit leptomeningeal contrast enhancement.
  - Other features may include vasculitis, hydrocephalus, or multiple cerebral infarctions with restricted diffusion in the basal ganglia, brainstem, or other locations.
- Examination of CSF:
  - Increased opening pressure.
  - Elevated concentration of protein and lactate.
  - Lymphocytic pleocytosis (range 10–140 cells/mm^3) and often also CSF-restricted OCB (57%) or identical OCB in CSF and serum (52%).
- Diagnosis
  - Through direct microscopic examination, cultures from blood, CSF, or urine. Cryptococcal antigen serological detection has very high sensitivity and specificity (both 90–100%).

- Treatment and prognosis:
  - Usually not considered in the differential diagnosis for patients with MS presenting with newly occurred non-specific neurologic manifestations, which may lead to delayed diagnosis and treatment of cryptococcal neuroinfections, which may be associated with high mortality. For treatment, amphotericin B, flucytosine, or fluconazole are used [264–271].

5.15.4 Cysticercosis

- The highest prevalence is in India, Asia, Africa, and South America. Patients with CNS involvement may exhibit brain calcifications resulting from resolved brain cysts, along with seizures and headaches. The cysts can resemble tumefactive lesions seen in MS. Brain lesions may also be in the subarachnoid space or basal cisterns, potentially causing obstructive hydrocephalus [272].

5.15.5 Leptospirosis

- Epidemiology:
  - Incidence 0.13/100.000/year (Europe).
  - Responsible for 60.000 deaths globally every year.
- Etiology:
  - Global zoonosis caused by pathogenic Leptospira species, which is transmitted via direct contact with infected animals or indirectly via soil or water contaminated by the urine of infected wild and domesticated animals (rats are the most important source).
  - Pathophysiological changes are driven by the direct effect of leptospires, or by an immune-mediated response against the bacterium.
- Disease course:
  - Initial (septicaemic) phase of leptospiremia with hematological, pulmonary, neurological, liver, or kidney involvement (3–14 days after infection).
  - This is followed by an immune phase (4–30 days) associated with the immune response against the bacteria, which may affect any body tissue.
- Non-neurological clinical features:
  - Disease presents with a wide range of clinical phenotypes, ranging from asymptomatic or mild self-limiting infection to fatal hepatorenal syndrome.
  - Anicteric leptospirosis (the more severe form)
  - Icteric leptospirosis.
  - Severe complications may include acute renal failure, liver failure, shock, or pulmonary infiltration.
  - Typical Weil's syndrome consists of conjunctival injection, jaundice, acute kidney injury and bleeding diathesis with thrombocytopenia.

- Neurological clinical features (in 10–15% of infected patients)
  - Neurological involvement might be present in both septicaemic (acute) phase and immune (delayed) phase.
  - Usually present together with other systemic manifestations, but isolated neurological involvement may also occur making diagnosis challenging.
  - Most common neurological complications include:
  - Aseptic meningitis (25%; the most common complication)
  - Encephalitis
  - ADEM (rare)
  - Cranial neuropathy (unilateral or bilateral)
  - Ischemic stroke, subarachnoid or intraparenchymal brain haemorrhage
  - Myelitis
  - Guillain–Barré-like syndrome; Mononeuritis.
- Imaging:
  - Normal or with non-specific white matter hyperintensities in brain.
  - May be present ischemic or hemorrhagic lesions.
- Examination of CSF:
  - Vast majority of patients exhibit elevated concentration of protein and marked mononuclear pleocytosis (>90%).
- Diagnosis:
  - Although, culture of Leptospira is the gold standard for diagnosis, it is technically difficult, time consuming and has low sensitivity.
  - PCR detecting bacterial DNA in blood is useful only during the acute septic phase, typically within the first 5–10 days of infection. However, it has higher specificity and sensitivity compared to IgM ELISA, which can become positive 6–8 days after infection.
  - A positive IgM ELISA is only a screening test requiring confirmation with microscopic agglutination test (MAT), which is positive 10–12 days after infection.
- Differential diagnosis:
  - Neurological manifestations are often misdiagnosed.
  - Diagnosis can be challenging if it is not suspected early, because the sensitivity of culture and PCR may be affected by preceding antibiotic use. Additionally, false-negative results can occur if the causative serovar is not included in the test.
  - CSF findings might mimic viral and bacterial meningo-encephalitis.
- Treatment and prognosis:
  - Early antibiotic treatment is associated with good outcomes [256, 273–279].

5.15.6 Listeria Monocytogenes

- Epidemiology:
  - Incidence 0.01–1/100.000/year.

- Definition:
  - A foodborne bacterium with a high affinity for the CNS affecting particularly in immunosuppressed (mainly with impaired cell-mediated immunity), pregnant, neonatal, or older patients, but may occur also in immunocompetent adults.
  - Immuno-modulatory treatments in MS may be associated with an increased risk of this infection (sphingosine-1-phosphate [S1P] inhibitors or alemtuzumab).
- Clinical features and imaging:
  - Immunocompetent individuals typically have only a self-limited febrile gastroenteritis with diarrhea.
  - Meningitis or meningo-encephalitis
    - Manifestations are often atypical for bacterial meningitis caused by other agents (for example often without meningeal signs)
    - Rarely may be complicated with ventriculitis causing elevated intracranial pressure.
  - Rhombencephalitis (rare; 10–17%)
    - Typically, a prodromal symptom such as vomiting, headache, and fever for many days, during which the infection moves from the gastroenteric tract to the CNS
    - Lesion in brainstem and cerebellum, but also in supratentorial region, where often show mass effect and ring contrast enhancement and
    - Rarely may be complicated with intracranial hemorrhage
    - Has very poor prognosis with high mortality rate and often neurological residuum
    - May mimic demyelinating event in MS
  - Brain abscess (rare)
- Examination of blood and CSF:
  - At the onset of the disease, blood tests may not show signs of systemic infection. However, as the infection progresses, elevated CRP levels and leukocytosis typically become evident.
  - CSF frequently shows decreased glucose levels, elevated concentrations of protein and lactate (77%).
  - Usually severe neutrophil-predominant pleocytosis, but pleocytosis may be absent in 1–12% of bacterial meningitis cases, and neutrophil predominance has poor discriminator to distinguish bacterial vs. viral meningitis.
- Diagnosis:
  - CSF culture (result after 2–3 days) or PCR (result within 2 hours)
  - Although the sensitivity of cultures in patients with meningitis is suboptimal (CSF 83%; blood 46–64%), most cases have one or more of the diagnostic modalities positive for this bacterium (CSF Gram stain, CSF culture, and blood cultures).
  - Suspected newly diagnosed MS patients, who present with brainstem and systemic infection symptoms should be evaluated for possible Listeria infection.

- Treatment and prognosis:
  - Ampicillin or penicillin G, or alternatively trimethoprim-sulfamethoxazole or meropenem for at least 21 days
  - Dexamethasone is not recommended
  - Associated with high mortality rate (30%) [280–286].

5.15.7 Mediterranean Spotted Fever

- Synonyms: Boutonneuse fever; Marseilles fever
- Etiology:
  - Caused by Rickettsia conorii (intracellular bacteria) and transmitted to humans by tick bite.
  - Frequent in the summer in the Mediterranean basin (Spain, France, Italy)
- Non-neurological clinical features:
  - Usually a benign self-limited febrile illness with generalized maculopapular rash, myalgia, headache and sometime eschar "tache noir" at the site of the tick bite.
  - Severe complications such as acute renal failure, thrombocytopenia, myocarditis, pneumonitis, gastric hemorrhage, or organ failure are rare.
- Neurological clinical features (rare):
  - Meningitis

    May be with leptomeningeal enhancement and dura thickenning
  - Encephalitis

    MRI may show multiple large subcortical, corpus callosum or brainstem white matter lesions with or without contrast enhancement

    May be complicated with brain venous thrombosis
  - Myelitis
- CSF may show pleocytosis
- Diagnosis is confirmed by serological testing
- Treatment with antibiotics [256, 287–289].

5.15.8 Mycoplasma Pneumonia Infection

- Etiology:
  - Prokaryotic microorganism (not bacteria)
  - More often affects children and young adults
  - Pathogenesis of organ system manifestations include direct invasion of the tissue, toxins production and immune-mediated damage (autoimmunity; organism-induced immunosuppression; immune complex vasculopathy; or thrombosis of vessels).

- Non-neurological clinical features:
  - Asymptomatic infection is common
  - Typically, respiratory tract infections
  - In addition, a wide range of extra-pulmonary complications:
    Cardiac (pericarditis, myocarditis, endocarditis, cardiac thrombi, and conduction abnormalities)
    Dermatologic
    Musculoskeletal (arthralgias, myalgias, arthritis)
    Hematologic
    Gastrointestinal
- Neurological clinical features (0.1% of all cases; 7% of hospitalized cases):
  - Respiratory infection precedes CNS symptoms (by 9–10 days)
  - Neurological complications occur in the early or the late phase of infection because neurological manifestations are driven either by direct invasion of Mycoplasma or by immune-mediated pathology. This needs to be distinguished to guide antibiotic or immuno-modulatory therapy.
  - Acute encephalitis or meningo-encephalitis
    Most frequent neurological complication
    13% of pediatric and 7% of adult encephalitis cases
  - Aseptic meningitis
  - ADEM
  - Cerebral ataxia
  - Optic neuritis and other cranial nerve neuropathies
  - Stroke
  - Transverse myelitis (diffuse, transverse, or polio-like)
  - Polyradiculitis, Guillain–Barré syndrome, Peripheral neuropathy
  - Myositis
- Imaging features
  - A few case studies showed acute demyelinating brain lesions; brainstem encephalitis and myelitis.
  - Lesions often show focal diffuse edema and may resolve after treatment
- Examination of blood and CSF:
  - Leukocytosis and high CRP in severe cases
  - CSF may show lymphocytic pleocytosis (around 33–66%) and CSF-restricted OCB, but many patients have normal CSF findings or only mildly elevated concentration of protein.
- Diagnosis:
  - PCR from nasopharyngeal swab, sputum, bronchoalveolar lavage fluid
  - However, PCR-based assays cannot distinguish between active infection, asymptomatic carriage, or co-infection.
  - Serology is used as an alternative when a PCR-based assay is not available. It is required to obtain serologies during acute infection and recovery after 4 weeks to show four-fold rise in IgG titers. The serology testing has low specificity because of the cross-reactivity with other bacterial species.

  - The combination of PCR plus serology yields the most reliable results. Direct detection of M. pneumoniae in CSF is extremely difficult and time consuming.
  - The patients with CNS manifestations of unknown cause, particularly if associated with atypical pneumonias should be screened for M. pneumoniae infection.
- Treatment and prognosis:
  - Macrolides or beta-lactam antibiotics
  - CNS complications may be life-threatening (mortality 10.3%), and around 30% of patients have resisual neurological deficit [290–298].

5.15.9 Schistosomiasis

- Synonym: Bilharziasis
- Epidemiology:
  - >230 million people worldwide are infected in 74 endemic areas.
  - Prevalence is increased in children, peaks in adolescents and declines in adult age.
  - Neuroschistosomiasis is underrecognized cause of acute myelopathy and encephalopathy in the tropical regions.
- Etiology:
  - Neuroschistosomiasis is a helminthic infection of the CNS by Schistosoma species
- Non-neurological clinical features:
  - Acute (early postinfective) phase

    Usually asymptomatic; symptoms are more likely to occur in travelers and non-immune people.

    Symptoms usually include a skin rash or cercarial dermatitis, headache, fever, dry cough, abdominal and muscle pain, bloody diarrhea, hepatosplenomegaly, and eosinophilia, sometime also myocarditis, pericarditis, septic meningitis, or interstitial pneumonitis.
  - Asymptomatic (latent) phase
  - Chronic phase

    Intestinal infection is the most frequent phenotype (abdominal pain and discomfort, diarrhea).

    Hepatointestinal schistosomiasis can be associated with hepatomegaly and portal hypertension.

    Fibrosis and calcification of the urinary tract with an obstructive uropathy.

    Other organ systems involvement.
- Neurological clinical features:
  - CNS involvement may occur in all three disease stages but are more frequent in the early postinfective phase.
  - Brain involvement:

    Encephalopathy, headache, seizures, and focal neurological deficit depending on the location of Schistosome granulomas.

59% of patients with hepatosplenic schistosomiasis without neurological manifestations shown MRI pathology (small focal T2 hyperintensities in white matter or symmetric hyperintense basal ganglia on T1-weighted images).

May occur tumor-like lesion surrounded by edema, cerebral vasculitis, or obstructive hydrocephalus.

- Spinal cord involvement:

  Often underrecognized cause of acute myelopathy in endemic areas.

  Mainly in young people exposed to freshwater.

  Usually occurs in the early stage of the disease, often without any systemic symptoms.

  Acute myelopathy, conus medullaris syndrome or acute/subacute lower limb myeloradiculopathy.

  Symptoms caused either by the immune reaction of the host around the eggs or by the formation of granulomatous masses in conus medullaris, lower spinal cord, or sacral roots.

  MRI features are unspecific and include swelling of conus medullaris, enlargement of the spinal cord at the lower thoracic level, thickening of spinal roots and cauda equine, and T2 hyperintensities in the spinal cord. Granulomas may show contrast enhancement.

- Examination of blood and CSF:

  Increased eosinophil counts in bone marrow and peripheral blood

  Elevated concentration of protein; lymphocytic pleocytosis; and raised IgG index are unspecific and found in only some patients with schistosomal myelopathy (50%).

  Often positive CSF-restricted OCB (>50%).

- Diagnosis:

  May be challenging while symptoms are unspecific, and blood eosinophilia, antibody levels or the presence of parasite ova in urine and/or stool may not be present at the disease onset.

  Used several serological techniques in serum and CSF (ELISA, hemagglutination and/or indirect immunofluorescence).

- Differential diagnosis:

  Spinal neuroschistosomiasis may mimic a chronic progressive paraparesis (based on clinical features) or spinal tumor (based on MRI features).

  Pseudotumoral brain schistosomiasis must be distinguished from neurocysticercosis, gliomas, cerebral tuberculomas, mycosis of the CNS or brain abscesses.

• Treatment and prognosis:
  - Antischistosomal drugs [299–301].

5.15.10 Toxocarosis

• Epidemiology:
  - One of the most prevalent helminthic infections in industrialized countries, but the exact prevalence is unknown.

- Seroprevalence varies widely (2.4–31% Europe; 13.9–37% USA; 39–93% tropical regions).
- Symptomatic disease occurs most often in children.

- Etiology:
  - Zoonosis caused by the Toxocara canis (host are dogs), or less frequently by the Toxocara cati (host are cats). Humans acquire the infection through accidental ingestion of eggs excreted in dog or cat feces or through consumption of contaminated meat.
- Non-neurological clinical features:
  - Usually asymptomatic infection.
  - Potential symptoms depend on affected organ, number of ingested larvae, age, and immune status of the human.
  - Typically, malaise, pruritic rash, dyspnea, or abdominal pain.
  - Productive cough, bronchospasm, recurrent pneumonia, hepatomegaly, diarrhea, nausea, vomiting, angioedema, pruritic rash, cardiac conduction, and muscle abnormalities.
  - Ocular larva migrans manifests with uni-lateral progressive vision loss over a period of days to weeks, due to larvae migration to the eye causing uveitis, endophthalmitis, granulomatous retinitis, or papillitis.
- Neurological clinical features (Neurotoxocariasis):
  - Rare and unpredictable complication.
  - May be the only organ complication of toxocarosis.
  - Caused by the presence of Toxocara larvae in the leptomeninges, brain, cerebellum, or spinal cord.
  - The spectrum of clinical manifestations is wide including mass lesion, cerebral vasculitis, seizures, and eosinophilic meningitis (36%) or encephalitis (62%), myelitis (28%), or obstructive hydrocephalus, stroke, unspecific white matter lesions, epidural abscess, or cluster-like headache.
  - Unilateral optic neuropathy with retinal damage.
  - Myelitis (sometime transverse myelitis) has usually subacute or slow progression, sometime with relapsing-remitting pattern and with mild to moderate neurological deficits. May mimic disease course in MS.
- Brain imaging:
  - In patients with Toxocara myelitis brain MRI is frequently normal.
  - However, patients with brain Toxocarosis may exhibit non-specific subcortical T2 hyperintense lesions.
- Spinal cord imaging:
  - Typically, single T2 hyperintense (T1 iso-intense) short length lesions located in the posterior and posterio-lateral segments of cervical spinal cord (lumbar region is usually not affected).
  - Lesions often show focal nodular contrast enhancement, focal swelling and enlarge.
  - MRI pattern often mimics findings seen in MS.
  - Imaging abnormalities disappear after successful treatment.

- Examination of CSF:
  - Neurotoxocariasis is commonly associated with elevated concentration of protein (54.5%), pleocytosis (62.5%) with a predominance of eosinophils, and positive anti-Toxocara IgG in the CSF (93.4%).
  - CSF eosinophilia is less common than peripheral eosinophilia, which occurs only in some patients.
- Diagnosis:
  - Clinical suspicion together with leukocytosis, eosinophilia, and the detection of specific IgG in blood and CSF using ELISA (might remain elevated over 5 years) is sufficient for diagnosing Toxocariasis. Positive results should be confirmed using the Western blot.
  - Toxocariasis should be considered particularly in differential diagnosis of myelopathy.
- Treatment and prognosis:
  - No consensus on the treatment of Neurotoxocariasis, but usually used anti-helminthic treatment (most often used albendazole) and corticosteroids.
  - Mortality is low, but some cases may have residual deficit [302–304].

5.16 Other Viral Infections

5.16.1 Acute Flaccid Myelitis

- Epidemiology:
  - Very rare.
  - Typically affects children and occurs in outbreaks.
- Etiology:
  - A number of viruses might be involved in pathogenesis (West Nile virus; Adenoviruses; Wild-type poliovirus, Japanese encephalitis virus Picornaviruses such as Enterovirus D68 and 71 or Coxsackie virus A and B, Rhinovirus, Mycoplasma pneumoniae).
- Clinical features:
  - A polio-like phenotype with sudden onset of asymmetric limb weakness.
  - Upper limbs may be more severely affected.
  - Can progress to the brainstem syndrome or respiratory failure requiring mechanical ventilation.
  - Commonly preceded by respiratory illness, gastrointestinal symptoms and/or fever strongly suggesting an infectious etiology (80%).
- Imaging:
  - Transverse myelitis restricted the gray matter of the spinal cord (particularly affected the motor neurons of the anterior horns), spanning one or more segments.
  - Commonly longitudinally extensive transverse myelitis (LETM), which is most pronounced in the cervical segments and is initially associated with diffuse cord edema.
  - Sometime can be seen contrast enhancement of the caudal roots and/or the cranial nerves.

- Examination of CSF:
  - Elevated protein levels are present in only some patients (about 50%), but the levels tend to increase over time.
  - Lymphocytic pleocytosis.
  - CSF-restricted OCB are usually negative and viral agents can be detected in the CSF in only a small minority of patients.
- Diagnosis:
  - Must be distinguished from Guillain–Barré syndrome and acute transverse myelitis.
  - The presence of a prodromal illness, along with hypo/areflexia, often neck weakness, asymmetric weakness, cranial neuropathy, and the absence of encephalopathy and sensory loss in acute flaccid myelitis can assist in the differential diagnosis.
- Treatment and prognosis:
  - There is no virus-specific causative treatment.
  - Some children fully recover, whereas others may remain quadriplegic and/or tracheostomy dependent [305, 306].

5.16.2 Cytomegalovirus (CMV) Infection

- Etiology:
  - Approximately 45–100% adults are affected with persistent or latent CMV infection in mononuclear lymphocytes, macrophages, bone marrow stroma, epithelial cells and other cell populations.
- Non-neurological clinical features:
  - CMV may cause severe systemic diseases in immunocompromised patients associated with marked morbidity and mortality through reactivation of the latent virus or primary infection (encephalopathy, hepatitis, retinitis, gastrointestinal disorders, cardiovascular diseases, pneumonia, or hematological abnormalities).
  - In immunocompetent patients the infection is usually asymptomatic (80%) or associated with mononucleosis-like syndrome (20%).
- Neurological clinical features and imaging
  - CMV-associated CNS infections in immunocompetent patients are extremely rare.
  - Necrotizing ventricular encephalitis

    The ventriculitis is highly suggestive for CMV infection and is typically associated with contrast enhancement of the ependymal surface and sometime also hydrocephalus.

    Ventriculitis may occasionally occur also in tuberculosis, cryptococcosis, and toxoplasmosis.
  - Encephalitis

    Subacute cognitive decline, cortical dysfunction, seizures, or encephalopathy.

MRI shows typically multiple T2 hyperintense punctate lesions in the subependymal white matter, less frequently in subcortical white matter or infratentorial region.

Lesions often exhibit restricted diffusion for an extended period but typically do not cause mass effect.

MRI appearance may resemble the HIV encephalitis, PML or primary CNS lymphoma.

Corpus callosum and periventriculat white matter is usually spared.

- Myelitis and radiculomyelitis

  Very rare condition, often without systemic symptoms only rarely occurring in immunocompetent individuals.

  Can occur contrast enhancement and spinal cord hemorrhage.

  CSF shows polymorphonuclear pleocytosis with elevated protein and low glucose.
- Congenital CMV infection

  Often asymptomatic at birth, but children are at higher risk for neurologic impairment within the first years of life.

- Diagnosis:
  - PCR detection of CMV DNA in the CSF
- Treatment:
  - Corticosteroids and antiviral drugs (Foscarnet).
  - Prognosis is poor in immunosuppressed patients [42, 307–309].

5.16.3 Dengue Fever

- Epidemiology:
  - Incidence 100–400 million infections/worldwide/year (70% in Asia).
  - After malaria, the second most common mosquito (genus Aedes) borne disease in humans.
- Etiology:
  - Caused by single-stranded RNA dengue virus (Flavivirus).
- Non-neurological clinical features:
  - Typically, asymptomatic infection (80%).
  - Symptomatic infection includes the following phenotypes (20%):
  - Dengue Without Warning Signs

    Nausea/vomiting, rash, headache, eye pain, muscle aches, or joint pain, leukopenia, positive tourniquet test.
  - Dengue with Warning Signs

    Additionally, symptoms include abdominal pain or tenderness, persistent vomiting, ascites or pleural effusion, mucosal bleeding, lethargy or restlessness, hepatomegaly >2 cm, increase in the hematocrit concurrent with a rapid decrease in the platelet count.
  - Severe Dengue

    Additionally, symptoms include severe plasma leakage leading to shock, fluid accumulation with respiratory distress, severe bleeding, severe organ involvement, elevated aspartate aminotransferase or alanine aminotransferase ≥1000 units/L, impaired consciousness, organ failure.

Diagnosis of dengue hemorrhagic fever (according to the older classification) requires presence of fever, hemorrhagic manifestations, thrombocytopenia (<100.000 cells/mm^3), and evidence of plasma leakage (pleural effusion, ascites, or hemoconcentration, hypoproteinemia).

- Expanded Dengue Syndrome

  Affected multiple organ systems.

  Pregnant women, infants, older adults, or immunosuppressed patients are at higher risk.

  Dengue fever and multi-organ involving include cardiac (arrhythmias, myocarditis, pericarditis), gastrointestinal (acute liver failure, cholecystitis, acute pancreatitis, bleeding gastric ulcers), renal (acute kidney injury), respiratory (respiratory distress syndrome, pneumonitis/bronchiolitis, pulmonary hemorrhages), hematological (splenomegaly, hemophagocytic lymphohistiocytosis, aplastic anemia, and thrombotic thrombocytopenic purpura) complications.

• Neurological clinical features and imaging:
  - May occur in all disease phenotypes and stages
  - Encephalopathy (0.5%; CSF is usually normal)
  - Encephalitis (6.2%)

    Symptoms of dengue fever are often absent (>50%).

    T2 hyperintensities in deep gray matter, temporal lobes, hippocampus, subcortical white matter, rarely also in brainstem and cerebellum.

    In most cases present restricted diffusion, microhemorrhages and symmetric gyral edema; sometime leptomeningeal enhancement
  - Ischemic or hemorrhagi stroke
  - Posterior Reversible Encephalopathy Syndrome (rare)
  - ADEM (may mimic MS)
  - Cerebellar syndrome
  - Ocular complications

    Maculopathy, subconjunctival and retinal hemorrhages, uveitis, vitritis, acute macular neuroretinopathy, intra-retinal edema, retinochoroiditis, neuroretinitis, optic disc swelling, optic neuritis, oculomotor nerve palsy and many other complications.

    Usually resolve spontaneously; corticosteroids may be helpful.
  - Acute Transverse Myelitis

    Extremely rare

    Occurs within 1–2 weeks after the infection onset

    Typically, LETM, therefore NMOSD and MS need to excluded
  - PNS complications:

    Mononeuropathies (optic neuritis, oculomotor nerve palsy, isolated sixth nerve palsy, isolated Bell's palsy, long thoracic neuropathy, or isolated phrenic nerve palsy)

    Guillain-Barré Syndrome and variants

Dengue-associated hypokalemic paralysis
Myositis, rhabdomyolysis and myalgias
- Examination of CSF:
  - Patients with CNS complications typically show elevated concentration of protein and pleocytosis, but in some cases is the CSF normal.
  - Some patients with myelitis may exhibit CSF-restricted OCB.
- Diagnosis:
  - Directly by detection of viral RNA in serum (PCR) or by detection of viral antigen non-structural protein 1 (NS1).
  - Indirectly by serology (virus-specific IgM by ELISA; or a four-fold increase in IgG titer in paired serum samples at follow-up).
- Differential diagnosis:
  - Early clinical presentations of Dengue, Chikungunya, and Zika virus infection may be very similar, therefore laboratory diagnostic confirmation is neeed. However, the results are usually not available soon enough to guide initial clinical management.
  - Japanese Encephalitis has worse prognosis (third of hospitalized cases die, and half have residual neurological deficit). However, patients with Dengue infections usually recovery without any significant deficit.
- Treatment:
  - No specific curative treatment.
  - Mortality rate is 0.2–5.0% [310–316].

5.16.4 Enterovirus 71

- Acute flaccid myelitis in children and young adults.
- Brainstem encephalitis.
  - After Listeria monocytogenes, the second most common infectious cause of rhombencephalitis
  - Neurogenic pulmonary edema
  - Myoclonus and ataxia
  - Skin rash of hand, foot, and mouth
  - Can be combined with flaccid myelitis [317].

5.16.5 Hepatitis A (HAV) and B (HBV)

- Approximately 5% of patients with chronic HBV, and rarely those with acute HBV infection, develop peripheral neuropathy or Guillain–Barré syndrome. The pathogenesis of these neurological complications likely involves the deposition of immune complexes in nerves or blood vessel walls and molecular mimicry, rather than direct viral infection. Although there are well-documented cases of

transverse myelitis following HBV vaccination, instances of HBV-associated acute transverse myelitis are very rare.
- HAV is only very rarely associated with encephalitis, meningo-encephalitis, encephalomyelitis, or acute transverse myelitis [55, 318–322].

5.16.6 Hepatitis E (HEV)

- Epidemiology:
  - The seroprevalence: Africa (21.76%); Asia (15.80%); Europe (9.31%); America (7–8%).
- Etiology:
  - A single-stranded RNA transmitted via the fecal-oral route, often by ingestion of contaminated raw meat.
- Disease course:
  - Spontaneous recovery within 4–8 weeks.
  - Chronic infection, especially in immunosuppressed patients, which may result in liver fibrosis and cirrhosis.
- Non-neurological clinical features:
  - Asymptomatic infection (most often).
  - Acute hepatitis, whether anicteric or icteric, is usually mild and rarely leads to fulminant liver failure. However, it is associated with a high mortality rate during pregnancy (25%).
  - Cardiovascular or hematological (myocarditis, thrombocytopenia, monoclonal gammopathy of uncertain significance, cryoglobulinemia, hemolytic anemia and aplastic anemia occur in approximately 35% of cases).
  - Gastrointestinal (autoimmune hepatitis and acute pancreatitis occur in 7% of cases).
  - Renal (glomerulonephritis and IgA nephropathy occur in approximately 1.24% of cases).
  - Endocrine (thyroiditis), skin disease, respiratory, muscular, immune system (each 0.31% of all extrahepatic manifestations).
- Neurological clinical features:
  - Occurs in around 5–30% of acute HEV infections; most common extrahepatic complications, which can be explained by the neurotropism of some HEV viral strains.
  - Neuralgic amyotrophy
    Synonyms: Parsonage-Turner syndrome; brachial plexus neuritis
    Often bilateral
    The most common neurological complication
  - Guillain–Barré syndrome
  - CNS involvement
    Very rare; usually in immunosuppressed patients
    Meningoencephaltis
    Ischemic stroke

Seizure
Transverse myelitis
  - Peripheral neuropathy (Mononeuritis multiplex, peripheral neuropathy, small-fiber neuropathy)
  - Cranial neuropathy (very rare; reported only a few cases of facial and vestibular nerve involvement)
  - Myasthenia gravis or myositis (very rare)
  - Meningoradiculitis [55, 323–326].
- Examination of CSF:
  - In a rare case of HEV-associated myelitis, the CSF showed polymorphonuclear pleocytosis (79 cells/mm^3), elevated protein concentration (0.72 g/L), and the presence of OCB identical in serum and CSF [327].
- Diagnosis
  - Of acute HEV infection through the detection of serum and/or stool HEV RNA by PCR, serum anti-HEV immunoglobulin M, HEV antigen, and rising anti-HEV immunoglobulin G titer.
  - HEV RNA is detectable in the blood and stools during the incubation period and can persist for 4 weeks in the blood (6 weeks in the feces).
  - Anti-HEV IgM antibodies are positive at the same time as liver enzyme activities increase.
  - Considering that a negative PCR does not exclude acute infection, and serology might be false-negative in immunosuppressed patients, the serology and PCR testing are used in combination.
  - Testing for HEV should be considered in patients with unexplained neurological manifestations.
- Treatment and prognosis:
  - Usually, self-limited infection not requiring antiviral therapy.
  - Ribavirin may be used in severe acute or chronic HEV infections.
  - There is no sufficient data about the effect of ribavirin in patients with HEV-associated neurological complications [323–326].

5.16.7 Human Herpesvirus 6 (HHV-6)

- Primary infection is an acute self-limited disease during infancy or early childhood with fever, lymphadenopathy, pharyngitis, conjunctivitis, and tympanitis and morbilliform skin rash (roseola).
- Neurologic complications are rare during primary infection.
- HHV-6 reactivation in adults occurs primarily in immunosuppressed post transplantation patients such as those with a fulminant limbic encephalitis with status epilepticus and amnesia.
- MRI shows symmetric T2 hyperintensities in the medial temporal lobes.
- Assessment of viral load in blood and HHV-6 DNA PCR in the CSF may help to distinguish primary HHV-6 infection and reactivation.
- Treatment include antivirotics [42].

5.16.8 Human Parvovirus (B19V)

- Etiology:
  - B19V causes the erythema infectiosum (fifth disease).
  - Around 50–60% of adults are seropositive for the virus indicating prior symptomatic or asymptomatic infection.
  - Infection is transmitted via respiratory secretions, blood, or blood products. The incubation period is between 4 and 21 days.
  - Mechanisms by which B19V causes tissue damage are direct viral toxicity, dysregulated immune response with release of cytokines, immune complex deposition on the endothelial cells, or intracellular accumulation of toxic non-structural protein 1 (NS1) protein.
- Non-neurological clinical features:
  - The virus causes may not only cause the fifth disease with typical rash, malaise, and low-grade fever, but also asymptomatic infection, or less commonly anemia or pancytopenia in immunocompromised hosts, transient aplastic crisis in patients with hemoglobinopathies, non-immune hydrops-fetalis (if infection in pregnancy), chronic arthritis, myocarditis, hepatitis, vasculitis, renal disease, or idiopathic thrombocytopenic purpura.
  - The rash occurs more often in children, but arthritis is more frequent in adults.
- Neurological clinical features:
  - CNS involvement:
    Most often in children
    Encephalopathy/encephalitis (most common complication)
    Aseptic meningitis
    Cerebellar ataxia
    Stroke occurs typically in patients with sickle cell disease due to anemia during aplastic crisis and the following brain hypoxemia.
    Transverse myelitis
  - Peripheral involvement:
    Most often in older population
    Brachial plexitis
    Peripheral neuropathy, carpal tunnel syndrome
    Neuralgic amyotrophy
    Guillain–Barré syndrome
  - In some patients, neurological complications may occur without the typical rash. This is especially true for immunocompromised individuals, in whom the rash is often absent due to the immunopathological nature of the rash.
- Imaging:
  - Majority of the patients (70%) with encephalopathy/encephalitis show abnormal MRI findings including enlarged ventricles, brain edema, or brain lesions in white matter, basal ganglia, cerebellum or corpus callosum.
- Examination of CSF:
  - Elevated protein (40%)
  - Mild lymphocytic or monocytic pleocytosis (50%)

  - B19V-induced Guillain–Barré syndrome may be associated only with elevated concentration of protein without pleocytosis.
- Diagnosis:
  - PCR confirms presence of the virus DNA in blood (60%) and CSF (90%) of patients with encephalitis. However, low levels of the virus DNA may be detectable for extended periods also in healthy individuals.
  - Often positive B19-specific IgM in a serum (80%) and CSF (20%) of patients with encephalitis.
  - Therefore, serum anti-B19 IgM and CSF B19 DNA testing is useful for diagnosing of B19 infection in patients with encephalitis and encephalopathy. B19 infection is probably underdiagnosed infection and should be incorporated in the differential diagnosis of encephalitis cases.
- Treatment:
  - Intravenous immunoglobulin with or without corticosteroids
  - The outcomes of CNS involvement is poor in 31% of patients [328–331].

5.16.9 Subacute Sclerosing Panencephalitis (SSPE)

- Epidemiology:
  - 6.5–11 cases of SSPE for each 100.000 cases of measles
- Etiology:
  - Progressive neurodegenerative encephalitis caused by persistence of mutant measles virus (single-stranded RNA Morbillivirus) in the CNS, which affects children and young adults. The virus enters to the brain during the acute exanthematous phase. However, human neurons generally lack signaling lymphocytic activation molecule (SLAM) and nectin-4 receptors, preventing the wild measles virus from entering neuronal cells. Although, intact measles virus is not able to spread within the brain, mutated virus may spread within the brain through synapses.
- Clinical features:
  - A persistent brain infection manifests years after the acute infection (average 6 years).
  - At the symptoms onset subtle cognitive decline and behavioral changes.
  - Followed by generalized myoclonus and gait abnormalities.
  - As disease progresses, the patients become akinetic and mute with autonomic instability. The disease progresses to a vegetative state and death within 1–4 years (range days to 12 years), but around 6% of patients might have spontaneous remission.
  - Acute-fulminant SSPE with a rapid course leading to death within 6 months may occur in pregnancy or in the early postpartum period.
  - Ocular involvement (chorioretinitis or involvement of visual cortex) is often and may precede other symptoms.
- Imaging:
  - Normal MRI findings at early disease stages do not exclude the SSPE.
  - At advanced stages present bilateral asymmetric T2 hyperintensities in cortical gray matter, subcortical and periventricular white matter in the almost all patients.

  - Lesions in corpus callosum, basal ganglia, cerebellum, and brainstem are less frequent.
  - Imaging findings might not correlate with clinical manifestations.
  - Rarely dominant involvement of brainstem.
  - Spinal cord is not affected.
- Electrophysiology:
  - EEG sows periodic discharges
- Examination of blood and CSF:
  - CSF abnormalities are often present even in children with common acute uncomplicated measles.
  - During SSPE is typically found normal CSF or with mildly elevated protein. However, there is a high titer of measles IgM and IgG in the CSF and serum.
  - Elevated gamma-globulin (IgG index), which is much higher than that in MS, and positive CSF-restricted OCB (>90%).
  - ELISA of CSF for measles virus IgG has high sensitivity (100%) and specificity (93%). However, PCR results are usually negative because the virus is not typically released into the extracellular space.
- Diagnosis:
  - Dyken's modified criteria:
    1. Progressive mental decline and/or generalized myoclonus
    2. Periodic EEG discharges
    3. Elevated gamma-globulin or OCB in CSF
    4. Elevated titers of antimeasles antibodies in CSF (ELISA)
    5. Intranuclear and cytoplasmic inclusion bodies and/or measles virus RNA or antigen in brain biopsy
  - Definitive diagnosis: requires presence of elevated measles antibodies in the serum and CSF, elevated gamma globulin in the CSF or histopathological evidence (if biopsy is performed).
  - Probable diagnosis: not requires presence of elevated measles antibodies in the CSF or histopathological evidence from a brain biopsy.
- Differential diagnosis:
  - At disease onset mimics psychiatric diseases
  - MRI features may mimic childhood demyelinating diseases, including ADEM.
  - Other mimickers include Autoimmune encephalopathies (mimic acute-fulminant SSPE); vitamin B12 deficiency; HSV encephalitis; syphilis; PML; eclampsia; brain neoplasms or demyelinating diseases such as MS and NMOSD.
- Treatment:
  - Isoprinosine, interferon-alpha, ribavirin may have some effect.
  - Measles vaccine protects against SSPE by protecting against measles.

5.16.10 West Nile Virus

- Epidemiology:
  - Peak incidence from late July to early September.

- Etiology
  - Transmission of this RNA virus occurs through Culex mosquitoes that have bitten infected birds.
- Clinical features:
  - Asymptomatic infection (80%)
  - Mild febrile syndrome (20%)

    Flu-like illness with non-specific and nonpruritic generalized maculopapular rash lasting 1 week
  - Neuroinvasive disease (<1%)

    More common in patients over 50 years of age and with comorbidities such as diabetes, hypertension or immunosuppression

    Meningitis (40%)

    Encephalitis (60%)
    - Non-specific manifestations including fever, diffuse weakness, fatigue, and encephalopathy
    - Can affect cortical gray matter, basal ganglia, thalamus or brainstem

    Acute flaccid paralysis (polio-like syndrome)
    - Virus can infect motor neurons in the anterior horns of the spinal cord leading to the true poliomyelitis

    Mixed phenotype (encephalitis plus myelitis)

    Cranial nerve palsies (relatively often)
- Imaging:
  - At the beginning often normal MRI findings (30–80%)
  - Lesions are often symmetric and typically located in deep gray matter (basal ganglia and thalami), brainstem, and cerebellum.
  - Less often temporal and subcortical white matter or leptomeningeal enhancement.
  - Restricted diffusion is present in half of the patients and precede the development of T2 signal hyperintensities.
  - Lesions are usually iso-intense on T1 images and do not show contrast enhancement
  - The similar MRI finfings are also seen on other viral encephalitides including Japanese encephalitis (more aggressive disease), St. Louis encephalitis (same severity as West Nile virus encephalitis) or influenza virus A.
  - Spinal cord lesions are commonly seen in the anterior horns and anterior roots of cervical segments, conus or cauda equina and may show contrast enhancement
- Examination of CSF:
  - Non-specifical findings as seen in other viral encephalitides, including normal glucose level, elevated concentration of protein (99%) and lymphocytic pleocytosis (40–50% initial neutrophil followed by lymphocyte predominance; mean 226 cells/mm^3) (97%)
- Diagnosis:
  - Detection of serum IgM antibodies against to West Nile virus
  - The presence of IgM antibodies in CSF strongly suggest West Nile virus encephalitis

- Treatment:
  - No causal treatment, however interferon-alpha 2b, ribavirin and intravenous immunoglobulin may have a positive effect when used within 9–10 days from the symptoms onset [332–335].

References

1. Nicolosi A, Hauser WA, Musicco M, Kurland LT. Incidence and prognosis of brain abscess in a defined population: Olmsted County, Minnesota, 1935-1981. Neuroepidemiology. 1991;10(3):122–31.
2. Baddley JW, Salzman D, Pappas PG. Fungal brain abscess in transplant recipients: epidemiologic, microbiologic, and clinical features. Clin Transpl. 2002;16(6):419–24.
3. Brouwer MC, Coutinho JM, van de Beek D. Clinical characteristics and outcome of brain abscess: systematic review and meta-analysis. Neurology. 2014;82(9):806–13.
4. Brouwer MC, Tunkel AR, van de Beek D. Brain abscess. N Engl J Med. 2014;371(18):1758.
5. Desbarats LN, Herlidou S, de Marco G, Gondry-Jouet C, Le Gars D, Deramond H, et al. Differential MRI diagnosis between brain abscesses and necrotic or cystic brain tumors using the apparent diffusion coefficient and normalized diffusion-weighted images. Magn Reson Imaging. 2003;21(6):645–50.
6. Feraco P, Donner D, Gagliardo C, Leonardi I, Piccinini S, del Poggio A, et al. Cerebral abscesses imaging: a practical approach. J Popul Ther Clin Ph. 2020;27(3):E14–27.
7. Haimes AB, Zimmerman RD, Morgello S, Weingarten K, Becker RD, Jennis R, et al. Mr imaging of brain abscesses. Am J Roentgenol. 1989;152(5):1073–85.
8. Reddy JS, Mishra AM, Behari S, Husain M, Gupta V, Rastogi M, et al. The role of diffusion-weighted imaging in the differential diagnosis of intracranial cystic mass lesions: a report of 147 lesions. Surg Neurol. 2006;66(3):246–50; discussion 50–1.
9. Hartmann M, Jansen O, Heiland S, Sommer C, Münkel K, Sartor K. Restricted diffusion within ring enhancement is not pathognomonic for brain abscess. Am J Neuroradiol. 2001;22(9):1738–42.
10. Holmes TM, Petrella JR, Provenzale JM. Original report. Distinction between cerebral abscesses and high-grade neoplasms by dynamic susceptibility contrast perfusion MRI. Am J Roentgenol. 2004;183(5):1247–52.
11. Kim JH, Park SP, Moon BG, Kim DR. Brain abscess showing a lack of restricted diffusion and successfully treated with linezolid. Brain Tumor Res Treat. 2018;6(2):92–6.
12. Grimstad IA, Hirschberg H, Rootwelt K. Tc-99m-Hexamethylpropyleneamine oxime leukocyte scintigraphy and C-reactive protein-levels in the differential-diagnosis of brain abscesses. J Neurosurg. 1992;77(5):732–6.
13. Fritz DP, Nelson PB. Brain abscesses. In: Roos KL, editor. Central nervous system infectious diseases and therapy. New York: Marcel Dekker; 1997. p. 481–98.
14. Barutta L, Ferrigno D, Melchio R, Borretta V, Bracco C, Brignone C, et al. Hepatic brucelloma. Lancet Infect Dis. 2013;13(11):987–93.
15. Oueslati I, Berriche A, Ammari L, Abdelmalek R, Kanoun F, Kilani B, et al. Epidemiological and clinical characteristics of neurobrucellosis case patients in Tunisia. Med Mal Infect. 2016;46(3):123–30.
16. Shakir R. Brucellosis. J Neurol Sci. 2021;420:117280.
17. Dean AS, Crump L, Greter H, Hattendorf J, Schelling E, Zinsstag J. Clinical manifestations of human brucellosis: a systematic review and meta-analysis. PLoS Negl Trop Dis. 2012;6(12):e1929.
18. Guven T, Ugurlu K, Ergonul O, Celikbas AK, Gok SE, Comoglu S, et al. Neurobrucellosis: clinical and diagnostic features. Clin Infect Dis. 2013;56(10):1407–12.

19. Soares CN, Angelim AIM, Brandão CO, Santos RQ, Mehta R, Silva M. Neurobrucellosis: the great mimicker. Rev Soc Bras Med Trop. 2022;55:e05672021.
20. Naderi H, Sheybani F, Parsa A, Haddad M, Khoroushi F. Neurobrucellosis: report of 54 cases. Trop Med Health. 2022;50(1):77.
21. Dreshaj S, Shala N, Dreshaj G, Ramadani N, Ponosheci A. Clinical manifestations in 82 Neurobrucellosis patients from Kosovo. Materia Socio-Med. 2016;28(6):408–11.
22. Franco MP, Mulder M, Gilman RH, Smits HL. Human brucellosis. Lancet Infect Dis. 2007;7(12):775–86.
23. Ma X, Wang Y, Wu Q, Ma X, Wang Q, Guo Q. Brucellosis infection complicated with myelitis: a case report and literature review. Front Cell Infect Microbiol. 2024;14:1378331.
24. Yazdi NA, Moosavi NS, Alesaeidi S, Salahshour F, Ghaemi O. Diffuse neurobrucellosis of cerebellum, brainstem, spinal cord, and cauda Equina: a case report and literature review. J Radiol Case Reports. 2022;16(5):1–9.
25. Karaoglan I, Akcali A, Ozkur A, Namýdurua M. Neurobrucellosis mimicking demyelinizating disorders. Ann Saudi Med. 2008;28(2):148–9.
26. Bussone G, La Mantia L, Grazzi L, Lamperti E, Salmaggi A, Strada L. Neurobrucellosis mimicking multiple sclerosis: a case report. Eur Neurol. 1989;29(4):238–40.
27. Pascual J, Combarros O, Polo JM, Berciano J. Localized CNS brucellosis: report of 7 cases. Acta Neurol Scand. 1988;78(4):282–9.
28. Bektaş O, Ozdemir H, Yılmaz A, Fitöz S, Ciftçi E, Ince E, et al. An unusual case of neurobrucellosis presenting as demyelination disorder. Turk J Pediatr. 2013;55(2):210–3.
29. Abrahão A, de Aquino CC, Pedroso JL, Baiense RF, Oliveira RA, Jorge VM, et al. Teaching NeuroImages: brucellosis mimicking demyelinating disease. Neurology. 2011;76(11):e51.
30. al Deeb SM, Yaqub BA, Sharif HS, Phadke JG. Neurobrucellosis: clinical characteristics, diagnosis, and outcome. Neurology. 1989;39(4):498–501.
31. Pang Z, Tang A, He Y, Fan J, Yang Q, Tong Y, et al. Neurological complications caused by SARS-CoV-2. Clin Microbiol Rev. 2024;37(4):e0013124.
32. Ellul MA, Benjamin L, Singh B, Lant S, Michael BD, Easton A, et al. Neurological associations of COVID-19. Lancet Neurol. 2020;19(9):767–83.
33. Stastna D, Menkyova I, Drahota J, Hrnciarova T, Kubala Havrdova E, Vachova M, et al. To be or not to be vaccinated: the risk of MS or NMOSD relapse after COVID-19 vaccination and infection. Mult Scler Relat Disord. 2022;65:104014.
34. Prosperini L, Arrambide G, Celius EG, Goletti D, Killestein J, Kos D, et al. COVID-19 and multiple sclerosis: challenges and lessons for patient care. Lancet Reg Health Eur. 2024;44:100979.
35. Stastna D, Vachova M, Dusek P, Fistravec G, Drahota J, Menkyova I, et al. Effectiveness of tixagevimab/cilgavimab (Evusheld) in antiCD20-treated patients with multiple sclerosis and neuromyelitis optica spectrum disorder. Mult Scler Relat Disord. 2024;85:105523.
36. Pezzini A, Padovani A. Lifting the mask on neurological manifestations of COVID-19. Nat Rev Neurol. 2020;16(11):636–44.
37. Uher T. et al. SARS-CoV-2 is linked to brain volume loss in multiple sclerosis. Ann Clin Transl Neurol. 2025;12(8):1548–55. https://doi.org/10.1002/acn3.70091.
38. Srifuengfung G, Suppakitjanusant P, Chaisrimaneepan N. EBV-associated CNS infection in an immunocompetent adult: a case report and literature review. Clin Case Rep. 2024;12(3):e8568.
39. Portegies P, Corssmit N. Epstein-Barr virus and the nervous system. Curr Opin Neurol. 2000;13(3):301–4.
40. Soldan SS, Lieberman PM. Epstein-Barr virus infection in the development of neurological disorders. Drug Discov Today Dis Models. 2020;32(Pt A):35–52.
41. Tselis AC. Epstein-Barr virus infections of the nervous system. Handb Clin Neurol. 2014;123:285–305.
42. Baldwin KJ, Cummings CL. Herpesvirus infections of the nervous system. Continuum (Minneap Minn). 2018;24(5, Neuroinfectious Disease):1349–69.

43. Caldas C, Bernicker E, Nogare AD, Luby JP. Case report: transverse myelitis associated with Epstein-Barr virus infection. Am J Med Sci. 1994;307(1):45–8.
44. Mohd Hanafiah K, Groeger J, Flaxman AD, Wiersma ST. Global epidemiology of hepatitis C virus infection: new estimates of age-specific antibody to HCV seroprevalence. Hepatology. 2013;57(4):1333–42.
45. Faccioli J, Nardelli S, Gioia S, Riggio O, Ridola L. Neurological and psychiatric effects of hepatitis C virus infection. World J Gastroenterol. 2021;27(29):4846–61.
46. Forton DM, Thomas HC, Murphy CA, Allsop JM, Foster GR, Main J, et al. Hepatitis C and cognitive impairment in a cohort of patients with mild liver disease. Hepatology. 2002;35(2):433–9.
47. Yarlott L, Heald E, Forton D. Hepatitis C virus infection, and neurological and psychiatric disorders - a review. J Adv Res. 2017;8(2):139–48.
48. Lee MH, Yang HI, Wang CH, Jen CL, Yeh SH, Liu CJ, et al. Hepatitis C virus infection and increased risk of cerebrovascular disease. Stroke. 2010;41(12):2894–900.
49. Mariotto S, Ferrari S, Monaco S. HCV-related central and peripheral nervous system demyelinating disorders. Inflamm Allergy Drug Targets. 2014;13(5):299–304.
50. Sobukawa E, Sakimura K, Hoshino S, Hoshino M, Miyoshi K. Hepatic myelopathy: an unusual neurological complication of advanced hepatic disease. Intern Med. 1994;33(11):718–22.
51. Nolte CH, Endres AS, Meisel H. Sensory ataxia in myelopathy with chronic hepatitis C virus infection. Neurology. 2002;59(6):958.
52. Suzuki K, Takao M, Katayama Y, Mihara B. Acute myelitis associated with HCV infection. BMJ Case Rep. 2013;2013:bcr2013008934.
53. Grewal AK, Lopes MB, Berg CL, Bennett AK, Alves VA, Trugman JM. Recurrent demyelinating myelitis associated with hepatitis C viral infection. J Neurol Sci. 2004;224(1–2):101–6.
54. Aktipi KM, Ravaglia S, Ceroni M, Nemni R, Debiaggi M, Bastianello S, et al. Severe recurrent myelitis in patients with hepatitis C virus infection. Neurology. 2007;68(6):468–9.
55. Stübgen JP. Immune-mediated myelitis associated with hepatitis virus infections. J Neuroimmunol. 2011;239(1–2):21–7.
56. Adil M, Jensen-Fangel S, Gammelgaard L, Petersen T. Longitudinally extensive transverse myelitis and hepatitis C-a case report and literature review. Clin Case Rep. 2021;9(8):e04631.
57. Ferreira JD, Caldas AC, de Sá JC, Geraldes R. Longstanding spastic paraparesis in a patient infected with hepatitis C virus and seropositive for aquaporin-4 antibody - case report and review of the literature. Mult Scler Relat Disord. 2016;8:120–3.
58. Smith JS, Robinson NJ. Age-specific prevalence of infection with herpes simplex virus types 2 and 1: a global review. J Infect Dis. 2002;186(Suppl 1):S3–28.
59. Corey L, Spear PG. Infections with herpes simplex viruses (2). N Engl J Med. 1986;314(12):749–57.
60. Bradshaw MJ, Venkatesan A. Herpes simplex Virus-1 encephalitis in adults: pathophysiology, diagnosis, and management. Neurotherapeutics. 2016;13(3):493–508.
61. Bulakbasi N, Kocaoglu M. Central nervous system infections of herpesvirus family. Neuroimaging Clin N Am. 2008;18(1):53–84; viii.
62. Nardone R, Versace V, Brigo F, Tezzon F, Zuccoli G, Pikija S, et al. Herpes simplex virus type 2 myelitis: case report and review of the literature. Front Neurol. 2017;8:199.
63. Wasay M, Mekan SF, Khelaeni B, Saeed Z, Hassan A, Cheema Z, et al. Extra temporal involvement in herpes simplex encephalitis. Eur J Neurol. 2005;12(6):475–9.
64. Choudhury NA, Castrodad-Molina RM, Hutton GJ, Cuascut FX. Elsberg syndrome following acute immunosuppressive treatment for multiple sclerosis relapse. Mult Scler Relat Disord. 2022;58:103498.
65. Whitley RJ, Cobbs CG, Alford CA Jr, Soong SJ, Hirsch MS, Connor JD, et al. Diseases that mimic herpes simplex encephalitis. Diagnosis, presentation, and outcome. NIAD Collaborative Antiviral Study Group. JAMA. 1989;262(2):234–9.
66. Saraya AW, Wacharapluesadee S, Petcharat S, Sittidetboripat N, Ghai S, Wilde H, et al. Normocellular CSF in herpes simplex encephalitis. BMC Res Notes. 2016;9:95.
67. WHO. https://www.who.int/data/gho/data/themes/hiv-aids. 2022.

68. Sacktor N. The epidemiology of human immunodeficiency virus-associated neurological disease in the era of highly active antiretroviral therapy. J Neurovirol. 2002;8(Suppl 2):115–21.
69. McArthur JC. HIV dementia: an evolving disease. J Neuroimmunol. 2004;157(1–2):3–10.
70. McArthur JC, Brew BJ, Nath A. Neurological complications of HIV infection. Lancet Neurol. 2005;4(9):543–55.
71. Ho DD, Neumann AU, Perelson AS, Chen W, Leonard JM, Markowitz M. Rapid turnover of plasma virions and CD4 lymphocytes in HIV-1 infection. Nature. 1995;373(6510):123–6.
72. Tyor WR, Wesselingh SL, Griffin JW, McArthur JC, Griffin DE. Unifying hypothesis for the pathogenesis of HIV-associated dementia complex, vacuolar myelopathy, and sensory neuropathy. J Acquir Immune Defic Syndr Hum Retrovirol. 1995;9(4):379–88.
73. Bilgrami M, O'Keefe P. Neurologic diseases in HIV-infected patients. Handb Clin Neurol. 2014;121:1321–44.
74. Saylor D, Dickens AM, Sacktor N, Haughey N, Slusher B, Pletnikov M, et al. HIV-associated neurocognitive disorder - pathogenesis and prospects for treatment. Nat Rev Neurol. 2016;12(5):309.
75. Dore GJ, Correll PK, Li Y, Kaldor JM, Cooper DA, Brew BJ. Changes to AIDS dementia complex in the era of highly active antiretroviral therapy. AIDS. 1999;13(10):1249–53.
76. Dal Pan GJ, Glass JD, McArthur JC. Clinicopathologic correlations of HIV-1-associated vacuolar myelopathy: an autopsy-based case-control study. Neurology. 1994;44(11):2159–64.
77. Ayele BA, Amogne W, Gemechu L. HIV-associated neurocognitive disorder and HIV-associated myelopathy in a patient with a preserved CD4, but high viral load-a rarely reported phenomenon: a case report and literature review. BMC Infect Dis. 2020;20(1):574.
78. Iragui VJ, Kalmijn J, Thal LJ, Grant I. Neurological dysfunction in asymptomatic HIV-1 infected men: evidence from evoked potentials. HNRC Group. Electroencephalogr Clin Neurophysiol. 1994;92(1):1–10.
79. Barohn RJ, Gronseth GS, LeForce BR, McVey AL, McGuire SA, Butzin CA, et al. Peripheral nervous system involvement in a large cohort of human immunodeficiency virus-infected individuals. Arch Neurol. 1993;50(2):167–71.
80. Mwanza JC, Nyamabo LK, Tylleskar T, Plant GT. Neuro-ophthalmological disorders in HIV infected subjects with neurological manifestations. Brit J Ophthalmol. 2004;88(11):1455–9.
81. Sakai M, Higashi M, Fujiwara T, Uehira T, Shirasaka T, Nakanishi K, et al. MRI imaging features of HIV-related central nervous system diseases: diagnosis by pattern recognition in daily practice. Jpn J Radiol. 2021;39(11):1023–38.
82. Jung AC, Paauw DS. Diagnosing HIV-related disease - using the CD4 count as a guide. J Gen Intern Med. 1998;13(2):131–6.
83. Chan P, Moreland S, Sacdalan C, Kroon E, Colby D, Sriplienchan S, et al. Cerebrospinal fluid pleocytosis is associated with HIV-1 neuroinvasion during acute infection. AIDS. 2024;38(3):373–8.
84. Skotzek B, Sander T, Zimmermann J, Kolmel HW. Oligoclonal bands in serum and cerebrospinal-fluid of patients with Hiv infection. J Neuroimmunol. 1988;20(2–3):151–2.
85. Mir WAY, Shrestha DB, Fiumara F, Mohapatra S, Sullivan T, Adhikari A, et al. HIV encephalopathy mimicking acute demyelinating processes. Cureus. 2021;13(10):e18494.
86. De Almeida SM, Rotta I, Tang B, Vaida F, Letendre S, Ellis RJ. IgG intrathecal synthesis in HIV-associated neurocognitive disorder (HAND) according to the HIV-1 subtypes and pattern of HIV RNA in CNS and plasma compartments. J Neuroimmunol. 2021;355:577542.
87. Chiodi F, Keys B, Albert J, Hagberg L, Lundeberg J, Uhlen M, et al. Human immunodeficiency virus type 1 is present in the cerebrospinal fluid of a majority of infected individuals. J Clin Microbiol. 1992;30(7):1768–71.
88. Hagberg L, Gisslen M. Cohort profile: a longitudinal study of HIV infection in the central nervous system with focus on cerebrospinal fluid - the Gothenburg HIV CSF Study Cohort. BMJ Open. 2023;13(5):e070693.
89. Tagliati M, Di Rocco A, Danisi F, Simpson DM. The role of somatosensory evoked potentials in the diagnosis of AIDS-associated myelopathy. Neurology. 2000;54(7):1477–82.

90. Croxford S, Stengaard AR, Brännström J, Combs L, Dedes N, Girardi E, et al. Late diagnosis of HIV: an updated consensus definition. HIV Med. 2022;23(11):1202–8.
91. Stefanou MI, Krumbholz M, Ziemann U, Kowarik MC. Human immunodeficiency virus and multiple sclerosis: a review of the literature. Neurol Res Pract. 2019;1:24.
92. Heaton RK, Velin RA, McCutchan JA, Gulevich SJ, Atkinson JH, Wallace MR, et al. Neuropsychological impairment in human immunodeficiency virus-infection: implications for employment. HNRC Group. HIV Neurobehavioral Research Center. Psychosom Med. 1994;56(1):8–17.
93. Staudinger R, Henry K. Remission of HIV myelopathy after highly active antiretroviral therapy. Neurology. 2000;54(1):267–8.
94. Fauci AS, Marston HD. Ending the HIV-AIDS pandemic--follow the science. N Engl J Med. 2015;373(23):2197–9.
95. Eusebio-Ponce E, Anguita E, Paulino-Ramirez R, Candel FJ. HTLV-1 infection: an emerging risk. Pathogenesis, epidemiology, diagnosis and associated diseases. Rev Esp Quimioter. 2019;32(6):485–96.
96. Yoshida M, Osame M, Kawai H, Toita M, Kuwasaki N, Nishida Y, et al. Increased replication of HTLV-I in HTLV-I-associated myelopathy. Ann Neurol. 1989;26(3):331–5.
97. Yamauchi J, Araya N, Yagishita N, Sato T, Yamano Y. An update on human T-cell leukemia virus type I (HTLV-1)-associated myelopathy/tropical spastic paraparesis (HAM/TSP) focusing on clinical and laboratory biomarkers. Pharmacol Ther. 2021;218:107669.
98. Rosadas C, Taylor GP. Mother-to-child HTLV-1 transmission: unmet research needs. Front Microbiol. 2019;10:999.
99. Nakagawa M, Izumo S, Ijichi S, Kubota H, Arimura K, Kawabata M, et al. HTLV-I-associated myelopathy: analysis of 213 patients based on clinical features and laboratory findings. J Neurovirol. 1995;1(1):50–61.
100. Castro NM, Rodrigues W Jr, Freitas DM, Muniz A, Oliveira P, Carvalho EM. Urinary symptoms associated with human T-cell lymphotropic virus type I infection: evidence of urinary manifestations in large group of HTLV-I carriers. Urology. 2007;69(5):813–8.
101. Orland JR, Engstrom J, Fridey J, Sacher RA, Smith JW, Nass C, et al. Prevalence and clinical features of HTLV neurologic disease in the HTLV outcomes study. Neurology. 2003;61(11):1588–94.
102. Araujo AQ, Silva MT. The HTLV-1 neurological complex. Lancet Neurol. 2006;5(12):1068–76.
103. Bonnan M, Olindo S, Signate A, Lobjois Q, Stephant M, Boulos DD, et al. NMOSD-like and longitudinal extensive HTLV1-associated myelitis are extremes that flank an overlooked continuum. Mult Scler J Exp Transl Clin. 2021;7(3):20552173211037361.
104. Maloney EM, Cleghorn FR, Morgan OS, Rodgers-Johnson P, Cranston B, Jack N, et al. Incidence of HTLV-I-associated myelopathy/tropical spastic paraparesis (HAM/TSP) in Jamaica and Trinidad. J Acquir Immune Defic Syndr Hum Retrovirol. 1998;17(2):167–70.
105. Kondo T, Kono H, Miyamoto N, Yoshida R, Toki H, Matsumoto I, et al. Age- and sex-specific cumulative rate and risk of ATLL for HTLV-I carriers. Int J Cancer. 1989;43(6):1061–4.
106. Kaplan JE, Osame M, Kubota H, Igata A, Nishitani H, Maeda Y, et al. The risk of development of HTLV-I-associated myelopathy/tropical spastic paraparesis among persons infected with HTLV-I. J Acquir Immune Defic Syndr (1988). 1990;3(11):1096–101.
107. Kira J, Fujihara K, Itoyama Y, Goto I, Hasuo K. Leukoencephalopathy in HTLV-I-associated myelopathy/tropical spastic paraparesis: MRI analysis and a two year follow-up study after corticosteroid therapy. J Neurol Sci. 1991;106(1):41–9.
108. Milagres AC, Jorge ML, Marchiori PE, Segurado AA. Human T cell lymphotropic virus type 1-associated myelopathy in Sao Paulo, Brazil. Epidemiologic and clinical features of a university hospital cohort. Neuroepidemiology. 2002;21(3):153–8.
109. Bangham CR, Araujo A, Yamano Y, Taylor GP. HTLV-1-associated myelopathy/tropical spastic paraparesis. Nat Rev Dis Primers. 2015;1:15012.
110. Umehara F, Nose H, Saito M, Fukuda M, Ogino M, Toyota T, et al. Abnormalities of spinal magnetic resonance images implicate clinical variability in human T-cell lymphotropic virus type I-associated myelopathy. J Neurovirol. 2007;13(3):260–7.

111. Azodi S, Nair G, Enose-Akahata Y, Charlip E, Vellucci A, Cortese I, et al. Imaging spinal cord atrophy in progressive myelopathies: HTLV-I-associated neurological disease (HAM/TSP) and multiple sclerosis (MS). Ann Neurol. 2017;82(5):719–28.
112. Link H, Cruz M, Gessain A, Gout O, de The G, Kam-Hansen S. Chronic progressive myelopathy associated with HTLV-I: oligoclonal IgG and anti-HTLV-I IgG antibodies in cerebrospinal fluid and serum. Neurology. 1989;39(12):1566–72.
113. Saito T, Osame M, Usuku K, Matsumoto M, Igata A. Oligoclonal IgG bands in patients with HTLV-I associated myelopathy--detection by agarose isoelectric focusing, transfer to cellulose nitrate and immunoperoxidase staining. Rinsho Shinkeigaku. 1989;29(8):976–81.
114. Saeidi M, Sasannejad P, Foroughipour M, Shahami S, Shoeibi A. Prevalence of peripheral neuropathy in patients with HTLV-1 associated myelopathy/tropical spastic paraparesis (HAM/TSP). Acta Neurol Belg. 2011;111(1):41–4.
115. De Castro-Costa CM, Araujo AQ, Barreto MM, Takayanagui OM, Sohler MP, da Silva EL, et al. Proposal for diagnostic criteria of tropical spastic paraparesis/HTLV-I-associated myelopathy (TSP/HAM). AIDS Res Hum Retrovir. 2006;22(10):931–5.
116. Abrams A, Akahata Y, Jacobson S. The prevalence and significance of HTLV-I/II seroindeterminate Western blot patterns. Viruses. 2011;3(8):1320–31.
117. da Silva BV, Santos FLN, Goncalves NLS, Araujo THA, Nascimento DSV, Pereira FM, et al. Performance of commercially available serological screening tests for human T-cell Lymphotropic virus infection in Brazil. J Clin Microbiol. 2018;56(12):e00961.
118. Araujo A, Bangham CRM, Casseb J, Gotuzzo E, Jacobson S, Martin F, et al. Management of HAM/TSP: systematic review and consensus-based recommendations 2019. Neurol Clin Pract. 2021;11(1):49–56.
119. Olindo S, Cabre P, Lezin A, Merle H, Saint-Vil M, Signate A, et al. Natural history of human T-lymphotropic virus 1-associated myelopathy: a 14-year follow-up study. Arch Neurol. 2006;63(11):1560–6.
120. Halperin JJ. Lyme neuroborreliosis. Curr Opin Infect Dis. 2019;32(3):259–64.
121. Halperin JJ. Neuroborreliosis and neurosyphilis. Continuum (Minneap Minn). 2018;24(5, Neuroinfectious Disease):1439–58.
122. Burn L, Vyse A, Pilz A, Tran TMP, Fletcher MA, Angulo FJ, et al. Incidence of Lyme Borreliosis in Europe: a systematic review (2005-2020). Vector Borne Zoonotic Dis (Larchmont, NY). 2023;23(4):172–94.
123. Kugeler KJ, Schwartz AM, Delorey MJ, Mead PS, Hinckley AF. Estimating the frequency of Lyme disease diagnoses, United States, 2010-2018. Emerg Infect Dis. 2021;27(2):616–9.
124. TibblesCD,EdlowJA.DoesthispatienthaveerythemaMigrans?JAMA.2007;297(23):2617–27.
125. Nadelman RB, Nowakowski J, Forseter G, Goldberg NS, Bittker S, Cooper D, et al. The clinical spectrum of early Lyme borreliosis in patients with culture-confirmed erythema migrans. Am J Med. 1996;100(5):502–8.
126. Krause PJ, Bockenstedt LK. Cardiology patient pages. Lyme disease and the heart. Circulation. 2013;127(7):e451–4.
127. Forrester JD, Meiman J, Mullins J, Nelson R, Ertel SH, Cartter M, et al. Notes from the field: update on Lyme carditis, groups at high risk, and frequency of associated sudden cardiac death--United States. MMWR Morb Mortal Wkly Rep. 2014;63(43):982–3.
128. Radolf JD, Strle K, Lemieux JE, Strle F. Lyme disease in humans. Curr Issues Mol Biol. 2021;42:333–84.
129. Träisk F, Lindquist L. Optic nerve involvement in Lyme disease. Curr Opin Ophthalmol. 2012;23(6):485–90.
130. Sibony P, Halperin J, Coyle PK, Patel K. Reactive Lyme serology in optic neuritis. J Neuroophthalmol. 2005;25(2):71–82.
131. Mikkilä HO, Seppälä IJ, Viljanen MK, Peltomaa MP, Karma A. The expanding clinical spectrum of ocular Lyme borreliosis. Ophthalmology. 2000;107(3):581–7.
132. Jha P, Rodrigues Pereira SG, Thakur A, Jhaj G, Bhandari S. A case of optic neuritis secondary to Lyme disease. WMJ. 2018;117(2):83–7.

133. Knudtzen FC, Andersen NS, Jensen TG, Skarphédinsson S. Characteristics and clinical outcome of Lyme Neuroborreliosis in a high endemic area, 1995-2014: a retrospective cohort study in Denmark. Clin Infect Dis. 2017;65(9):1489–95.
134. Garcia-Monco JC, Benach JL. Lyme Neuroborreliosis: clinical outcomes, controversy, pathogenesis, and polymicrobial infections. Ann Neurol. 2019;85(1):21–31.
135. Krüger H, Kohlhepp W, König S. Follow-up of antibiotically treated and untreated neuroborreliosis. Acta Neurol Scand. 1990;82(1):59–67.
136. Ogrinc K, Lusa L, Lotrič-Furlan S, Bogovič P, Stupica D, Cerar T, et al. Course and outcome of early European Lyme Neuroborreliosis (Bannwarth syndrome): clinical and laboratory findings. Clin Infect Dis. 2016;63(3):346–53.
137. Garkowski A, Zajkowska J, Zajkowska A, Kułakowska A, Zajkowska O, Kubas B, et al. Cerebrovascular manifestations of Lyme Neuroborreliosis-a systematic review of published cases. Front Neurol. 2017;8:146.
138. Steere AC, Schoen RT, Taylor E. The clinical evolution of Lyme arthritis. Ann Intern Med. 1987;107(5):725–31.
139. De Guio F, Reyes S, Duering M, Pirpamer L, Chabriat H, Jouvent E. Decreased T1 contrast between gray matter and normal-appearing white matter in CADASIL. AJNR Am J Neuroradiol. 2014;35(1):72–6.
140. Mygland A, Ljøstad U, Fingerle V, Rupprecht T, Schmutzhard E, Steiner I. EFNS guidelines on the diagnosis and management of European Lyme neuroborreliosis. Eur J Neurol. 2010;17(1):8–16, e1–4.
141. Halperin JJ, Krupp LB, Golightly MG, Volkman DJ. Lyme borreliosis-associated encephalopathy. Neurology. 1990;40(9):1340–3.
142. Halperin JJ, Luft BJ, Anand AK, Roque CT, Alvarez O, Volkman DJ, et al. Lyme neuroborreliosis: central nervous system manifestations. Neurology. 1989;39(6):753–9.
143. Agarwal R, Sze G. Neuro-Lyme disease: MR imaging findings. Radiology. 2009;253(1):167–73.
144. Fernandez RE, Rothberg M, Ferencz G, Wujack D. Lyme disease of the CNS: MR imaging findings in 14 cases. AJNR Am J Neuroradiol. 1990;11(3):479–81.
145. Krüger H, Heim E, Schuknecht B, Scholz S. Acute and chronic neuroborreliosis with and without CNS involvement: a clinical, MRI, and HLA study of 27 cases. J Neurol. 1991;238(5):271–80.
146. Kalina P, Decker A, Kornel E, Halperin JJ. Lyme disease of the brainstem. Neuroradiology. 2005;47(12):903–7.
147. Aalto A, Sjöwall J, Davidsson L, Forsberg P, Smedby O. Brain magnetic resonance imaging does not contribute to the diagnosis of chronic neuroborreliosis. Acta Radiol (Stockholm, Sweden : 1987). 2007;48(7):755–62.
148. Hildenbrand P, Craven DE, Jones R, Nemeskal P. Lyme neuroborreliosis: manifestations of a rapidly emerging zoonosis. AJNR Am J Neuroradiol. 2009;30(6):1079–87.
149. Morgen K, Martin R, Stone RD, Grafman J, Kadom N, McFarland HF, et al. FLAIR and magnetization transfer imaging of patients with post-treatment Lyme disease syndrome. Neurology. 2001;57(11):1980–5.
150. Henriksson A, Link H, Cruz M, Stiernstedt G. Immunoglobulin abnormalities in cerebrospinal fluid and blood over the course of lymphocytic meningoradiculitis (Bannwarth's syndrome). Ann Neurol. 1986;20(3):337–45.
151. Hammers-Berggren S, Hansen K, Lebech AM, Karlsson M. Borrelia burgdorferi-specific intrathecal antibody production in neuroborreliosis: a follow-up study. Neurology. 1993;43(1):169–75.
152. Eckman EA, Pacheco-Quinto J, Herdt AR, Halperin JJ. Neuroimmunomodulators in Neuroborreliosis and Lyme encephalopathy. Clin Infect Dis. 2018;67(1):80–8.
153. John TM, Taege AJ. Appropriate laboratory testing in Lyme disease 2019;86(11):751–759.
154. Rauer S, Kastenbauer S, Hofmann H, Fingerle V, Huppertz HI, Hunfeld KP, et al. Guidelines for diagnosis and treatment in neurology - Lyme neuroborreliosis. German Med Sci. 2020;18:Doc03.

155. Patriquin G, LeBlanc J, Heinstein C, Roberts C, Lindsay R, Hatchette TF. Cross-reactivity between Lyme and syphilis screening assays: Lyme disease does not cause false-positive syphilis screens. Diagn Microbiol Infect Dis. 2016;84(3):184–6.
156. Thomas K, Schultheiss T, Ziemssen T. Neuroborreliosis during natalizumab treatment in multiple sclerosis. Neurology. 2013;81(11):1012–4.
157. Karussis D, Weiner HL, Abramsky O. Multiple sclerosis vs Lyme disease: a case presentation to a discussant and a review of the literature. Mult Scler. 1999;5(6):395–402.
158. Weigelt W, Schneider T, Lange R. Sequence homology between spirochaete flagellin and human myelin basic protein. Immunol Today. 1992;13(7):279–80.
159. Martin R, Gran B, Zhao Y, Markovic-Plese S, Bielekova B, Marques A, et al. Molecular mimicry and antigen-specific T cell responses in multiple sclerosis and chronic CNS Lyme disease. J Autoimmun. 2001;16(3):187–92.
160. Dattwyler RJ, Halperin JJ, Pass H, Luft BJ. Ceftriaxone as effective therapy in refractory Lyme disease. J Infect Dis. 1987;155(6):1322–5.
161. Strle F, Stupica D, Bogovič P, Visintainer P, Wormser GP. Is the risk of early neurologic Lyme borreliosis reduced by preferentially treating patients with erythema migrans with doxycycline? Diagn Microbiol Infect Dis. 2018;91(2):156–60.
162. Halperin JJ, Shapiro ED, Logigian E, Belman AL, Dotevall L, Wormser GP, et al. Practice parameter: treatment of nervous system Lyme disease (an evidence-based review): report of the Quality Standards Subcommittee of the American Academy of Neurology. Neurology. 2007;69(1):91–102.
163. Bozic C, Subramanyam M, Richman S, Plavina T, Zhang A, Ticho B. Anti-JC virus (JCV) antibody prevalence in the JCV epidemiology in MS (JEMS) trial. Eur J Neurol. 2014;21(2):299–304.
164. Cortese I, Reich DS, Nath A. Progressive multifocal leukoencephalopathy and the spectrum of JC virus-related disease. Nat Rev Neurol. 2021;17(1):37–51.
165. Sharma K, Tolaymat S, Yu H, Elkhooly M, Jaiswal S, Jena A, et al. Progressive multifocal leukoencephalopathy in anti-CD20 and other monoclonal antibody (mAb) therapies used in multiple sclerosis: a review. J Neurol Sci. 2022;443:120459.
166. Major EO, Yousry TA, Clifford DB. Pathogenesis of progressive multifocal leukoencephalopathy and risks associated with treatments for multiple sclerosis: a decade of lessons learned. Lancet Neurol. 2018;17(5):467–80.
167. Schweitzer F, Laurent S, Cortese I, Fink GR, Silling S, Skripuletz T, et al. Progressive multifocal leukoencephalopathy: pathogenesis, diagnostic tools, and potential biomarkers of response to therapy. Neurology. 2023;101(16):700–13.
168. Warnke C, Olsson T, Hartung HP. PML: the dark side of immunotherapy in multiple sclerosis. Trends Pharmacol Sci. 2015;36(12):799–801.
169. Brooks BR, Walker DL. Progressive multifocal leukoencephalopathy. Neurol Clin. 1984;2(2):299–313.
170. Schwab N, Schneider-Hohendorf T, Melzer N, Cutter G, Wiendl H. Natalizumab-associated PML: challenges with incidence, resulting risk, and risk stratification. Neurology. 2017;88(12):1197–205.
171. Koralnik IJ, Wüthrich C, Dang X, Rottnek M, Gurtman A, Simpson D, et al. JC virus granule cell neuronopathy: a novel clinical syndrome distinct from progressive multifocal leukoencephalopathy. Ann Neurol. 2005;57(4):576–80.
172. Wüthrich C, Cheng YM, Joseph JT, Kesari S, Beckwith C, Stopa E, et al. Frequent infection of cerebellar granule cell neurons by polyomavirus JC in progressive multifocal leukoencephalopathy. J Neuropathol Exp Neurol. 2009;68(1):15–25.
173. Lindå H, von Heijne A, Major EO, Ryschkewitsch C, Berg J, Olsson T, et al. Progressive multifocal leukoencephalopathy after natalizumab monotherapy. N Engl J Med. 2009;361(11):1081–7.
174. Cinque P, Koralnik IJ, Gerevini S, Miro JM, Price RW. Progressive multifocal leukoencephalopathy in HIV-1 infection. Lancet Infect Dis. 2009;9(10):625–36.

175. Tan IL, McArthur JC, Clifford DB, Major EO, Nath A. Immune reconstitution inflammatory syndrome in natalizumab-associated PML. Neurology. 2011;77(11):1061–7.
176. Wattjes MP, Barkhof F. Diagnosis of natalizumab-associated progressive multifocal leukoencephalopathy using MRI. Curr Opin Neurol. 2014;27(3):260–70.
177. Wijburg MT, Witte BI, Vennegoor A, Roosendaal SD, Sanchez E, Liu Y, et al. MRI criteria differentiating asymptomatic PML from new MS lesions during natalizumab pharmacovigilance. J Neurol Neurosurg Psychiatry. 2016;87(10):1138–45.
178. Wattjes MP, Wijburg MT, van Eijk J, Frequin S, Uitdehaag BMJ, Barkhof F, et al. Inflammatory natalizumab-associated PML: baseline characteristics, lesion evolution and relation with PML-IRIS. J Neurol Neurosurg Psychiatry. 2018;89(5):535–41.
179. Hodel J, Darchis C, Outteryck O, Verclytte S, Deramecourt V, Lacour A, et al. Punctate pattern: a promising imaging marker for the diagnosis of natalizumab-associated PML. Neurology. 2016;86(16):1516–23.
180. Vaneckova M, Martinkova A, Tupy R, Fiedler J, Stetkarova I, Medova E, et al. The spectrum of MRI findings of progressive multifocal leukoencephalopathy in patients with multiple sclerosis in The Czech Republic. Mult Scler J. 2019;25:473.
181. Bernal-Cano F, Joseph JT, Koralnik IJ. Spinal cord lesions of progressive multifocal leukoencephalopathy in an acquired immunodeficiency syndrome patient. J Neurovirol. 2007;13(5):474–6.
182. Outteryck O, Zéphir H, Salleron J, Ongagna JC, Etxeberria A, Collongues N, et al. JC-virus seroconversion in multiple sclerosis patients receiving natalizumab. Mult Scler. 2014;20(7):822–9.
183. Schwab N, Schneider-Hohendorf T, Pignolet B, Breuer J, Gross CC, Göbel K, et al. Therapy with natalizumab is associated with high JCV seroconversion and rising JCV index values. Neurol Neuroimmunol Neuroinflamm. 2016;3(1):e195.
184. McGuigan C, Craner M, Guadagno J, Kapoor R, Mazibrada G, Molyneux P, et al. Stratification and monitoring of natalizumab-associated progressive multifocal leukoencephalopathy risk: recommendations from an expert group. J Neurol Neurosurg Psychiatry. 2016;87(2):117–25.
185. Baber U, Bouley A, Egnor E, Sloane JA. Anti-JC virus antibody index changes in rituximab-treated multiple sclerosis patients. J Neurol. 2018;265(10):2342–5.
186. Möhn N, Luo Y, Skripuletz T, Schwenkenbecher P, Ladwig A, Warnke C, et al. Cerebrospinal fluid analysis in 108 patients with progressive multifocal leukoencephalopathy. Fluids Barriers CNS. 2020;17(1):65.
187. Wijburg MT, Kleerekooper I, Lissenberg-Witte BI, de Vos M, Warnke C, Uitdehaag BMJ, et al. Association of progressive multifocal leukoencephalopathy lesion volume with JC virus polymerase chain reaction results in cerebrospinal fluid of Natalizumab-treated patients with multiple sclerosis. JAMA Neurol. 2018;75(7):827–33.
188. Swinnen B, Saegeman V, Beuselinck K, Wouters A, Cypers G, Meyfroidt G, et al. Predictive value of JC virus PCR in cerebrospinal fluid in the diagnosis of PML. Diagn Microbiol Infect Dis. 2019;95(3):114859.
189. Berger JR, Aksamit AJ, Clifford DB, Davis L, Koralnik IJ, Sejvar JJ, et al. PML diagnostic criteria: consensus statement from the AAN Neuroinfectious disease section. Neurology. 2013;80(15):1430–8.
190. Berger JR. Progressive multifocal leukoencephalopathy. Handb Clin Neurol. 2014;123:357–76.
191. Foley JF, Defer G, Ryerson LZ, Cohen JA, Arnold DL, Butzkueven H, et al. Comparison of switching to 6-week dosing of natalizumab versus continuing with 4-week dosing in patients with relapsing-remitting multiple sclerosis (NOVA): a randomised, controlled, open-label, phase 3b trial. Lancet Neurol. 2022;21(7):608–19.
192. Scarpazza C, Prosperini L, De Rossi N, Moiola L, Sormani MP, Gerevini S, et al. To do or not to do? Plasma exchange and timing of steroid administration in progressive multifocal leukoencephalopathy. Ann Neurol. 2017;82(5):697–705.

193. Pavlovic D, Patera AC, Nyberg F, Gerber M, Liu M. Progressive multifocal leukoencephalopathy: current treatment options and future perspectives. Ther Adv Neurol Disord. 2015;8(6):255–73.
194. Dong-Si T, Richman S, Wattjes MP, Wenten M, Gheuens S, Philip J, et al. Outcome and survival of asymptomatic PML in natalizumab-treated MS patients. Ann Clin Transl Neurol. 2014;1(10):755–64.
195. Joly M, Conte C, Cazanave C, Le Moing V, Tattevin P, Delobel P, et al. Progressive multifocal leukoencephalopathy: epidemiology and spectrum of predisposing conditions. Brain. 2023;146(1):349–58.
196. de Souza RL, Dos Santos Madeira LDP, Pereira MVS, da Silva RM, de Luna Sales JB, Azevedo VN, et al. Prevalence of syphilis in female sex workers in three countryside cities of the state of Pará, Brazilian Amazon. BMC Infect Dis. 2020;20(1):129.
197. Chow F. Neurosyphilis. Continuum (Minneap Minn). 2021;27(4):1018–39.
198. Newman L, Rowley J, Vander Hoorn S, Wijesooriya NS, Unemo M, Low N, et al. Global estimates of the prevalence and incidence of four curable sexually transmitted infections in 2012 based on systematic review and global reporting. PLoS One. 2015;10(12):e0143304.
199. Workowski KA, Bachmann LH, Chan PA, Johnston CM, Muzny CA, Park I, et al. Sexually transmitted infections treatment guidelines, 2021. MMWR Recomm Rep. 2021;70(4):1–187.
200. Lukehart SA, Hook EW 3rd, Baker-Zander SA, Collier AC, Critchlow CW, Handsfield HH. Invasion of the central nervous system by Treponema pallidum: implications for diagnosis and treatment. Ann Intern Med. 1988;109(11):855–62.
201. Chapel TA. The signs and symptoms of secondary syphilis. Sex Transm Dis. 1980;7(4):161–4.
202. Wu Y, Wu W. Neurosyphilis presenting with myelitis-case series and literature review. J Infect Chemother. 2020;26(2):296–9.
203. Timmermans M, Carr J. Neurosyphilis in the modern era. J Neurol Neurosurg Psychiatry. 2004;75(12):1727–30.
204. Kodama T, Sato H, Osa M, Fujikura Y, Kawana A. Cerebral syphilitic gumma in immunocompetent man. Japan Emerg Infect Dis. 2018;24(2):395–6.
205. Corrêa DG, de Souza SR, Freddi TAL, Fonseca APA, Dos Santos RQ, Hygino da Cruz LC Jr. Imaging features of neurosyphilis. J Neuroradiol. 2023;50(2):241–52.
206. Kodama K, Okada S, Komatsu N, Yamanouchi N, Noda S, Kumakiri C, et al. Relationship between MRI findings and prognosis for patients with general paresis. J Neuropsychiatry Clin Neurosci. 2000;12(2):246–50.
207. Pesaresi I, Sabato M, Doria R, Desideri I, Guida M, Giorgi FS, et al. Susceptibility-weighted imaging in parenchymal neurosyphilis: identification of a new MRI finding. Sex Transm Infect. 2015;91(7):489–92.
208. Nagappa M, Sinha S, Taly AB, Rao SL, Nagarathna S, Bindu PS, et al. Neurosyphilis: MRI features and their phenotypic correlation in a cohort of 35 patients from a tertiary care university hospital. Neuroradiology. 2013;55(4):379–88.
209. Chen YY, Zhang YF, Qiu XH, Zhang Q, Chen FY, Liu L, et al. Clinical and laboratory characteristics in patients suffering from general paresis in the modern era. J Neurol Sci. 2015;350(1–2):79–83.
210. Jones HD, Urquhart N, Mathias RG, Banerjee SN. An evaluation of oligoclonal banding and CSF IgG index in the diagnosis of neurosyphilis. Sex Transm Dis. 1990;17(2):75–9.
211. Davis LE, Schmitt JW. Clinical significance of cerebrospinal fluid tests for neurosyphilis. Ann Neurol. 1989;25(1):50–5.
212. Tuddenham S, Katz SS, Ghanem KG. Syphilis laboratory guidelines: performance characteristics of Nontreponemal antibody tests. Clin Infect Dis. 2020;71(Suppl 1):S21–s42.
213. Marra CM, Maxwell CL, Smith SL, Lukehart SA, Rompalo AM, Eaton M, et al. Cerebrospinal fluid abnormalities in patients with syphilis: association with clinical and laboratory features. J Infect Dis. 2004;189(3):369–76.
214. Liao H, Zhang Y, Yue W. Case report: a case report of neurosyphilis mimicking limbic encephalitis. Front Neurol. 2022;13:862175.

215. Shi M, Luo D, Li Z, Li M, Jin S, Yang D, et al. A case report of neurosyphilis coexisting with a positive MOG antibody manifested as optic neuritis. Front Neurol. 2023;14:1258043.
216. World Health O. Global tuberculosis report 2018. Geneva: World Health Organization; 2018. p. 2018.
217. Donovan J, Thwaites GE, Huynh J. Tuberculous meningitis: where to from here? Curr Opin Infect Dis. 2020;33(3):259–66.
218. Cherian A, Ajitha KC, Iype T, Divya KP. Neurotuberculosis: an update. Acta Neurol Belg. 2021;121(1):11–21.
219. Rajasekaran S, Soundararajan DCR, Shetty AP, Kanna RM. Spinal tuberculosis: current concepts. Global Spine J. 2018;8(4 Suppl):96s–108s.
220. Sanei Taheri M, Karimi MA, Haghighatkhah H, Pourghorban R, Samadian M, Delavar KH. Central nervous system tuberculosis: an imaging-focused review of a reemerging disease. Radiol Res Pract. 2015;2015:202806.
221. Dodd PJ, Osman M, Cresswell FV, Stadelman AM, Lan NH, Thuong NTT, et al. The global burden of tuberculous meningitis in adults: a modelling study. PLOS Glob Public Health. 2021;1(12):e0000069.
222. Synmon B, Phukan P, Sharma SR, Hussain M. Etiological and radiological spectrum of longitudinal myelitis: a hospital-based study in north East India. J Neurosci Rural Pract. 2021;12(4):739–44.
223. Mazurek GH, Villarino ME. Guidelines for using the QuantiFERON-TB test for diagnosing latent mycobacterium tuberculosis infection. Centers for Disease Control and Prevention. MMWR Recomm Rep. 2003;52(Rr-2):15–8.
224. Bélard E, Semb S, Ruhwald M, Werlinrud AM, Soborg B, Jensen FK, et al. Prednisolone treatment affects the performance of the QuantiFERON gold in-tube test and the tuberculin skin test in patients with autoimmune disorders screened for latent tuberculosis infection. Inflamm Bowel Dis. 2011;17(11):2340–9.
225. Dian S, Ganiem AR, Te Brake LH, van Laarhoven A. Current insights into diagnosing and treating neurotuberculosis in adults. CNS Drugs. 2023;37(11):957–72.
226. Sharma SK, Ryan H, Khaparde S, Sachdeva KS, Singh AD, Mohan A, et al. Index-TB guidelines: guidelines on extrapulmonary tuberculosis for India. Indian J Med Res. 2017;145(4):448–63.
227. Trbojevic-Cepe M. Detection of Oligoclonal Ig bands: clinical significance and trends in methodological improvement. Ejifcc. 2004;15(3):86–94.
228. Fragoso YD, Elso FG, Carrá A. Differential diagnosis of multiple sclerosis in Latin America. Mult Scler J Exp Transl Clin. 2017;3(3):2055217317714279.
229. Khan MI, Garg RK, Rizvi I, Malhotra HS, Kumar N, Jain A, et al. Tuberculous myelitis: a prospective follow-up study. Neurol Sci. 2022;43(9):5615–24.
230. Roca B, Tornador N, Tornador E. Presentation and outcome of tuberculous meningitis in adults in the province of Castellon, Spain: a retrospective study. Epidemiol Infect. 2008;136(11):1455–62.
231. Garg RK, Malhotra HS, Kumar N. Paradoxical reaction in HIV negative tuberculous meningitis. J Neurol Sci. 2014;340(1–2):26–36.
232. Nagel MA, Cohrs RJ, Mahalingam R, Wellish MC, Forghani B, Schiller A, et al. The varicella zoster virus vasculopathies: clinical, CSF, imaging, and virologic features. Neurology. 2008;70(11):853–60.
233. Insinga RP, Itzler RF, Pellissier JM, Saddier P, Nikas AA. The incidence of herpes zoster in a United States administrative database. J Gen Intern Med. 2005;20(8):748–53.
234. Nagel MA, Gilden D. Neurological complications of varicella zoster virus reactivation. Curr Opin Neurol. 2014;27(3):356–60.
235. Hart MN, Earle KM. Haemorrhagic and perivenous encephalitis: a clinical-pathological review of 38 cases. J Neurol Neurosurg Psychiatry. 1975;38(6):585–91.
236. Takami K, Kenzaka T, Kumabe A, Fukuzawa M, Eto Y, Nakata S, et al. Varicella-zoster virus-associated meningitis, encephalitis, and myelitis with sporadic skin blisters: a case report. World J Clin Cases. 2022;10(2):717–24.

237. Gilden D, Cohrs RJ, Mahalingam R, Nagel MA. Varicella zoster virus vasculopathies: diverse clinical manifestations, laboratory features, pathogenesis, and treatment. Lancet Neurol. 2009;8(8):731–40.
238. Sweeney CJ, Gilden DH. Ramsay hunt syndrome. J Neurol Neurosurg Psychiatry. 2001;71(2):149–54.
239. Bert RJ, Samawareerwa R, Melhem ER. CNS MR and CT findings associated with a clinical presentation of herpetic acute retinal necrosis and herpetic retrobulbar optic neuritis: five HIV-infected and one non-infected patients. AJNR Am J Neuroradiol. 2004;25(10):1722–9.
240. Friedman DP. Herpes zoster myelitis: MR appearance. AJNR Am J Neuroradiol. 1992;13(5):1404–6.
241. Polat YB, Kula AY, Balsak S, Oran Z, Alkan A. MR features of varicella-zoster myelitis in an immunocompetent patient. Curr Med Imaging. 2023;19(4):394–7.
242. Wanninayake L, Rajapaksha D, Nair N, Gunarathne K, Ranawaka U. Guillain-Barre syndrome of acute motor axonal neuropathy (AMAN) type associated with herpes zoster: a case report. BMC Neurol. 2024;24(1):109.
243. Sieracki JC. Whipple's disease-observation on systemic involvement. I Cytologic observations. AMA Arch Pathol. 1958;66(4):464–7.
244. Schneider T, Moos V, Loddenkemper C, Marth T, Fenollar F, Raoult D. Whipple's disease: new aspects of pathogenesis and treatment. Lancet Infect Dis. 2008;8(3):179–90.
245. El-Abassi R, Soliman MY, Williams F, England JD. Whipple's disease. J Neurol Sci. 2017;377:197–206.
246. Samuels T, Hamilton P, Shaw P. Whipple disease of the mediastinum. AJR Am J Roentgenol. 1990;154(6):1187–8.
247. Anderson M. Neurology of Whipple's disease. J Neurol Neurosurg Psychiatry. 2000;68(1):2–5.
248. Panegyres PK, Edis R, Beaman M, Fallon M. Primary Whipple's disease of the brain: characterization of the clinical syndrome and molecular diagnosis. Qjm-Int J Med. 2006;99(9):609–23.
249. Compain C, Sacre K, Puechal X, Klein I, Vital-Durand D, Houeto JL, et al. Central nervous system involvement in Whipple disease: clinical study of 18 patients and long-term follow-up. Medicine (Baltimore). 2013;92(6):324–30.
250. Kundu A, Sen P, Khurana S. Isolated CNS Whipple's disease: a diagnostic dilemma. BMJ Case Rep. 2015;2015:bcr2015211784.
251. Clarke CE, Falope ZF, Abdelhadi HA, Franks AJ. Cervical myelopathy caused by Whipple's disease. Neurology. 1998;50(5):1505–6.
252. Messori A, Di Bella P, Polonara G, Logullo F, Pauri P, Haghighipour R, et al. An unusual spinal presentation of Whipple disease. AJNR Am J Neuroradiol. 2001;22(5):1004–8.
253. Balasa M, Gelpi E, Rey MJ, Vila J, Ramio-Torrenta L, Quiles Granado AM, et al. Clinical and neuropathological variability in clinically isolated central nervous system Whipple's disease. Brain Pathol. 2014;24(3):230–8.
254. Podsiadły E, Chmielewski T, Tylewska-Wierzbanowska S. Bartonella henselae and Borrelia burgdorferi infections of the central nervous system. Ann N Y Acad Sci. 2003;990:404–6.
255. Klotz SA, Ianas V, Elliott SP. Cat-scratch disease. Am Fam Physician. 2011;83(2):152–5.
256. Brinar VV, Habek M. Rare infections mimicking MS. Clin Neurol Neurosurg. 2010;112(7):625–8.
257. Zangwill KM, Hamilton DH, Perkins BA, Regnery RL, Plikaytis BD, Hadler JL, et al. Cat scratch disease in Connecticut. Epidemiology, risk factors, and evaluation of a new diagnostic test. N Engl J Med. 1993;329(1):8–13.
258. Hopkins KL, Simoneaux SF, Patrick LE, Wyly JB, Dalton MJ, Snitzer JA. Imaging manifestations of cat-scratch disease. AJR Am J Roentgenol. 1996;166(2):435–8.
259. Dietmann A, Colin-Benoit E, Tinkhauser G, Meinel TR, Scheidegger O. Pearls & Oy-sters: bilateral mononeuropathic neuralgic Amyotrophy triggered by Bartonella henselae infection responsive to immunoglobulin. Neurology. 2022;98(14):597–600.
260. Sendi P, Hirzel C, Bloch A, Fischer U, Jeannet N, Berlinger L, et al. Bartonella-associated transverse myelitis. Emerg Infect Dis. 2017;23(4):712–3.

261. Baylor P, Garoufi A, Karpathios T, Lutz J, Mogelof J, Moseley D. Transverse myelitis in 2 patients with Bartonella henselae infection (Cat Scratch Disease). Clin Infect Dis. 2007;45(4):e42–e5.
262. Py MO. Neurologic manifestations of Chagas disease. Curr Neurol Neurosci Rep. 2011;11(6):536–42.
263. Useche Y, Pérez AR, de Meis J, Bonomo A, Savino W. Central nervous system commitment in Chagas disease. Front Immunol. 2022;13:975106.
264. Del Poeta M, Ward BJ, Greenberg B, Hemmer B, Cree BAC, Komatireddy S, et al. Cryptococcal meningitis reported with Fingolimod treatment: case series. Neurol Neuroimmunol Neuroinflamm. 2022;9(3):e1156.
265. Valenzuela RM, Pula JH, Garwacki D, Cotter J, Kattah JC. Cryptococcal meningitis in a multiple sclerosis patient taking natalizumab. J Neurol Sci. 2014;340(1–2):109–11.
266. Panackal AA, Wuest SC, Lin YC, Wu T, Zhang N, Kosa P, et al. Paradoxical immune responses in non-HIV cryptococcal meningitis. PLoS Pathog. 2015;11(5):e1004884.
267. Kaur P, Lewis A, Basit A, Cyr NS, Muhammad Z. Increased risk of disseminated cryptococcal infection in a patient with multiple sclerosis on fingolimod. IDCases. 2020;22:e00961.
268. Iyer KR, Revie NM, Fu C, Robbins N, Cowen LE. Treatment strategies for cryptococcal infection: challenges, advances and future outlook. Nat Rev Microbiol. 2021;19(7):454–66.
269. Maziarz EK, Perfect JR. Cryptococcosis. Infect Dis Clin N Am. 2016;30(1):179–206.
270. Qu J, Jiang J, Lv X. The utility of cerebrospinal fluid white cell count during the prognostic assessment for cryptococcal meningitis patients: a retrospective study. BMC Infect Dis. 2020;20(1):571.
271. Skripuletz T, Schwenkenbecher P, Pars K, Stoll M, Conzen J, Bolat S, et al. Importance of follow-up cerebrospinal fluid analysis in cryptococcal meningoencephalitis. Dis Markers. 2014;2014:162576.
272. Correale J, Solomon AJ, Cohen JA, Banwell BL, Gracia F, Gyang TV, et al. Differential diagnosis of suspected multiple sclerosis: global health considerations. Lancet Neurol. 2024;23(10):1035–49.
273. Bismaya K, Dev P, Favas TT, Pathak A. Neuro-leptospirosis: experience from a tertiary center of North India. Rev Neurol. 2023;179(3):238–43.
274. Nguyen L, Chimunda T. Neuro-leptospirosis - A batty diagnostic enigma. IDCases. 2023;32:e01731.
275. Xucla-Ferrarons T, Turon-Sans J, Caballero-Avila M, Cortes-Vicente E, Rojas-Garcia R. Leptospirosis-induced acute acquired inflammatory neuropathy. J Peripher Nerv Syst. 2023;28(1):125–9.
276. Bhatt M, Rastogi N, Soneja M, Biswas A. Uncommon manifestation of leptospirosis: a diagnostic challenge. BMJ Case Rep. 2018;2018:bcr2018225281.
277. Dupouey J, Faucher B, Edouard S, Richet H, Kodjo A, Drancourt M, et al. Human leptospirosis: an emerging risk in Europe? Comp Immunol Microbiol Infect Dis. 2014;37(2):77–83.
278. van Samkar A, van de Beek D, Stijnis C, Goris M, Brouwer MC. Suspected leptospiral meningitis in adults: report of four cases and review of the literature. Neth J Med. 2015;73(10):464–70.
279. Chen SX, Han DK, Liu Y, Ye ZH, Lu K, Xu B, et al. Leptospira infection complicated by demyelinating disease: a case report. Front Neurol. 2022;13:1021364.
280. Zhao CW, Dai S, Wu Q. Pearls & Oy-sters: diagnosis and subtyping of listeria ventriculitis in an immunocompetent host. Neurology. 2022;99(3):123–6.
281. Benninger F, Steiner I. CSF in acute and chronic infectious diseases. Handb Clin Neurol. 2017;146:187–206.
282. Brouwer MC, van de Beek D, Heckenberg SG, Spanjaard L, de Gans J. Community-acquired listeria monocytogenes meningitis in adults. Clin Infect Dis. 2006;43(10):1233–8.
283. Garrì F, Puthenparampil M, Simonato D, Rinaldi F, Gallo P. A rare case of listeria rhombencephalitis with a sudden onset and unusual brain MRI features. Neurol Sci. 2024;45(1):353–5.

284. Pelegrín I, Moragas M, Suárez C, Ribera A, Verdaguer R, Martínez-Yelamos S, et al. Listeria monocytogenes meningoencephalitis in adults: analysis of factors related to unfavourable outcome. Infection. 2014;42(5):817–27.
285. Tecellioglu M, Kamisli O, Kamisli S, Erdogmus UA, Özcan C. Listeria monocytogenes rhombencephalitis in a patient with multiple sclerosis during fingolimod therapy. Mult Scler Relat Disord. 2019;27:409–11.
286. Décard BF, Thöne J, Haghikia A, Börnke C, Anders A, Lukas C, et al. Listeria rhombencephalitis mimicking a demyelinating event in an immunocompetent young patient. Mult Scler. 2017;23(1):123–5.
287. Spernovasilis N, Markaki I, Papadakis M, Mazonakis N, Ierodiakonou D. Mediterranean spotted fever: current knowledge and recent advances. Trop Med Infect Dis. 2021;6(4):172.
288. Del Prete E, Pizzanelli C, Moretti P, Cosottini M, Bonuccelli U. Mediterranean spotted fever: an unusual clinical and neuroradiological presentation. Neurol Sci. 2015;36(11):2141–3.
289. Aliaga L, Sánchez-Blázquez P, Rodríguez-Granger J, Sampedro A, Orozco M, Pastor J. Mediterranean spotted fever with encephalitis. J Med Microbiol. 2009;58(Pt 4):521–5.
290. Tran H, Allworth A, Bennett C. A case of mycoplasma pneumoniae-associated encephalomyelitis in a 16-year-old female presenting to an adult teaching hospital. Clin Med Insights Case Rep. 2013;6:209–11.
291. Francis DA, Brown A, Miller DH, Wiles CM, Bennett ED, Leigh N. MRI appearances of the CNS manifestations of mycoplasma pneumoniae: a report of two cases. J Neurol. 1988;235(7):441–3.
292. Guleria R, Nisar N, Chawla TC, Biswas NR. Mycoplasma pneumoniae and central nervous system complications: a review. J Lab Clin Med. 2005;146(2):55–63.
293. Taylor-Robinson D. Infections due to species of mycoplasma and Ureaplasma: an update. Clin Infect Dis. 1996;23(4):671–82; quiz 83–4.
294. Maida E, Kristoferitsch W. Cerebrospinal fluid findings in mycoplasma pneumoniae infections with neurological complications. Acta Neurol Scand. 1982;65(5):524–38.
295. Smith R, Eviatar L. Neurologic manifestations of mycoplasma pneumoniae infections: diverse spectrum of diseases. A report of six cases and review of the literature. Clin Pediatr. 2000;39(4):195–201.
296. Woo MH, Shin JW. Acute brainstem encephalitis associated with mycoplasma pneumoniae in an adult: a case report. Encephalitis (Seoul, Korea). 2021;1(4):120–3.
297. de Groot RCA, Meyer Sauteur PM, Unger WWJ, van Rossum AMC. Things that could be mycoplasma pneumoniae. J Infect. 2017;74(Suppl 1):S95–s100.
298. Ueda N, Minami S, Akimoto M. Mycoplasma pneumoniae-associated mild encephalitis/encephalopathy with a reversible splenial lesion: report of two pediatric cases and a comprehensive literature review. BMC Infect Dis. 2016;16(1):671.
299. Carod Artal FJ. Cerebral and spinal schistosomiasis. Curr Neurol Neurosci Rep. 2012;12(6):666–74.
300. Ross AG, McManus DP, Farrar J, Hunstman RJ, Gray DJ, Li YS. Neuroschistosomiasis. J Neurol. 2012;259(1):22–32.
301. Pammenter MD, Haribhai HC, Epstein SR, Rossouw EJ, Bhigjee AI, Bill PL. The value of immunological approaches to the diagnosis of schistosomal myelopathy. Am J Trop Med Hyg. 1991;44(3):329–35.
302. Cicero CE, Allibrio FE, Giuliano L, Luna J, Preux PM, Nicoletti A. Toxoplasma gondii and multiple sclerosis: a systematic review and meta-analysis. Eur J Neurol. 2021;28(12):4251–7.
303. Helsen G, Vandecasteele SJ, Vanopdenbosch LJ. Toxocariasis presenting as encephalomyelitis. Case Rep Med. 2011;2011:503913.
304. Lee IH, Kim ST, Oh DK, Kim HJ, Kim KH, Jeon P, et al. MRI findings of spinal visceral larva migrans of Toxocara canis. Eur J Radiol. 2010;75(2):236–40.
305. Uprety P, Graf EH. Enterovirus infection and acute flaccid myelitis. Curr Opin Virol. 2020;40:55–60.

306. Helfferich J, Knoester M, Van Leer-Buter CC, Neuteboom RF, Meiners LC, Niesters HG, et al. Acute flaccid myelitis and enterovirus D68: lessons from the past and present. Eur J Pediatr. 2019;178(9):1305–15.
307. Merchan-Del Hierro X, Halalau A. Cytomegalovirus-related transverse myelitis in an immunocompetent host: a subacute onset of an immune-mediated disease? BMJ Case Rep. 2017;2017:bcr2017220563.
308. Tetsuka S, Suzuki T, Ogawa T, Hashimoto R, Kato H. Encephalopathy associated with severe cytomegalovirus infection in an immunocompetent young woman. Case Rep Infect Dis. 2021;2021:5589739.
309. Holland NR, Power C, Mathews VP, Glass JD, Forman M, McArthur JC. Cytomegalovirus encephalitis in acquired immunodeficiency syndrome (AIDS). Neurology. 1994;44(3 Pt 1):507–14.
310. Trivedi S, Chakravarty A. Neurological complications of dengue fever. Curr Neurol Neurosci Rep. 2022;22(8):515–29.
311. Guzman MG, Gubler DJ, Izquierdo A, Martinez E, Halstead SB. Dengue infection. Nat Rev Dis Primers. 2016;2:16055.
312. Kumar N, Mishra R, Bargali A, Bhavana RI. Dengue-associated longitudinally extensive transverse myelitis. BMJ Case Rep. 2024;17(3):e259388.
313. Comtois J, Camara-Lemarroy CR, Mah JK, Kuhn S, Curtis C, Braun MH, et al. Longitudinally extensive transverse myelitis with positive aquaporin-4 IgG associated with dengue infection: a case report and systematic review of cases. Mult Scler Relat Disord. 2021;55:103206.
314. Weerasinghe WS, Medagama A. Dengue hemorrhagic fever presenting as encephalitis: a case report. J Med Case Rep. 2019;13(1):278.
315. Carod-Artal FJ, Wichmann O, Farrar J, Gascón J. Neurological complications of dengue virus infection. Lancet Neurol. 2013;12(9):906–19.
316. Viswanathan S, Botross N, Rusli BN, Riad A. Acute disseminated encephalomyelitis complicating dengue infection with neuroimaging mimicking multiple sclerosis: a report of two cases. Mult Scler Relat Disord. 2016;10:112–5.
317. Jubelt B, Mihai C, Li TM, Veerapaneni P. Rhombencephalitis/brainstem encephalitis. Curr Neurol Neurosci Rep. 2011;11(6):543–52.
318. Stübgen JP. Neuromuscular disorders associated with hepatitis B virus infection. J Clin Neuromuscul Dis. 2011;13(1):26–37.
319. Basheer A, Mookkappan S, Shanmugham V, Natarajan N. Hepatitis-B associated acute transverse myelitis mimicking syringomyelia. J Case Rep. 2014;4(1):77–81.
320. Mekki M, Eley B, Hardie D, Wilmshurst JM. Subacute sclerosing panencephalitis: clinical phenotype, epidemiology, and preventive interventions. Dev Med Child Neurol. 2019;61(10):1139–44.
321. Bellini WJ, Rota JS, Lowe LE, Katz RS, Dyken PR, Zaki SR, et al. Subacute sclerosing panencephalitis: more cases of this fatal disease are prevented by measles immunization than was previously recognized. J Infect Dis. 2005;192(10):1686–93.
322. Yilmaz K, Yilmaz M, Mete A, Celen Z. A correlative study of FDG PET, MRI/CT, electroencephalography, and clinical features in subacute sclerosing panencephalitis. Clin Nucl Med. 2010;35(9):675–81.
323. Jha AK, Kumar G, Dayal VM, Ranjan A, Suchismita A. Neurological manifestations of hepatitis E virus infection: an overview. World J Gastroenterol. 2021;27(18):2090–104.
324. Lhomme S, Abravanel F, Cintas P, Izopet J. Hepatitis E virus infection: neurological manifestations and pathophysiology. Pathogens. 2021;10(12):1582.
325. Ripellino P, Pasi E, Melli G, Staedler C, Fraga M, Moradpour D, et al. Neurologic complications of acute hepatitis E virus infection. Neurol Neuroimmunol Neuroinflamm. 2020;7(1):e643.
326. Mclean BN, Gulliver J, Dalton HR. Hepatitis E virus and neurological disorders. Pract Neurol. 2017;17(4):282–8.
327. Sarkar P, Morgan C, Ijaz S. Transverse myelitis caused by hepatitis E: previously undescribed in adults. BMJ Case Rep. 2015;2015:bcr2014209031.

328. Douvoyiannis M, Litman N, Goldman DL. Neurologic manifestations associated with parvovirus B19 infection. Clin Infect Dis. 2009;48(12):1713–23.
329. Barah F, Whiteside S, Batista S, Morris J. Neurological aspects of human parvovirus B19 infection: a systematic review. Rev Med Virol. 2014;24(3):154–68.
330. Bale JF Jr. Measles, mumps, rubella, and human parvovirus B19 infections and neurologic disease. Handb Clin Neurol. 2014;121:1345–53.
331. Watanabe T, Kawashima H. Acute encephalitis and encephalopathy associated with human parvovirus B19 infection in children. World J Clin Pediatr. 2015;4(4):126–34.
332. Dervisoglu E, Altintas Taslicay C, Alparslan B, Anik Y. Progressive MRI findings of West Nile virus encephalitis in a patient with diabetes mellitus. BMJ Case Rep. 2022;15(5):e249142.
333. Jehan F, Sazawal S, Baqui AH, Nisar MI, Dhingra U, Khanam R, et al. Multiomics characterization of preterm birth in low- and middle-income countries. JAMA Netw Open. 2020;3(12):e2029655.
334. Davis LE, DeBiasi R, Goade DE, Haaland KY, Harrington JA, Harnar JB, et al. West Nile virus neuroinvasive disease. Ann Neurol. 2006;60(3):286–300.
335. Petersen LR, Brault AC, Nasci RS. West Nile virus: review of the literature. JAMA. 2013;310(3):308–15.

Acquired Metabolic and Nutritional Diseases

6

6.1 Central Pontine Myelinolysis

6.1.1 Epidemiology

- The precise incidence remains unclear owing to underdiagnosis. However, it is estimated that osmotic demyelination syndrome affects approximately 2.5% of patients in intensive care units [1].

6.1.2 Etiology and Definition

- The osmotic demyelination syndrome results from damage to the myelin sheaths. Although pontine white matter tracts are frequently impacted, leading to central pontine myelinolysis (CPM), extrapontine myelinolysis also occurs commonly (6–13% without pontine CPM; 25–31% combined with CPM). The precise pathogenesis remains unclear, but the rapid correction of chronic hyponatremia is recognized as the most common trigger [2, 3].
- Most affected patients are alcoholics (>50%), as well as individuals with malnutrition, cancer, cirrhosis, or after liver transplantation.
- Less common causes of CPM include severe hypophosphatemia and hypokalemia, diabetes mellitus (resulting in hyperglycemia), renal failure, hemodialysis, hyperemesis gravidarum, anorexia nervosa, Wilson disease, severe burns, or systemic lupus erythematosus (SLE) [4].

T. Uher, *Mimics and Red Flags of Multiple Sclerosis*,
https://doi.org/10.1007/978-3-031-98945-2_6

6.1.3 Clinical Features

- The typical course is biphasic, but the manifestations can vary greatly.
- Initially, patients experience seizures (12.5–25%) or encephalopathy (37.1–44.5%), which gradually improves, or are followed by progression with:
  - Dysarthria, dysphagia, oculomotor dysfunction (one of those in 10–20%)
  - Hemi/quadriparesis (33%)
  - Coma (7.1–14.1%) or locked-in syndrome in the most severe cases [4].
- Some patients may show mild symptoms or may even be asymptomatic [5].

6.1.4 Brain Imaging

- Lesions' location:
  - Remarkable symmetry of magnetic resonance imaging (MRI) pathology
  - T2 hyperintense lesions in the central pons ("trident," "batwing," or "pig's snout" shaped) or in extrapontine structures including midbrain, cerebellum, thalamus, basal ganglia, lateral geniculate body, external and extreme capsule, gray-white matter junction of the cerebral cortex, and the hippocampus. Rarely might be lesions in mammillary bodies, columns of the fornix, amygdala, anterior commissure, optic tracts, and the subthalamic nuclei (Fig. 6.1).

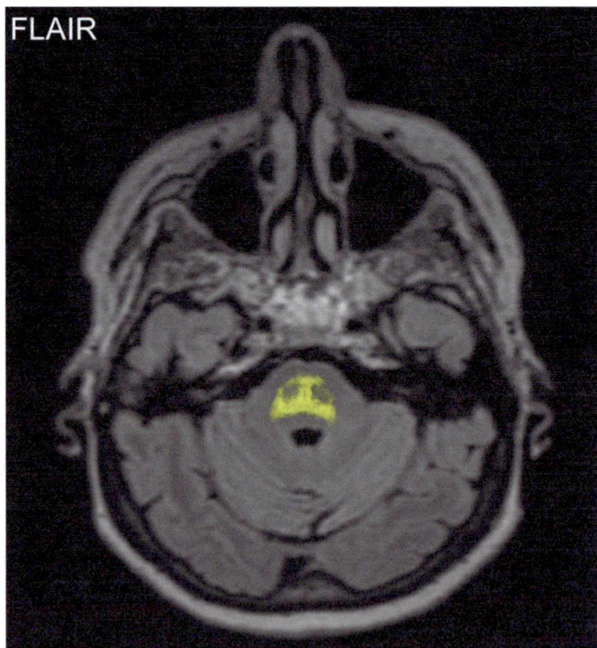

Fig. 6.1 Trident/batwing/pig's snout-shaped lesion in the central pons in central pontine myelinolysis

- Lesions' appearance
  - Restricted diffusion with increased signal on diffusion-weighted imaging (DWI) and decreased apparent diffusion coefficient (ADC) values (indicative of cytotoxic edema) is one of the earliest imaging features and is present in approximately 50% of cases. This typically normalizes within 3–4 weeks.
  - Changes on DWI are followed by T2 hyperintensities after 7–10 days.
  - T2 lesions, which can be large, are sharply defined and without mass effect.
  - T1 lesions are present only occasionally, particularly in later stages.
  - Lesion type, volume, location, or enhancement do not affect the prognosis.
- Contrast enhancement
  - Occasionally at the periphery of the lesions (<21%).
- Evolution over time:
  - Initially, MRI might be normal despite severe clinical deterioration.
  - T2 lesions may resolve completely or incompletely with residual gliosis [4, 6–11].

6.1.5 Spinal Cord Imaging

- Rare case studies of patients with centrally located T2 hyperintense lesions in the cervical and thoracic segments that are longitudinally extensive, as in longitudinally extensive transverse myelitis (LETM) [10, 12, 13].

6.1.6 Blood Work

- Hyponatremia (in 60% severe hyponatremia <120 mmol/L) [4].

6.1.7 Examination of CSF

- Although routine cerebrospinal fluid (CSF) tests are usually normal, some patients might have elevated concentrations of protein and mild pleocytosis [12, 13].

6.1.8 Diagnosis

- Based on laboratory testing, clinical, and MRI features.

6.1.9 Differential Diagnosis

- Posterior reversible encephalopathy syndrome (PRES); Wernicke's encephalopathy; calcineurin inhibitor toxicity; multiple sclerosis (MS); brainstem stroke or metastasis; neoplasm (associated with a mass effect and the asymmetry); central nervous system (CNS) lymphoma; Progressive multi-focal leukoencephalopathy (PML); Acute autoimmune or infectious encephalitis; mitochondrial encephalopathies or CNS vasculitis [11].

6.1.10 Treatment and Prognosis

- Only symptomatic treatment
- Although some patients experience a poor outcome, others achieve a good or nearly complete recovery. Even individuals with severe deterioration at the onset of the disease may show significant improvement over time [4, 14].

6.2 Cobalamin and Folate Deficiency

6.2.1 Epidemiology

- Cobalamin (vitamin B12) deficiency is relatively common, especially in older age.
- Folate (vitamin B19) deficiency usually does not occur in isolation but is associated with multiple nutrient deficiencies.

6.2.2 Etiology

- In many patients, these deficiencies are associated with malnutrition, atrophic gastritis, pernicious anemia, gastrointestinal conditions, or surgery, H2 antagonists, or alcoholism. In the case of folate deficiency, folate antagonists such as methotrexate or trimethoprim may also be the cause.
- Vitamin B12 deficiency can lead to lowered levels of methionine synthetase, which results in a functional folate deficiency. Therefore, deficits of both vitamins share common clinical and imaging features.
- Nutritional deficits often occur together with infectious diseases.

6.2.3 Non-neurological Clinical Features

- Gastrointestinal manifestations
- Hematologic manifestations (see Sect. 6.2.8)
- Systemic manifestations including orthostatic hypotension, fatigue, pallor, palpitations, or lightheadedness.

6.2.4 Neurological Clinical Features

- May occur without hematologic abnormalities and vice versa
- Myelopathy (subacute combined degeneration)
  - Affected dorsal columns and lateral corticospinal tract with combined motor pyramidal and sensory manifestations.
  - Symmetrical motor weakness of lower limbs.
  - Symmetrical distal paresthesia progressing into sensory loss (numbness) with distal-to-proximal progression and later to sensory ataxia and sphincter dysfunction.
  - Myelopathy usually has more sensory than motor deficit and affects deeper than superficial sensory loss.
  - In patients with folic acid deficiency, myelopathy is less frequent.
- Visual symptoms (can be bilateral) or diplopia
- Cognitive impairment and psychiatric syndromes
- Myeloneuropathy
- Peripheral neuropathy in some patients

6.2.5 Brain Imaging

- Rarely leukoencephalopathy-like pattern with diffuse T2 lesions in the subcortical white matter, brainstem, and cerebellum.

6.2.6 Spinal Cord Imaging

- T2-lesions in the posterior and lateral columns, rarely in the anterior parts of the spinal cord.
- T2-hyperintensities with a shape of “an inverted V sign” (axial plane)
- Only rarely with mild contrast enhancement
- Might be mild cord expansion
- B12 deficiency must be excluded in human immunodeficiency virus (HIV) patients with myelopathy, because B12 deficiency is often present in HIV patients and B12 deficit associated myelopathy may mimic vacuolar myelopathy in HIV patients (Fig. 6.2).

6.2.7 Electrophysiology

- Electromyography (EMG) may show mild axonal neuropathy
- Visual evoked potentials (VEP) have often delayed latencies (60%)

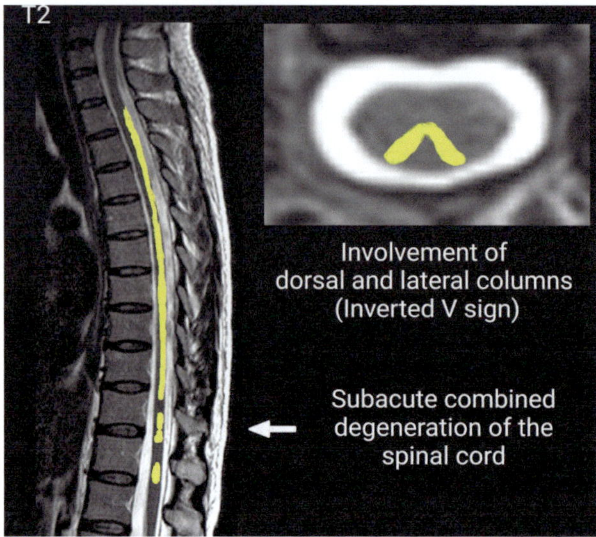

Fig. 6.2 MRI characteristics of cobalamin and folate deficiency

6.2.8 Blood Work

- Megaloblastic macrocytic anemia
- Neutrophil hypersegmentation and neutropenia
- Rarely isolated thrombocytopenia, neutropenia, pancytopenia, or hemolytic anemia
- Decreased concentrations of vitamin B12 and increased concentrations of methylmalonic acid and homocysteine.

6.2.9 Examination of CSF

- Case studies show normal findings without CSF-restricted oligoclonal bands (OCB)

6.2.10 Diagnosis

- B12 levels are usually decreased, and blood count usually exhibits characteristic changes.
- If B12 levels are in normal ranges, but a deficit is suspected, it is recommended to examine levels of homocysteine and methylmalonic acid, which should be increased and serve as sensitive markers of vitamin B12 deficiency.
- Remember that elevated homocysteine and methylmalonic acid levels may also be higher in familial hyperhomocysteinemia, levodopa administration, renal insufficiency, and volume depletion.
- A low serum folate level establishes the diagnosis of folate deficiency. Increased homocysteine level confirms folate deficiency.

6.2.11 Treatment and Prognosis

- B12 and folate acid supplementation [15, 16].

6.3 Cooper Deficiency and Zinc Overload

6.3.1 Etiology

- Often associated with stomach or duodenal malabsorption resulting from gastrointestinal surgery or diseases, it can also be caused by high zinc intake. However, in some patients, the underlying cause remains unidentified.
- Conversely, zinc deficiency may be associated with a higher risk of neurodegenerative and affective disorders, because of decreased neurogenesis.

6.3.2 Clinical Features

- Asymptomatic cases may occur.
- Manifestations resemble the subacute combined degeneration of the spinal cord (SACD) in vitamin B12 deficiency because copper is also involved in the methylation cycle.
- Present combined upper and lower motor neuron syndrome (absent ankle jerks, positive Babinski sign).
- Dorsal columns syndrome with sensory ataxia, decreased vibration and proprioception, and numbness or paresthesia.
- Bilateral optic neuropathy with visual loss and retinal nerve fiber layer (RNFL) thinning on optical coherence tomography (OCT) and slowed conduction velocities on VEP.
- Cognitive impairment
- Peripheral neuropathy
- Patients have insidious onset with progression of symptoms.
- Neurological symptoms may manifest even years after gastrointestinal surgery.

6.3.3 Brain Imaging

- Normal or shows non-specific T2 hyperintensities in white matter.
- Without contrast enhancement and restricted diffusion.

6.3.4 Spinal Cord Imaging

- Myelopathy with features resembling those in B12 deficiency.
- T2 hyperintensities in the dorsal columns of the cervical and thoracic cord at multiple segments.

- Can be longitudinally extensive transverse myelitis (LETM) mimicking neuromyelitis optica spectrum disorders (NMOSD).
- Differential diagnosis includes: B12 deficiency, nitrous oxide toxicity, HIV vacuolar myelopathy, herpes virus infection (HSV), syphilis (tabes dorsalis), acute disseminated encephalomyelitis (ADEM), or MS.

6.3.5 Blood Work

- Copper levels can be undetectable in blood and urine
- Can be anemia and neutropenia

6.3.6 Examination of CSF

- Rare case studies showed normal findings without CSF-restricted OCB

6.3.7 Treatment and Prognosis

- Copper supplementation and treatment of the primary cause of malabsorption or cessation of high zinc intake.
- Treatment may prevent further neurologic deterioration, but improvement of neurologic impairment can be absent [15–21].

6.4 Lathyrism

- Highest prevalence in India, Pakistan, Bangladesh, and Ethiopia.
- Caused by the excessive consumption of grass (chickling) peas containing the neurotoxin l-α, β-diamino propionic acid.
- Results in irreversible but non-progressive spastic paraparesis (upper motor neuron syndrome), vascular damage (e.g., aneurysms), and abnormal bone growth (skeletal deformities, particularly in the knees and feet).
- There are no diagnostic criteria for neurolathyrism, and diagnosis is based on clinical features, epidemiology, and the exclusion of other diagnoses [22].

6.5 Marchiafava–Bignami Disease

6.5.1 Epidemiology

- Rare disorder with unknown prevalence, with female/male ratio of 1/1 [23].

6.5.2 Etiology and Definition

- Occurs worldwide in patients with a history of chronic alcoholism (especially wine) and non-drinkers with malnutrition.
- Rarely can be associated with cancer (paraneoplastic etiology), major surgery, osmotic myelinolysis syndrome [23], or Wernicke's disease [24–26].
- Although the precise mechanism of the disease remains unclear, it is considered to be caused by a deficit of vitamin B complex, particularly thiamine (B1), leading to demyelination and necrosis of the corpus callosum [26].

6.5.3 Clinical Features

- Age of symptom onset varies (range, 14–79 years).
- There are no typical features, but two distinct subtypes are recognized:
- Type A is characterized by:
  - Major impairment of consciousness, confusion, delirium, and seizures.
  - Interhemispheric disconnection syndromes.
  - Expressive aphasia, dysarthria, hemiparesis, impaired walking, incontinence, sensory symptoms, gaze palsy, or diplopia.
- Type B is characterized by:
  - Mild impairment of consciousness [23–25].

6.5.4 Brain Imaging

- Lesions' location and appearance:
  - Symmetrically increased T2 and decreased T1 signal in either the entire corpus callosum (type A) or only a portion of it (type B).
  - Less frequently, extracallosal brain lesions may occur in the middle cerebellar peduncles, the internal capsule, and cerebral cortex (47% type A; 17% type B) (Fig. 6.3).
  - Often restricted diffusion of the corpus callosum extending into the adjacent white matter but usually sparing the subcortical U-fibers. DWI shows the lesions earliest and can identify more extensive callosal involvement than fluid-attenuated inversion recovery (FLAIR) sequences. ADC maps show decreased signal consistent with the presence of cytotoxic edema.
- Contrast enhancement:
  - Temporary contrast enhancement of the corpus callosum may occur
- Perilesional changes:
  - Edema of corpus callosum

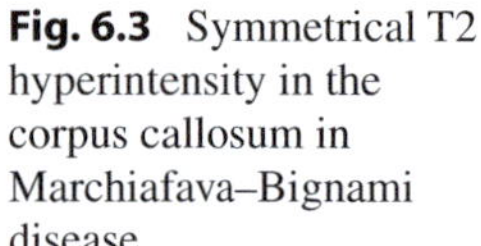

Fig. 6.3 Symmetrical T2 hyperintensity in the corpus callosum in Marchiafava–Bignami disease

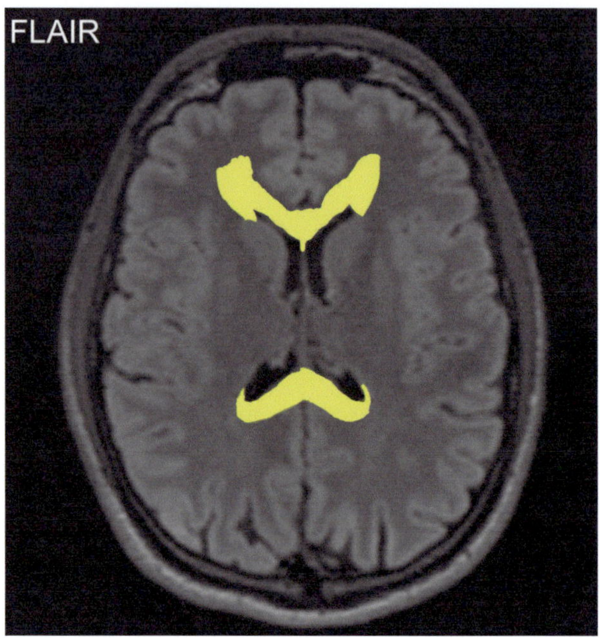

- Evolution over time:
  - In the chronic stages symmetric atrophy of the corpus callosum, focal T2 hyperintensities, T1 hypointensities, and cysts can be observed.
- Associated Findings:
  - Rarely seen microhemorrhages in the corpus callosum [23, 26, 27].

6.5.5 Spinal Cord Imaging

- A case study revealed a patient with a spinal cord involvement exhibiting longitudinally extensive, non-enhancing short tau inversion recovery (STIR)-hyperintense lesion extending from spinal C2 to T1 spinal segment with mild edema. The authors hypothesized an association between the spinal cord pathology and the coexistent B12 deficiency in this patient [28].

6.5.6 Examination of Blood and CSF

- Low serum levels of B vitamins occur often [28].
- Elevated concentration of protein or pleocytosis is rare (8.1%)
- There is a lack of data regarding the presence of CSF-restricted OCB, but they are anticipated to be negative [23, 28].

6.5.7 Diagnosis

- Based on patients' history and imaging

6.5.8 Differential Diagnosis

- The number of other disorders may mimic imaging features of this condition:
- Wernicke encephalopathy (usually with lesions of the mammillary bodies, periaqueductal region, and the walls of the third ventricle)
- Toxic leukoencephalopathy (for example, after chemotherapy)
- Para-infectious encephalitis (pathological CSF)
- Paraneoplastic leukoencephalopathy
- Neuroinfections including HIV-related encephalopathy, multifocal leukoencephalopathy, cytomegalovirus infection, or others [23, 26].

6.5.9 Treatment and Prognosis

- The treatment is similar to that used for Wernicke–Korsakoff syndrome.
- Early thiamine (B1) replacement therapy together with administration of other vitamins such as folate (B9), vitamin B12, and other B vitamins. Some authors also reported a positive effect of a high-dose corticosteroids.
- Long-term disability (61%) and dead (8%) frequently occur.
- Type B typically carries a better prognosis compared to type A [23, 25, 26].

6.6 Nitrous Oxide-Induced Myeloneuropathy

6.6.1 Synonyms

- Nitrous oxide (N_2O) is a sweet-smelling gas also known as "laughing gas," "nangs," "whippets," or "balloons."

6.6.2 Epidemiology

- Prevalence of lifetime use varies between 11% and 38.6% [29].

6.6.3 Etiology and Definition

- Inhalation of N_2O causes euphoria, relaxation, and anesthesia; therefore, it is used as an anesthetic but also misused as a recreational psychoactive substance.

- Chronic abuse of N_2O cause oxidation of vitamin B12. Subsequent functional depletion of vitamin B12 can become symptomatic in some patients.
- There is very high variability in the deleterious effects of N_2O on individuals [30, 31].

6.6.4 Clinical Features

- Depletion of B12 can cause a myeloneuropathy, an encephalopathy, or both.
- Most common neurological manifestations include:
- Sensory ataxia/dorsal column syndrome (58%)
- Altered distal sensation with paresthesia (80%)
- Peripheral (potentially also central) motor weakness (43%)
- Lhermitte's sign (15%)
- Urinary retention or incontinence (5–8%).
- In a small proportion of patients, encephalopathy with headache, lethargy, and cognitive symptoms is observed. Other symptoms, such as cerebellar syndrome or cranial neuropathy, are rare [30, 31].

6.6.5 Brain Imaging

- Normal [32].

6.6.6 Spinal Cord Imaging

- Normal (60–85%) [33] or shows T2 hyperintensities in the dorsal columns. Axial plane: inverted "V" shaped lesions; sagittal plane: longitudinally extensive T2 lesions in the dorsal columns (68–95%).
- Lesions are usually in cervical, thoracic, or both spinal cord segments.
- Lateral tracts of the spinal cord (lateral corticospinal tracts or lateral spinothalamic tracts) may also be affected, but involvement of the anterior part of the cord is very rare [30, 31].

6.6.7 Blood Work

- Decreased concentration of vitamin B12 (71%).
- The B12 levels do not correlate with the severity of clinical manifestations, because N_2O causes only functional B12 deficiency through irreversible inactivation of B12 from its active form to its inactive form. Therefore, users often have neurological symptoms mimicking nutritional B12 deficiency but with normal B12 levels in the blood.

- In cases of N_2O abuse, elevated concentrations of homocysteine may serve as a more useful marker for functional B12 deficiency (homocysteine levels can also rise in folate deficiency).
- High proportion of patients have pernicious anemia [30, 31].

6.6.8 Examination of CSF

- Normal findings or occasionally mild pleocytosis [30].

6.6.9 Electrophysiology

- Nerve conduction studies show demyelinating (23%) or axonal (11%) sensorimotor peripheral neuropathy [30, 31].

6.6.10 Diagnosis

- Based on the history of N_2O abuse and typical clinical and imaging features

6.6.11 Treatment and Prognosis

- Complete abstinence from N_2O and high-dose parenteral vitamin B12 supplementation, which is also recommended for patients with normal B12 levels.
- Some authors also recommend oral methionine.
- Supplementing with B12 while abusing N_2O does not prevent myeloneuropathy.
- Complete remission of clinical manifestations and MRI pathology may occur after a few months, but incomplete recovery is the most common outcome [30, 31, 34, 35].

6.7 Vitamin E Deficiency

6.7.1 Etiology

- Vitamin E protects tissues from oxidative stress, and its deficiency may be associated with a wide range of systemic and neurological manifestations.
- Vitamin E deficiency can be caused by rare genetic autosomal recessive disorders as well as various acquired conditions.

- The genetic disease associated with vitamin E deficiency:
  - Ataxia with Vitamin E Deficiency (AVED), also known as Ataxia with Isolated Vitamin E Deficiency, is caused by mutations in the tocopherol (alpha) transfer protein (*TTPA*) gene. This gene encodes the alpha-tocopherol transfer protein, and mutations lead to impaired distribution of vitamin E.
  - Abetalipoproteinemia results from mutations in the microsomal triglyceride transfer protein (*MTTP*) gene, which disrupts the absorption and transport of fat-soluble vitamins, including vitamin E.
  - Homozygous hypobetalipoproteinemia is caused by mutations in the Apolipoprotein B (*APOB*) gene, leading to very low levels of apolipoprotein B and consequently low levels of low-density lipoprotein (LDL). The reduced LDL levels impair the absorption of fat-soluble vitamins, including vitamin E.
  - Familial Isolated Vitamin E Deficiency is a disorder similar to AVED, characterized by an isolated deficiency of vitamin E despite normal lipid levels.
- Diseases associated with less severe vitamin E deficiency are associated with chronic fat malabsorption:
  - Short-bowel syndromes, intestinal lymphangiectasia, cholestatic liver diseases, celiac disease (CD), Crohn's disease, chronic pancreatitis, cystic fibrosis, systemic sclerosis, common variable immunodeficiency associated enteropathy.
- Other conditions potentially associated with asymptomatic vitamin E deficiency:
  - Malnutrition; alcoholism, hemolytic anemia; renal failure and hemodialysis.

6.7.2 Clinical Features

- Cereberall ataxia
  - One of the first manifestations. Some patients are asymptomatic, others have a variable severity of cerebellar syndrome.
  - Severe gait disturbances may result in a wheelchair bound state.
  - Often head tremor (28–73%).
- Sensory manifestations:
  - Dorsal column syndrome
  - Touch, pinprick, and temperature sensation are usually normal
- Upper motor neuron syndrome:
  - Initially, motor symptoms only poorly expressed, with motor strength typically remaining unaffected until the late stages. In late stages of the disease, spastic gait may be observed.
  - Babinski is often positive (66–100%), but the tendon reflexes are usually decreased or absent.
- Eye symptoms:
  - Retinitis pigmentosa with progressive impairment of visual acuity and night blindness.
  - Eye movement abnormalities with gaze paralysis, saccadic eye movements, bilateral, and horizontal nystagmus.

- Other less frequent neurological complications:
  - Distal amyotrophy (asymmetric lower limb motor neuropathy)
  - Focal or generalized dystonia
  - Myoclonus
  - Deafness and tinnitus
  - Urinary urgency or incontinence
- Usually, no mental retardation or cognitive dysfunction
- Non-neurological manifestations
  - Skeletal abnormalities (pes cavus, kyphoscoliosis)
  - Cardiac involvement (left ventricular hypertrophy, mild dilated cardiomyopathy, abnormal electrocardiography (ECG), or congestive heart failure)

6.7.3 Disease Course

- Age of symptom onset is 5–15 years, less frequently later in adulthood

6.7.4 Brain Imaging

- Normal

6.7.5 Spinal Cord Imaging

- Normal findings or bilateral T2 lesions in the posterior and lateral columns of the spinal cord, which may mimic findings observed in MS.

6.7.6 Electrophysiology

- Often moderate sensory axonal neuropathy with reduced amplitudes but normal nerve conduction velocities.

6.7.7 Blood Work

- Except for severely decreased vitamin E concentration (<2 mg/L), routine blood testing may show anemia and acanthocytosis.

6.7.8 Examination of CSF

- Normal

6.7.9 Diagnosis

- Assessment of serum vitamin E concentration and genetic testing

6.7.10 Treatment and Prognosis

- Vitamin E supplementation is usually effective and may prevent clinical manifestations in presymptomatic patients of affected family members [15, 16, 36–38].

6.8 Wernicke Encephalopathy

6.8.1 Epidemiology

- Common but greatly underdiagnosed disorder in adults and children
- Prevalence 40–130/100.000 (clinical studies) and 800–2800/100.000 (autopsy studies) [39].

6.8.2 Etiology and Definition

- Wernicke encephalopathy (WE) is caused by deficiency in vitamin B1 (thiamine), which frequently occurs in alcoholism and malnutrition but also in patients after gastrointestinal and bariatric surgery, recurrent vomiting, chronic diarrhea, use of chemical compounds and drugs, cancer and chemotherapeutic treatments, acquired immunodeficiency syndrome (AIDS), renal diseases, thyrotoxicosis, or magnesium depletion.
- Associated with brain lesions that are confined to regions with high thiamine content within 2–3 weeks.
- In Asian populations, a deficit in vitamin B1 is typically associated with cardiovascular (wet) beriberi disease, whereas in Europeans, it is usually linked to dry beriberi with polyneuropathy and WE [39–41].
- Severe, short-term B1 deficiency usually results in WE, whereas a chronic mild deficiency is frequently associated with peripheral neuropathy [39, 42, 43].

6.8.3 Clinical Features

- Acute syndrome
  - A. Mental-status changes ranging from confusion to coma resulting from involvement of thalamic or mamillary bodies (82%).
  - B. Ocular abnormalities with nystagmus, symmetrical or asymmetrical incomplete ophthalmoplegia, or conjugate-gaze palsies resulting from involvement of pontine tegmentum and oculomotor nuclei (29%).

  - C. Gait and trunk ataxia result from involvement of the cerebellar vermis and vestibular dysfunction (23%). The WE frequently coexists with polyneuropathy, which may also contribute to gait instability.
  - Complete triad (A. + B. + C.) seen in only 10–16% of patients.
  - Around 19% of patients do not have any of the symptoms from the classic triad at the disease onset, but at least one of the typical features occurs in the later disease course.
- Uncommon early manifestations may include:
  - Stupor
  - Hypotension and tachycardia
  - Hypothermia
  - Bilateral visual disturbances and papilloedema
  - Seizures
  - Hearing loss
  - Hallucinations and behavioural disturbances
- Late-stage symptoms
  - Hyperthermia
  - Increased muscular tone and spastic paresis
  - Choreic dyskinesias
  - Coma
- Approximately 80% of WE survivors develop Korsakoff's syndrome, which is characterized by severe working memory deficit, a relatively mild deficit of reference memory, and confabulations.
- Extraneural manifestations include heart failure, orthopnea, pulmonary and peripheral edema, severe hypotension, and lactic acidosis
- Age of onset between 30 and 70 years [39, 42, 43].

6.8.4 Brain Imaging

- Symmetrical T2 hyperintensities in the para-ventricular regions of the thalamus, the hypothalamus, the mamillary bodies, the periaqueductal region, the floor of the fourth ventricle, and midline cerebellum.
- This typical MRI pattern is present in only a proportion of patients (58%).
- Sensitivity of MRI findings for diagnosis of WE is low (53%), but the specificity is relatively high (93%).
- Sometimes might occur lesions in atypical locations such as the cortex or the splenium of the corpus callosum, show contrast enhancement (especially in mamillary bodies) or restricted diffusion [39, 44–46] (Fig. 6.4).

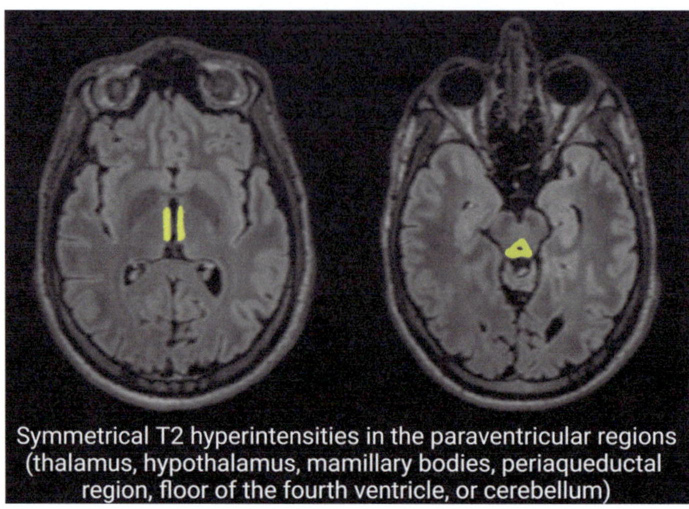

Fig. 6.4 MRI characteristics of Wernicke encephalopathy

6.8.5 Spinal Cord Imaging

- A case study reported a patient with WE and a long hyperintense T2 lesion in the central gray matter of the cervical cord without restricted diffusion, possibly due to vasogenic edema [47].

6.8.6 Blood Work

- Thiamin levels are decreased.

6.8.7 Examination of CSF

- Typically normal, although elevated protein may occur in later stages [39].

6.8.8 Diagnosis

- Often missed by routine clinical examination in the vast majority of cases, owing to a non-specific clinical manifestation in many patients or poorly recognized clinical features. The signs of WE are difficult or often impossible to differentiate from drunkenness.
- There is no specific laboratory, imaging or other paraclinical test available; therefore, diagnosis of WE should be clinical. However, MRI is considered as a valuable tool to confirm its diagnosis. The diagnosis is mainly supported by the response to thiamin [39].

6.8.9 Differential Diagnosis

- Differential diagnosis include mainly: paramedian thalamic infarction (top-of-the-basilar syndrome); ventriculo-encephalitis; Miller–Fisher syndrome; primary CNS lymphoma; Behçet's disease; MS; Leigh's disease; variant Creutzfeldt-Jakob disease; paraneoplastic encephalitis; severe hypophosphatasemia; acute intoxication from methyl bromide (fumigant and pesticide); or chronic intoxication from bromvalerylurea (old sedative drug) [39, 45, 48, 49].
- Acute hypophosphatemia commonly occurs in patients with alcohol abuse, burns, or starvation. It can lead to severe neuromuscular disturbances, including rhabdomyolysis, seizures, coma, and, in extreme cases, death. Patients may also exhibit hemolytic anemia, reduced oxygen release from hemoglobin, and impaired leukocyte and platelet function [50, 51].
- Cases of misdiagnosis of WE as MS have been reported, [52] as well as instances of the coexistence of WE with MS [53].

6.8.10 Treatment and Prognosis

- WE is medical emergency requiring immediate administration of parenteral thiamin before or concomitantly with intravenous glucose, because glucose alone can precipitate the WE in patients with thiamine deficiency.
- Recommended to administer parenteral thiamine to all patients with coma or a stuporous state, hypothermia or hyperthermia of unknown nature, or tachycardia and intractable hypotension of unknown cause, regardless of the symptoms, and particularly in patients from high-risk populations for WE.
- Therapeutic delay may result in irreversible neurological damage. In contrast, early treatment may be life-saving [39].
- The mortality rate is 17% [54].

References

1. Rao PB, Azim A, Singh N, Baronia AK, Kumar A, Poddar B. Osmotic demyelination syndrome in intensive care unit. Indian J Crit Care Med. 2015;19(3):166–9.
2. Brown WD. Osmotic demyelination disorders: central pontine and extrapontine myelinolysis. Curr Opin Neurol. 2000;13(6):691–7.
3. Sterns RH, Riggs JE, Schochet SS. Osmotic demyelination syndrome following correction of hyponatremia. N Engl J Med. 1986;314(24):1535–42.
4. Singh TD, Fugate JE, Rabinstein AA. Central pontine and extrapontine myelinolysis: a systematic review. Eur J Neurol. 2014;21(12):1443–50.
5. Newell KL, Kleinschmidt-DeMasters BK. Central pontine myelinolysis at autopsy; a twelve year retrospective analysis. J Neurol Sci. 1996;142(1):134–9.
6. Kallakatta RN, Radhakrishnan A, Fayaz RK, Unnikrishnan JP, Kesavadas C, Sarma SP. Clinical and functional outcome and factors predicting prognosis in osmotic demyelination syndrome (central pontine and/or extrapontine myelinolysis) in 25 patients. J Neurol Neurosurg Psychiatry. 2011;82(3):326–31.

7. Graff-Radford J, Fugate JE, Kaufmann TJ, Mandrekar JN, Rabinstein AA. Clinical and radiologic correlations of central pontine Myelinolysis syndrome. Mayo Clin Proc. 2011;86(11):1063–7.
8. Förster A, Nölte I, Wenz H, Al-Zghloul M, Kerl HU, Brockmann C, et al. Value of diffusion-weighted imaging in central pontine and extrapontine myelinolysis. Neuroradiology. 2013;55(1):49–56.
9. Ruzek KA, Campeau NG, Miller GM. Early diagnosis of central pontine myelinolysis with diffusion-weighted imaging. Am J Neuroradiol. 2004;25(2):210–3.
10. Kleinschmidt-DeMasters BK, Rojiani AM, Filley CM. Central and extrapontine myelinolysis: then…and now. J Neuropathol Exp Neurol. 2006;65(1):1–11.
11. Alleman AM. Osmotic demyelination syndrome: central pontine myelinolysis and extrapontine myelinolysis. Semin Ultrasound CT MR. 2014;35(2):153–9.
12. Jacob S, Gupta H, Nikolic D, Gundogdu B, Ong S. Central pontine and extrapontine myelinolysis: the great masquerader—an autopsy case report. Case Rep Neurol Med. 2014;2014:745347.
13. Biller J, Hornik A, Rodriguez-Porcel F, Agha C, Flaster M, Morales Vidal SG, et al. Central and extrapontine myelinolysis affecting the brain and spinal cord. An unusual presentation of pancreatic encephalopathy. Front Neurol. 2012:3.
14. Louis G, Megarbane B, Lavoué S, Lassalle V, Argaud L, Poussel J-F, et al. Long-term outcome of patients hospitalized in intensive care units with central or extrapontine myelinolysis*. Crit Care Med. 2012;40(3):970–2.
15. Goodman BP. Metabolic and toxic causes of myelopathy. Continuum (Minneap Minn). 2015;21(1 Spinal Cord Disorders):84–99.
16. Corrêa DG, da LCH C Jr, da Rocha AJ, Pacheco FT. Imaging aspects of toxic and metabolic myelopathies. Semin Ultrasound CT MR. 2023;44(5):452–63.
17. King D, Siau K, Senthil L, Kane KF, Cooper SC. Copper deficiency myelopathy after upper gastrointestinal surgery. Nutr Clin Pract. 2018;33(4):515–9.
18. Yarandi SS, Griffith DP, Sharma R, Mohan A, Zhao VM, Ziegler TR. Optic neuropathy, myelopathy, anemia, and neutropenia caused by acquired copper deficiency after gastric bypass surgery. J Clin Gastroenterol. 2014;48(10):862–5.
19. Pineles SL, Wilson CA, Balcer LJ, Slater R, Galetta SL. Combined optic neuropathy and myelopathy secondary to copper deficiency. Surv Ophthalmol. 2010;55(4):386–92.
20. Hedera P, Peltier A, Fink JK, Wilcock S, London Z, Brewer GJ. Myelopolyneuropathy and pancytopenia due to copper deficiency and high zinc levels of unknown origin II. The denture cream is a primary source of excessive zinc. Neurotoxicology. 2009;30(6):996–9.
21. Choi S, Hong DK, Choi BY, Suh SW. Zinc in the brain: friend or foe? Int J Mol Sci. 2020;21(23)
22. Correale J, Solomon AJ, Cohen JA, Banwell BL, Gracia F, Gyang TV, et al. Differential diagnosis of suspected multiple sclerosis: global health considerations. Lancet Neurol. 2024;23(10):1035–49.
23. Hillbom M, Saloheimo P, Fujioka S, Wszolek ZK, Juvela S, Leone MA. Diagnosis and management of Marchiafava-Bignami disease: a review of CT/MRI confirmed cases. J Neurol Neurosurg Psychiatry. 2014;85(2):168–73.
24. Rosa A, Demiati M, Cartz L, Mizon JP. Marchiafava-Bignami disease, syndrome of interhemispheric disconnection, and right-handed agraphia in a left-hander. Arch Neurol. 1991;48(9):986–8.
25. Heinrich A, Runge U, Khaw AV. Clinicoradiologic subtypes of Marchiafava-Bignami disease. J Neurol. 2004;251(9):1050–9.
26. Wenz H, Eisele P, Artemis D, Förster A, Brockmann MA. Acute Marchiafava-Bignami disease with extensive diffusion restriction and early recovery: case report and review of the literature. J Neuroimaging. 2014;24(4):421–4.
27. Chang KH, Cha SH, Han MH, Park SH, Nah DL, Hong JH. Marchiafava-Bignami disease: serial changes in corpus callosum on MRI. Neuroradiology. 1992;34(6):480–2.

28. Perea J, Luis MB, Lázaro LG, Scollo S, Tamargo A, Crespo J, et al. Marchiafava-Bignami disease associated with spinal involvement. Case Rep Neurol Med. 2020;2020:8867383.
29. De Halleux C, Juurlink DN. Diagnosis and management of toxicity associated with the recreational use of nitrous oxide. Can Med Assoc J. 2023;195(32):E1075–e81.
30. Swart G, Blair C, Lu Z, Yogendran S, Offord J, Sutherland E, et al. Nitrous oxide-induced myeloneuropathy. Eur J Neurol. 2021;28(12):3938–44.
31. Oussalah A, Julien M, Levy J, Hajjar O, Franczak C, Stephan C, et al. Global burden related to nitrous oxide exposure in medical and recreational settings: a systematic review and individual patient data meta-analysis. J Clin Med. 2019;8(4)
32. Trowbridge P, Poland C. Missing a case of nitrous oxide toxicity. Ther Adv Infect Dis. 2022;9:20499361221104377.
33. Holroyd KB, Berkowitz AL. Metabolic and toxic myelopathies. Continuum (Minneap Minn). 2024;30(1):199–223.
34. Noh T, Osman G, Chedid M, Hefzy H. Nitrous oxide-induced demyelination: clinical presentation, diagnosis and treatment recommendations. J Neurol Sci. 2020;414:116817.
35. Zheng D, Ba F, Bi G, Guo Y, Gao Y, Li W. The sharp rise of neurological disorders associated with recreational nitrous oxide use in China: a single-center experience and a brief review of Chinese literature. J Neurol. 2020;267(2):422–9.
36. Yokota T, Wada Y, Furukawa T, Tsukagoshi H, Uchihara T, Watabiki S. Adult-onset spinocerebellar syndrome with idiopathic vitamin E deficiency. Ann Neurol. 1987;22(1):84–7.
37. Hentati F, El-Euch G, Bouhlal Y, Amouri R. Ataxia with vitamin E deficiency and abetalipoproteinemia. Handb Clin Neurol. 2012;103:295–305.
38. Jung JB, Kim Y, Oh K, Kim SA, Doh JH, Oh HJ, et al. Subacute combined degeneration associated with vitamin E deficiency due to small bowel obstruction: a case report. Medicine (Baltimore). 2019;98(36):e17052.
39. Sechi G, Serra A. Wernicke's encephalopathy: new clinical settings and recent advances in diagnosis and management. Lancet Neurol. 2007;6(5):442–55.
40. Blass JP, Gibson GE. Abnormality of a thiamine-requiring enzyme in patients with Wernicke-Korsakoff syndrome. N Engl J Med. 1977;297(25):1367–70.
41. Schenker S, Henderson GI, Hoyumpa AM Jr, McCandless DW. Hepatic and Wernicke's encephalopathies: current concepts of pathogenesis. Am J Clin Nutr. 1980;33(12):2719–26.
42. Harper CG, Giles M, Finlay-Jones R. Clinical signs in the Wernicke-Korsakoff complex: a retrospective analysis of 131 cases diagnosed at necropsy. J Neurol Neurosurg Psychiatry. 1986;49(4):341–5.
43. Sinha S, Kataria A, Kolla BP, Thusius N, Loukianova LL. Wernicke encephalopathy—clinical pearls. Mayo Clin Proc. 2019;94(6):1065–72.
44. Degnan AJ, Levy LM. Neuroimaging of rapidly progressive dementias, part 2: prion, inflammatory, neoplastic, and other etiologies. AJNR Am J Neuroradiol. 2014;35(3):424–31.
45. Weidauer S, Nichtweiss M, Lanfermann H, Zanella FE. Wernicke encephalopathy: MR findings and clinical presentation. Eur Radiol. 2003;13(5):1001–9.
46. Antunez E, Estruch R, Cardenal C, Nicolas JM, Fernandez-Sola J, Urbano-Marquez A. Usefulness of CT and MR imaging in the diagnosis of acute Wernicke's encephalopathy. AJR Am J Roentgenol. 1998;171(4):1131–7.
47. Ishikawa S, Ando K, Katakami T, Kawamoto M. Cervical cord lesions in Wernicke's encephalopathy. Radiol Case Rep. 2022;17(7):2424–7.
48. Brechtelsbauer DL, Urbach H, Sommer T, Blümcke I, Woitas R, Solymosi L. Cytomegalovirus encephalitis and primary cerebral lymphoma mimicking Wernicke's encephalopathy. Neuroradiology. 1997;39(1):19–22.
49. Squier MV, Thompson J, Rajgopalan B. Case report: neuropathology of methyl bromide intoxication. Neuropathol Appl Neurobiol. 1992;18(6):579–84.

50. Berger MM, Appelberg O, Reintam-Blaser A, Ichai C, Joannes-Boyau O, Casaer M, et al. Prevalence of hypophosphatemia in the ICU – results of an international one-day point prevalence survey. Clin Nutr (Edinburgh, Scotland). 2021;40(5):3615–21.
51. Diringer M. Neurologic manifestations of major electrolyte abnormalities. Handb Clin Neurol. 2017;141:705–13.
52. Lal D, Farrell MC, Krishnamurthy M. Wernicke's encephalopathy mimicking multiple sclerosis in a young female patient post-bariatric gastric sleeve surgery. J Community Hosp Intern Med Perspect. 2021;11(5):658–61.
53. Geny C, Pradat PF, Yulis J, Walter S, Cesaro D, Degos JD. Hypothermia, Wernicke encephalopathy and multiple sclerosis. Acta Neurol Scand. 1992;86(6):632–4.
54. Victor M, Adams RD, Collins GH. The Wernicke-Korsakoff syndrome. A clinical and pathological study of 245 patients, 82 with post-mortem examinations. Contemp Neurol Ser. 1971;7:1–206.

Inherited Metabolic Diseases 7

7.1 Biotinidase Deficiency

7.1.1 Epidemiology

- Prevalence 1/60.000 [1].
- Higher prevalence in Turkey (1/11.614).
- In some countries incorporated into the newborn screening [2].

7.1.2 Etiology and Definition

- Biotinidase deficiency (BTD) is an autosomal recessive metabolic disease associated with dysfunctional cleaving and recycling of biotin resulting in keto-lactic acidosis and organic acidemia. It is hypothesized that having some residual enzymatic activity may be responsible for the later onset of symptoms.
- BTD is often associated with a later onset of symptoms, whereas the holocarboxylase synthetase deficiency (multiple carboxylase deficiency) is associated with neonatal presentations [1, 3].

7.1.3 Clinical Features

- BTD in adults usually manifests as myelopathy, with or without optic neuropathy.
- Myelopathy and optic neuropathy occur gradually or simultaneously.
- Symptoms may worsen by stressful events, infection, or surgery [3, 4].

T. Uher, *Mimics and Red Flags of Multiple Sclerosis*,
https://doi.org/10.1007/978-3-031-98945-2_7

- Neurological features:
  - Hypotonia, growth retardation, seizures; hearing loss, ataxia; pallhypesthesia, myelopathy with motor deficit, stroke-like episodes, autonomic involvement
- Skin/mucosal features:
  - Alopecia, skin rash
- Ocular features:
  - Optic nerve atrophy, visual loss, bilateral central scotoma, conjunctivitis
- Systemic features:
  - Immunodeficiency (T and B-lymphocytes dysfunction) is associated with a greater risk of severe infections and sepsis.
  - If untreated, risk of severe metabolic acidosis with coma [1, 3–6].
- Symptom onset is in childhood, only rarely in adolescence or adulthood [6].

7.1.4 Brain Imaging

- Imaging can be normal [7–9].
- Magnetic resonance imaging (MRI) abnormalities are often clinically asymptomatic [10].
- Bilateral symmetric T2 hyperintensities located particularly in:
  - Optic nerve, optic chiasm, tectum, fornix, mammillary bodies, and
  - Medulla oblongata, periependymal regions at the fourth ventricle level, periaqueductal region, or anterior commissure level
- Lesions might show contrast enhancement [8, 11, 12].

7.1.5 Spinal Cord Imaging

- Imaging can be normal.
- If T2 hyperintensities are present, they often resemble longitudinally extensive transverse myelitis (LETM) and may encompass almost the entire spinal cord, from the cervicomedullary junction to the conus medullaris, mimicking neuromyelitis optica spectrum disorders (NMOSD) or myelin oligodendrocyte glycoprotein antibody-associated disease (MOGAD) [8, 13].
- The abnormal signal is typically located in the anterior or central part of the spinal cord [8]. However, some patients may also exhibit hyperintensities in the lateral and posterior columns [13].
- Lesions might show a mild contrast enhancement [11] or edema [12].
- MRI abnormalities are often clinically asymptomatic [10] (Fig. 7.1).

7.1.6 Blood Work

- Blood testing shows metabolic acidosis, elevated lactate, and pyruvate levels.

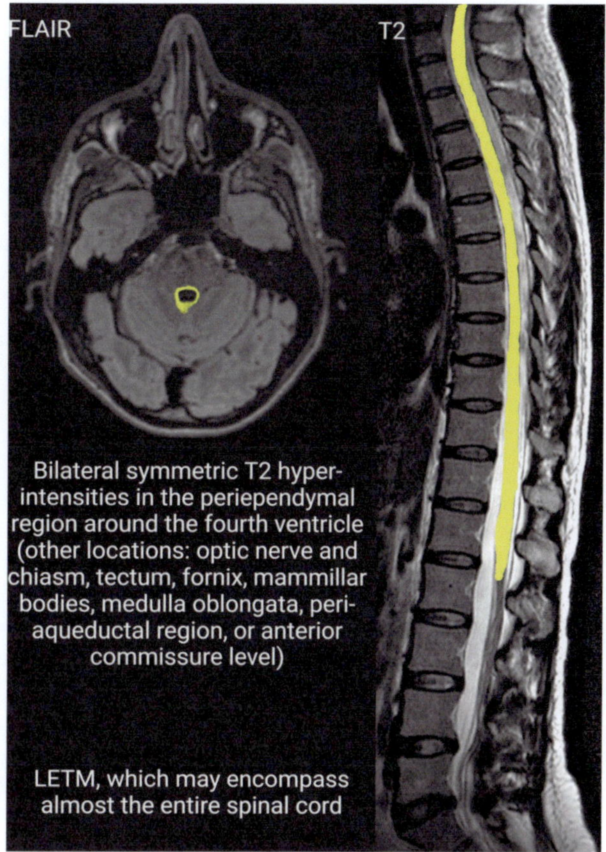

Fig. 7.1 MRI characteristics of biotinidase deficiency

7.1.7 Urine Analysis

- Contains abnormal organic acids (such as acylcarnitine)

7.1.8 Examination of CSF

- Elevated concentration of lactate, other parameters should be normal.
- Several case reports showed cerebrospinal fluid (CSF)-restricted oligoclonal bands (OCB) and elevated immunoglobulin G (IgG) index [14].

7.1.9 OCT

- Optical coherence tomography (OCT) may show marked retinal nerve fiber layer (RNFL) thinning in all quadrants [4].

7.1.10 Electrophysiological Studies

- Visual evoked potentials (VEP) are sometimes abnormal [7].

7.1.11 Diagnosis

- Easily diagnosed through assessment of blood biotinidase activity. Levels below 10% indicate profound deficiency, whereas those between 10% and 30% suggest partial BTD.
- Genetic testing (whole-exome sequencing) can confirm the presence of a homozygous mutation in the *BTD* gene [1].

7.1.12 Differential Diagnosis

- Owing to the heterogeneous phenotype of late-onset BTD and lack of awareness among most physicians regarding its manifestation in adults, the disorder is often overlooked in the differential diagnosis of multiple sclerosis (MS) and NMOSD.
- Adult-onset BTD with central paresis and optic nerve involvement may mimic NMOSD, MOGAD, or MS. Several case reports document patients initially misdiagnosed with MS or NMOSD who are having BTD [3, 5–8, 11–13, 15–17].
- Hence, it is advisable to consider screening for BTD in the differential diagnosis of MS and other demyelinating disorders, particularly in patients presenting with spinal and optic features. This is especially true for those who do not respond to immunomodulatory treatment [3].

7.1.13 Treatment and Prognosis

- Early diagnosis and treatment with biotin supplementation (5–10 mg/day) are crucial for preventing neurological and other systemic complications. If diagnosed and supplemented early enough, manifestations of the deficiency might significantly improve or completely resolve. Delayed initiation of treatment is often associated with irreversible neuronal damage [3, 16].

7.2 Cerebrotendinous Xanthomatosis

7.2.1 Epidemiology

- Prevalence (depends on geographical region) 0.4–2.2/100.000
- Likely significantly underdiagnosed, as genetic studies suggest a prevalence several times higher than the number of diagnosed patients [18, 19].

7.2.2 Etiology and Definition

- Inherited autosomal recessive neurodegenerative disorder linked to mutations in the *CYP27A1* gene, which result in a deficiency of 27-sterol hydroxylase. This enzyme plays a crucial role in converting cholesterol into bile acids. There is an accumulation of cholestanol and other bile acid precursors in the plasma and tissues, alongside increased urinary excretion of bile alcohols. Subsequently, abnormal lipid deposits (xanthomatous lesions) accumulate in various tissues, notably in tendons as well as in the central and peripheral nervous system [19–23].

7.2.3 Non-neurological Clinical Features

- Tendon xanthomas (70%)
  - Usually movable, nontender subcutaneous nodules.
  - Often in Achilles tendons, either symmetrically or asymmetrically. Other areas include the extensor surface of the metacarpophalangeal and interphalangeal joints, olecranon, or knees.
  - They are not specific to cerebrotendinous xanthomatosis (CTX); they may also manifest in sitosterolemia, familial hypercholesterolemia, or cholestatic liver disease.
  - Might be absent (30%) or develop in later disease stages after the onset of neurological symptoms. They usually occur after the age of 40 years (rarely before 20 years of age).
- Juvenile cataracts (89%)
  - Often present already in the early stages of the disease, typically between 5 and 15 years of age, and usually precedes the onset of central nervous system (CNS) symptoms by several years.
  - It is also typical for conditions such as galactosemia, Sjögren's syndrome, or myotonic dystrophy type 1.
- Intractable chronic diarrhea (40–50%)
  - Often earliest symptom of CTX manifests in early childhood.
  - Almost always manifests before or simultaneously with neurologic symptoms.
- Premature osteoporosis/osteopenia (67%)
  - Often, but usually mild, subclinical form diagnosed by densitometry.
- Prolonged unexplained neonatal jaundice or cholestasis
  - May also occur in other autosomal recessive lipid storage disorders.
- Other
  - Might occur pes cavus, pulmonary insufficiency, cardiovascular pathology (25%), endocrinopathy, renal and hepatic calculi.

7.2.4 Neurological Clinical Features

- CNS involvement usually dominates the clinical phenotype:
  - Spastic paraparesis (64%)
  - Cognitive impairment (often present already at school age) (60%)
  - Psychiatric symptoms (44%)
  - Ataxia (36%)
  - Seizures (33%)
  - Parkinsonism (9%)
  - Sensory deficit (rare)
- Peripheral neuropathy is often, but usually, subclinical (24–70%)
- Although the majority of clinical features are present in most patients, the age of onset and severity can vary substantially [19–21, 23–25].

7.2.5 Disease Course

- The mean age of symptom onset is around 25–36 years.
- Jaundice, diarrhea, cognitive impairment and cataract may occur in children.
- Xanthomas and neurological manifestations usually occur in young adulthood, and their prevalence increases with disease duration.
- Although cognitive or psychiatric manifestations might be present already at the diagnosis (30%), they typically develop later in the disease course.
- Course is progressive [21, 23, 24].

7.2.6 Brain Imaging

- Lesions' location:
  - Brain imaging in early disease stages or patients with spinal cord phenotype may be normal [26, 27].
  - However, most patients show a symmetric distribution of lesions in the gray matter structures, particularly in the basal ganglia and infratentorially [28].
  - Most patients also exhibit bilateral non-homogeneous T2 hyperintensities of the dentate nuclei and surrounding cerebellar white matter (in 75% on T2 and 100% on fluid-attenuated inversion recovery [FLAIR]). However, this characteristic feature might appear relatively late in the disease progression [29]. Dentate nuclei pathology consists of crystalline clefts embedded in a fibrous tissue and lipid and hemosiderin depositions [30] (Fig. 7.2)
  - Other less frequent locations include globus pallidus abutting the lateral border of the posterior limb of the internal capsula, cerebral peduncles extending into the substantia nigra, and inferior olives [28].
  - In addition, there are typically nonspecific focal or diffuse T2 lesions in the deep white matter, along with brain atrophy [28, 29].

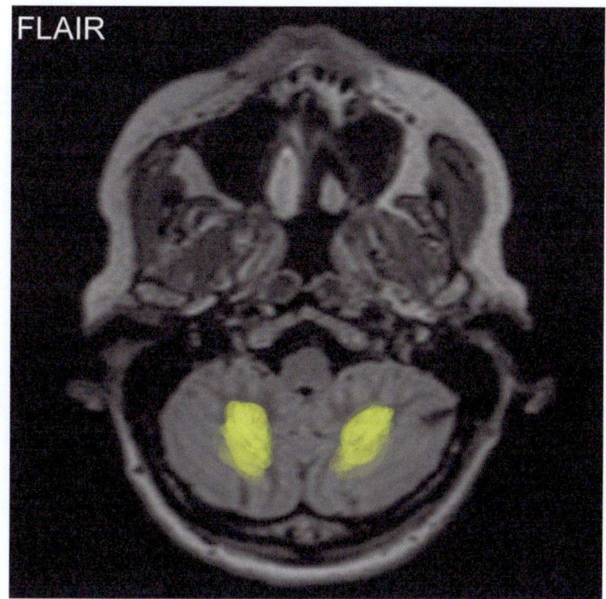

Fig. 7.2 Bilateral non-homogeneous T2 hyperintensities of the dentate nuclei and surrounding cerebellar white matter in cerebrotendinous xanthomatosis

- Lesions' appearance:
  - Lesions are hyperintense on T2-weighted images and iso-intense or hypo-intense (when extensive) on T1-weighted images [28].
  - Leukodystrophy-like pattern is rare [18].

7.2.7 Spinal Cord Imaging

- Spinal cord lesions are often, usually symmetric (suggesting metabolic etiology) and located typically in lateral and posterior columns [28].
- Some patients with progressive myelopathy may present with extensive white matter cord lesions resembling longitudinally extensive transverse myelitis (LETM), while showing a normal brain MRI and an absence of cerebral or cerebellar symptoms or tendon xanthomas ("spinal xanthomatosis") [26, 27, 31].
- Occasionally, brain and spinal cord MRI may appear normal. However, this should not discourage consideration of a possible diagnosis of spinal CTX [31].

7.2.8 Blood Work

- Elevated concentrations of plasma and bile cholestanol
- Elevated concentrations of urinary bile alcohol glucuronides
- Decreased concentration of biliary chenodeoxycholic acid [20].

7.2.9 Examination of CSF

- Protein concentration might be elevated, but routine testing should otherwise yield normal results, including the absence of CSF-restricted OCB [26, 31].

7.2.10 Electrophysiological Studies

- VEP are usually normal, [26] but electromyography (EMG) shows abnormalities in patients with peripheral neuropathy [23].

7.2.11 Diagnosis

- Early diagnosis before neurological damage occurs is important. But considering the heterogeneous phenotypes, early diagnosis can be challenging, and misdiagnoses occur often [23, 28].
- A "suspicion index" was developed to enhance early diagnosis of CTX.
  - Very strong (score = 100)
    - Sibling with CTX
    - Tendon xanthomas (their presence is not obligatory for the diagnosis)
  - Strong (score = 50)
    - Consanguineous parents (when parents share a common ancestor)
    - Juvenile cataract
    - Childhood-onset chronic diarrhea
    - Prolonged unexplained neonatal jaundice or cholestasis
    - Ataxia and/or spastic paraparesis
    - Dentate nuclei hyperintensities at brain magnetic resonance imaging (MRI)
    - Intellectual disability and/or psychiatric disturbances
  - Moderate (score = 25)
    - Early osteoporosis
    - Epilepsy
    - Parkinsonism
    - Polyneuropathy
- A total score of ≥100 indicates the need for assessment of serum cholestanol concentrations, [23] which must be measured in the absence of treatment with bile acids, statins, and corticosteroids, which can lower plasma cholestanol [32].
- Normal serum cholestanol levels indicate an alternative diagnosis.
- In case of increased plasma *cholestanol* level, diagnosis of CTX is confirmed by molecular analysis of the CYP27A1 gene.
- Family members of diagnosed patients should also undergo examination [23].

7.2.12 Differential Diagnosis

- CTX should be considered and excluded in children and young individuals presenting with unexplained bilateral cataracts accompanied by chronic diarrhea [20].
- Spinal xanthomatosis can be easily misdiagnosed as primary progressive MS, cervical myelopathy or hereditary spastic paraparesis. Therefore, some authors suggest screening all patients suspected of having primary progressive MS for the presence of chronic diarrhea or early-onset bilateral cataracts [26, 27].
- Although the symmetric involvement of gray matter structures (basal ganglia and infra-tentorial) may suggest a metabolic disorder like CTX, similar patterns are also observed in other rare conditions such as Langerhans cell histiocytosis, Erdheim–Chester disease, adreno-myeloneuropathy, or Refsum disease [28].

7.2.13 Treatment and Prognosis

- Oral chenodeoxycholic acid (CDCA) decreases synthesis of toxic bile acid (lower cholestanol levels) and limits the synthesis of cholesterol by the liver.
- Long-term treatment aims to stabilize or improve clinical and laboratory parameters, potentially preventing neurological impairment, particularly when initiated early. However, the effectiveness of treatment on neurological involvement may diminish if initiated during later disease stages.
- Despite treatment, some patients still experience disease progression [19–21, 23].
- Untreated CTX is associated with premature death [23].

7.3 Fabry Disease

7.3.1 Epidemiology

- Prevalence of mutations associated with classic (symptomatic or asymptomatic) phenotype: 2.5–4.5/100.000 (males), very rare in females.
- Prevalence of mutations associated with atypical ("late-onset") phenotype: 30–100/100.000 (males) and 2.5–17/100.000 (females).
- All races and ethnic groups are equally affected.
- Female/male ratio 1/2, but males are more severely affected [33–35].

7.3.2 Etiology and Definition

- Metabolic lysosomal storage disease (glycosphingolipidosis) associated with deficiency of the lysosomal hydrolase alpha-galactosidase A (alpha-Gal A), resulting in accumulation of globotriaosylceramide (Gb3) within lysosomes of different cells.

- X-linked inheritance of mutation in the α-galactosidase A (*GLA*) gene causes males to be more often and severely affected.
- Described >1.000 disease-associated mutations in the alpha-Gal A gene [35, 36]

7.3.3 Subtypes

- Classic Fabry disease: less common, more severe, onset of symptoms in childhood or adolescence, males are more frequently affected.
- Late-onset Fabry disease: ten-fold more often than classic phenotype; begins between 30 and 50 years of age; both sexes are affected [34, 35].

7.3.4 Neurological Clinical Features

- Neurological signs and symptoms may be the first and only manifestations of Fabry disease.
- Central nervous system (CNS)
  - Caused mainly by cerebral vasculopathy and a dilative arteriopathy
  - Mechanism is embolic or micro/macroangiopathic.
  - Large vessel pathology results in ischemic strokes, particularly in young adults (median age of the first stroke: 39 years in males and 46 years in females).
  - Small vessel pathology (microangiopathy) results in the progressive occurrence of white matter lesions, which are initially asymptomatic.
  - In progressed cases, can develop multi-infarct dementia.
- Peripheral nervous system
  - Peripheral small-fiber neuropathy with intermittent acroparesthesia (burning pain) or chronic pain. Therefore, distinguishing Fabry disease from other mostly autoimmune disorders in patients with painful small-fiber neuropathy remains a major challenge [34].
  - May be present recurrent painful episodes triggered by stress, fever, or exercise.
  - Decreased cold/warm perception manifesting first in the feet.
  - Autonomic symptoms from sympathetic nerve system involvement.
- Other neurological symptoms:
  - Around 40% patients have tinnitus. But the presence of pain, angiokeratomas, and proteinuria may help to distinguish Fabry disease from Meniere disease and other types of vestibular syndromes.

7.3.5 Non-neurological Clinical Features

- Skin: cutaneous vascular lesions (angiokeratomas, which are benign capillary ectasia in the superficial dermis); or hypo/anhidrosis
- Cardiac: left ventricular hypertrophy or arrhythmias in young adults

- Renal: chronic kidney disease; proteinuria of unknown etiology; multiple incidental renal sinuses; renal pelvis cysts
- Abdominal: pain; nausea; diarrhea; or irritable bowel syndrome in young adults
- Eye: typical corneal and lenticular opacities
- Rheumatologic: arthritis without synovial inflammation; fever of unknown origin; or muscle pain
- Others: osteopenia and osteoporosis; poor exercise tolerance
- In general, there are variable phenotypes ranging from severe manifestations in some males to asymptomatic presentation in some females.
- Patients have a positive family history of suspected symptoms [34, 35, 37, 38].

7.3.6 Brain Imaging

- Lesions' location and appearance:
  - Young adults may exhibit normal MRI findings. Conversely, brain pathology may be detected in asymptomatic patients.
  - Usually widespread brain involvement (80%)
  - Cortical or lacunar infarcts
  - T2 hyperintensities in deep white matter, particularly in frontal and parietal lobes
  - Higher frequency of ischemic lesions in the vertebrobasilar territory
  - Corpus callosum lesions are rare, and "Dawson fingers" are absent
  - T2 hyperintensities often correspond to hypointensities on T1 images
- Lesions' patterns:
  - A. Punctate subcortical white matter lesions or
  - B. Asymmetric and confluent white matter lesions or
  - C. Combination of both types (a + b)
- Contrast enhancement:
  - Absent
- Associated Findings:
  - Lesions are ischemic rather than inflammatory; therefore, central vein sign (CVS) typically yields negative results
  - Restricted diffusion may precede the formation of new white matter lesions
  - Presence of ecstatic (abnormally dilatated) mostly vertebral or basilar arteries (less frequently other arteries) may predict ischemic strokes
  - T1 hyperintensities of the pulvinar ("pulvinar sign") are rare (3%) and probably unrelated to Fabry disease
  - Microhemorrhages might occur [34, 35, 37–45] (Fig. 7.3)

7.3.7 Spinal Cord Imaging

- Typically, normal findings, but data are scarce, and the prevalence of cord pathology may be underestimated [37].
- Rare cases of spinal cord ischemic lesions have been documented [46, 47].

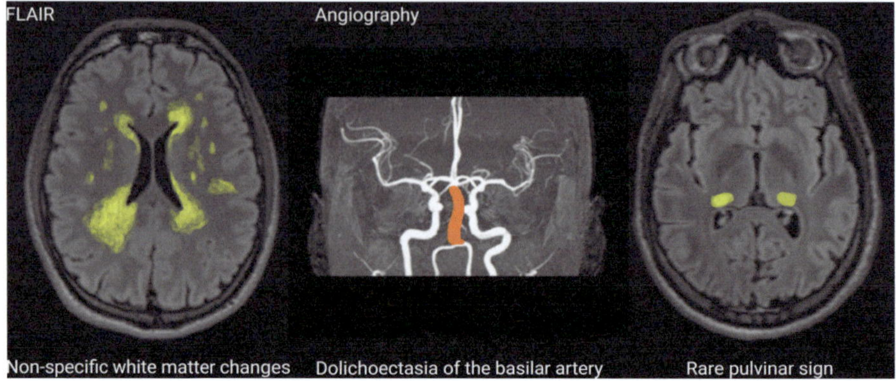

Fig. 7.3 MRI characteristics of Fabry disease

7.3.8 Blood Work

- Decreased alpha-Gal A activity (more details below).

7.3.9 Examination of CSF

- Mildly elevated concentration of protein (<0.8 g/L) and mild to moderate pleocytosis (<76 cells/mL) (30–40%).
- Some patients may exhibit a high proportion of neutrophils (>30%).
- Evidence of aseptic meningitis may indicate either an inflammatory reaction to stored lipids or brain ischemic injury.
- CSF-restricted OCB are rare (9%) [37].

7.3.10 Electrophysiology

- Conduction studies are normal because only small fibers are affected [35].
- VEP can be abnormal [48].

7.3.11 Diagnosis in Males

- Measurement of alpha-Gal A activity in leukocytes, plasma, fibroblasts, or dried blood spots.
- Undetectable activity (<3%) enables diagnosis of classic Fabry disease.
- If the alpha-Gal A activity falls within the range of 3–35%, genetic testing is indicated to search for a disease-causing mutation in the *GLA* gene.

- If no disease-causing mutation is found and suspicion remains high, gene-targeted deletion/duplication assays are indicated.
- If all tests are negative or if alpha-Gal A activity exceeds 35%, a diagnosis of Fabry disease cannot be established.
- Alpha-Gal A activity >30–35% is typically asymptomatic [34, 35, 37, 38].

7.3.12 Diagnosis in Females

- The measurement of alpha-Gal A activity in heterozygous females is unreliable, as their activity levels can overlap with those of healthy controls.
- The sensitivity and specificity of the alpha-Gal A assay are almost 100% in classically affected males, but only 50% in female carriers.
- Therefore, the initial step is to search for a disease-causing mutation in the *GLA* gene. If no disease-causing mutation is identified, a diagnosis of Fabry disease can be ruled out.
- Biopsy of affected organs with the demonstration of elevated globotriaosylceramide by electron microscopy or mass spectroscopy may be helpful in confirming the diagnosis [34, 35, 37, 38].

7.3.13 Differential Diagnosis

- Misdiagnosis or significant diagnostic delays are common, primarily due to the non-specific symptoms and the rarity of Fabry disease [49].
- Many misdiagnosed Fabry disease patients have transient cerebellar and brainstem symptoms attributable to vertebrobasilar transient ischemic attacks. In most cases, these symptoms appear intermittently and often coincide with symptoms of small-fiber neuropathy.
- Typical manifestations of MS, such as optic neuritis or internuclear ophthalmoplegia, are usually absent. Although brain MRI findings may resemble those seen in MS, the presence of CSF-restricted OCB and involvement of the spinal cord are rare, and the response to corticosteroids is usually poor [37].
- It is possible for MS and Fabry disease to coexist. There is a higher prevalence of autoimmune disorders in patients with Fabry disease. It is hypothesized that glycosphingolipid tissue deposition may represent a continuous pro-inflammatory stimulus, resulting in tissue epitope exposure and subsequent auto-reactive T-cell activation and inflammation [50].
- Although the prevalence of Fabry disease in the population of suspected or definite MS patients does not appear to be high, a delay in diagnosis may have serious consequences. Therefore, screening for Fabry disease should be indicated in atypical cases [37, 51].

7.3.14 Treatment and Prognosis

- Enzyme replacement or oral chaperone therapy.
- Diagnosis should be established as soon as possible, because the treatment response depends on the severity of organ involvement.
- Symptomatic treatment, including pharmacologic management of chronic neuropathic pain.
- With advancing age, Fabry disease can be linked to life-threatening complications such as heart disease, stroke, kidney disease, and kidney failure, ultimately leading to a reduced life expectancy, especially among men [34, 35, 38].

7.4 Homocysteine Remethylation Disorders

7.4.1 Etiology

- Rare inherited disorders caused by a decreased activity of the enzymes involved in the remethylation pathway.
- There are several different subtypes of this disorder, including disorders of cobalamin metabolism or methylenetetrahydrofolate reductase (MTHFR) deficiency, but all share similar phenotype.

7.4.2 Clinical Features

- Most patients experience symptom onset in infancy, characterized by poor feeding, hypotonia, seizures, coma, or death.
- In the rare late-onset phenotype, symptoms typically begin around the age of 21 years (range, 14–40 years).
- The clinical features of the late-onset phenotype are different from early-onset phenotype and are characterized by:
  - Gait disturbances due to:
    - Upper neuron syndrome from involvement of the lateral columns of the spinal cord
    - Dorsal column syndrome with sensory deficit
    - Asymmetric lower limb motor demyelinating neuropathy (amyotrophy) in the distal muscles of the legs with steppage gait
  - Cognitive impairment and psychiatric syndromes
  - Encephalopathy
  - Thrombotic events
  - Other rare manifestations include tremor, dysarthria, anorexia, cataract, epilepsy, or dermatitis.
- Symptoms are frequently exacerbated suddenly following triggers such as flu, dietary changes, or psychological stress.

7.4.3 Brain Imaging

- Can be normal, but many patients have symmetrical T2 lesions in periventricular and subcortical white matter and the terminal areas of the white matter, suggesting delayed/impaired myelination
- Often signal changes of basal ganglia in children, but rare in adults
- Brain atrophy
- Rarely, reversibly increased signal in the dorsal portions of the cerebellar hemispheres (Fig. 7.4)

7.4.4 Spinal Cord Imaging

- Normal or present bilateral T2 hyperintensities in the posterior and lateral columns and spinal cord atrophy

7.4.5 Electrophysiology

- EMG often shows demyelinating sensori-motor peripheral neuropathy of the lower limbs, which may be subclinical or symptomatic.

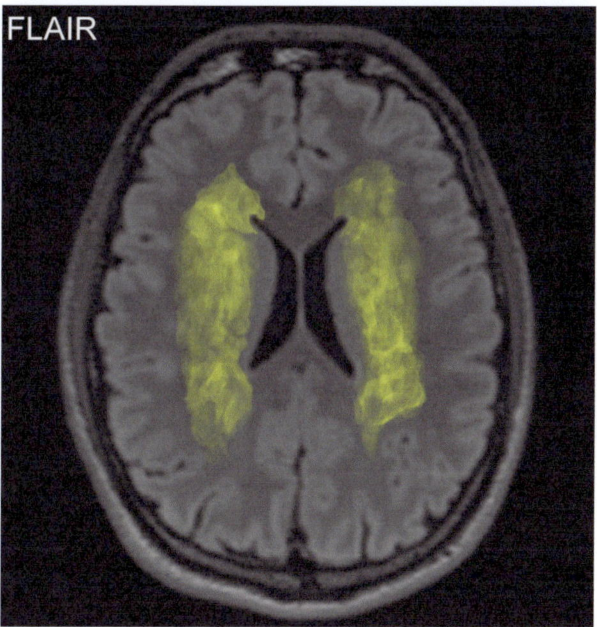

Fig. 7.4 Symmetrical lesions in the periventricular and subcortical white matter in homocysteine remethylation disorders

7.4.6 Blood Work

- Increased concentration of homocysteine
- Ketoacidosis (common in children bur rare in adults)
- Anemia
- B12 and folic acid concentrations are typically normal

7.4.7 Examination of Urine

- Methylmalonic acid levels are increased or normal

7.4.8 Examination of CSF

- No data

7.4.9 Diagnosis

- Misdiagnosis or delayed diagnosis by many years is often. Differential diagnosis includes vitamin B12 deficiency, hereditary spastic paraparesis, hereditary, or immune peripheral neuropathy but also MS.
- In patients with unexplained psychiatric symptoms should be assessed concentration of serum homocysteine. In suspected patients with levels >50 μmol/L, should be performed organic acid screening and next-generation genetic sequencing.

7.4.10 Treatment and Prognosis

- Treatable disease by a mixture of vitamins and other supplements such as hydroxycobalamin, betaine, folic acid, L-carnitine, and other B vitamins.
- Unlike early-onset patients, late-onset patients usually respond promptly to the treatment [52–54].

7.5 Hyperornithinemia-Hyperammonemia-Homocitrullinuria (HHH) Syndrome and Other Disorders of Glutamate and Urea Cycle Metabolism

7.5.1 Epidemiology

- Incidence 2.9/100.000 live births.
- Accounts for 1–3.8% of all urea cycle disorders.
- Female/male ratio 1/2 [55].

7.5.2 Etiology and Definition

- An autosomal recessive genetic disorder of the urea cycle caused by mutations in genes encoding the mitochondrial ornithine carrier [56].
- CNS pathology involves demyelination, atrophy, and stroke-like lesions induced by the toxic effects of ammonia and glutamine on astrocytes [57].

7.5.3 Clinical Features

- Acute non-neurological:
  - More common in infancy and presents with hyperammonemia, tachypnea, respiratory alkalosis, gastrointestinal problems, and liver failure.
- Neurological:
  - Severity may vary widely, ranging from neurologically asymptomatic patients to severe cases with coma and seizures.
  - Disease is typically slowly progressive, commonly associated with an aversion to protein-rich foods and recurrent vomiting.
  - Pyramidal tract signs encompass lower limb hyperreflexia, positive Babinski sign, and, less frequently, severe spastic paraparesis (66%).
  - Cerebellar symptoms.
  - Myoclonic seizures (35%).
  - Progressive encephalopathy with cognitive impairment.
  - Other neurological features include involuntary hand movements, buccofaciolingual dyspraxia, psychiatric disorders, dysmorphic features, cerebral dysplasia and microcephaly, dysphasia, or drop-attacks.
- Ocular:
  - Photophobia, hemeralopia, tapetoretinal degeneration, cataract, and abnormal electroretinogram might be present [56, 58, 59].

7.5.4 Disease Course

- Although the age of symptom onset varies, it typically occurs in early infancy; however, it can rarely manifest in adolescence or adulthood (9%).
- No correlation between the age of onset and disease severity, except for the severe neonatal phenotypes [58–61].

7.5.5 Brain Imaging

- MRI findings may be normal, or show wide range of pathologies such as:
- Multiple non-specific focal T2 hyperintensities in the subcortical white matter [56, 58, 59, 61].

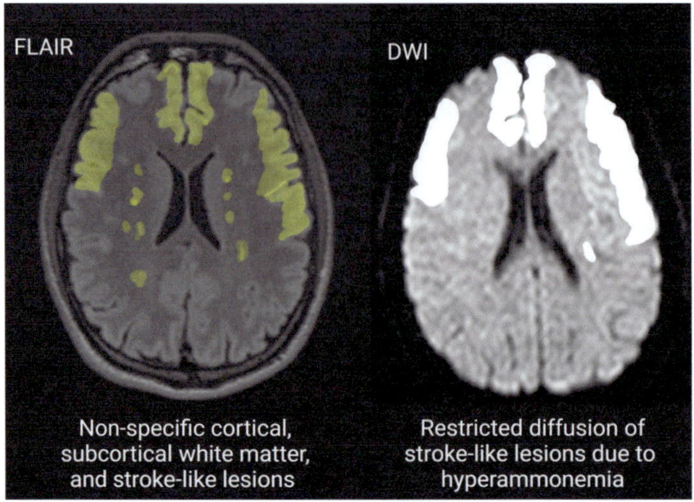

Fig. 7.5 MRI characteristics of hyperornithinemia-hyperammonemia-homocitrullinuria (HHH) syndrome and other disorders of glutamate and urea cycle metabolism

- Multiple stroke-like lesions with restricted diffusion in the cingulate gyrus, insular cortex, or other cortical regions may be present, which are considered specific to hyperammonemia, regardless of the cause [60] (Fig. 7.5).
- Stroke-like lesions may also be observed in children [62].
- Mild subcortical, cortical, and cerebellar atrophy.
- Cystic lesions and calcifications in basal ganglia.
- Subdural hematoma.
- Diffuse brain edema in acute stages [56, 58, 59, 61].

7.5.6 Spinal Cord Imaging

- Cord atrophy in some patients [63].

7.5.7 Examination of Blood and CSF

- Blood: see Sect. 7.5.9.
- CSF: Insufficient data.

7.5.8 Electrophysiology

- Often abnormal motor evoked potentials (MEP) affecting the pyramidal tract of lower but not upper limbs. Somatosensory evoked potentials are normal.
- EMG may show abnormal nerve conduction and signs of spinal anterior horn cells degeneration [64, 65].

7.5.9 Diagnosis

- Established based on the combination of the metabolic triad of hyperammonemia, hyperornithinemia, and urinary excretion of homocitrulline. However, some patients may not present with a complete metabolic triad.
- Genetic testing is the gold standard to confirm the diagnosis [56, 58].

7.5.10 Differential Diagnosis

- Hyperammonemia is also associated with a wide range of other inborn errors of metabolism, including organic acidemias or fatty acid oxidation defects [58].
- Similarly to HHH syndrome, other treatable complex disorders of glutamate and urea cycle metabolism, such as delta-1-pyrroline-5-carboxylate synthetase (P5CS) deficiency and arginase deficiency (ARG1 deficiency) may also be associated with spastic paraparesis. Their presentations may resemble cerebral palsy or hereditary spastic paraparesis [66].

7.5.11 Treatment and Prognosis

- Long-term treatment involves low-protein diet supplemented with citrulline or arginine. In some patients, sodium benzoate and/or sodium phenylbutyrate are also used to decrease blood ammonia levels.
- The prognosis varies widely, but early diagnosis and treatment may improve clinical outcomes [56, 58].

7.6 Lysosomal Storage and Peroxisomal Function Disorders

7.6.1 Epidemiology

- Rare and underdiagnosed diseases
- Subtypes that can potentially mimic the clinical and imaging features of MS include the following disorders [67, 68], along with their incidence rates in newborns:
  - X-linked adrenoleukodystrophy: 1 in 15–17.000 [69, 70]
  - Krabbe disease: 1 in 100.000 (late adolescent-form <5% of cases) [71]
  - Metachromatic leukodystrophy: 1 in 40–160.000 [72]
  - Fabry disease: see Sect. 7.3
  - Chédiak–Higashi disease: <1 in 1.000.000 [73]
  - Niemann–Pick disease type C: 1 in 120.000 [74]
  - Tay-Sachs: 1 in 320.000 [75]

7.6.2 Cause and Definition

- Inherited metabolic disorders associated with abnormal catabolism of complex molecules (lipids, glycoproteins, or oligosaccharides) resulting in toxic accumulation of cellular debris.

7.6.3 X-Linked Adrenoleukodystrophy (X-ALD)

- Synonyme: Adrenomyeloneuropathy
- Cause:
  - X-linked recessive disorder (therefore more severe in males)
  - Disorder of peroxisomal fatty acid beta oxidation resulting in the accumulation of very long chain fatty acids in the adrenal glands, testes, central, and peripheral nervous system (causing demyelination and/or axonopathy).
- Diagnosis:
  - Very long chain fatty acids analysis of plasma and genetic testing
- Clinical course is unpredictable and consists of several variants:
  1. Childhood-onset adrenoleukodystrophy (most severe form)
     - Progressive severe disease beginning between ages 4 and 10 presenting with pseudobulbar palsy, cognitive deficit, psychiatric symptoms, cortical blindness, deafness, and ataxia.
     - MRI shows bilateral white matter changes.
     - Adrenal insufficiency with failure of steroid synthesis.
  2. Isolated primary adrenal insufficiency (Addison's disease)
     - Should be suspected in boys and men with primary adrenal insufficiency with no detectable steroid-21-hydroxylase antibodies or other organ-specific antibodies.
  3. Adult-onset adrenoleukodystropy (rare, rapidly progressive)
     - Occurs in males between 10 and 21 years of age.
     - Manifests after the onset of adrenomyeloneuropathy with involvement of the spinal cord and peripheral nerves. If it occurs before adrenomyeloneuropathy (only rarely), it is associated with an elevated risk of misdiagnosis.
     - Usually less severe and progresses slower as compared with the childhood-onset variant. But severe inflammatory reaction and fulminant disease course mimicking tumoriform demyelination (MS, acute disseminated encephalomyelitis [ADEM], MOGAD) may be devastating and rapidly progressive as is in the childhood-onset variant.
  4. (Adult-onset) adrenomyeloneuropathy—slowly progressive
     - Only this form affects females (other forms are extremely rare in females).
     - Myeloneuropathy includes simultaneous damage of the spinal cord and peripheral nerves in the lower limbs.
     - Although peripheral neuropathy is common, it is rarely symptomatic or dominating symptom.

- Patients usually have spastic paraparesis resembling primary progressive MS or hereditary spastic paraparesis.
- Symptoms onset is between 20 and 50 years of age.
- Life expectancy is normal.
- Hemizygous females.
  - Asymptomatic or slowly progressive adrenal, brain, and spinal involvement. Myelopathy with spastic paraparesis or only mild symptoms (20–50%).
  - Brain involvement and adrenocortical deficiency are rare.
  - A case study reported patient with transient unilateral blurred vision at disease onset.
- Hemizygous males:
  - Often spinal cord but also brain invovement.
  - Patients have progressive spastic paraparesis, marked bowel/bladder disturbance, dorsal collumns syndrome, and/or peripheral neuropathy usually after 35–40 years of age, which may mimic progressive MS.
  - Adrenal insufficiency may precede years or even decades before the onset of neurological symptoms.
  - Head trauma and stroke may precipitate the onset of brain manifestations [67, 76–83].

- Brain imaging:
  - MRI may be normal in early disease stages
  - Only 4–20% of females have typical white matter lesions in the brain
  - T2 hyperintensities and T1 hypointensities mostly in periventricular white matter
  - There are five patterns of the brain white matter involvement:
    - Pattern 1: parieto-occipital white matter (66%).
    - Pattern 2: frontal white matter or genu of corpus callosum (15.5%).
    - Pattern 3: corticospinal tract (frontopontine or corticospinal projection fibers) (12%).
    - pattern 4: cerebellar white matter or brainstem (1%).
    - pattern 5: concomitant parieto-occipital and frontal white matter (2.5%).
  - Cortical gray matter and subcortical U-fiber are usually spared.
  - Males may show curvilinear contrast enhancement outlining the boundaries of demyelination areas and restricted diffusion.
  - Patients, particularly males exhibiting the suspected MRI patterns, whether or not they show cognitive and neurological symptoms, should be evaluated for X-ALD (Fig. 7.6).
- Spinal cord imaging
  - Cord atrophy (mostly in thoracic segments) without T2 lesions is usually present in adrenomyeloneuropathy.
  - Therefore, X-ALD-related myelopathy should be considered in symptomatic adults with a normal MRI.
  - Only rarely longitudinally extensive transverse myelitis (LETM) [78, 81, 84, 85].

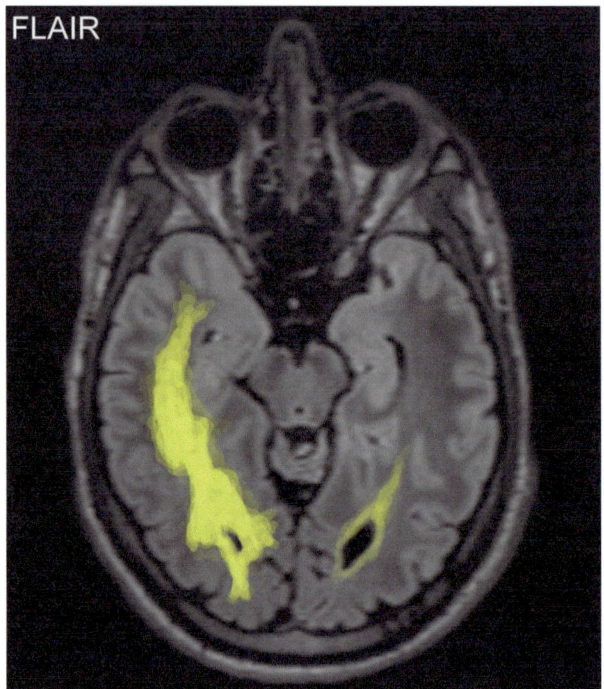

Fig. 7.6 Parieto-occipital white matter involvement (Pattern 1) in X-linked adrenoleukodystrophy (X-ALD)

- EMG may show demyelinating or axonal peripheral neuropathy
- Laboratory:
  - Blood: should be examined for adrenocortical function.
  - CSF shows elevated concentration of protein.
  - Occasionally (prevalence is unclear) CSF-restricted OCB [67, 76–81, 83].

7.6.4 Krabbe Disease

- Synonyme: globoid cell leukodystrophy
- Cause:
  - Autosomal recessive disorder with a deficiency of galactocerebrosidase, resulting in the accumulation of galactolipids.
- Diagnosis:
  - Assessment of the amount of galactosyl-ceramidase enzyme in the lymphocytes and genetic testing.
- Clinical:
  - The adolescent-onset (between 10 and 20 years of age) is very rare
  - Large number of asymptomatic individuals
  - Insidiously progressive symmetric or asymmetric paraparesis, but some patient may have subacute disease onset
  - Cognitive impairment and peripheral neuropathy

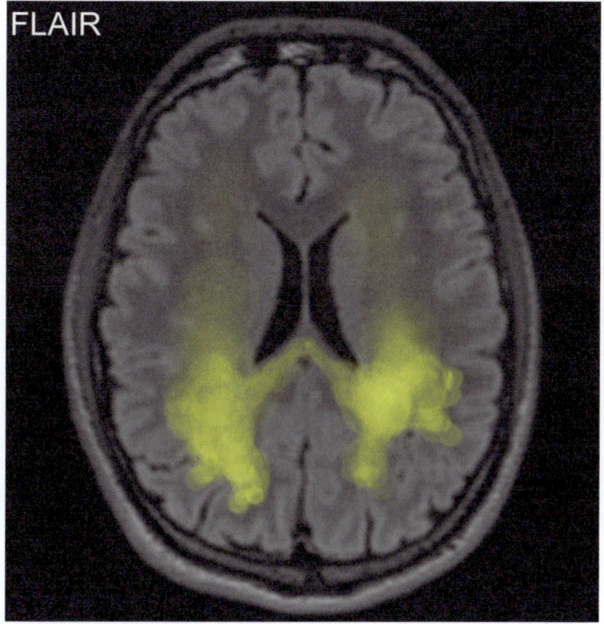

Fig. 7.7 Prominent, symmetric involvement of the posterior white matter and the splenium of the corpus callosum in Krabbe disease

  - Less frequently, paresthesia on lower limbs and visual loss
  - May mimic primary progressive MS
- Imaging:
  - Imaging "red flags" suggesting the Krabbe disease not MS are:
  - Prominent symmetric posterior white matter hyperintensities along the corticospinal (pyramidal) tracts
  - Symmetric or confluent involvement of the periventricular mainly posterior white matter
  - Involvement of splenium of the corpus callosum
  - U-fibers are usually spared (Fig. 7.7)
- EMG may show demyelinating or axonal neuropathy
- CSF is normal, but some patients have elevated concentration of protein or CSF-restricted OCB [67, 86, 87].

7.6.5 Metachromatic Leukodystrophy

- Cause:
  - Autosomal recessive disorder with an arylsulphatase A (ARSA) deficiency resulting in lysosomal accumulation of sulphatides.
- Diagnosis:
  - Assessment of increased urinary sulphatide level and decreased ARSA activity in lymphocytes.
  - Sural nerve or brain biopsy shows metachromatic deposits.
  - Genetic testing.

- Clinical:
  - There are four variants:
    - Late infantile (before the age of 4 years)
    - Early juvenile (ages 4–6 years)
    - Late juvenile (ages 6–16 years) and
    - Adult-type (after the age of 16 years)—only 10–20% of cases
  - Most patients with adult-onset variant have psychiatric symptoms, schizophrenia-like manifestations and cognitive impairment progressing in dementia.
  - Some patients have epilepsy, spastic paresis, visual loss, dystonia or peripheral neuropathy.
  - The patients are often misdiagnosed as having schizophrenia, affective disorder, or personality disorder.
- Imaging:
  - MRI "red flags" to suggest this disorder rather than MS are:
    - Symmetric or confluent "sheet-like" involvement of the periventricular mainly frontal WM progressing to subcortical white matter.
    - Almost all patients have increased T2 signal and atrophy of the corpus callosum. Splenium may sometime show restricted diffusion.
    - Involvement of the corticospinal tracts in the supratentorial white matter and the brainstem.
    - U-fibers are usually spared.
    - In advanced disease stages can be seen tigroid appearance of the white matter (better seen on T2-weighed images than FLAIR).
    - In advanced stages may be also signal changes and atrophy in cerebellum and thalamus.
    - There is contrast enhancement.
    - Spinal cord is usually normal (Fig. 7.8).
- EMG may show demyelinating peripheral neuropathy.
- CSF shows elevated concentration of protein.
- Opthalmological examination shows foveal white patches [67, 72, 79, 88, 89].

7.6.6 Fabry Disease

- For more details, see Sect. 7.3.
- Cause
  - X chromosome-linked recessive disorder (more severe in males).
  - Deficiency of alpha-galactosidase A results in accumulation of globotriasylceramide in vascular endothelial cells, cardio-myocytes, and renal podocytes.
- Diagnosis:
  - Evaluation of decreased activity of alpha-galactosidase A in leukocytes and genetic testing.

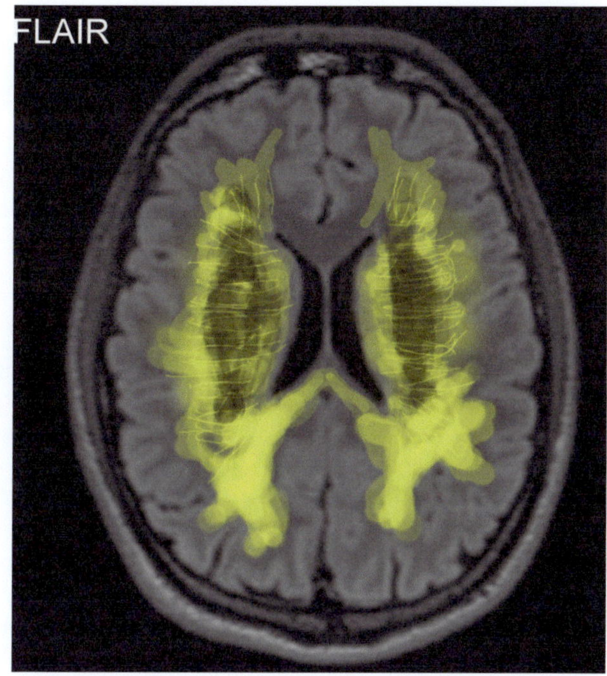

Fig. 7.8 Confluent involvement of the periventricular white matter and corpus callosum, occasionally exhibiting a tigroid appearance in metachromatic leukodystrophy

- Clinical:
  - Temperature-sensitive acroparaesthesias, anhidrosis, abdominal pain, cerebrovascular events, fatigue, psychiatric symptoms.
  - Can be relapsing-remitting disease course mimicking MS.
- Imaging
  - MRI "red flags" to suggest this disorder rather than MS are:
    - Progressive non-specific, multi-focal, asymmetric T2 lesions in deep and subcortical white matter.
    - Ectatic vertebrobasilar arteries.
    - Normal spinal cord imaging.
- Laboratory
  - Urine analysis may show proteinuria.
  - CSF shows elevated protein and rarely also CSF-restricted OCB.
- Slit-lamp ophthalmologic exam shows lenticular opacities in 30% of males.
- Skin exam may show angiokeratomas [37, 51, 67].

7.6.7 Niemann–Pick Disease Type C

- Cause
  - Autosomal recessive disorder with excessive low-density lipoprotein-cholesterol (LDL-C) uptake, deficient cholesterol biosynthesis, and trafficking resulting in endosomal accumulation and excessive cholesterol storage in lysosomes.

- Diagnosis
  - Cholesterol esterification studies, quantification of oxysterols in plasma, and genetic testing.
- Clinical
  - May be symptoms onset in adolescence or adulthood (27%).
  - Specific features include (often missing in adult forms):
    - Partial/generalized seizures with gelastic cataplexy (brief episodes of generalized loss of muscle tone without alteration in consciousness triggered by laughter).
    - Vertical supranuclear gaze ophthalmoplegia.
  - Other unspecific features include:
    - Ataxia, dysarthria, dystonia, cognitive impairment, psychiatric symptoms and central palsy.
- Imaging
  - Non-enhancing T2 hyperintense periventricular (mainly parieto-occipital) lesions in white matter.
  - T2 lesions and atrophy of corpus callosum.
  - Brain atrophy: frontal lobe, deep gray matter, hippocampus, and cerebellum
  - MRI findings may mimic MS.
  - Abdominal ultrasound may show subclinical hepatosplenomegaly.
- Laboratory
  - Routine blood tests are normal.
  - Case studies reported normal protein and cytology, but presence of CSF-restricted OCB [67, 74, 90, 91].

7.6.8 Chédiak–Higashi Disease

- Cause:
  - Autosomal recessive disorder with mutation of the lysosomal trafficking regulator (*LYST*) gene associated with abnormal lysosomal trafficking.
- Diagnosis
  - Peripheral blood smear shows neutrophils with enlarged granules and decreased function of natural killer cells.
  - Genetic testing.
  - Skin biopsy shows amyloid depositions and abnormal pigmentation.
- Clinical:
  - Immune dysfunction and repeated pyogenic infections in early childhood due to decreased phagocytosis.
  - Pigmentary abnormalities (albinism, solar sensitivity, and photophobia).
  - 10–15% of patients have an attenuated late (adult-onset) variant of the disease with only subtle pigmentary abnormalities, absent or subclinical immunologic abnormalities, but present neurological manifestations such as peripheral neuropathy, progressive spastic paraparesis, spinocerebellar degeneration, movement disorders (dystonia, parkinsonism), and cognitive impairment.

- Imaging
  - Progressing periventricular T2 hyperintensities in white matter.
  - Brain and spinal cord atrophy [67, 73, 92, 93].

7.6.9 Tay-Sachs Disease

- Cause
  - Autosomal recessive disorder.
  - Heterozygous or homozygous mutations leading to decreased Beta-hexosaminidase A activity and intracellular accumulation of CNS gangliosides (lipids).
  - Sandhoff and Tay-Sachs disease are very similar disorders (GM2-gangliosidoses), but Tay-Sachs disease has the highest incidence in among Ashkenazi Jews. Sandhoff disease is not associated with any specific ethnicity.
- Diagnosis
  - Assessment of the hexosaminidase activity in serum, fibroblasts, or leukocytes and genetic testing.
- Clinical
  - Disease onset is in childhood, adolescence, or early adulthood (late-onset form).
  - Some adults present with progressive upper and lower motor neuronopathy without sensory involvement, mimicking amyotrophic lateral sclerosis (ALS).
  - Characteristic vertical supranuclear gaze palsy may be missing.
  - Often tremor and extrapyramidal symptoms (dystonia, myoklonus, etc.)
  - Additional manifestations may include peripheral sensory neuropathy, ataxia, psychiatric symptoms (>30%), or proximal pattern of muscle weakness.
- Imaging
  - Initially, T2 hyperintensities in basal ganglia and thalamus.
  - Later also lesions in deep white matter, cortical gray matter or cerebellum are associated with marked whole brain and cerebellar atrophy.
  - May be thalamic calcifications.
  - Spinal cord is normal [87, 94–96].

7.6.10 Pompe Disease

- Autosomal recessive disorder caused by the decreased degradation of lysosomal glycogen.
- Clinical manifestations usually begin after birth or in childhood and include myopathic syndrome, hypertrophic cardiomyopathy, and respiratory difficulties (recurrent pulmonary infections, dyspnea after exercise).
- Often present increased levels of muscle and hepatic enzymes.
- There are rare adult forms, but differential diagnosis from MS should not be difficult.
- A few case studies documented comorbid Pompe disease and MS [97, 98].

7.6.11 Blood Work (in General)

- Routine blood tests are typically normal, except for some cases where muscle or liver enzymes may be elevated.

7.6.12 Examination of CSF (in General)

- May be an elevated concentration of protein
- CSF-restricted OCB were reported mostly in patients with:
  - Fabry disease.
  - X-linked adrenoleukodystrophy and adrenomyeloneuropathy.
  - Metachromatic leukodystrophy.
  - Niemann–Pick disease type C [37, 67, 91].

7.6.13 Diagnosis (in General)

- Many case studies have reported cases of misdiagnosis as MS.
- Established through biochemical analysis of plasma and genetic testing.
- Be aware that routine panels may not identify some types of mutations (large deletions, duplications, expansions, or mutations in mitochondrial deoxyribonucleic acid [mtDNA]). In some cases, may be required whole-exome or genome sequencing.
- It is also important to note that a delay between blood or CSF withdrawal and sample processing may result in falsely low enzyme activity. Additionally, hyperlipidemia (particularly very-long-chain fatty acids) can affect results, so a fasting sample and lipid profile may be necessary for accurate interpretation of metabolic testing.
- Several clinical and imaging features may help to narrow down the spectrum of diagnoses considered in differential diagnosis.
- Clues to diagnosis of Lysosomal storage and peroxisomal function disorders (LSPFD) in patients with "MS-like" presentations include:
  - Presence of peripheral neuropathy (frequently in Krabbe disease, metachromatic leukodystrophy, and X-linked adrenoleukodystrophy spectrum disorders).
  - Extra-neurological manifestations, such as cardiac, renal and skin manifestations of Fabry disease; splenomegaly in Niemann–Pick disease type C (and rarely in Fabry disease); or immunodeficiency and pigmentary abnormalities in Chédiak–Higashi disease.
  - Absence of CSF-restricted OCB.
  - Progressive clinical course.
  - Marked cognitive deterioration, dementia or psychiatric symptoms.

- Myelopathy without focal spinal cord lesions (in X-ALD).
- Symmetric confluent posterior white matter lesions in the brain, sparing U-fibers [67, 76–78, 86, 88, 94, 99].

- There are case reports of patients with coexisting LSPFD and MS [12].

7.6.14 Treatment and Prognosis (in General)

- Several LSPFD can be treated with hematopoietic stem cell transplantation.
- For some subtypes is available systemic enzyme replacement or gene therapy
- In general, treatment is reserved for children and young adults in pre- or early-symptomatic disease stages [67, 68]

7.7 Mitochondrial Disorders

7.7.1 Epidemiology

- Prevalence 20–25/100.000 [100, 101].

7.7.2 Cause and Definition

- A heterogeneous group of genetic multisystem disorders resulting from dysfunction in the mitochondria [102].
- The absence of a family history does not rule out the diagnosis, since mitochondrial disorders (MD) may exhibit incomplete penetrance and heteroplasmy (the presence of two or more mtDNA variants within the same cell).
- Individuals with these mutations may remain clinically asymptomatic unless exposed to certain environmental factors or have a low mutation load [67, 100].
- Mitochondrial dysfunction is associated with increased production of the reactive oxygen species and oxidative stress, which leads to microglial activation, neuronal injury, and neurodegeneration.
- MD share some pathophysiological features with MS, which may explain the increased coexistence of some MD with demyelinating diseases.
- MD can mimic diseases such as MS, NMOSD, or MOGAD [67, 103, 104].

7.7.3 Subtypes

- MD variants that can manifest with symptoms beginning in adulthood include:
  - Alpers–Huttenlocher disease (Progressive infantile poliodystrophy; Polymerase gamma gene [POLG1] mutation; AHS).

- Kearns–Sayre syndrome (Chronic external ophthalmoplegia plus with retinal pigment abnormalities; KSS).
- Leber's hereditary optic neuropathy (LHON).
- Leigh's syndrome/disease (Subacute necrotizing encephalomyelitis; LS).
- Leukoencephalopathy with brain stem and spinal cord involvement and lactic acidosis (LBSL).
- Mitochondrial encephalomyopathy, lactic acidosis, and stroke-like episodes (MELAS).
- Myoclonic epilepsy with and ragged red fibers (MERRF).

* Pediatric variants of MD that occasionally allow for survival into adulthood include:
  - KSS; LBSL; LHON; LS; MELAS; MERRF
  - Chronic progressive external ophthalmoplegia (CPEO)
  - Dominant optic atrophy (DOA)
  - Maternally inherited Leigh syndrome (MILS)
  - Mitochondrial depletion syndrome (MDS)
  - Mitochondrial membrane protein associated neurodegeneration (MPAN)
  - Mitochondrial multiorgan disorder syndrome (MIMODS)
  - Mitochondrial neuro-gastro-intestinal encephalopathy (MNGIE)
  - Neurogenic muscle weakness, ataxia, and retinitis pigmentosa (NARP)
  - Other POLG-related disorders (POLG)
  - Pearson syndrome (PS)
  - Primary coenzyme-Q (CoQ) deficiency
  - Pyruvate dehydrogenase (PDH) deficiency
  - Sensory ataxic neuropathy, dysarthria, and ophthalmoparesis (SANDO)
  - Wolfram syndrome (DIDMOAD) [105]

7.7.4 Non-neurological Clinical Features

* The phenotypes are highly variable and may affect any organ system, either clinically or subclinically: muscles (97%), CNS (72%), endocrine glands (69%), heart (58%), intestines (55%), peripheral nerves (50%).
* The organ system features suggesting MD include:
* Short stature, facial dysmorphism.
* Hypertrophic cardiomyopathy, atrial fibrillation, cardiac conduction abnormalities, and arterial hypertension.
* Hepatopathy, diverticulosis, nephrolithiasis, renal insufficiency, anemia.
* Endocrinopathy:
  - Diabetes, thyroid dysfunction, hypogonadism
  - Hypothalamic-Hypophysial-Adrenal Axis dysfunction
    * May lead to hypopituitarism associated with short stature, hypothyroidism, hypocorticism, hypogonadism, polydipsia, or arterial hypotonia.
    * For example, in MELAS, KSS, or mutations in the isoleucyl transfer ribonucleic acid (tRNA) synthetase gene.

- The key ocular features suggesting MD include:
  - Optic neuropathy, which is usually severe and does not improve after corticosteroids. It may occur in MELAS, MERRF, DOA, and LHON and may be associated with optic neuropathy, spasticity, and ataxia.
  - Pigmentary retinopathy.

7.7.5 Neurological Clinical and Imaging Features

- Although MD are typically multisystem diseases, CNS involvement may occur without manifestations in other organs.
- Clinical manifestations may occur without abnormalities on imaging, and vice versa abnormal MRI or functional studies may not have clinical manifestations.
- Symptoms may be caused directly by the metabolic defect or secondary from involvement of other organs (e.g., stroke from atrial fibrillation).
- Stroke-like episodes:
  - Often in MELAS, but also in MERRF, KSS, LS or coenzyme-Q deficiency
  - Frequently secondary to cardiac involvement
  - The common symptom is cortical blindness
  - MRI shows the stroke-like ischemic lesions
- Epileptic seizures:
  - Adult-onset epilepsy in MELAS, LHON, NARP, and SANDO
- Headache:
  - Migraine-like (often), cluster, noncalcified, or tension headache
  - Isolated, dominant, or nondominant clinical feature.
  - Mostly in AHD, MELAS, MERRF, CPEO, LHON, LS, Mitochondrial recessive ataxia syndrome (MIRAS), cyclic vomiting syndrome, or Mitochondrial DNA Depletion Syndrome (MDS).
- Ataxia:
  - A dominant feature in X-linked Sideroblastic Anemia (XLSA), PDH deficiency, NARP, or MIRAS.
  - XLSA has additional lower limb spasticity.
  - NARP has additional muscle weakness and retinitis pigmentosa.
  - A non-dominant feature in MELAS, MERRF, KSS, LS, Multiple systemic lipomatosis, MDS, SANDO, or Pontocerebellar Hypoplasia (PCH).
- Hearing loss:
  - Often bilateral and progressive.
- Movement disorders:
  - Any type of hypo and hyperkinetic disorder.
- Muscle Weakness:
  - Involvement of upper or lower motor neurons.
- Psychiatric manifestations:
  - May be present without neurological manifestations and include cognitive impairment, mood and anxiety disorders, or psychosis.

  - Less frequently, bipolar disorder, attention deficit hyperactivity disorder, or autism spectrum disorders.
  - Cognitive impairment is the most common in MELAS, but also occurs in MERRF, NARP, LHON, CPEO, KSS, MNGIE, LS, and AHS.
- Nystagmus:
  - Mostly in LS, less frequent in LHON, MELAS, MDS, and AHS.
- Peripheral nervous system involvement:
  - Peripheral neuropathy.
  - Myopathy of extra-ocular (external ophthalmoplegia), facial, bulbar, axial, respiratory, or limb muscles [67, 106, 107].

7.7.6 Disease Course

- Age of symptoms onset ranges between birth and adolescence or early adulthood.
- Clinical course is usually slowly progressive, but some patients may have acute or relapsing-remitting phenotype.
- CNS symptoms may be permanent (e.g. cognitive impairment, motor deficit) or transient (e.g. seizure, stroke, migraine) [67, 106, 107].

7.7.7 Brain Imaging

- May appear normal.
- May present clinically asymptomatic imaging findings.
- MRI features are highly variable and may mimic a wide range of diseases.
- Lesions' location:
  - Typically, bilateral, and symmetric, but some cases may have asymmetric or rarely unilateral involvement.
  - White matter:
    - Periventricular and deep white matter.
    - Most common in MELAS, MNGIE, KSS, LS, LHON, LBSL, LS, NARP, MIMODS, and PCH.
  - Gray matter:
    - Either in isolation or together with white matter lesions.
    - Cortex, subcortical region, basal ganglia, thalamus, midbrain, brainstem, cerebellum.
    - Rarely diffuse brainstem involvement.
    - Most common in LS (basal ganglia and brainstem), less frequently in LHON, CoQ-deficiency, MIMODS, MELAS (cortical lesions) or MERRF (periaqueductal gray matter).
  - Stroke-like lesions:
    - Typically, not confined to a vascular territory. All brain regions can be involved, but the occipito-temporal lobe is most often affected.

- Optic nerve:
  - Bilateral thinning, increased T2 signal or contrast enhancement of the prechiasmatic optic nerve and chiasm may be present
  - Typical for LHON and DOA, MIMODS, and other optic atrophy spectrum disorders.
- Lesions' appearance:
  - Single, multifocal, confluent, diffuse, small or large, solid or cystic (chronic lesions with cavities), homogeneous or inhomogeneous T2 hyperintense and T1 hypointense lesions.
  - Leukoencephalopathy-like pattern can be seen in various subtypes of MD. It is characterized by a diffuse T2 signal in the white matter, involving the corpus callosum and cerebellar white matter. Subcortical U-fibers may be affected, whereas the periventricular white matter may be spared. Focal areas of restricted diffusion and contrast enhancement can be present.
  - Stroke-like lesions are heterogeneous in morphology and dynamics, making them difficult to identify as such. They are usually symptomatic.
  - In the acute stage, lesions appear as T2 hyperintensities, occasionally with restricted diffusion and hyperperfusion on perfusion-weighted imaging (PWI). Magnetic resonance spectroscopy (MRS) may indicate a lactate peak.
    - In the chronic stage, lesions may progress or regress (even completely). T2 signal intensity can be hyper-, iso-, or hypointense, whereas diffusion-weighted imaging (DWI) is usually normal. PWI or single-photon emission computed tomography (SPECT) may reveal hypoperfusion. Ultimately, these lesions can evolve into normal brain tissue, white matter lesions, cystic lesions, focal atrophy, or laminar cortical necrosis.
- Contrast enhancement:
  - Usually without enhancement, but may be present.
- Evolution over time:
  - New and enlarging lesions typically occur, but occasionally regression or even resolution of lesions may be observed.
- Associated Findings:
  - Brain atrophy:
    - Whole brain or regional (for example, cerebellar) is seen in half of the cases. Especially in advanced disease stages of CPEO, MELAS, MERRF, PDH deficiency, KSS, LHON, or PCH (which can be combined with a complete agenesis of the corpus callosum).
  - Calcifications:
    - Symmetric or asymmetric, particularly in basal ganglia or less frequently in dentate nucleus and cerebellum.
    - Often in MELAS, LS, and KSS.
  - 18-fludeoxyglucose positron emission tomography (FDG-PET)
    - Regional hypometabolism in the cerebellum, the basal ganglia, and the temporal lobes or other regions may be present.
  - Ischemic and hemorrhagic strokes [105, 106, 108]

7.7.8 Spinal Cord Imaging

- Cord lesions are present in considerable proportion of pediatric and adult patients. Spinal cord pathology is usually accompanied by brain changes, and isolated symptomatic spinal cord involvement is rare.
- The imaging and histopathological features are variable, including ischemia, necrosis, edema of the gray matter, vascular congestion, or demyelination around the central canal and dorsal columns.
- There are two distinct subtypes of the spinal cord involvement. In general, the A pattern involves mostly cervical lesions in the white matter or sometimes also gray matter. However, the B pattern involves mostly lesions in the lower spinal cord segments (thoracic or thoracolumbar) and has ischemic features with selective gray matter involvement.
- A. subtypes overlap with demyelinating disorders:
  - Lesions are often in the cervical and thoracic cords.
  - Pathology is restricted only to the white matter or also to the gray matter.
  - Half of the patients have tumefactive lesions or longitudinally extensive transverse myelitis (LETM) mimicking NMOSD or MOGAD (but all these patients with MD are seronegative for anti-aquaporin-4 [AQP4] and anti-myelin oligodendrocyte glycoprotein [MOG] IgG).
  - Lesions may affect the whole cross-section area of the cord.
  - May occur "H-sign" appearance with the most pronounced signal abnormality in the central gray matter.
  - Some patients have short peripheral white matter lesions mimicking MS.
  - Leukoencephalopathy with brainstem and spinal cord involvement and lactate elevation (LBSL) subtype is associated with cervical spinal lesions affecting the posterior columns and lateral corticospinal tracts.
- B. subtype overlaps with the spinal cord ischemia:
  - Mitochondrial dysfunction impairing cellular energy metabolism may cause or contribute to tissue ischemia.
  - The ischemic origin of these lesions supports their location within the lower thoracolumbar spine and conus medullaris and has the classic ischemic "snake-eye" appearance.
  - The Leigh syndrome (LS) is the most frequent disease with this pattern (75%).
  - In both patterns, contrast enhancement is typically absent, and in chronic stages, regression of signal changes can occur [103, 109] (Fig. 7.9).

7.7.9 Other Organ Systems Imaging

- Muscles pathology can be determined by ultrasound, computed tomography (CT), or MRI by measuring the muscle volume, amount of connective tissue, or amount of fat.
- Cardiac MRI shows abnormality in about half of the patients [110].

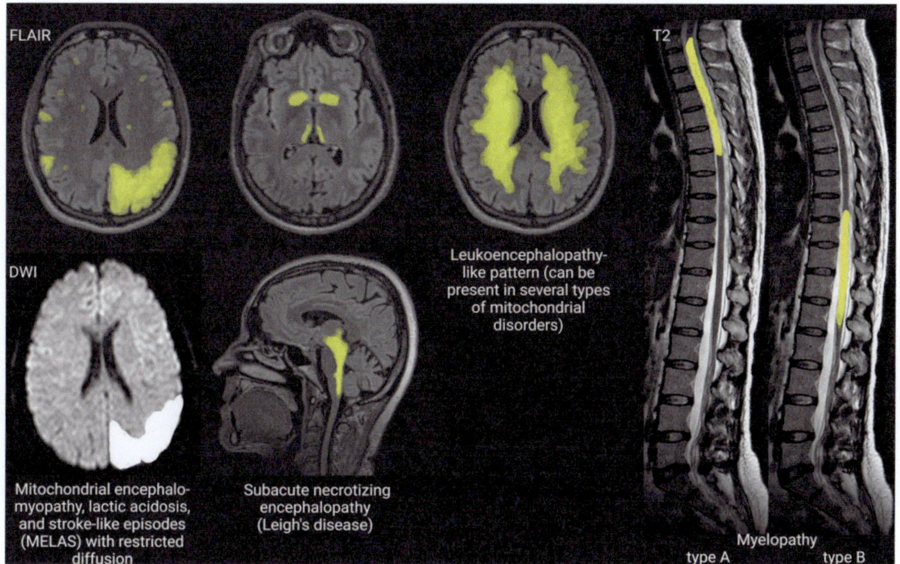

Fig. 7.9 MRI characteristics of mitochondrial disorders

7.7.10 Blood Work

- Elevated lactate level
  - Not limited to MD but can be caused by a wide range of conditions, such as ischemia, exercise, or hypoglycemia.
  - The sensitivity for diagnosing MD ranges from 34% to 62%, whereas the specificity is between 83% and 100% (with cut-off >27 mg/dL = >3.0 mmol/L)
  - The sensitivity of the lactate stress test (assessment of serum lactate level during exercise) is 66% and specificity is 84%.
- Elevated pyruvate level
  - Can be caused by MD, as well as other conditions such as pyruvate dehydrogenase complex deficiency, pyruvate carboxylase deficiency, or biotinidase deficiency.
  - The sensitivity for diagnosing MID ranges from 35% to 88%, whereas the specificity is between 81% and 87%.
- Elevated lactate/pyruvate ratio (>20)
  - The most useful biomarker, with a sensitivity of 77% and specificity of 91% for diagnosing MD.
- Other markers, such as elevated levels of creatine kinase, creatinine, or various amino acids, have a low diagnostic value [110–114].

7.7.11 Examination of CSF

- May show elevated concentration of protein and mild pleocytosis.
- CSF-restricted OCB is usually absent [103, 115–118].
- An elevated lactate level in the CSF (>19.9 mg/dL = 2.21 mmol/L) likely exhibits greater specificity for diagnosing MD compared to blood levels. Increased lactate CSF/blood ratio (>0.91) may also provide diagnostic information [113, 114].

7.7.12 OCT

- Patients with optic neuropathy may show severe bilateral temporal or diffuse thinning of the retinal nerve fiber layer (RNFL) [119].

7.7.13 Electrophysiology

- Peripheral neuropathy is associated with abnormalities on conduction studies.
- Patients with optic neuropathy may show delayed latencies in VEP [107].

7.7.14 Diagnosis

- There is no single biomarker for detection of all different MD variants.
- Diagnostic accuracy of biochemical biomarkers is limited because muscle, myocardium, and brain may not be affected in every patient, and levels of the biomarkers depend on the timing of the exam (rest or during exercise).
- Although biopsy (skeletal muscle, the myocardium, liver, or the skin) is invasive, it is one of the best instruments to diagnose MD.
- MD are frequently multisystem diseases; therefore, all potentially affected organs need to be prospectively investigated, irrespective of clinical manifestations [110].
- Clues to diagnosis of MD are:
  - Non-Mendelian/maternal transmission.
  - Typical systemic and neurological clinical features (see above).
  - Symmetric bilateral T2 hyperintense lesions in the basal ganglia, or multifocal gray matter involvement on brain MRI.
  - Increased lactate and pyruvate levels and absence of clear inflammatory pattern in CSF [67].

7.7.15 Differential Diagnosis

- MD often shows imaging phenotypes mimicking MS, NMOSD, or MOGAD [103].
- MS-like manifestations occur mainly in LHON, MELAS, MERRF, LS, POLG-related disorders (but not AHS) [100, 105].

7.7.16 Treatment and Prognosis

- Some patients may have a surprisingly good response to immunomodulating therapy [118, 120].
- For the majority of MD, only symptomatic treatment is available, as specific therapies exist for only a few subtypes.
- Pediatric disease onset is associated with poorer prognosis [100, 121].

7.8 Wilson's Disease

7.8.1 Epidemiology

- Prevalence 3/100.000

7.8.2 Etiology

- Inherited disorder with copper overload due to reduced copper excretion secondary to genetic mutations in the ATPase, copper transporting, beta polypeptide (*ATP7B*) gene.

7.8.3 Clinical Features

- Systemic manifestations:
  - Wide range of symptoms.
  - Hepatic manifestations are the most often and range from asymptomatic subtle morphological changes to severe hepatitis and cirrhosis.
  - Slit-lamp examination may show Kayser–Fleischer rings.
- Neurological and psychiatric manifestations:
  - Movement disorders (most often), speech disturbances, drooling, psychiatric syndromes, gait and balance disturbance.
  - Less often, olfactory dysfunction, peripheral neuropathy, restless leg syndrome, rapid eye movement, sleep abnormalities, tics, myoclonus, headache, pyramidal signs, oculomotor impairment, and taste impairment.

7.8.4 Brain Imaging

- Symmetric T2 hyperintense changes in the basal ganglia (mainly the putamen and caudate nuclei), but also thalami, midbrain, cerebral peduncles, and pons.
- In advanced stages, lesions are hypointense on T1-weighted images.
- T2 hyperintensities are partially reversible after anti-copper treatment.
- MRI changes are found in almost 100% of treatment-naive patients with neurological manifestations; in 40–75% of patients with hepatic manifestations; and in 20–30% of presymptomatic patients (Fig. 7.10).

7.8.5 Spinal Cord Imaging

- Normal

7.8.6 Blood Work

- Serum ceruloplasmin level is decreased.
- Cooper concentration is increased.

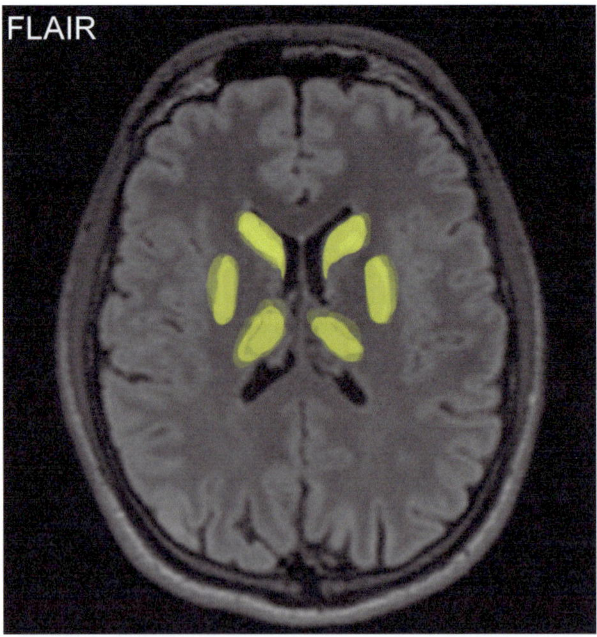

Fig. 7.10 Symmetric T2 hyperintense changes in the basal ganglia, thalami, and brainstem in Wilson's disease

7.8.7 Urine

- Increased urinary copper excretion.

7.8.8 Liver Biopsy

- Increased concentration of copper (in the absence of cholestasis).

7.8.9 Examination of CSF

- Normal

7.8.10 Treatment and Prognosis

- Lifelong pharmacological therapy with:
  - Chelators: increase urinary copper excretion.
  - Zinc salts: decrease copper absorption.
- Liver transplantation [122, 123]
- There are a few case reports of patients with co-existing Wilson's disease and MS. [124]

7.9 Other Rare Inherited Metabolic Diseases

7.9.1 Acute Intermittent Porphyria

- An autosomal dominant disease linked with a deficiency of enzymes in the heme biosynthetic pathway leads to the accumulation of heme precursors. Typically, disease onset occurs in the second or third decade of life. Patients experience acute neurovisceral attacks characterized by abdominal pain; some may also exhibit mental changes, seizures, and peripheral neuropathy. MRI findings reveal diffuse, patchy periventricular T2 hyperintensities in white matter. Diagnosis is supported by elevated levels of porphobilinogen in the urine (which may cause the urine to appear reddish-brown or red) and confirmed through genetic molecular testing [125].

7.9.2 Alpha-Methylacyl-CoA Racemase Deficiency

- Autosomal recessive peroxisomal disorder characterized by impaired oxidation of the pristanic acid. Disease onset is in adulthood. Patients present with peripheral neuropathy, epilepsy, relapsing encephalopathy, type 2 diabetes mellitus, cataracts, pigmentary retinopathy, and tremors. MRI reveals bilateral acute and chronic lesions in the thalamus, midbrain, and pons. Encephalopathic episodes are associated with acute stroke-like lesions. Diagnosis is confirmed by markedly elevated levels of pristanic acid in the blood and genetic molecular testing. Patients may benefit from a restricted diet low in phytanic and pristanic acid intake and possibly plasmapheresis. Pristanic acid stored in the adipose tissue, however, may be released during the acute illness phase [126, 127].

7.9.3 Adult Polyglucosan Body Disease

- An autosomal recessive disorder primarily affecting individuals of Ashkenazi Jewish descent. This glycogen storage disease type IV is characterized by a deficiency in glycogen branching enzyme, resulting in the abnormal intracellular accumulation of polyglucosan bodies in the central and peripheral nervous system, and various other organs. Onset typically occurs in older age, usually in the fifth or sixth decade of life, and manifests as a combination of myelopathy and peripheral neuropathy. Patients exhibit progressive paraparesis (from lower to upper extremities), a mix of upper and lower motor neuron palsy, distal sensory deficits in the legs, neurogenic bladder, and mild cognitive impairment. MRI findings often include T2 hyperintensities in periventricular and subcortical white matter, as well as in the posterior limb of the internal capsule, the external capsule, and the pyramidal tracts and medial lemniscus of the pons and medulla. Additionally, atrophy of the medulla oblongata and spinal cord may be observed. Diagnosis is established through genetic molecular testing [67, 128].

7.9.4 Aicardi–Goutières Syndrome

- A genetically determined encephalopathy, typically inherited in an autosomal recessive manner, resulting from dysfunctional sensing and/or metabolism of nucleic acids. This dysfunction triggers an autoimmune response characterized by increased production of the interferon-α (IFN-α; type I interferonopathy). The clinical phenotype is variable and may include systemic manifestations affecting the skin, thyroid, eyes, and blood vessels, as well as manifestations within the CNS. Many patients experience severe intellectual and physical disabilities. There are variants with early and late onset. Some patients present with spastic paraparesis, whereas others may exhibit brain vasculopathy. Brain MRI findings can vary, ranging from normal to those showing calcifications, white matter hyperintensities, and cerebral atrophy. CSF analysis typically reveals pleocytosis and elevated levels of IFN-α and neopterin. Treatment options are currently limited to symptomatic management [129].

7.9.5 Arginase 1 Deficiency

- A rare autosomal recessive inborn error of the urea cycle, occurring in approximately 0.14 per 100,000 births, results in elevated arginine levels, potentially leading to the accumulation of toxic arginine metabolites and ammonia. Symptoms typically emerge in late infancy or early childhood and include lower limb spasticity, developmental delay, cognitive impairment, and seizures. The presentation may mimic cerebral palsy or hereditary spastic paraparesis. Brain atrophy is evident on MRI scans, whereas spinal cord imaging is typically normal. Diagnosis involves plasma amino acid analysis, erythrocyte arginase 1 enzymatic activity assays, and genetic testing. The primary goal of treatment is to reduce plasma arginine levels through dietary adjustments or nitrogen scavengers. Human enzyme therapies are currently being investigated as potential treatment options [130–132].

7.9.6 Brown-Vialetto-Van Laere and Fazio Londe Syndrome

- Also called Fazio-Londe syndrome, this rare neurodegenerative genetic disorder (with only dozens of cases reported) can present at any age. It is caused by mutations in the riboflavin transporter genes, which encode the intestinal riboflavin transporter, resulting in riboflavin deficiency. Common manifestations include ponto-bulbar neuropathy, sensorineural deafness, and respiratory compromise. Less frequent features are progressive muscle weakness, hypotonia, or diaphragm paralysis. However, abnormalities in plasma flavin levels and/or plasma acylcarnitine profiles are not observed in all patients. Therefore, diagnosis requires genetic testing of all three transporter genes. Riboflavin supplementation should be started immediately, even before the results of genetic testing are available. This treatment is lifesaving and typically leads to rapid or gradual clinical improvement [133, 134].

7.9.7 Canavan Disease (Aspartoacylase Deficiency)

- An autosomal recessive spongiform leukodystrophy particularly prevalent among Ashkenazi Jews. The deficiency of aspartoacylase leads to the accumulation of N-acetylaspartic acid in the brain, resulting in oligodendrocyte dysfunction, spongiform changes, and the absence of myelin. The disease typically manifests in infancy, with rare occurrences in early childhood. Clinical symptoms include lethargy, weak cry and suck, poor head control, macrocephaly, and hypotonia. As the disease progresses, spasticity, cerebellar syndrome, or blindness may develop. Brain MRI often reveals multiple round or oval cystic changes, which are dilated Virchow-Robin spaces associated with spongiform degeneration. Additionally, restricted diffusion in the deep white matter and the brainstem due to cytotoxic brain edema may be observed. Currently, only supportive care is available for this condition [135, 136].

7.9.8 Coenzyme Q10 Deficiency

- A rare autosomal recessive mitochondrial disorder characterized by defects in Coenzyme Q10 (CoQ10) biosynthesis. Secondary CoQ10 deficiency can also result from factors such as statin use or fibromyalgia. The disorder presents with five major clinical phenotypes: (1) encephalomyopathy (manifesting as seizures, pyramidal signs, mental retardation, and delayed motor development, along with progressive external ophthalmoplegia and ptosis); (2) severe infantile multisystemic disease; (3) nephropathy; (4) cerebellar ataxia; and (5) isolated myopathy (with symptoms including muscle weakness, myoglobinuria, exercise intolerance, cramps, myalgia, and elevated creatine kinase levels). Clinical onset typically occurs during childhood, with cerebellar ataxia and atrophy being predominant manifestations. Diagnosis is established by assessing decreased concentrations of CoQ10 in muscle biopsy or skin fibroblasts. Patients often exhibit increased blood lactate levels. Treatment options include supplementation with CoQ10 [137].

7.9.9 Delta-1-Pyrroline-5-Carboxylase Synthetase Deficiency

- A rare autosomal recessive or dominant genetic disorder, which disrupts glutamate and urea cycle metabolism in mitochondria and results in mild hyperammonemia. Clinical manifestations include hyperelastic skin, joint hyperlaxity, epilepsy, cataracts, developmental delay, short stature, microcephaly, and spastic paraparesis. The presentation may resemble cerebral palsy or hereditary spastic paraplegia. Treatment typically involves amino acid supplementation [66, 138].

7.9.10 Glut1 Deficiency Syndrome

- A rare genetic disorder (prevalence 2/100.000) characterized by decreased glucose transport across the blood–brain barrier and astrocyte plasmatic membrane into the CNS due to dysfunction of glucose transporter type 1 (Glut1). Diagnosis is based on establishing low glucose concentration in the CSF simultaneously with normal glucose concentration in the blood and genetic molecular testing. Symptoms typically onset in early childhood, although rare late-onset cases have been described. Clinical features include early-onset drug-resistant epilepsy, unexplained paroxysmal events, movement disorders (such as spasticity, dystonia, and ataxia), stroke-like episodes, hemiplegic migraine, and developmental delay. Some children may exhibit T2 hyperintensities in subcortical U-fibers, prominence of perivascular Virchow spaces, or delayed myelination on brain MRI. This disorder is treated with a ketogenic diet [139, 140].

7.9.11 Pelizaeus–Merzbacher Disease

- A rare X-linked genetic leukodystrophy (prevalence of 0.2–0.5/100.000) attributed to pathogenic variants of the gene encoding proteolipid protein 1. This condition is characterized by dysmyelination or hypomyelination of the CNS, with normal myelination never occurring in affected individuals. Onset of the disease typically occurs in early childhood, although instances of onset in early adulthood are exceedingly rare. Clinical manifestations encompass nystagmus, spasticity, athetosis, tremor, and ataxia. Pathogenic variants may lead to severe congenital forms or relatively milder presentations, such as spastic paraplegia type 2 (SPG2), which is considered a subtype of hereditary spastic paraparesis. Brain MRI findings commonly reveal a lack of myelination (manifesting as low T1 but high T2 signal in white matter) alongside diffuse or patchy T2 hyperintensities, often presenting a tigroid appearance. Additionally, patients may exhibit patchy and confluent T2 hyperintensity of the spinal cord white matter. Some individuals may also display CSF-restricted OCB. Rare late-onset forms of this condition may present diagnostic challenges, resembling MS. [141–143]

7.9.12 Pseudoxanthoma Elasticum

- Rare autosomal recessive disorder characterized by ectopic mineralization and fragmentation of the elastic fibers within connective tissues. Clinical suspicion typically arises from skin and/or eye lesions, which are present in 90% of cases. Patients often exhibit yellowish papules and plaques, alongside retinal changes leading to central vision loss, and accelerated atherosclerosis with vascular complications such as ischemic strokes. Neurological complications occur in 10% of patients, with progressive spastic paraplegia being a common feature. Brain MRI may reveal an increasing number and volume of white matter lesions, calcifications, and atrophy over time [144].

References

1. Wolf B. Biotinidase: its role in biotinidase deficiency and biotin metabolism. J Nutr Biochem. 2005;16(7):441–5.
2. Baykal T, Huner G, Sarbat G, Demirkol M. Incidence of biotinidase deficiency in Turkish newborns. Acta Paediatr. 1998;87(10):1102–3.
3. Wolf B. Biotinidase deficiency should be considered in individuals thought to have multiple sclerosis and related disorders. Mult Scler Relat Disord. 2019;28:26–30.

4. Radelfahr F, Riedhammer KM, Keidel LF, Gramer G, Meitinger T, Klopstock T, et al. Biotinidase deficiency: a treatable cause of hereditary spastic paraparesis. Neurol Genet. 2020;6(6):e525.
5. Bilge N, Yevgi R. Biotinidase deficiency in differential diagnosis of neuromyelitis optica spectrum disorder. Mult Scler Relat Disord. 2020;44:102280.
6. Wolf B. Biotinidase deficiency should be considered in individuals exhibiting myelopathy with or without and vision loss. Mol Genet Metab. 2015;116(3):113–8.
7. Wolf B, Pomponio RJ, Norrgard KJ, Lott IT, Baumgartner ER, Suormala T, et al. Delayed-onset profound biotinidase deficiency. J Pediatr. 1998;132(2):362–5.
8. Deschamps R, Savatovsky J, Vignal C, Fisselier M, Imbard A, Wolf B, et al. Adult-onset biotinidase deficiency: two individuals with severe, but reversible optic neuropathy. J Neurol Neurosurg Psychiatry. 2018;89(9):1009–10.
9. Ferreira CR, Whitehead MT, Leon E. Biotin-thiamine responsive basal ganglia disease: identification of a pyruvate peak on brain spectroscopy, novel mutation in SLC19A3, and calculation of prevalence based on allele frequencies from aggregated next-generation sequencing data. Am J Med Genet A. 2017;173(6):1502–13.
10. Wolf B. The neurology of biotinidase deficiency. Mol Genet Metab. 2011;104(1–2):27–34.
11. Yilmaz S, Serin M, Canda E, Eraslan C, Tekin H, Ucar SK, et al. A treatable cause of myelopathy and vision loss mimicking neuromyelitis optica spectrum disorder: late-onset biotinidase deficiency. Metab Brain Dis. 2017;32(3):675–8.
12. Bottin L, Prud'hon S, Guey S, Giannesini C, Wolf B, Pindolia K, et al. Biotinidase deficiency mimicking neuromyelitis optica: initially exhibiting symptoms in adulthood. Mult Scler. 2015;21(12):1604–7.
13. Bhat MD, Bindu PS, Christopher R, Prasad C, Verma A. Novel imaging findings in two cases of biotinidase deficiency-a treatable metabolic disorder. Metab Brain Dis. 2015;30(5):1291–4.
14. Yang Y, Li C, Qi Z, Xiao J, Zhang Y, Yamaguchi S, et al. Spinal cord demyelination associated with biotinidase deficiency in 3 Chinese patients. J Child Neurol. 2007;22(2):156–60.
15. Ramaekers VT, Suormala TM, Brab M, Duran R, Heimann G, Baumgartner ER. A biotinidase km variant causing late onset bilateral optic neuropathy. Arch Dis Child. 1992;67(1):115–9.
16. Ferreira P, Chan A, Wolf B. Irreversibility of symptoms with biotin therapy in an adult with profound Biotinidase deficiency. JIMD Rep. 2017;36:117–20.
17. Girard B, Bonnemains C, Schmitt E, Raffo E, Bilbault C. Biotinidase deficiency mimicking neuromyelitis optica beginning at the age of 4: a treatable disease. Mult Scler. 2017;23(1):119–22.
18. Lorincz MT, Rainier S, Thomas D, Fink JK. Cerebrotendinous xanthomatosis: possible higher prevalence than previously recognized. Arch Neurol. 2005;62(9):1459–63.
19. Duell PB, Salen G, Eichler FS, DeBarber AE, Connor SL, Casaday L, et al. Diagnosis, treatment, and clinical outcomes in 43 cases with cerebrotendinous xanthomatosis. J Clin Lipidol. 2018;12(5):1169–78.
20. Moghadasian MH, Salen G, Frohlich JJ, Scudamore CH. Cerebrotendinous xanthomatosis: a rare disease with diverse manifestations. Arch Neurol. 2002;59(4):527–9.
21. Wong JC, Walsh K, Hayden D, Eichler FS. Natural history of neurological abnormalities in cerebrotendinous xanthomatosis. J Inherit Metab Dis. 2018;41(4):647–56.
22. Cali JJ, Russell DW. Characterization of human sterol 27-hydroxylase. A mitochondrial cytochrome P-450 that catalyzes multiple oxidation reaction in bile acid biosynthesis. J Biol Chem. 1991;266(12):7774–8.
23. Mignarri A, Gallus GN, Dotti MT, Federico A. A suspicion index for early diagnosis and treatment of cerebrotendinous xanthomatosis. J Inherit Metab Dis. 2014;37(3):421–9.
24. Degos B, Nadjar Y, Amador Mdel M, Lamari F, Sedel F, Roze E, et al. Natural history of cerebrotendinous xanthomatosis: a paediatric disease diagnosed in adulthood. Orphanet J Rare Dis. 2016;11:41.
25. Federico A, Gallus GN. Cerebrotendinous Xanthomatosis. In: Adam MP, Feldman J, Mirzaa GM, Pagon RA, Wallace SE, Bean LJH, et al., editors.. Seattle (WA): GeneReviews((R)); 1993.

26. Bartholdi D, Zumsteg D, Verrips A, Wevers RA, Sistermans E, Hess K, et al. Spinal phenotype of cerebrotendinous xanthomatosis–a pitfall in the diagnosis of multiple sclerosis. J Neurol. 2004;251(1):105–7.
27. Verrips A, Nijeholt GJ, Barkhof F, Van Engelen BG, Wesseling P, Luyten JA, et al. Spinal xanthomatosis: a variant of cerebrotendinous xanthomatosis. Brain. 1999;122(Pt 8):1589–95.
28. Barkhof F, Verrips A, Wesseling P, van Der Knaap MS, van Engelen BG, Gabreels FJ, et al. Cerebrotendinous xanthomatosis: the spectrum of imaging findings and the correlation with neuropathologic findings. Radiology. 2000;217(3):869–76.
29. De Stefano N, Dotti MT, Mortilla M, Federico A. Magnetic resonance imaging and spectroscopic changes in brains of patients with cerebrotendinous xanthomatosis. Brain. 2001;124(Pt 1):121–31.
30. Soffer D, Benharroch D, Berginer V. The neuropathology of cerebrotendinous xanthomatosis revisited: a case report and review of the literature. Acta Neuropathol. 1995;90(2):213–20.
31. Nicholls Z, Hobson E, Martindale J, Shaw PJ. Diagnosis of spinal xanthomatosis by next-generation sequencing: identifying a rare, treatable mimic of hereditary spastic paraparesis. Pract Neurol. 2015;15(4):280–3.
32. Siman-Tov T, Meiner V, Gadoth N. Could steroids mask the diagnosis of cerebrotendinous xanthomatosis? J Neurol Sci. 2006;243(1–2):83–6.
33. Spada M, Pagliardini S, Yasuda M, Tukel T, Thiagarajan G, Sakuraba H, et al. High incidence of later-onset fabry disease revealed by newborn screening. Am J Hum Genet. 2006;79(1):31–40.
34. El-Abassi R, Singhal D, England JD. Fabry's disease. J Neurol Sci. 2014;344(1–2):5–19.
35. Germain DP. Fabry disease. Orphanet J Rare Dis. 2010;5:30.
36. Kint JA. Fabry's disease: alpha-galactosidase deficiency. Science. 1970;167(3922):1268–9.
37. Bottcher T, Rolfs A, Tanislav C, Bitsch A, Kohler W, Gaedeke J, et al. Fabry disease – underestimated in the differential diagnosis of multiple sclerosis? PLoS One. 2013;8(8):e71894.
38. Desnick RJ, Brady R, Barranger J, Collins AJ, Germain DP, Goldman M, et al. Fabry disease, an under-recognized multisystemic disorder: expert recommendations for diagnosis, management, and enzyme replacement therapy. Ann Intern Med. 2003;138(4):338–46.
39. Buechner S, Moretti M, Burlina AP, Cei G, Manara R, Ricci R, et al. Central nervous system involvement in Anderson-Fabry disease: a clinical and MRI retrospective study. J Neurol Neurosurg Psychiatry. 2008;79(11):1249–54.
40. Burlina AP, Manara R, Caillaud C, Laissy JP, Severino M, Klein I, et al. The pulvinar sign: frequency and clinical correlations in Fabry disease. J Neurol. 2008;255(5):738–44.
41. Fellgiebel A, Muller MJ, Ginsberg L. CNS manifestations of Fabry's disease. Lancet Neurol. 2006;5(9):791–5.
42. Cocozza S, Olivo G, Riccio E, Russo C, Pontillo G, Ugga L, et al. Corpus callosum involvement: a useful clue for differentiating Fabry disease from multiple sclerosis. Neuroradiology. 2017;59(6):563–70.
43. Cocozza S, Russo C, Pisani A, Olivo G, Riccio E, Cervo A, et al. Redefining the Pulvinar sign in Fabry disease. AJNR Am J Neuroradiol. 2017;38(12):2264–9.
44. Maggi P, Absinta M, Grammatico M, Vuolo L, Emmi G, Carlucci G, et al. Central vein sign differentiates multiple sclerosis from central nervous system inflammatory vasculopathies. Ann Neurol. 2018;83(2):283–94.
45. Baas K, Everard A, Körver S, van Dussen L, Coolen B, Strijkers G, et al. Progressive changes in cerebral apparent diffusion values in Fabry disease: a 5-year follow-up MRI study. Am J Neuroradiol. 2023;44:1157.
46. Kramer J, Glaser F, Hasselblatt M, Brand E, Pogoda C, Lenders M, et al. Case report: a spinal ischemic lesion in a 24-year-old patient with Fabry Disease. Front Immunol. 2020;11:595514.
47. Invernizzi P, Bonometti MA, Turri E, Benedetti MD, Salviati A. A case of Fabry disease with central nervous system (CNS) demyelinating lesions: a double trouble? Mult Scler. 2008;14(7):1003–6.
48. Hajas A, Grubits J, Varga Z. P04—neurophysiologic examinations in patients with Fabry-Anderson disease. Clin Ther. 2012;34(4, Supplement):e19–20.

49. Lidove O, Kaminsky P, Hachulla E, Leguy-Seguin V, Lavigne C, Marie I, et al. Fabry disease 'the new great imposter': results of the French Observatoire in Internal Medicine Departments (FIMeD). Clin Genet. 2012;81(6):571–7.
50. Russo C, Riccio E, Pontillo G, Cocozza S, Tedeschi E, Centonze D, et al. Multiple sclerosis and Fabry disease, two sides of the coin? The case of an Italian family. Mult Scler Relat Disord. 2018;26:164–7.
51. Rekova P, Kovarova I, Uher T, Srpova B, Dostalova G, Linhart A, et al. Missed diagnosis of Fabry disease: should we screen patients with multiple sclerosis? Neurol Sci. 2024;45(1):231–9.
52. Chang KJ, Zhao Z, Shen HR, Bing Q, Li N, Guo X, et al. Adolescent/adult-onset homocysteine remethylation disorders characterized by gait disturbance with/without psychiatric symptoms and cognitive decline: a series of seven cases. Neurol Sci. 2021;42(5):1987–93.
53. Gales A, Masingue M, Millecamps S, Giraudier S, Grosliere L, Adam C, et al. Adolescence/adult onset MTHFR deficiency may manifest as isolated and treatable distinct neuro-psychiatric syndromes. Orphanet J Rare Dis. 2018;13(1):29.
54. Huemer M, Diodato D, Schwahn B, Schiff M, Bandeira A, Benoist JF, et al. Guidelines for diagnosis and management of the cobalamin-related remethylation disorders cblC, cblD, cblE, cblF, cblG, cblJ and MTHFR deficiency. J Inherit Metab Dis. 2017;40(1):21–48.
55. Summar ML, Koelker S, Freedenberg D, Le Mons C, Haberle J, Lee HS, et al. The incidence of urea cycle disorders. Mol Genet Metab. 2013;110(1–2):179–80.
56. Haberle J, Boddaert N, Burlina A, Chakrapani A, Dixon M, Huemer M, et al. Suggested guidelines for the diagnosis and management of urea cycle disorders. Orphanet J Rare Dis. 2012;7:32.
57. Braissant O. Current concepts in the pathogenesis of urea cycle disorders. Mol Genet Metab. 2010;100(Suppl 1):S3–S12.
58. Martinelli D, Diodato D, Ponzi E, Monne M, Boenzi S, Bertini E, et al. The hyperornithinemia-hyperammonemia-homocitrullinuria syndrome. Orphanet J Rare Dis. 2015;10:29.
59. Tezcan K, Louie KT, Qu Y, Velasquez J, Zaldivar F, Rioseco-Camacho N, et al. Adult-onset presentation of a hyperornithinemia-hyperammonemia-homocitrullinuria patient without prior history of neurological complications. JIMD Rep. 2012;3:97–102.
60. Moien-Afshari F, Mirhosseini NZ, Lemire EG, Voll CL. An acute encephalopathy accelerated by a large amount of milk consumption. Can J Neurol Sci. 2016;43(2):345–6.
61. Filosto M, Alberici A, Tessa A, Padovani A, Santorelli FM. Hyperornithinemia-hyperammonemia-homocitrullinuria (HHH) syndrome in adulthood: a rare recognizable condition. Neurol Sci. 2013;34(9):1699–701.
62. Al-Hassnan ZN, Rashed MS, Al-Dirbashi OY, Patay Z, Rahbeeni Z, Abu-Amero KK. Hyperornithinemia-hyperammonemia-homocitrullinuria syndrome with stroke-like imaging presentation: clinical, biochemical and molecular analysis. J Neurol Sci. 2008;264(1–2):187–94.
63. Olivieri G, Pro S, Diodato D, Di Capua M, Longo D, Martinelli D, et al. Corticospinal tract damage in HHH syndrome: a metabolic cause of hereditary spastic paraplegia. Orphanet J Rare Dis. 2019;14(1):208.
64. Lemay JF, Lambert MA, Mitchell GA, Vanasse M, Valle D, Arbour JF, et al. Hyperammonemia-hyperornithinemia-homocitrullinuria syndrome: neurologic, ophthalmologic, and neuropsychologic examination of six patients. J Pediatr. 1992;121(5 Pt 1):725–30.
65. Shigeto H, Yamada T, Kobayashi T, Goto I. A case of hyperornithinemia-hyperammonemia-homocitrullinuria (HHH) syndrome with spastic paraparesis and severe distal muscle atrophy of lower limbs. Rinsho Shinkeigaku. 1992;32(7):729–32.
66. Teive HAG, Camargo CHF, Pereira ER, Coutinho L, Munhoz RP. Inherited metabolic diseases mimicking hereditary spastic paraplegia (HSP): a chance for treatment. Neurogenetics. 2022;23(3):167–77.
67. Weisfeld-Adams JD, Katz Sand IB, Honce JM, Lublin FD. Differential diagnosis of Mendelian and mitochondrial disorders in patients with suspected multiple sclerosis. Brain. 2015;138(Pt 3):517–39.

68. Parenti G, Medina DL, Ballabio A. The rapidly evolving view of lysosomal storage diseases. EMBO Mol Med. 2021;13(2):e12836.
69. Moser AB, Jones RO, Hubbard WC, Tortorelli S, Orsini JJ, Caggana M, et al. Newborn screening for X-linked Adrenoleukodystrophy. Int J Neonatal Screen. 2016;2(4)
70. Engelen M, Kemp S, de Visser M, van Geel BM, Wanders RJ, Aubourg P, et al. X-linked adrenoleukodystrophy (X-ALD): clinical presentation and guidelines for diagnosis, follow-up and management. Orphanet J Rare Dis. 2012;7:51.
71. Wenger DA, Rafi MA, Luzi P. Molecular genetics of Krabbe disease (globoid cell leukodystrophy): diagnostic and clinical implications. Hum Mutat. 1997;10(4):268–79.
72. Gieselmann V, Krägeloh-Mann I. Metachromatic leukodystrophy–an update. Neuropediatrics. 2010;41(1):1–6.
73. Kaplan J, De Domenico I, Ward DM. Chediak-Higashi syndrome. Curr Opin Hematol. 2008;15(1):22–9.
74. Vanier MT. Niemann-Pick disease type C. Orphanet J Rare Dis. 2010;5:16.
75. Frisch A, Colombo R, Michaelovsky E, Karpati M, Goldman B, Peleg L. Origin and spread of the 1278insTATC mutation causing Tay-Sachs disease in Ashkenazi Jews: genetic drift as a robust and parsimonious hypothesis. Hum Genet. 2004;114(4):366–76.
76. Stöckler S, Millner M, Molzer B, Ebner F, Körner E, Moser HW. Multiple sclerosis-like syndrome in a woman heterozygous for adrenoleukodystrophy. Eur Neurol. 1993;33(5):390–2.
77. Zwetsloot CP, Padberg GW, van Seters AP, Maaswinkel-Mooy PD, Onkenhout W. Adult adrenoleukodystrophy: the clinical spectrum in a large Dutch family. J Neurol. 1992;239(2):107–11.
78. Carra-Dalliere C, Scherer C, Ayrignac X, Menjot de Champfleur N, Bellesme C, Labauge P, et al. Adult-onset cerebral X-linked adrenoleukodystrophy with major contrast-enhancement mimicking acquired disease. Clin Neurol Neurosurg. 2013;115(9):1906–7.
79. Kazibutowska Z, Bal A, Gołba A, Ługowska A. Metachromatic leukodystrophy in adult patient initially diagnosed as multiple sclerosis. Neurol Neurochir Pol. 2002;36(6):1209–19.
80. Raymond GV, Seidman R, Monteith TS, Kolodny E, Sathe S, Mahmood A, et al. Head trauma can initiate the onset of adreno-leukodystrophy. J Neurol Sci. 2010;290(1–2):70–4.
81. Engelen M, van Ballegoij WJC, Mallack EJ, Van Haren KP, Köhler W, Salsano E, et al. International recommendations for the diagnosis and management of patients with Adrenoleukodystrophy: a consensus-based approach. Neurology. 2022;99(21):940–51.
82. Resende LL, de Paiva ARB, Kok F, da Costa LC, Lucato LT. Adult Leukodystrophies: a step-by-step diagnostic approach. Radiographics. 2019;39(1):153–68.
83. Jenkins T, Sarasamma P, Gillett G, Coley S, Sharrack B. Multiple sclerosis in an adrenoleukodystrophy carrier. Clin Pract. 2011;1(4):e125.
84. Fatemi A, Smith SA, Dubey P, Zackowski KM, Bastian AJ, van Zijl PC, et al. Magnetization transfer MRI demonstrates spinal cord abnormalities in adrenomyeloneuropathy. Neurology. 2005;64(10):1739–45.
85. Loes DJ, Fatemi A, Melhem ER, Gupte N, Bezman L, Moser HW, et al. Analysis of MRI patterns aids prediction of progression in X-linked adrenoleukodystrophy. Neurology. 2003;61(3):369–74.
86. Tomás J, Durães J, Lacerda L, Macário MC. Adolescent-onset Krabbe disease with an initial diagnosis of multiple sclerosis and a novel mutation. BMJ Case Rep. 2015;2015:bcr2015210625.
87. Sedel F, Tourbah A, Fontaine B, Lubetzki C, Baumann N, Saudubray JM, et al. Leukoencephalopathies associated with inborn errors of metabolism in adults. J Inherit Metab Dis. 2008;31(3):295–307.
88. Chebel S, Barboura I, Boughammoura-Bouatay A, Ammar M, Ferchichi S, Miled A, et al. Adult-type metachromatic leukodystrophy mimicking multiple sclerosis. Can J Neurol Sci. 2009;36(4):521–3.
89. Martin A, Sevin C, Lazarus C, Bellesme C, Aubourg P, Adamsbaum C. Toward a better understanding of brain lesions during metachromatic leukodystrophy evolution. AJNR Am J Neuroradiol. 2012;33(9):1731–9.

90. Patterson MC, Mengel E, Wijburg FA, Muller A, Schwierin B, Drevon H, et al. Disease and patient characteristics in NP-C patients: findings from an international disease registry. Orphanet J Rare Dis. 2013;8:12.
91. Grau AJ, Brandt T, Weisbrod M, Niethammer R, Forsting M, Cantz M, et al. Adult Niemann-Pick disease type C mimicking features of multiple sclerosis. J Neurol Neurosurg Psychiatry. 1997;63(4):552.
92. Weisfeld-Adams JD, Mehta L, Rucker JC, Dembitzer FR, Szporn A, Lublin FD, et al. Atypical Chédiak-Higashi syndrome with attenuated phenotype: three adult siblings homozygous for a novel LYST deletion and with neurodegenerative disease. Orphanet J Rare Dis. 2013;8:46.
93. Karim MA, Suzuki K, Fukai K, Oh J, Nagle DL, Moore KJ, et al. Apparent genotype-phenotype correlation in childhood, adolescent, and adult Chediak-Higashi syndrome. Am J Med Genet. 2002;108(1):16–22.
94. Godeiro-Junior C, Felicio AC, Benites V, Chieia MA, Oliveira AS. Late-onset hexosaminidase A deficiency mimicking primary lateral sclerosis. Arq Neuropsiquiatr. 2009;67(1):105–6.
95. Barritt AW, Anderson SJ, Leigh PN, Ridha BH. Late-onset Tay-Sachs disease. Pract Neurol. 2017;17(5):396–9.
96. Mugikura S, Takahashi S, Higano S, Kurihara N, Kon K, Sakamoto K. MR findings in Tay-Sachs disease. J Comput Assist Tomogr. 1996;20(4):551–5.
97. Winkel LP, Hagemans ML, van Doorn PA, Loonen MC, Hop WJ, Reuser AJ, et al. The natural course of non-classic Pompe's disease; a review of 225 published cases. J Neurol. 2005;252(8):875–84.
98. Sepulveda M, Munteis E, Rubio MA, Pascual J, Roquer J. Adult onset Pompe disease associated with multiple sclerosis. J Neurol. 2011;258(12):2286–7.
99. Williams T, Houlden H, Murphy E, John N, Fox NC, Schott JM, et al. How to diagnose difficult white matter disorders. Pract Neurol. 2020;20(4):280–6.
100. Ng YS, Turnbull DM. Mitochondrial disease: genetics and management. J Neurol. 2016;263(1):179–91.
101. Buajitti E, Rosella LC, Zabzuni E, Young LT, Andreazza AC. Prevalence and health care costs of mitochondrial disease in Ontario, Canada: a population-based cohort study. PLoS One. 2022;17(4):e0265744.
102. Finsterer J, Zarrouk-Mahjoub S. Cerebral involvement in mitochondrial disorders on imaging. Childs Nerv Syst. 2016;32(11):2059–60.
103. Alves C, Goldstein A, Teixeira SR, Martin-Saavedra JS, de Barcelos IP, Fadda G, et al. Involvement of the spinal cord in primary mitochondrial disorders: a neuroimaging mimicker of inflammation and ischemia in children. AJNR Am J Neuroradiol. 2021;42(2):389–96.
104. Iñiguez C, Arenas J, Montoya J, Mostacero E, López del Val J, Morales F. Mitochondrial respiratory chain deficiency may present as multiple sclerosis. Neurologia (Barcelona, Spain). 1998;13(4):199–203.
105. Finsterer J. Cerebral imaging in adult mitochondrial disorders. J Neurol Sci. 2019;404:29–35.
106. Finsterer J, Carvalho EHT. Cerebral manifestations of mitochondrial disorders. Can J Neurol Sci. 2017;44(6):654–63.
107. Finsterer J, Zarrouk-Mahjoub S. Biomarkers for detecting mitochondrial disorders. J Clin Med. 2018;7(2)
108. Mascalchi M, Montomoli M, Guerrini R. Neuroimaging in mitochondrial disorders. Essays Biochem. 2018;62(3):409–21.
109. Finsterer J, Leutmezer F. Celiac disease with cerebral and peripheral nerve involvement mimicking multiple sclerosis. J Med Life. 2014;7(3):440–4.
110. Finsterer J, Zarrouk-Mahjoub S. Involvement of the spinal cord in mitochondrial disorders. J Neurosci Rural Pract. 2018;9(2):245–51.
111. Shayota BJ. Biomarkers of mitochondrial disorders. Neurotherapeutics. 2024;21(1):e00325.
112. Jeppesen TD, Schwartz M, Frederiksen AL, Wibrand F, Olsen DB, Vissing J. Muscle phenotype and mutation load in 51 persons with the 3243A>G mitochondrial DNA mutation. Arch Neurol. 2006;63(12):1701–6.

113. Yamada K, Toribe Y, Yanagihara K, Mano T, Akagi M, Suzuki Y. Diagnostic accuracy of blood and CSF lactate in identifying children with mitochondrial diseases affecting the central nervous system. Brain Dev. 2012;34(2):92–7.
114. Parikh S, Goldstein A, Koenig MK, Scaglia F, Enns GM, Saneto R, et al. Diagnosis and management of mitochondrial disease: a consensus statement from the mitochondrial medicine society. Genet Med. 2015;17(9):689–701.
115. Palace J. Multiple sclerosis associated with Leber's hereditary optic neuropathy. J Neurol Sci. 2009;286(1–2):24–7.
116. Degos B, Laforêt P, Jardel C, Sedel F, Jossay-Winter M, Romero NB, et al. POLG mutations associated with remitting/relapsing neurological events. J Clin Neurosci. 2014;21(1):186–8.
117. Hacohen Y, Narula S, Waldman A, Hopkins S, Brenton J, Bar-Or A, et al. Acute evidence of CNS inflammation in patients with mitochondrial diseases (P4.053). Neurology. 2015;84(14_supplement):P4.053.
118. Della Marina A, Bertolini A, Wegener-Panzer A, Flotats-Bastardas M, Reinhardt T, El Naggar I, et al. Mitochondrial diseases mimicking autoimmune diseases of the CNS and good response to steroids initially. Eur J Paediatr Neurol. 2022;41:27–35.
119. Chen BS, Harvey JP, Gilhooley MJ, Jurkute N, Yu-Wai-Man P. Mitochondria and the eye-manifestations of mitochondrial diseases and their management. Eye (Lond). 2023;37(12):2416–25.
120. Echaniz-Laguna A, Chassagne M, de Sèze J, Mohr M, Clerc-Renaud P, Tranchant C, et al. POLG1 variations presenting as multiple sclerosis. Arch Neurol. 2010;67(9):1140–3.
121. Wortmann SB, Mayr JA. Choline-related-inherited metabolic diseases-a mini review. J Inherit Metab Dis. 2019;42(2):237–42.
122. Członkowska A, Litwin T, Dusek P, Ferenci P, Lutsenko S, Medici V, et al. Wilson disease. Nat Rev Dis Primers. 2018;4(1):21.
123. Dusek P, Litwin T, Członkowska A. Neurologic impairment in Wilson disease. Ann Transl Med. 2019;7(Suppl 2):S64.
124. Despotov K, Klivényi P, Nagy I, Pálvölgyi A, Vécsei L, Rajda C. Rare co-occurrence of multiple sclerosis and Wilson's disease – case report. BMC Neurol. 2022;22(1):178.
125. Sardh E, Barbaro M. Acute intermittent porphyria. In: Adam MP, Feldman J, Mirzaa GM, Pagon RA, Wallace SE, Bean LJH, et al., editors. GeneReviews(®). Seattle: University of Washington, Seattle Copyright © 1993–2024, University of Washington, Seattle. GeneReviews is a registered trademark of the University of Washington, Seattle. All rights reserved; 1993.
126. Clarke CE, Alger S, Preece MA, Burdon MA, Chavda S, Denis S, et al. Tremor and deep white matter changes in alpha-methylacyl-CoA racemase deficiency. Neurology. 2004;63(1):188–9.
127. Haugarvoll K, Johansson S, Tzoulis C, Haukanes BI, Bredrup C, Neckelmann G, et al. MRI characterisation of adult onset alpha-methylacyl-coA racemase deficiency diagnosed by exome sequencing. Orphanet J Rare Dis. 2013;8:1.
128. Mochel F, Schiffmann R, Steenweg ME, Akman HO, Wallace M, Sedel F, et al. Adult polyglucosan body disease: natural history and key magnetic resonance imaging findings. Ann Neurol. 2012;72(3):433–41.
129. Dell'Isola GB, Dini G, Culpepper KL, Portwood KE, Ferrara P, Di Cara G, et al. Clinical spectrum and currently available treatment of type I interferonopathy Aicardi-Goutières syndrome. World J Pediatr. 2023;19(7):635–43.
130. McNutt MC, Foreman N, Gotway G. Arginase 1 deficiency in patients initially diagnosed with hereditary spastic paraplegia. Mov Disord Clin Pract. 2023;10(1):109–14.
131. Bin Sawad A, Jackimiec J, Bechter M, Trucillo A, Lindsley K, Bhagat A, et al. Epidemiology, methods of diagnosis, and clinical management of patients with arginase 1 deficiency (ARG1-D): a systematic review. Mol Genet Metab. 2022;137(1–2):153–63.
132. Carvalho DR, Farage L, Martins BJ, Brum JM, Speck-Martins CE, Pratesi R. Brain MRI and magnetic resonance spectroscopy findings in patients with hyperargininemia. J Neuroimaging. 2014;24(2):155–60.

133. Camargos S, Guerreiro R, Bras J, Mageste LS. Late-onset and acute presentation of Brown-Vialetto-Van Laere syndrome in a Brazilian family. Neurol Genet. 2018;4(1):e215.
134. Bosch AM, Stroek K, Abeling NG, Waterham HR, Ijlst L, Wanders RJ. The Brown-Vialetto-Van Laere and Fazio Londe syndrome revisited: natural history, genetics, treatment and future perspectives. Orphanet J Rare Dis. 2012;7:83.
135. Nagy A, Bley AE, Eichler F. Canavan Disease. In: Adam MP, Feldman J, Mirzaa GM, Pagon RA, Wallace SE, Bean LJH, et al., editors. GeneReviews(®). Seattle (WA): University of Washington, Seattle Copyright © 1993–2024, University of Washington, Seattle. GeneReviews is a registered trademark of the University of Washington, Seattle. All rights reserved; 1993.
136. Wei H, Moffett JR, Amanat M, Fatemi A, Tsukamoto T, Namboodiri AM, et al. The pathogenesis of, and pharmacological treatment for, Canavan disease. Drug Discov Today. 2022;27(9):2467–83.
137. Emmanuele V, López LC, Berardo A, Naini A, Tadesse S, Wen B, et al. Heterogeneity of coenzyme Q10 deficiency: patient study and literature review. Arch Neurol. 2012;69(8):978–83.
138. Martinelli D, Haberle J, Rubio V, Giunta C, Hausser I, Carrozzo R, et al. Understanding pyrroline-5-carboxylate synthetase deficiency: clinical, molecular, functional, and expression studies, structure-based analysis, and novel therapy with arginine. J Inherit Metab Dis. 2012;35(5):761–76.
139. Klepper J, Akman C, Armeno M, Auvin S, Cervenka M, Cross HJ, et al. Glut1 Deficiency Syndrome (Glut1DS): state of the art in 2020 and recommendations of the international Glut1DS study group. Epilepsia Open. 2020;5(3):354–65.
140. De Vivo DC, Trifiletti RR, Jacobson RI, Ronen GM, Behmand RA, Harik SI. Defective glucose transport across the blood-brain barrier as a cause of persistent hypoglycorrhachia, seizures, and developmental delay. N Engl J Med. 1991;325(10):703–9.
141. Pizzini F, Fatemi AS, Barker PB, Nagae-Poetscher LM, Horská A, Zimmerman AW, et al. Proton MR spectroscopic imaging in Pelizaeus-Merzbacher disease. AJNR Am J Neuroradiol. 2003;24(8):1683–9.
142. Rubegni A, Battisti C, Tessa A, Cerase A, Doccini S, Malandrini A, et al. SPG2 mimicking multiple sclerosis in a family identified using next generation sequencing. J Neurol Sci. 2017;375:198–202.
143. Singh R, Samanta D. Pelizaeus-Merzbacher Disease. StatPearls. Treasure Island (FL) ineligible companies. Disclosure: Debopam Samanta declares no relevant financial relationships with ineligible companies.: StatPearls Publishing Copyright © 2024, StatPearls Publishing LLC.; 2024.
144. Legrand A, Pujol C, Durand CM, Mesnil A, Rubera I, Duranton C, et al. Pseudoxanthoma elasticum overlaps hereditary spastic paraplegia type 56. J Intern Med. 2021;289(5):709–25.

Neurodegenerative Hereditary Diseases

8

8.1 Autosomal Recessive Cerebellar Ataxias (ARCA)

8.1.1 Epidemiology

- Friedreich's ataxia (FRDA): prevalence 2–4/100.000 (heterozygous carrier frequency is 1 in 85 Caucasians).
- Ataxia telangiectasia (TA): prevalence 1–2.5/100.000.
- Autosomal recessive spastic ataxia of Charlevoixe-Saguenay (ARSACS) is the third most prevalent type of ARCA. Other types of ARCA are less common [1, 2].

8.1.2 Etiology and Definition

- A heterogeneous group of inherited autosomal recessive cerebellar ataxias characterized by the degeneration or abnormal development of the cerebellum and spinal cord.
- There are various classifications of ARCA:
- Based on disease course:
  - Progressive.
  - Non-progressive with impaired development of the cerebellum and its connections (congenital ataxias).
  - Metabolic with progressive or intermittent natural history [1]
- Based on the topography of the manifestations:
  - Sensory and spinocerebellar ataxias.
  - Cerebellar ataxias with sensory-motor peripheral neuropathy.
  - Pure cerebellar ataxia (rare) [3]
- Clinically oriented:
  - Congenital or developmental ataxias.
    - Joubert syndrome.
    - Cayman cerebellar ataxia.

T. Uher, *Mimics and Red Flags of Multiple Sclerosis*, https://doi.org/10.1007/978-3-031-98945-2_8

- Metabolic ataxias (caused by enzymatic defects).
  - Ataxia with isolated vitamin E deficiency (AVED).
    - For further details, please refer to the dedicated chapter.
  - Abetalipoproteinemia.
    - Malabsorption, pigmentary degeneration of the retina, and progressive ataxic neuropathy are caused by a deficiency of vitamin E. Total cholesterol levels are markedly low (<70 mg/dL or 1.8 mmol/L) and triglycerides and low-density lipoprotein cholesterol (LDL-C) are nearly undetectable.
  - Cerebrotendinous xanthomatosis.
    - For further details, please refer to the dedicated chapter.
  - Refsum disease.
    - Retinitis pigmentosa, chronic polyneuropathy, and cerebellar ataxia. Sometime also anosmia, deafness, cardiac arrhythmias, bony and skin abnormalities.
- Ataxia due to DNA repair defects.
  - Ataxia telangiectasia (AT).
  - Ataxia with oculomotor apraxia 1 (AOA1) and 2 (AOA2).
  - Ataxia-telangiectasia-like disorder (ATLD).
  - Spinocerebellar ataxia with axonal neuropathy type 1 (SCAN1).
  - Xeroderma pigmentosum (XP).
- Degenerative and progressive ataxic disorders.
  - Friedreich ataxia (FRDA).
    - The expanded GAA repeat results in inhibition of the FRDA gene expression and decreased production of frataxin, which plays a role in mitochondrial function.
  - Mitochondrial recessive ataxic syndrome (MIRAS).
  - Charlevoix-Saguenay spastic ataxia (ARSACS).
  - Early-onset cerebellar ataxia with retained tendon reflexes.
  - Infantile-onset spinocerebellar ataxia.
  - Marinesco–Sjögren syndrome.
  - Coenzyme Q10 (CoQ10) deficiency with cerebellar ataxia.
  - Posterior column ataxia and retinitis pigmentosa.
- Ataxias of unknown etiology.
- ARCA with additional features [1].

8.1.3 Clinical Features

- ARCA manifests in childhood, although there are late-onset cases as well.
- FRDA.
  - The following central and peripheral nervous system structures are affected:
  - Dentate nucleus of the cerebellum.
    - Progressive gait and limb ataxia.
    - Dysarthria.

- Proprioceptive system (degeneration of sensory ganglion cells, the posterior columns, and spino-cerebellar tracts).
  - Sensory ataxia.
  - Sensory loss.
- Corticospinal tracts.
  - Motor weakness.
  - Extensor plantar responses.
  - Spasticity and sphincter disturbances (less frequent).
- Peripheral nerves (axonal neuropathy).
  - Motor weakness.
  - Hyporeflexia.
- The phenotype of FRDA can vary, but ataxia, dysarthria, areflexia on lower limb, and deep sensory loss are consistently observed.
- Ataxia often results from a combination of peripheral sensory neuropathy, degeneration of the spinocerebellar tracts, cerebellar pathology, and involvement of the vestibular nerve.
- Typically, motor weakness predominantly affects the lower limbs. Initially, it is primarily attributed to peripheral neuropathy, characterized by diminished tendon reflexes and distal wasting. In later stages, it becomes more intertwined with pyramidal (central) motor weakness, accompanied by spasticity, and the extensor plantar responses. Contractures and painful muscle spasms may develop as the condition progresses.
- Other manifestations may include dysphagia, nystagmus, optic atrophy with visual loss, deafness, scoliosis, foot deformity (pes cavus), hypertrophic cardiomyopathy, diabetes mellitus or glucose intolerance.
- The age of symptoms onset is 10–16 years (rarely after 40 years).
- Majority of patients are wheelchair bound within 10–15 years.
- Cardiac disease is the most common cause of death [1, 4, 5].

- AT
  - Progressive cerebellar ataxia.
  - Oculocutaneous telangiectasia.
  - Variable immunodeficiency with recurrent infections.
  - Radiosensitivity (patients should not undergo X-ray or computed tomography [CT] scan).
  - Susceptibility to malignancies.
  - Some patients may exhibit movement disorders (dystonia, tremor, chorea), cognitive deficit, peripheral neuropathy, and eye movement disorders (oculomotor apraxia, slow saccades, and nystagmus).
  - The age of symptom onset is 2–4 years; however, late-onset cases have also been documented [1, 6].
- ARSACS
  - Slowly progressive course with wheelchair bound in adulthood.
  - Some patients may have paroxysmal/relapsing-remitting symptoms.
  - Patients exhibit a clinical triad comprising:
  - (A) Early-onset cerebella ataxia

  - (B) Central lower limb motor weakness with spasticity, increased tendon reflexes, and extensor plantar response. Upper limbs may also be affected to a lesser extent.
  - (C) Peripheral neuropathy with progressive distal wasting, reduced vibratory and positional senses, and decreased ankle reflexes.
  - Other features may include dysarthria, nystagmus, impaired ocular pursuit, and hypermyelination of the retinal fibers.
  - Mental retardation is rare, and cognitive function typically remains within the normal range.
  - The age of symptom onset is in childhood; however, rare late-onset cases have also been documented [1, 2, 7].
- AOA1 and 2 AOA2.
  - Progressive gait ataxia, dysarthria, distal muscle weakness and wasting, mild loss of vibration and position sense.
  - Some patients may present with additional symptoms such as dystonia, mental retardation, oculomotor apraxia, or choreoathetosis.
  - The age of symptom onset is in early childhood. In type 2, onset usually occurs between 11 and 22 years [1].

8.1.4 Brain and Spinal Cord Imaging

- Most patients exhibit cerebellar atrophy, with some also showing atrophy in the brainstem and spinal cord. Supratentorial brain regions typically remain unaffected.
- FRDA.
  - In contrast to other ARCA, there is either no cerebellar atrophy or only mild atrophy of the upper vermis or the medulla oblongata.
  - Sometime present T2 hyperintensities in the posterior or lateral spinal cord columns and atrophy of cervical spinal cord.
- AT:
  - Progressive cerebellar atrophy, particularly affecting the vermis and to a lesser extent, the hemispheres.
  - In some cases, T2 and susceptibility weighted imaging (SWI) hypointensities in deep white matter, indicating the presence of hemosiderin deposits and telangiectatic vessels (Fig. 8.1).
  - Older patients may exhibit diffuse T2 hyperintensities in deep white matter and rarely also microbleeds attributed to vascular damage.
- ARSACS.
  - Early progressive atrophy of the superior cerebellar vermis.
  - Symmetrical linear T2 hypointensities (without corresponding findings on T1 images) in the pons near the pyramidal tracts.
  - Cervical spinal cord atrophy.
- AOA1 and AOA2.
  - Diffuse cerebellar atrophy, particularly of the anterior vermis.
  - Sometimes brainstem atrophy.
  - Disappearance of hypointensity in the dentate nuclei on SWI [7–9].

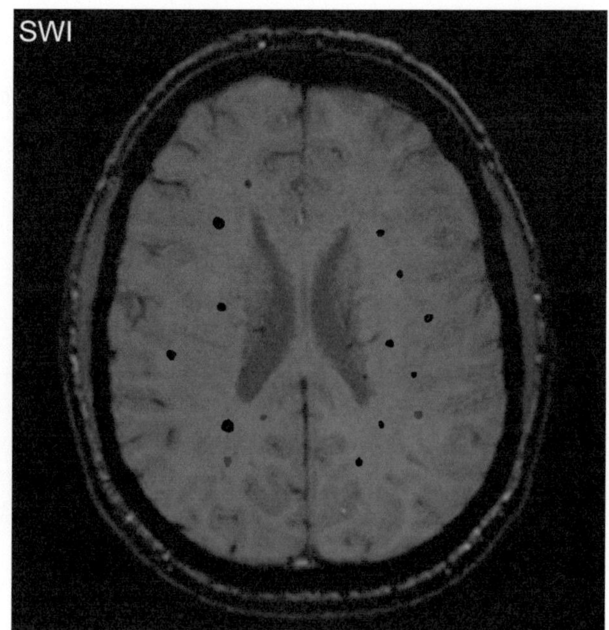

Fig. 8.1 Hemosiderin deposits and telangiectatic vessels in ataxia telangiectasia

8.1.5 Blood Work

- Most patients with AT exhibit elevated concentrations of alpha-fetoprotein levels.
- Patients with AOA1 typically present with hypoalbuminemia and hypercholesterolemia.
- Patients with AOA2 often display elevated levels of gamma globulin, alpha-protein, and creatine kinase.
- Otherwise, routine blood testing yields normal results [1, 6].

8.1.6 Examination of CSF

- A limited number of small sample size studies showed normal findings, including negative oligoclonal bands (OCB) in cerebrospinal fluid (CSF) [10, 11].

8.1.7 OCT

- Optical coherence tomography (OCT) shows a decrease in retinal nerve fiber layer (RNFL) thickness is observed in patients with FRDA [12].

8.1.8 Electrophysiology

- FRDA and ARSACS are associated with axonal peripheral neuropathy, primarily affecting sensory fibers and, to a lesser extent, motor fibers.
- AT is associated with demyelinating and axonal neuropathy [1, 7].

8.1.9 Diagnosis

- Given that ARCA are autosomal recessive diseases, the familial history is typically negative.
- In suspected cases (determined by disease course and clinical manifestations), the diagnosis is established through neuroimaging (to differentiate from developmental and degenerative diseases), electromyography, biochemical, and genetic molecular testing [1].

8.1.10 Treatment

- Omaveloxolon (antioxidant inflammation modulator) for FRDA [13].
- Apart from treatments targeting deficiencies in vitamin E, CoQ10, and cerebrotendinous xanthomatosis, there are no other specific treatments available for most patients with ARCA [1].

8.2 Cerebellar Ataxia with Neuropathy and Vestibular Areflexia Syndrome (CANVAS)

8.2.1 Epidemiology

- Prevalence 5–16/100.000 [14].

8.2.2 Etiology and Definition

- CANVAS is autosomal recessive disorder caused by a biallelic expansion of an intronic AAGGG repeat in the replication factor C subunit 1 (*RFC1*) gene [15].
- This leads to cerebellar atrophy primarily affecting the vermian Purkinje cells while preserving the brainstem neurons. Additionally, there is atrophy of the vestibular, geniculate, and trigeminal ganglia, as well as atrophy of the sensory ganglia and dorsal columns of the spinal cord [16]. The precise mechanism underlying neurodegeneration remains unknown [17].

- If both parents are heterozygous carriers of the AAGGG repeat expansion, the child has a 25% chance of being affected, a 50% chance of being an asymptomatic carrier, and a 25% chance of being unaffected and not a carrier.
- Prenatal genetic testing for pregnancies at increased risk, as well as preimplantation testing, are available [18].

8.2.3 Core Clinical Features

- Sensory symptoms (75%).
  - Hypesthesia, pins, needles, and neuropathic pain.
  - Often attacks of sudden neuropathic pain or trigeminal neuralgia.
  - In the early stages, sensory symptoms can be asymmetrical.
  - Length-dependent sensory neuronopathy:
    - The involvement of large, myelinated fibers leads to impaired vibration and joint position sense. This impairment follows a length-dependent pattern, starting in the distal parts of the limbs and being most severe there.
  - Non-length-dependent sensory neuronopathy:
    - Affects all types of sensory fibers, including large and small myelinated and unmyelinated fibers. Therefore, impaired pinprick sensation (pain sensation), indicating involvement of small unmyelinated fibers, can also occur [17, 19–21].
- Vestibulopathy (90%).
  - An abnormal head impulse test (HIT), indicating bilateral vestibular areflexia, is almost always present and should therefore be examined in every older patient with ataxia [22].
  - The vestibular areflexia syndrome with reduced visually enhanced vestibulo-ocular reflex is also very common and suggests the coexistence of vestibular and cerebellar pathology.
  - Nystagmus with oscillopsia may be sometime present. (30%).
  - Vertigo is rare and probably unrelated to CANVAS [17–19].
- Progressive imbalance (100%).
  - A relatively early feature, driven by a combination of sensory neuropathy, cerebellar ataxia, and vestibulopathy.
  - Often worsens in the dark, suggesting a contribution from peripheral large-fiber sensory neuropathy [17–19].

8.2.4 Additional Clinical Features

- Chronic dry spasmodic cough. (65%).
  - May occur up to 30 years before the onset of the neurological symptoms.
  - Might be disabling and together with neuropathic pain represent major sources of discomfort.

  - The cause remains unclear, but it is suggested that small-fiber involvement within the sensory pathways responsible for regulating cough may be a factor [17–20].
- Abnormal eye movements of cerebellar origin.
  - Might occur in the early stages of the disease and often includes downbeat nystagmus (28–65%), along with other disturbances such as broken pursuit, square wave jerks, dysmetric saccades, or impaired velocity and/or latency [17, 21–23].
- Autonomic dysfunction (>50%).
  - Postural hypotension; lightheadedness (65%); dry mouth/eyes (52%); pale or blue feet (39%); feet colder than rest of body (78%); reduced feet sweating compared to rest of body (48%); reduced feet sweating during exercise or warm weather (35%); increased sweating in hands compared to rest of body (0%); nausea, vomiting or bloating after a small meal (26%); persistent diarrhea (4%); persistent constipation (65%); leakage of urine (39%); or erectile dysfunction (78%) [22].
- Tendon reflexes and motor functions.
  - The partial or complete sparing of tendon reflexes (reduced, normal, or brisk) despite sensory neuropathy is typical for CANVAS. The conservation of deep tendon reflexes and H reflexes is hypothesized to be due to the selective impairment of small and large sensory fibers, whereas the muscle spindle fibers (Aα and Aβ) are preserved [19, 24].
  - The muscle strength is always normal [17, 18].
- Dysarthria and dysphagia:
  - Attributable to cerebellar dysfunction.
  - Frequent in later disease stages.
  - Blink and masseter reflexes can be decreased due to sensory neuropathy affecting also trigeminal nerve [17].
- Cognitive impairment (25%) [17].
- The clinical presentation is complete in two-thirds and incomplete in one-third of cases. For example, isolated sensory neuropathy is observed (15%), whereas isolated cerebellar syndrome has not been described [17, 19].
- CANVAS is likely underdiagnosed in patients presenting with ataxia, particularly when vestibular function is not assessed [22]. Conversely, approximately 30% of patients with 'idiopathic' bilateral vestibulopathy have CANVAS. This condition may be overlooked in differential diagnoses due to the absence of ataxia and neuropathy [25].

8.2.5 Disease Course

- The mean age of symptom onset is 52 years. (range, 19–76).
- Slowly progressive course [19].
- There is a pattern of spatial progression from the early involvement of sensory neurons to the vestibular system and later the cerebellum [17].

8.2.6 Brain Imaging

- Cerebellar atrophy, mainly in the vermis and the hemispheric crus (70%).
- Whole brain atrophy can also be present [22, 23].
- Small non-enhancing T2 hyperintense lesions in the supratentorial white matter or brainstem are non-specific and are typically attributed to age-related small vessel disease in older patients [18].

8.2.7 Spinal Cord Imaging

- Symmetric non-enhancing T2 hyperintense lesions may occur in the dorsal columns and roots of the spinal cord. This can be explained by centripetal Wallerian degeneration of the sensory tracts stemming from dorsal root ganglionopathy [26].
- Rarely, patients exhibit spinal cord lesions typical of multiple sclerosis (MS). In such cases, it is essential to exclude the comorbidity of CANVAS and MS. [26, 27].
- Spinal cord atrophy can be present [22, 23].

8.2.8 Peripheral Nerve Ultrasound

- The decreased cross-sectional area of peripheral nerves is driven by axonal loss secondary to ganglion cell loss, which could help narrow down the differential diagnosis before undergoing genetic testing [26].

8.2.9 Skin Biopsy

- A severe, non-length-dependent loss of intraepidermal nerve fibers [18].

8.2.10 Examination of Blood and CSF

- Typically normal [20].
- Similarly, as with spinal cord lesions, there are few case studies describing patients with CANVAS and positive CSF-restricted OCB, suggesting possible comorbidity between CANVAS and MS. [26, 27].

8.2.11 Electrophysiology

- Pathology in dorsal columns of the spinal cord is associated with major reduction or complete loss of sensory action potentials on conduction studies (sensory axonal neuronopathy). Motor conduction studies are normal (90%) or with only minor reduction of motor action potentials (10%). As noted above, muscle strength is preserved [16, 17, 26].

- The H reflex testing integrity of peripheral motor fibers and muscle spindle afferent fibers is normal and is in agreement with frequently observed normoreflexia [17, 28].

8.2.12 Diagnosis

- Molecular genetic testing detects biallelic intronic AAGGG expansions in *RFC1* gene. This cannot be identified using sequence-based multigene panels or exome sequencing but may be suspected through genome sequencing. It's important to note that CANVAS exhibits incomplete penetrance. Therefore, the discovery of biallelic *RFC1* AAGGG repeat expansions does not necessarily indicate a diagnosis of CANVAS [18].

8.2.13 Differential Diagnosis

- MS:
  - There are a few reported cases of patients with positive genetic testing for CANVAS and a phenotype typical for MS, including CSF-restricted OCB, typical spinal cord lesions, and response to corticosteroids. It remains unclear whether these patients have a co-occurrence of CANVAS and MS, or if CANVAS can be associated with susceptibility to autoimmune demyelination [18, 19].
  - Therefore, in general, the presence of CSF-restricted OCB should not automatically lead to the exclusion of non-inflammatory neurological diseases [29].
  - Features suggesting a possible diagnosis of MS include not only CSF-restricted OCB but also clearly upper motor neuron symptoms, rapid disease progression, relapsing course, or a typical magnetic resonance imaging (MRI) pattern [27].
- Acquired sensory neuronopathies:
  - Positive sensory symptoms such as paresthesia, pins and needles, or neuropathic pain are typically not present in other hereditary neuropathies. Therefore, patients with CANVAS are often misdiagnosed with acquired immune-mediated sensory neuronopathy associated with, for example, Sjögren's or paraneoplastic syndrome, and may receive immunomodulatory treatments as a result [20].
- Friedreich's ataxia (FRDA):
  - Shares a similar phenotype with CANVAS but typically manifests at a younger age (<25 years). Unlike CANVAS, FRDA is associated with prominent motor signs and symptoms such as muscle atrophy, spasticity, and skeletal deformities (pes cavus and scoliosis). Additionally, FRDA is often

accompanied by cardiomyopathy, diabetes mellitus, and involvement of vision and hearing. However, like CANVAS, FRDA can also be associated with sensory neuropathy, cerebellar dysfunction, and vestibular areflexia, with the exception of dry cough, which is not seen in FRDA [17, 23].

- Mitochondrial diseases:
  - Can present with a similar phenotype to CANVAS, but they typically manifest at an earlier age and often exhibit chronic external ophthalmoplegia or multisystem organ involvement [17, 30].
- Multiple system atrophy (MSA):
  - Differentiating CANVAS from MSA may pose a diagnostic challenge in patients with late-onset cerebellar ataxia. CANVAS differs from MSA in several key aspects: it lacks rapid clinical progression; it lacks rapid eye movement (REM) sleep behavior disorder; and Parkinson's syndrome. Additionally, brainstem atrophy on MRI and "hot cross-bun" signs, which manifest as cruciform T2 hyperintensity in the pons, are absent in CANVAS. Downbeat nystagmus (28–65%) and bilateral vestibulopathy are observed in CANVAS, but rarely occurring in MSA [17, 31]. Sphincter symptoms tend to be more severe in MSA [21, 22]. Autonomic failure is a primary cause of morbidity in MSA, whereas in CANVAS, ataxia is the main cause of morbidity [32]. Furthermore, CANVAS is associated with non-length-dependent sensory neuronopathy, which is not typically seen in MSA, where motor axonopathy is rarely observed [33].

8.2.14 Treatment and Prognosis

- Only symptomatic.
- Patients should avoid agents/circumstances of known toxicity for peripheral nerves (e.g., neurotoxic chemotherapy agents, pyridoxine), the cerebellum (e.g., phenytoin), or the vestibular system (e.g., aminoglycosides); and chronic alcohol consumption [34].
- Disease progression typically occurs at a very slow pace, and life expectancy is usually not affected. After 10 years, approximately 50% of patients require one-sided support when walking, and 25% become wheelchair-dependent within the subsequent 5 years [17–19].

8.3 Charcot-Marie-Tooth Neuropathy

8.3.1 Epidemiology

- Prevalence 40/100.000.
- Second most common form of hereditary motor and sensory neuropathy.
- Female/male ratio 1/1.

8.3.2 Etiology and Definition

- Charcot-Marie-Tooth (CMT) neuropathy is a group of inherited X-linked dominant diseases characterized by exclusive or predominant involvement of the peripheral nervous system and usually associated with a positive family history.
- It is caused by hundreds of different mutations in the Gap junction beta-1 (*GJB1*) gene, which encodes the gap junction protein connexin 32. This protein is expressed in Schwann cells and oligodendrocytes. Mutations in this gene cause the most common X-linked form of CMT (CMT1X). Consequently, patients with CMT1X exhibit involvement of both the peripheral and central nervous system.

8.3.3 Clinical Features

- Peripheral motor and sensory neuropathy characterized by progressive muscle atrophy, weakness, areflexia, and variable sensory manifestations.
- Familial ataxia.
- Self-limited stroke-like episodes lasting hours to weeks, presenting as transient neurological dysfunction (mainly central palsy and dysarthria) with either acute or slow evolution.
- In rare cases, these recurrent attacks in children and adults may be associated with transient leukoencephalopathy resembling acute disseminated encephalomyelitis (ADEM).
- Although stroke-like episodes typically have a full remission, some patients may experience persistent (fixed) central nervous system (CNS) manifestations, such as dysarthria, spasticity, hyperreflexia, extensor plantar response, hearing loss, dysphonia, or dysphagia.
- Women tend to be less severely affected, and some may even remain asymptomatic.

8.3.4 Disease Course

- Progressive disease.
- Symptoms onset typically occurs between 5 and 25 years of age. Initial symptoms usually include peripheral neuropathy, while stroke-like episodes are less common as an initial feature.
- Some female patients develop symptoms later in life.

8.3.5 Brain and Spinal Imaging

- Brain MRI is only rarely normal during exacerbations of stroke-like episodes.
- Stroke-like episodes are typically associated with symmetric, non-enhancing, confluent (or diffuse) T2 lesions in the subcortical white matter (often involving the posterior centrum semiovale) and the splenium of the corpus callosum.

- These lesions typically spare the subcortical U fibers and exhibit restricted diffusion.
- While diffusion-weighted imaging (DWI) abnormalities usually resolve within weeks, T2 hyperintensities tend to persist longer, sometimes even in already asymptomatic patients.
- Unilateral or bilateral symmetric involvement of the cerebellar peduncles or periventricular white matter is rare but can occur.
- Can occur bilateral corticospinal tract hyperintensities.

8.3.6 Electrophysiology

- Pathological nerve conduction studies are characterized by slowed conduction and distal axonal loss.
- Pathological findings are commonly observed in visual, brainstem auditory, somatosensory, and motor evoked responses.

8.3.7 Nerve Biopsy

- Axonal loss predominates over demyelination and remyelination.

8.3.8 Examination of Blood and CSF

- Except for a possible mild elevation in CSF protein, routine testing is expected to yield normal results.

8.3.9 Diagnosis

- Genetic testing is recommended for suspected patients (e.g., those with familial ataxia and peripheral neuropathy).
- Prenatal and preimplantation genetic diagnoses are feasible for families with a diagnosed case of CMT.

8.3.10 Differential Diagnosis

- There is an increased number of patients with both CMT and MS, particularly those with mutations affecting the CNS, suggesting a potential causal relationship. CMT with CNS manifestations may mimic MS and ADEM.
- Cerebral autosomal dominant arteriopathy with subcortical infarcts and leukoencephalopathy (CADASIL) usually does not present with peripheral neuropathy.
- Chronic inflammatory demyelinating polyneuropathy (CIDP).
- Fabry disease with ischemic stroke and small fiber neuropathy.
- Leukodystrophies.

- Mitochondrial encephalomyopathy, lactic acidosis and stroke-like episodes (MELAS).
- Metabolic encephalopathy or ischemia due to complications of diabetes mellitus, kidney disease, or liver disease.
- Polymerase gamma gene (POLG)-related disorders.
- Sarcoidosis.
- SLE and other collagen vascular diseases.
- Stroke.
- Systemic vasculitis.

8.3.11 Treatment

- Only symptomatic treatment.
- Corticosteroids have no effect on stroke-like episodes.

8.3.12 Prognosis

- Disease progression is generally slow, and patients have a normal life expectancy. Although patients often require walking aids, complete loss of ambulation is rare, except in male patients with CMTX3, who may experience a more severe course and require a wheelchair at an early stage [35–41].

8.4 Dopa-Responsive Dystonia

8.4.1 Synonym

- Segawa disease [42].

8.4.2 Epidemiology

- Prevalence 0.05/100.000.
- 5–10% of all primary dystonias [43].

8.4.3 Etiology and Definition

- A group of genetic neurodegenerative diseases with autosomal dominant, or less frequently, autosomal recessive heredity. Only 30% of patients have a positive family history, mostly due to incomplete penetrance, with sporadic cases also occurring. The disease is characterized by nigrostriatal dopamine deficiency due to dysfunction in catecholaminergic biosynthesis, which can be caused by various enzymatic defects [44, 45].

8.4.4 Clinical Features of Classical Dopa-Responsive Dystonia (DRD)

- Phenotypes are highly variable.
- Unilateral or asymmetric lower (or upper) limb action dystonia causing equinovarus posture of the foot during walking.
- Dystonia often progresses to segmental or generalized dystonia.
- Marked diurnal fluctuation with a benefit of rest and exacerbation by physical activity (80–94%).
- Dystonia responses well to L-3,4-dihydroxyphenylalanine (L-Dopa).
- Although tendon reflexes may be increased, there are no other signs of pyramidal, sensory, cerebellar, autonomic, or cognitive dysfunction.
- Age of symptom onset is usually in childhood or adolescence, but late-onset cases in adulthood may also occur.

8.4.5 Clinical Features of DRD-Plus Variant

- Young age onset.
- Additional atypical features include spasticity, a sensation of rigidity, and pain in the lower limbs while walking; as well as spastic paraparesis; ataxia; and autonomic dysfunction. These symptoms can mimic other CNS diseases.
- Other atypical features include may encephalopathy, psychomotor retardation, psychiatric symptoms, microcephaly, hypotonia, eating disorders, epilepsy, sleep disorders, hyperthermia, ptosis; oculogyric crises, ocular flutter, striatal foot, laryngeal dystonia, myoclonus, tics, various types of focal dystonia, childhood-onset parkinsonism, L-Dopa–induced dyskinesia, or poor response to L-Dopa [42, 44, 46].

8.4.6 Brain and Spinal Cord Imaging

- Normal [42, 44].

8.4.7 Examination of Blood and CSF

- Normal [42, 44].

8.4.8 Diagnosis

- Diagnosis is based on clinical features, family history, genetic testing and L-Dopa test which is recommended in all patients with early-onset focal dystonia of unclear etiology [42, 44].

8.4.9 Differential Diagnosis

- Atypical DRD-Plus cases may mimic spastic paraplegia 11 (SPG11)-related hereditary spastic paraparesis [42], spinocerebellar ataxia (SCA) types 2 and 3 [6], Glucose transporter 1 (GLUT1) deficiency, ataxia-telangiectasia (AT) [48], Wilson's disease, Niemann–Pick disease type C, or other diseases associated with dystonia [44].
- MRI might help to exclude excessive brain iron accumulation associated with neurodegenerative diseases such as SPG11-related hereditary spastic paraparesis, Wilson's disease, or SCA [44].
- Some authors suggest that a trial of levodopa should be offered to every patient upon clinical suspicion of hereditary spastic paraparesis/paraplegia, which can mimic DRD [49].
- Evaluation of alpha-fetoprotein, ceruloplasmin levels, acanthocytes, and liver function tests may also aid in revealing alternative diagnoses [44].

8.4.10 Treatment

- Symptomatic treatment involves L-Dopa therapy and physical therapy [42, 44].

8.4.11 Other Dopamine Synthesis Defects

- GTP Cyclohydrolase 1-Deficient Dopa-Responsive Dystonia.
  - Rare childhood-onset dystonia with a robust response to levodopa, gait disturbance due to foot dystonia, and diurnal fluctuation [50].
- Other tetrahydrobiopterin (BH4) deficiencies.
  - The group of six rare disorders (including subtypes of Dopa-responsive dystonia) is characterized by insufficient synthesis of dopamine and serotonin. The majority of patients present with hyper-phenylalaninemia, although it is not observed in patients with Dopa-responsive dystonia. Patients exhibit heterogeneous phenotypes, including hypotonia, hypersalivation, ataxia, coordination and movement disorders, or delayed motor development. Supplementation of neurotransmitter precursors and treatment of hyperphenylalaninemia may improve the symptoms [51].
- Sepiapterin reductase deficiency.
  - Phenotypes vary widely, ranging from severe motor and cognitive deficits to minimal clinical symptoms. Most patients exhibit motor and speech delay, axial hypotonia, dystonia, weakness, oculogyric crises, and diurnal fluctuation. Additionally, some patients may present with Parkinsonism, limb hypertonia, hyperreflexia, cognitive impairment, psychiatric symptoms, somnolence, and autonomic dysfunction [52].

8.5 Episodic Ataxias

8.5.1 Epidemiology

- Prevalence <1/100.000 (but may be underestimated).

8.5.2 Etiology and Definition

- A heterogeneous group of inherited channelopathies, mostly autosomal dominant, characterized by relapses of cerebral syndrome.

8.5.3 Clinical Features

- Clear clinical onset and resolution of cerebellar syndrome.
- In addition to the relapses, many patients also experience interictal progression of ataxia, which may resemble progressive ataxias.
- Episodic ataxia 1 (EA1) subtype:
  - Typically begins in childhood and is characterized by brief (minutes, rarely days) relapses of ataxia and dysarthria. Episodes are triggered by physical, emotional stress, or abrupt movements. There is often interictal myokymia (neuromyotonia), muscle stiffness, twitching, flickering, and muscle hypertrophy. Around 20% of patients experience chronic residual ataxia. Some patients may also exhibit distal motor weakness, tremor, tinnitus, epilepsy, choreoathetosis, a spinning sensation, or cognitive dysfunction.
- Episodic ataxia 2 (EA2) subtype:
  - Most common variant, which can begin at any time of the entire lifespan. Episodes take longer (hours). Children may initially present with a paroxysmal tonic upward gaze usually lasting minutes, which is during time replaced by cerebellar syndrome. Patients may show interictal nystagmus. Otherwise, may be free of symptoms or can have residual symptoms with mildly progression.
- EA3-7 subtypes.
  - Very rare subtypes exhibiting similar phenotypes to EA1 and EA2 [53, 54].

8.5.4 Brain and Spinal Cord Imaging

Some patients exhibit atrophy of the cerebellar vermis [55].

8.5.5 Examination of Blood and CSF

Routine blood testing is normal [55].

There are no available data regarding the CSF findings.

8.5.6 Diagnosis

Based on clinical features and genetic testing.

8.5.7 Treatment and Prognosis

Acetazolamide or, alternatively, aminopyridine can reduce the frequency of relapses [53, 54].

8.6 Fragile X-Associated Tremor/Ataxia Syndrome (FXTAS)

8.6.1 Etiology and Definition

- Fragile X Syndrome (FXS) and FXTAS are inherited disorders caused by a trinucleotide expansion in the Fragile X mental retardation 1 (*FMR1*) gene.
- FXS is caused by a complete loss of function of the FMR1 gene (expansion CGG repeats >200) resulting in developmental delay, mental retardation, seizures, and autism in affected children.
- FXATS is associated with a premutation of the FMR1 gene (expansion 55–199 CGG repeats; the normal range is 5–40 repeats) resulting in adult late-onset phenotype [56].

8.6.2 Epidemiology

- Prevalence of the FXTAS in population over the age of 55 years is 25/100.000 (men) and 13/100.000 (women), but the disease is probably underdiagnosed.
- FXTAS is less common than FXS, and there are often diagnosed multiple cases within the same family [57–59].

8.6.3 Clinical Features

- Cerebellar syndrome.
  - Intention tremor, limb, and gait ataxia.
  - Together with cognitive impairment the core clinical feature.
  - May be isolated feature, without other manifestations (20%).

- Cognitive impairment (50%).
  - Mild subclinical deficit may occur early, whereas more severe cognitive dysfunctions typically manifest later than ataxia. In advanced stages progresses to dementia.
  - Initially affected executive functions and memory.
  - May be present also anxiety, depression, irritability, agitation, or apathy.
- Other less frequent neurological features:
  - Parkinson syndrome or hyperkinetic movement disorders.
  - Peripheral neuropathy and autonomic dysfunction (bowel/bladder and erectile dysfunction, orthostatic hypotension).
  - Rarely pyramidal signs and symptoms; fatigue; chronic pain due to small-fiber painful neuropathy; insomnia; REM sleep behavior disorder or hearing loss.
- Gonadal failure is very common in females [56, 59–61].

8.6.4 Disease Course

- The age of symptoms onset is late, usually after 50–60 years of age.
- The progression is slow, taking more than 15 years to lead to severe disability, and it does not involve relapses.
- Women tend to have more variable and less severe disease [56, 59–61].

8.6.5 Brain Imaging

- Most typical features are T2 hyperintense lesion in the middle cerebellar peduncles (MCP sign; present in 60% of affected males and 13% females). In advanced stages of the disease, these lesions may become symmetrical, which is uncommon in MS.
- The next typical imaging feature represents T2 hyperintensity in the splenium of the corpus callosum. It is as common as the MCP sign and more prevalent in males (Fig. 8.2).
- Other features:
  - T2 hyperintensities in periventricular white matter, pons, or insula.
  - T2 hyperintensities in the afferent projections of the middle and superior cerebellar peduncles.
  - Whole brain, corpus callosum, and cerebellar atrophy [56, 59, 60, 62].

8.6.6 Spinal Cord Imaging

- Normal.

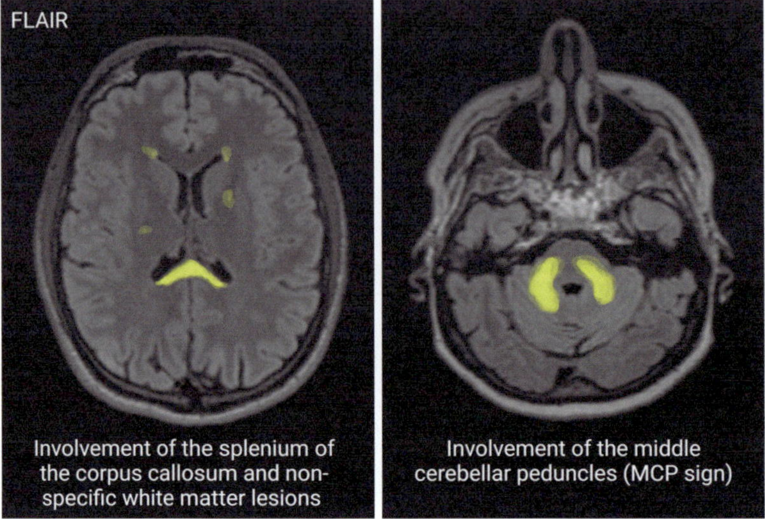

Fig. 8.2 MRI characteristics of fragile X-associated tremor/ataxia syndrome (FXTAS)

8.6.7 Blood Work

- Normal.

8.6.8 Examination of CSF

- Elevated concentration of protein [63].
- CSF-restricted OCB are absent [64].

8.6.9 Diagnosis

- Diagnosis is confirmed by genetic testing.

8.6.10 Differential Diagnosis

- FXTAS should be excluded in older patients with unexplained cerebellar syndrome and family history of cerebellar or psychiatric diseases.
- Differential diagnosis may be challenging due to overlapping manifestations with many other neurological diseases such as SCA, MSA, Parkinson disease, essential tremor or also MS [59, 60].
- Indeed, some patients initially diagnosed with MS are later found to have FXTAS. Therefore, screening patients diagnosed with atypical MS for the FMR1 premutation is recommended, particularly if there is a family history of primary

ovarian insufficiency, developmental delay, autism, cerebellar syndrome, cognitive impairment, or peripheral neuropathy [65, 66].
- Cases studies reported patients diagnosed with FXTAS and MS. This was interpreted as a possible coincidence of FXTAS and MS, or that FXTAS may manifest clinically as MS, or that FXTAS may stimulate the pathophysiology of MS. [67].
- Although late-onset Neuronal Intranuclear Inclusion Disease may present with restricted diffusion on diffusion-weighted imaging (DWI) in the corticomedullary junction, it shares similar clinical and imaging features with FXTAS. Therefore, genetic testing is crucial for distinguishing between these two diseases [68, 69].

8.6.11 Treatment

- Only symptomatic [60].

8.7 Hereditary Spastic Paraplegias (HSP)

8.7.1 Epidemiology

- Prevalence 1–10/100.000 [70].

8.7.2 Etiology and Definition

- A heterogeneous group of genetic monogenic neurodegenerative diseases affecting length-dependent corticospinal tracts and dorsal columns.
- Primarily associated with degeneration of the upper motor neurons, but often also present muscle atrophy and fasciculations associated with lower motor neuron involvement.
- Variable modes of inheritance including autosomal dominant, autosomal recessive, X-linked or mitochondrial maternal.
- Around 13–40% of cases sporadic (without positive family history) [70, 71].
- Described over 80 causative genes and the list is growing steadily [72, 73].
- Molecular mechanisms are variable and involve mitochondrial dysfunction, axonal transport, membrane trafficking and organelle shaping, myelination abnormalities, and lipid metabolism disturbances [70, 74, 75].

8.7.3 Clinical Features of Pure (Uncomplicated) Form

- Slowly progressive spasticity of the lower limbs, which may exhibit slight asymmetry and could manifest without obvious paraparesis.

- Upper limb hyperreflexia may occur without spasticity or motor weakness.
- Sphincter symptoms are common but manifest in later stages of the disease.
- Mild decrease of vibration sense may also occur [70, 71, 74].

8.7.4 Clinical Features of Complex (Complicated) Form

- Patients do not only present with spastic paraparesis but also exhibit other neurological or non-neurological features.
- Neurological:
  - Cognitive and psychiatric disturbances; cerebellar syndrome, dysarthria, peripheral neuropathy, or seizures.
  - Less frequent manifestations include movement disorders (chorea, parkinsonism, dystonia), myopathic features (ptosis and ophthalmoparesis), and autonomic dysfunction.
  - Silver syndrome includes paraparesis and muscle atrophy in the hands.
- Non-neurological.
  - Ocular pathology (optic neuropathy, pigmentary retinal degeneration, and cataracts).
  - Dysmorphic features (macrocephaly, microcephaly, short stature, facial dysmorphisms, or other deformative syndromes) and orthopedic anomalies (scoliosis; hip dislocation; or foot deformities) [70, 71, 74].

8.7.5 Disease Course

- The onset of symptoms is in infancy, childhood, adolescence, adulthood, or rarely in older individuals.
- Disease progression is slow, without relapses [70, 71, 73, 76].

8.7.6 Autosomal Recessive Subtypes of HSP (More Frequent)

- Spastic paraplegia type 11 (SPG11) accounts for 8% of all HSP cases, with onset occurring between 4 and 36 years of age. It usually presents as a complex phenotype with cognitive dysfunction, dysarthria, ataxia, axonal motor neuropathy, and urinary symptoms. Some patients may experience progression to upper limb involvement, levodopa-responsive parkinsonism, oromandibular dystonia, seizures, and visual symptoms due to optic atrophy.
- SPG15: presents with a phenotype like that of SPG11.
- SPG7 exhibit a later disease onset compared to other subtypes (mean age of onset 41.7 years). It is characterized by a combination of lower limb spasticity, cerebellar ataxia, and dysarthria. Some patients may exhibit a waddling gait due to proximal myopathic-like weakness, external ophthalmoplegia, and optic neu-

ropathy, which is often asymptomatic and detectable only on OCT. Mitochondrial dysfunction can be confirmed through muscle biopsy.
- Other autosomal recessive variants are rare [70, 71].

8.7.7 Autosomal Dominant Subtypes of HSP (Less Frequent)

- SPG4 accounts for >30% of all HSP cases (the most common subtype). The mean age of symptom onset is 31 years, although onset as late as 70 years has been observed. It can present as a complex phenotype, not limited to lower limb spasticity, and may include bladder or sensory dysfunction, cognitive impairment, extrapyramidal symptoms, dysarthria, or dysphagia.
- SPG3A accounts for 5–10% of all HSP cases. It typically presents as a pure phenotype with isolated lower limb spasticity, sometimes accompanied by bladder dysfunction. Although like SPG4 in some features, around 25% of cases exhibit axonal motor neuropathy. Onset of the disease is usually in childhood (mean age 5.6 years).
- SPG31 presents with a phenotype like that of SPG3A, characterized by isolated lower limb spasticity, often with axonal neuropathy (50%).
- Pure forms of HSP often exhibit autosomal dominant inheritance [70, 71].

8.7.8 Brain Imaging

- Mostly normal findings, age-related changes, or nonspecific T2 hyperintensities in the white matter, which may be mistaken for lesions seen in MS [77, 78].
- Only some patients with certain HSP subtypes exhibit specific imaging features.
- SPG1 (rare X-linked) may exhibit aquaductal stenosis and hydrocephalus [79].
- SPG2 (rare X-linked) may present with leukoencephalopathy [77, 78].
- Particularly, SPG11 and SPG15 frequently exhibit the "Ears of the lynx" sign visible on axial fluid-attenuated inversion recovery (FLAIR) images. It corresponds to bilateral T2 hyperintensities in the frontal corners of the lateral ventricles (sensitivity 79–97%; specificity 91–100% for diagnosis of SPG11 and 15). This sign can be mistaken for gliosis at the calloso-caudate angle observed in the healthy population, which exhibits a rounded, not flaming capping and is smaller than the ears of the lynx [77] (Fig. 8.3).
- SPG7 and some other subtypes exhibit atrophy of cerebellar vermis and iso/hyper-intense dentate nucleus (normally hypointense) on T2 images [80].
- Some subtypes exhibit corpus callosum atrophy and iron deposition in basal ganglia [78].

8.7.9 Spinal Cord Imaging

- Often spinal cord atrophy (not always visually evident).

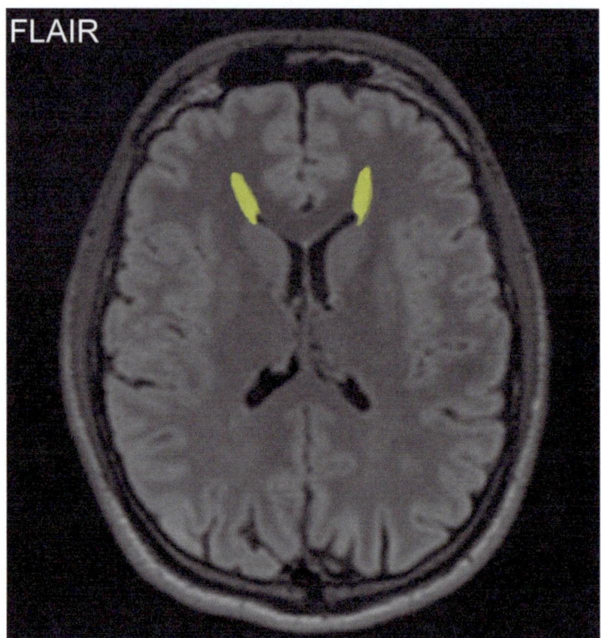

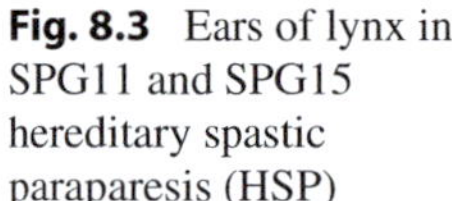
Fig. 8.3 Ears of lynx in SPG11 and SPG15 hereditary spastic paraparesis (HSP)

- No specific features; therefore, rarely helpful in differential diagnosis [78, 81].
- Only SPG2 (rare X-linked leukodystrophy) may exhibit diffuse T2 hyperintensities [82].

8.7.10 Examination of Blood and CSF

- Routine blood tests are normal.
- The CSF may only exhibit mildly elevated concentration of protein, with normal cytology, and likely without CSF-restricted OCB (lack of data) [83].

8.7.11 OCT

- Some patients exhibit a reduction of the retinal nerve fiber layer (RNFL) in the temporal region, resembling findings seen in MS [84].

8.7.12 Electrophysiology

- Abnormal findings are frequently observed in the lower limbs, but to a lesser extent, they may also affect the upper limbs. Electromyography (EMG) commonly reveals distal axonal motor neuropathy accompanied by associated neurogenic changes.

- Motor evoked potentials (MEP) and somatosensory evoked potentials (SSEP) often show abnormal central conduction times [85].

8.7.13 Diagnosis

- Diagnosis requires the identification of pathogenic mutations in a SPG-designated gene.
- Genetic testing presents challenges, and a genetic diagnosis remains elusive in 50–70% of patients suspected to have HSP [70–72, 86].
- Genetic testing encompasses various options. Targeted sequencing gene panels offer a cost-effective solution but come with the risk of missing a diagnosis if the mutation lies outside the panel's coverage. If this initial step yields inconclusive results, conducting whole-exome sequencing (WES) is recommended. However, WES may lack reliability in detecting copy number variants, mutations in promoter or deep intronic regions, and triplet repeat disorders. Whole-genome sequencing stands as the most comprehensive approach but is associated with a high cost and challenges in interpreting the amounts of data involved [72].
- Next-generation sequencing (NGS) is utilized in clinical practice [86]. However, the expanding list of genes associated with HSP poses challenges in keeping gene testing panels up to date. Moreover, there exists a significant phenotypic overlap between HSP and other disorders, such as peripheral neuropathies, amyotrophic lateral sclerosis (ALS), hereditary ataxias, or Parkinson's disease. This overlap complicates the selection of the appropriate panel for analysis. For instance, whereas an SPG11 mutation may cause HSP, it can also manifest as Charcot-Marie-Tooth neuropathy (CMT). Similarly, mutations in ATP13A2 can lead to various conditions including neuronal ceroid lipofuscinosis, neurodegeneration with brain iron accumulation, Kufor–Rakeb syndrome, and complicated HSP with cognitive impairment, ataxia, and polyneuropathy (SPG78). Furthermore, distinguishing when to classify a disorder as HSP can be challenging. However, if spastic paraparesis is the predominant clinical feature, a diagnosis of HSP is typically warranted [75].
- Although effective treatment for HSP is not available, obtaining a genetic diagnosis offers several advantages. These include providing prognostic insights, facilitating genetic counseling, and aiding in family planning or prenatal genetic diagnosis [72].

8.7.14 Differential Diagnosis

- The differential diagnosis of HSP encompasses a broad spectrum of structural, inflammatory, and infectious diseases. It should entail comprehensive assessments such as imaging studies, CSF analysis, neurophysiological evaluations, ophthalmologic examinations, metabolic screening, and genetic testing [74].

- MS:
  - HSP can present with features that mimic primary progressive MS. Therefore, it is crucial to search for red flags of MS, such as the absence of spinal cord lesions, normal CSF findings, lack of response to immuno-modulatory treatments, or the presence of confluent symmetrical lesions in the brain during the early stages of the disease [87, 88].
  - Cases of patients with comorbid HSP and MS have been described, with over 20 cases published, the majority of which are related to the most common SPG4 subtype [89].
- Metabolic diseases:
  - In contrast to typical HSP, metabolic mimics often exhibit a more accelerated disease course and are more likely to present with cognitive impairment, epilepsy, visual symptoms, deafness, or movement disorders [49].
  - It has been suggested that a trial of levodopa should be offered to patients upon clinical suspicion of HSP, which it can mimic dopa-responsive dystonia [49].
  - Early-onset forms of HSP and inborn metabolic diseases with motor involvement are the most common "mimics" of cerebral palsy in children [73].
- Treatable metabolic mimics of HSP or cerebral palsy:
  - Attention should be given to atypical presentations of treatable mimickers of HSP such as adrenoleukodystophy, arginase deficiency, cerebrotendinous xanthomatosis (CTX), dopa-responsive dystonia, phenyl-ketonuria, biotinidase deficiency, cobalamin-related remethylation disorders, hyperornithinemia-hyperammonemia-homocitrullinuria (HHH) syndrome, methylenetetrahydrofolate reductase (MTHFR)-related disorders, or primary CoQ10 deficiencies [70, 73].
- Several of these diseases are triplet repeat disorders (such as SCA type 1 and 3, or FRDA) and might not be covered by some next-generation sequencing panels [70].

8.7.15 Treatment and Prognosis

- Only symptomatic; genotype-specific therapies are not available yet [70].
- Data on prognosis are scarce, but progression is typically slow. The median duration of the disease until the loss of independent walking is approximately 22 years. Onset of the disease at an older age is associated with earlier loss of independent walking. Earlier disease onset and pure (uncomplicated) subtypes are associated with less severe disease [71].

8.7.16 Spastic Paraplegia, Optic Atrophy, and Neuropathy (SPOAN) Syndrome

- Rare autosomal recessive neurodegenerative disorder that is considered as a complicated form of hereditary spastic paraparesis. Patients typically experience progressive spastic paraplegia from infancy. As they enter later childhood, they develop motor and sensory axonal peripheral neuropathy, leading to severe mobility limitations by the age of 15 years. By the third decade, dysarthria and an exacerbation of the acoustic startle response emerge. Additionally, patients commonly experience visual impairment due to non-progressive congenital optic atrophy, with some exhibiting fixation nystagmus and retinopathy. Normal nerve conduction studies rule out this disease. Cognitive functioning typically remains within normal range [90, 91].

8.8 Kennedy's Disease

8.8.1 Synonym

- Spinal and bulbar muscular atrophy (SBMA); X-linked bulbospinal neuronopathy.

8.8.2 Epidemiology

- Prevalence 1–2/100.000 (very rare disease; higher prevalence in Japan).
- Often underdiagnosed (prevalence is around four times lower than expected).

8.8.3 Etiology and Definition

- X-linked hereditary lower motor neuron disease with sex-linked recessive pattern of inheritance.
- Caused by CAG repeat expansion in the androgen receptor (*AR*) gene.
- Although a positive family history is common, a negative family history does not exclude the diagnosis.

8.8.4 Clinical Features

- Lower motor neuron syndrome (muscle weakness, wasting of the limbs, bulbar weakness, tremor, cramps, fasciculations).
- Sensory neuropathy.
- Gynecomastia, sexual/erectile dysfunction, testicular atrophy, reduced fertility (all may precede motor deficit).

- Women are typically asymptomatic and only rarely report mild cramping or tremors.
- Rare manifestations, such as jaw drop, myotonia-like symptoms, a pure bulbar phenotype, sphincter dysfunction, or autonomic dysfunction, may complicate the differential diagnosis.

8.8.5 Disease Course

- Mean age of symptoms onset is between 35 and 40 years of age (rarely in adolescence or elderly).
- Slowly progressive disease course.

8.8.6 Brain and Spinal Imaging

- Aside from spinal cord atrophy, findings are generally expected to be normal.

8.8.7 Examination of Blood and CSF

- Frequently (80%) elevated concentrations of serum creatine kinase.
- Can be elevated liver enzymes and dyslipidemia.

8.8.8 Electrophysiology

- Acute and chronic diffuse denervation atrophy with low sensory nerve action potentials (SNAP) amplitudes and sensory neuropathy.

8.8.9 Diagnosis

- Genetic testing.

8.8.10 Differential Diagnosis

- Kennedy's disease is often misdiagnosed as ALS. Approximately 2% of patients initially diagnosed with ALS are later found to have Kennedy's disease. ALS typically progresses more rapidly, genetic testing for SBMA is negative, and there is also upper motor neuron involvement, characterized by hyperreflexia and spasticity. Additionally, ALS presents with greater asymmetry in its manifestations.
- Spinal muscular atrophy (SMA) type IV.

- Distal hereditary motor neuropathies.
- Metabolic myopathies and polymyositis.
- Myasthenia gravis.
- Progressive muscular atrophy.
- Post-polio syndrome (neuroinfections).
- Spinal cord pathology.
- Paraneoplastic syndromes.
- Chronic intoxications (for example chronic lead poisoning).

8.8.11 Treatment

- Only symptomatic treatment.

8.8.12 Prognosis

- Good ambulation is typically preserved until the late stages of the disease, with wheelchair use generally becoming necessary around the age of 60. Life expectancy remains unaffected [92–94].

8.9 Nonmetabolic Inherited Leukodystrophies and Leukoencephalopathies

- Heterogeneous group of rare inherited diseases that are not strictly classifiable as metabolic diseases. Their diagnosis is based on genetic testing [95].

8.9.1 Adult-Onset Alexander Disease

- Etiology and definition:
  - Autosomal dominant.
  - Missense mutations in glial fibrillary acidic protein (GFAP) causes abnormal modulation of mophology and motility of astrocytes.
- Clinical features and subtypes:
  - Infantile-onset form.
    - Macrocephaly, growth failure, seizures, and progressive neurological impairment.
  - Juvenile-onset form.
  - Late-onset form (>25% of cases).
    - Progressive gait ataxia, spasticity, pyramidal signs, bulbar signs, singultus, vomiting, epilepsy and autonomic features.
    - 35% patients may have palatal myoclonus, which is rarely seen in other disorders and help with differential diagnosis.

- Macrocephaly and mental retardation is not frequent.
- Can mimic primary progressive MS [95–97].

- Brain and spinal cord imaging:
  - Rarely normal findings.
  - Progressive atrophy and T2 hyperintensities of the medulla oblongata and upper cervical spinal cord ("Tadpole brainstem") are highly suggestive (almost in 100%).
  - Brainstem lesions may be tumefactive and show contrast enhancement.
  - May be increased T2 signal in the hilum of the dentate, the medial lemniscus and the corticospinal tracts of the brainstem.
  - Some patients have midbrain dorsal peripheral T2 hyperintese rim.
  - T2 hyperintensities in periventricular and deep white matter (65–75%).
  - In general, MRI findings may be easily mistaken for MS [95, 97, 98] (Fig. 8.4).
- Diagnosis.
  - Based on genetic testing.
  - The Alexander disease can be suspected based on:
    - MRI findings (brainstem/cervical cord).
    - Association of ataxia with palatal tremor.
    - Absence of response to corticosteroids and immunosupression.
    - Absent CSF-restricted OCB (although in some cases may be present).
- Differential diagnosis:
  - Brainstem glioma, viral encephalomyelitis, granulomatous or histiocytic disorders, Behçet's disease, mitochondrial disorders and MS [96–98].

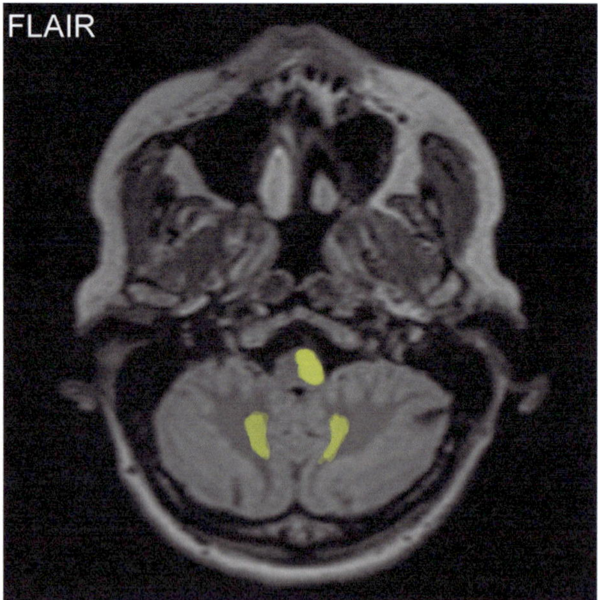

Fig. 8.4 Lesions in the medulla oblongata and upper cervical spinal cord (tadpole brainstem) along with increased T2 signal in the hilum of the dentate nuclei in adult-onset Alexander disease

8.9.2 Autosomal Dominant Leukodystrophy

- Etiology and definition:
  - Autosomal dominant.
  - Duplications of the lamin B1 (*LMNB1*) gene causes lamin B1 overexpression associated with abnormal oligodendroglial differentiation and demyelination.
- Clinical features:
  - Early autonomic dysfunction, cognitive impairment, pyramidal signs and symptoms, cerebellar dysfunction with age of symptoms onset at 30–50 years.
- Brain and spinal cord imaging:
  - Subtle or extensive symmetrical T2 hyperintensities in white matter (leukodystrophy-like pattern).
  - Periventricular white matter is preserved or less affected than other white matter regions.
  - Lesions may be also in middle cerebellar peduncles and brainstem.
  - Often atrophy of corpus callosum and brainstem [95, 99].

8.9.3 Leukoencephalopathy with Brainstem and Spinal Cord Involvement and Lactate Elevation

- Etiology and definition:
  - Autosomal recessive.
  - Caused by mutations in dysfunctional mitochondrial aspartyl tRNA synthetase (*DARS2*) gene.
- Clinical features:
  - Slowly progressive pyramidal, cerebellar, and dorsal column syndrome particularly on lower extremities, dysarthria, and epilepsy.
  - Symptoms onset in adolescence or early adulthood.
- Brain and spinal cord imaging:
  - Confluent or patchy T2 hyperintensities in white matter (leukodystrophy-like), dorsal columns and lateral corticospinal tracts of the medulla oblongata and the spinal cord.
  - U-fibers are relatively spared.
  - Lesions may show contrast enhancement.
  - Signal changes can be seen also in corpus callosum, internal capsule, cerebellar peduncles, spinocerebellar tracts and cerebellar white matter.
  - MRI spectrocopy often show increased lactate in abnormal white matter [95, 100].

8.9.4 Adult-Onset Leukoencephalopathy with Axonal Spheroids and Pigmented Glia (ALSP)

- Etiology and definition:
  - Autosomal dominant.

  - Caused by mutations in colony stimulating factor 1 receptor (*CSF1R*) gene associated with dysregulation of survival, proliferation, differentiation and function of CNS microglia.
- Clinical features:
  - Typically dominating psychiatric and cognitive symptoms.
  - May be present also motor deficit and epilepsy.
  - Symptoms onset in early adulthood (24–45 years).
- Brain and spinal cord imaging:
  - Often asymmetric and patchy white matter lesions.
  - In later stages become confluent white matter lesions (leukodystrophy-like pattern).
  - Involvement of corpus callosum, cortical gray matter and corticospinal tracts.
  - May be present brainstem atrophy and contrast enhancement [95, 101].

8.9.5 ClC-2 Chloride Channel Deficiency Leukoencephalopathy

- Etiology and definition:
  - Caused by biallelic autosomal recessive.
  - Abnormal chloride ion and water homeostasis causing white matter edema.
- Clinical features:
  - Cerebellar ataxia, tremor, spastic paraparesis, ataxia, optic neuropathy (macular atrophy), chorioretinopathy, nystagmus, cognitive deficit, headache, tinnitus, dizziness.
  - Symptoms onset in 30–57 years of age.
- Brain and spinal cord imaging:
  - Confluent, symmetric T2 hyperintensities along the fiber tracts, without contrast enhancement.
  - Typically located in midbrain, middle cerebellar peduncles, and posterior limb of internal capsule. The periventricular white matter is relatively spared.
  - Lesions may exhibit restricted diffusion [95, 102].

8.9.6 Adult-Onset Neuronal Intranuclear Inclusion Disease

- Rare but underdiagnosed disorder.
- Etiology and definition:
  - Slowly progressive inherited (sporadic or familial) neurodegenerative disease characterized by eosinophilic hyaline intranuclear inclusions in the central and peripheral nervous systems and in visceral organs.
  - The CGG repeat length in the fragile X messenger ribonucleoprotein 1 (*FMR1*) gene is expanded.
- Clinical features:
  - A wide range of clinical manifestations, but dementia is usually the dominant and initial symptom (94.7%).
  - Other manifestations include miosis, ataxia, bladder dysfunction, unconsciousness, movement disorders, muscle weakness and sensory disturbance.

- May occur a subacute encephalitic episode, sometime with focal brain edema and contrast enhancement. In these cases, pulses of corticosteroids can be effective to reduce brain edema and improve consciousness in the short term.
- The symptoms onset is between infancy and sixth decade (2/3 of cases has infantile or juvenile onset).

- Brain imaging.
  - Typically, increased signal in corticomedullary junction on DWI and leukoencephalopathy on T2-weighted images with confluent and bilaterally symmetrical lesions.
  - Can be also involvement of cortical gray matter.
- Examination of CSF:
  - Elevated concentration of protein in CSF (65.5%).
- Electrophysiology:
  - Abnormal nerve conduction studies.
- Diagnosis:
  - Histopathology (intranuclear inclusions in the skin, rectum, or CNS tissue) and genetic testing [69].

8.10 Presenilin-1-Related Familial Alzheimer's Disease

8.10.1 Epidemiology

- Late-onset Alzheimer's disease (AD) (94–95%); early-onset AD (5–6%).
- Prevalence of early-onset AD (onset before 65 years of age) is 24.2/100.000.
  - Presenilin-1 (*PSEN1*) gene mutations (70–75% of all cases; >300 mutations).
  - Presenilin-2 (*PSEN2*) gene mutations (5% of all cases).
  - Amyloid protein precursor (*APP*) gene mutations (<1% of all cases) [103–106].

8.10.2 Clinical Features

- Spastic paraplegia.
  - Pure spastic paraplegia develops in 13.7% of patients with PSEN1-related familial AD at some point of the disease (driven by shared vulnerability of corticospinal tract axons and cortical neurons toward disturbances of the same molecular pathways).
  - Might precedes the clinical onset of dementia by several years (7.5%), thus the phenotype may mimic hereditary spastic paraplegia.
  - Age of onset of spastic paraparesis is 20–55 years [105, 107–109].
- Cognitive impairment.
  - Progressive amnestic syndrome in familial AD is similar to that seen in sporadic late-onset but onset of symptoms occurs in earlier age (20–65 years) and disease progress faster than in late-onset AD [105, 107–109].

  - Some patients do not fulfill the diagnostic criteria for AD, but present with other phenotypes, such as frontotemporal dementia, progressive non-fluent aphasia or Pick's disease, Parkinson's disease, or dementia with Lewy bodies [105, 110].
- Other neurological and non-neurological manifestations.
  - Except of spastic paraplegia, several other manifestations were related to *PSEN1* mutations such as ataxia, myoclonus, seizures, movement disorders, behavioral and language dysfunctions, acne inversa or dilated cardiomyopathy [105, 110].

8.10.3 Brain and Spinal Cord Imaging

- Brain MRI may show diffuse brain atrophy (particularly in the parietal lobes and hippocampal nuclei) and unspecific focal changes in deep white matter.
- Compared to typical late-onset AD, early-onset variant has relative hippocampal sparing and a greater regional accumulation of amyloid and tau.
- Imaging of the spinal cord is usually normal [105, 109, 111–113].

8.10.4 Examination of Blood and CSF

- CSF shows decreased levels of amyloid-ß (Aß42) and increased levels of phosphorylated tau which is consistent with AD [109].
- Routine CSF testing is usually normal [112, 113].

8.10.5 Diagnosis

- Genetic testing [114].

8.10.6 Differential Diagnosis

- *PSEN1* genetic testing is recommended to be included in the differential diagnosis of spastic paraparesis, especially when associated with a family history of cognitive decline [107].
- However, considerable proportion of *PSEN1* mutations occur de novo [114].
- PSEN1-related spastic paraplegia can be considered as a form of hereditary spastic paraplegia [109].

8.10.7 Treatment

- Considering emerging disease-modifying therapies for familial and sporadic AD, early genetic diagnosis for the patients is important [107].

8.11 Spinal Muscular Atrophy Type 4 (SMA-4)

8.11.1 Synonyms

- Adult spinal muscular atrophy; Kugelberg–Welander disease.

8.11.2 Epidemiology

- Rarest (<5% of SMA cases) and mildest type of SMA.
- Prevalence: 0.3/100.000.

8.11.3 Etiology and Definition

- SMA is a progressive, autosomal recessive genetic disorder resulting in the degeneration of anterior horn cells in the spinal cord (i.e., lower motor neurons) and the brainstem nuclei.
- Most forms of SMA are caused by mutations in the survival motor neuron 1 (SMN1) gene.
- Four distinct types of SMA are described, classified by age of onset and length of survival.

8.11.4 Clinical Features

- Patients with SMA type 4 typically experience mild to moderate symmetric muscle weakness, atrophy, and fasciculations, which are more pronounced proximally than distally, with no respiratory issues or, in some cases, only mild ones.
- Symptom onset typically occurs in early adulthood, primarily in the second or third decade of life.
- Some patients may present with atypical clinical features, such as oculomotor palsy, epilepsy, deafness, tremor, olivopontocerebellar atrophy, or multiple arthrogryposis, which are collectively referred to as the "SMA plus" phenotype.

8.11.5 Brain and Spinal Cord Imaging

- Patients with infantile-onset SMA often exhibit signal changes in the cortical gray matter, subcortical white matter, basal ganglia, thalamus, hippocampus, and periventricular regions. In contrast, adult-onset SMA (such as SMA-4) is typically not associated with white matter changes but may present with reduced cerebellar volume.

8.11.6 Examination of Blood and CSF

- Some adult patients with SMA types 2 and 3 may exhibit an increased albumin quotient, indicating blood-brain barrier dysfunction.
- CSF-restricted OCB is rare but can occur (11% in SMA-3); however, many patients show corresponding OCB in both serum and CSF.
- Other blood and CSF markers are typically normal.
- There is a lack of information regarding findings in patients with SMA-4.

8.11.7 Diagnosis

- Based on clinical features, electrophysiological studies (fibrillation potentials, denervation, and increased amplitude), and genetic testing.

8.11.8 Treatment and Prognosis

- Nusinersen is a synthetic antisense oligonucleotide that enables the *SMN2* gene to produce a full-length protein, which functions normally. This drug may slow the progression of SMA.
- There is a normal life expectancy; however, some patients may lose their ability to walk and have decreased quality of life [115–118].

8.12 Spinocerebellar Ataxias (SCA)

8.12.1 Epidemiology

- Prevalence 2.7 (range 0–5.6)/100.000; but marked geographical differences [76].
- The most common variants:
  - SCA3 (20–50% of all SCA subtypes).
  - SCA2 (13–18%).
  - SCA6 (13–15%) [119].

8.12.2 Etiology and Definition

- A group of autosomal dominantly hereditary cerebellar ataxias exhibiting highly heterogeneous phenotypes and pathophysiology.
- These progressive inherited neurodegenerative diseases entail the degeneration of the cerebellum but may also impact other brain regions.
- In Europe, repeat expansions account for nearly half of the cases of SCA. The remainder is attributed to non-repeat mutations [120, 121].
- The term spino-cerebellar reflects the concomitant involvement of the spinal cord and the cerebellum. However, the spinal cord is unaffected in many SCA subtypes. Conversely, many SCA subtypes have pathology in brainstem, basal ganglia, or peripheral nerves [121].

8.12.3 Clinical Features

- Phenotypes vary widely even within families or individuals with a certain subtype of SCA, partly because many SCA are caused by dynamic repeat expansions.
- The core clinical feature is progressive ataxia, which has mainly cerebellar origin, but afferent and vestibular ataxia also contribute to the clinical manifestations:
  - Gait ataxia is usually one of the first symptoms.
  - Limb ataxia occurs with disease progression.
  - Almost all patients with have dysarthria and dysphagia.
  - Many patients have oculomotor abnormalities associated with cerebellar dysfunction, such as disturbed pursuit eye movements, gaze-evoked nystagmus, and inaccuracy of fast saccadic eye movements or subjective double vision.
- Non-ataxia features may also occur, albeit rarely preceding ataxia or dominating the clinical presentation:
  - Motor (pyramidal signs, motor weakness, spasticity; amyotrophy).
  - Extrapyramidal (parkinsonism, dystonia, chorea).
  - Other ocular (gaze palsy, ophthalmoplegia, visual loss due to retinal degeneration).
  - Mild cognitive impairment and psychiatric symptoms.
  - Sensory symptoms.
  - Urinary dysfunction.
  - Sleep disorders (restless leg syndrome, rapid eye movement sleep behavior disorder, hypersomnia, insomnia or sleep apnea) (Table 8.1) [120–122].

8.12.4 Disease Course

- The age of onset of ataxia is usually in mid-adulthood but can occur at any age.
- Course is slowly progressive [121].

Table 8.1 Clinical features and associated genetic subtypes in SCA (adapted and modified from recent systematic reviews) [120, 123]

Additional clinical feature	Genetic subtypes
Peripheral neuropathy	1, 2, 3, 4, 18, 25, 38, 43, 46
Pyramidal signs	1, 3, 7, 8, 10, 14, 15, 17, 35, 40, 43
Dystonia	3, 14, 17, 20, 35
Myoclonus	14
Parkinsonism	2, 3, 10, 14, 17, 19/22, 21
Tremor	12, 15, 27
Chorea	17, 27, DRPLA (Dentatorubral-pallidoluysian atrophy)
Cognitive impairment	2, 8, 13, 17, 19/22, 21, 36, 44, DRPLA
Psychiatric symptoms	2, 17
Ophthalmoplegia	2, 3, 28, 40
Visual impairment	7
Face/tongue fasciculation	36
Ichthyosiform plaques	34
Seizures	10, 19/22, ATN1 (atrophin 1)
Narcolepsy	DNMT1 (DNA methyltransferase 1)
Hearing loss	31, 36, DNMT1

8.12.5 Brain Imaging

- Findings display significant variability, with cerebellar atrophy being a prevalent feature. Additionally, many patients exhibit brainstem atrophy or whole brain atrophy in the advanced disease stages.
- Case studies have reported nonspecific subcortical white matter lesions in some patients with SCA 1 and 8, which may mimick MS.
- Some patients with SCA 1, 2, 3, 7, and 8 have selective degeneration of transverse pontocerebellar tracts and median pontine raphe nuclei creating cross-shaped T2 hyperintensity on axial images in the pons, which is called "hot cross bun" sign or lesions in middle cerebral peduncles [9, 124–128] (Fig. 8.5).

8.12.6 Spinal Cord Imaging

- Spinal cord atrophy in some SCA subtypes [9].

8.12.7 Blood Work

- Normal.

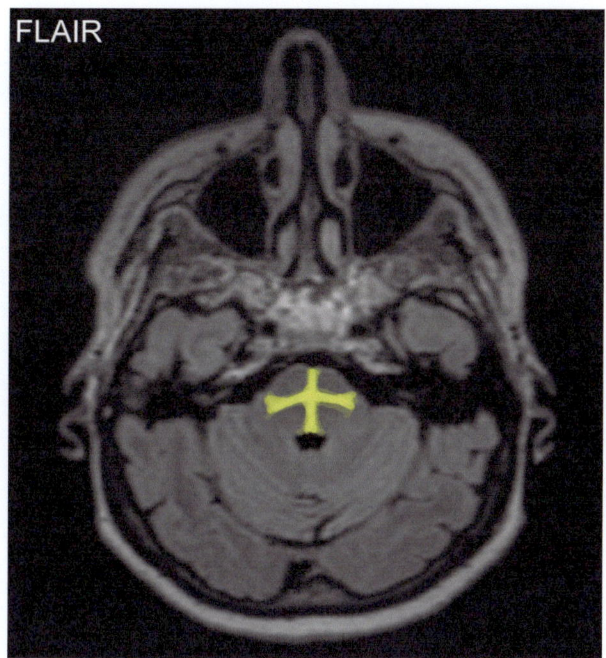

Fig. 8.5 The "hot cross bun" sign in spinocerebellar ataxias (SCA)

8.12.8 Examination of CSF

- Only a very limited number of case studies have been reported, which may not fully represent the entire population of patients with SCA. CSF analyses typically did not reveal any pathological findings, although detailed information about CSF-restricted OCB was not provided in these studies.
- However, some patients with SCA can have CSF-restricted OCB [127, 129, 130].

8.12.9 OCT

- A mild and progressive decrease in retinal nerve fiber layer (RNFL) thickness with preservation of the temporal sector was observed in SCA 3 patients [131].

8.12.10 Electrophysiology

- Frequently mixed (axonal and demyelinating) sensory and motor peripheral neuropathy in all common SCA subtypes [132, 133].

8.12.11 Diagnosis

- In suspected cases presenting with progressive ataxia, a positive family history, and lacking evidence of acquired etiology, genetic testing is typically employed for diagnosis.
- Additional assessments such as MRI, EMG, or neuropsychology may aid in ruling out alternative diagnoses. However, they typically do not significantly contribute to the selection of the molecular genetic test. Therefore, a systematic approach is recommended for the diagnosis of SCA [120, 121].
- Advances in NGS increase the success of molecular diagnosis for patients currently undiagnosed by standard genetic testing. For example, exome sequencing has an average diagnostic rate of 36% compared to a target resequencing panel with a rate only 17% [134].

8.12.12 Differential Diagnosis

- There are case studies reporting the extremely rare, possibly incidental, coexistence of different subtypes of SCA with MS [135–138] or neuromyelitis optica spectrum disorders (NMOSD) [139, 140].
- In most of these cases, MS was diagnosed after the established diagnosis of SCA.

8.12.13 Treatment and Prognosis

- No causal treatment, but an effect of several drugs including riluzole, valproic acid, varenicline and lithium carbonate is being investigated.
- Many patients with SCA have premature death [121].

References

1. Palau F, Espinós C. Autosomal recessive cerebellar ataxias. Orphanet J Rare Dis. 2006;1:47.
2. Bereznyakova O, Dupré N. Spastic ataxias. Handb Clin Neurol. 2018;155:191–203.
3. Koenig M. Rare forms of autosomal recessive neurodegenerative ataxia. Semin Pediatr Neurol. 2003;10(3):183–92.
4. Keita M, McIntyre K, Rodden LN, Schadt K, Lynch DR. Friedreich ataxia: clinical features and new developments. Neurodegener Dis Manag. 2022;12(5):267–83.
5. Cook A, Giunti P. Friedreich's ataxia: clinical features, pathogenesis and management. Br Med Bull. 2017;124(1):19–30.
6. Tiet MY, Horvath R, Hensiek AE. Ataxia telangiectasia: what the neurologist needs to know. Pract Neurol. 2020;20(5):404–14.
7. Bouchard JP, Richter A, Mathieu J, Brunet D, Hudson TJ, Morgan K, et al. Autosomal recessive spastic ataxia of Charlevoix-Saguenay. Neuromuscular Disorder: NMD. 1998;8(7):474–9.
8. Martin MH, Bouchard JP, Sylvain M, St-Onge O, Truchon S. Autosomal recessive spastic ataxia of Charlevoix-Saguenay: a report of MR imaging in 5 patients. AJNR Am J Neuroradiol. 2007;28(8):1606–8.

9. Cocozza S, Pontillo G, De Michele G, Di Stasi M, Guerriero E, Perillo T, et al. Conventional MRI findings in hereditary degenerative ataxias: a pictorial review. Neuroradiology. 2021;63(7):983–99.
10. Keogh MJ, Steele H, Douroudis K, Pyle A, Duff J, Hussain R, et al. Frequency of rare recessive mutations in unexplained late onset cerebellar ataxia. J Neurol. 2015;262(8):1822–7.
11. Imbault V, Dionisi C, Naeije G, Communi D, Pandolfo M. Cerebrospinal fluid proteomics in Friedreich ataxia reveals markers of neurodegeneration and neuroinflammation. Front Neurosci. 2022;16:885313.
12. Fortuna F, Barboni P, Liguori R, Valentino ML, Savini G, Gellera C, et al. Visual system involvement in patients with Friedreich's ataxia. Brain. 2009;132(Pt 1):116–23.
13. Boesch S, Indelicato E. Experimental drugs for Friedrich's ataxia: progress and setbacks in clinical trials. Expert Opin Investig Drugs. 2023;32(11):967–9.
14. Cortese A, Simone R, Sullivan R, Vandrovcova J, Tariq H, Yau WY, et al. Biallelic expansion of an intronic repeat in RFC1 is a common cause of late-onset ataxia. Nat Genet. 2019;51(4):649–58.
15. Szmulewicz DJ, Waterston JA, MacDougall HG, Mossman S, Chancellor AM, McLean CA, et al. Cerebellar ataxia, neuropathy, vestibular areflexia syndrome (CANVAS): a review of the clinical features and video-oculographic diagnosis. Ann N Y Acad Sci. 2011;1233:139–47.
16. Szmulewicz DJ, McLean CA, Rodriguez ML, Chancellor AM, Mossman S, Lamont D, et al. Dorsal root ganglionopathy is responsible for the sensory impairment in CANVAS. Neurology. 2014;82(16):1410–5.
17. Cortese A, Curro R, Vegezzi E, Yau WY, Houlden H, Reilly MM. Cerebellar ataxia, neuropathy and vestibular areflexia syndrome (CANVAS): genetic and clinical aspects. Pract Neurol. 2022;22(1):14–8.
18. Cortese A, Reilly MM, Houlden H. In: Adam MP, Mirzaa GM, Pagon RA, Wallace SE, Bean LJH, Gripp KW, et al., editors. RFC1 CANVAS/Spectrum disorder. Seattle (WA): GeneReviews((R)); 1993.
19. Cortese A, Tozza S, Yau WY, Rossi S, Beecroft SJ, Jaunmuktane Z, et al. Cerebellar ataxia, neuropathy, vestibular areflexia syndrome due to RFC1 repeat expansion. Brain. 2020;143(2):480–90.
20. Magy L, Chazelas P, Richard L, Deschamps N, Frachet S, Vallat JM, et al. Early diagnosis in Cerebellar Ataxia, Neuropathy, Vestibular Areflexia Syndrome (CANVAS) by focusing on major clinical clues: beyond ataxia and vestibular impairment. Biomedicines. 2022;10(8)
21. Szmulewicz DJ, Waterston JA, Halmagyi GM, Mossman S, Chancellor AM, McLean CA, et al. Sensory neuropathy as part of the cerebellar ataxia neuropathy vestibular areflexia syndrome. Neurology. 2011;76(22):1903–10.
22. Wu TY, Taylor JM, Kilfoyle DH, Smith AD, McGuinness BJ, Simpson MP, et al. Autonomic dysfunction is a major feature of cerebellar ataxia, neuropathy, vestibular areflexia 'CANVAS' syndrome. Brain. 2014;137(Pt 10):2649–56.
23. Huin V, Coarelli G, Guemy C, Boluda S, Debs R, Mochel F, et al. Motor neuron pathology in CANVAS due to RFC1 expansions. Brain. 2022;145(6):2121–32.
24. Burke D, Halmagyi GM. Normal tendon reflexes despite absent sensory nerve action potentials in CANVAS: a neurophysiological study. J Neurol Sci. 2018;387:75–9.
25. Strupp M, Dieterich M, Brandt T. The treatment and natural course of peripheral and central vertigo. Dtsch Arztebl Int. 2013;110(29–30):505–15. quiz 15–6
26. El Houjeiry E, Coudray S, Thouvenot E, Ion IM. Spinal cord lesion mimicking a dysimmune myelitis revealing CANVAS syndrome. J Spinal Cord Med. 2023;46(2):332–6.
27. Azzimonti M, Fazio R, Giordano A, Tagliapietra M, Ferrarini M, Rocca MA, et al. Association between inflammatory central nervous system lesions and Cerebellar Ataxia, Neuropathy and Vestibular Areflexia Syndrome (CANVAS): a case series. J Neurol. 2022;269(10):5668–73.
28. Infante J, Garcia A, Serrano-Cardenas KM, Gonzalez-Aguado R, Gazulla J, de Lucas EM, et al. Cerebellar ataxia, neuropathy, vestibular areflexia syndrome (CANVAS) with chronic cough and preserved muscle stretch reflexes: evidence for selective sparing of afferent Ia fibres. J Neurol. 2018;265(6):1454–62.

29. Pannewitz-Makaj K, Wurster U, Jendretzky KF, Gingele S, Suhs KW, Stangel M, et al. Evidence of oligoclonal bands does not exclude non-inflammatory neurological diseases. Diagnostics (Basel). 2020;11(1)
30. Rahman S, Copeland WC. POLG-related disorders and their neurological manifestations. Nat Rev Neurol. 2019;15(1):40–52.
31. Chelban V, Bocchetta M, Hassanein S, Haridy NA, Houlden H, Rohrer JD. An update on advances in magnetic resonance imaging of multiple system atrophy. J Neurol. 2019;266(4):1036–45.
32. Lipp A, Sandroni P, Ahlskog JE, Fealey RD, Kimpinski K, Iodice V, et al. Prospective differentiation of multiple system atrophy from Parkinson disease, with and without autonomic failure. Arch Neurol. 2009;66(6):742–50.
33. Gawel M, Jamrozik Z, Szmidt-Salkowska E, Slawek J, Rowinska-Marcinska K. Is peripheral neuron degeneration involved in multiple system atrophy? A clinical and electrophysiological study. J Neurol Sci. 2012;319(1–2):81–5.
34. Cortese A, Simone R, Sullivan R, Vandrovcova J, Tariq H, Yau WY, et al. Author correction: Biallelic expansion of an intronic repeat in RFC1 is a common cause of late-onset ataxia. Nat Genet. 2019;51(5):920.
35. Abrams CK. GJB1 Disorders: Charcot-Marie-Tooth Neuropathy (CMT1X) and Central Nervous System Phenotypes. In: Adam MP, Feldman J, Mirzaa GM, Pagon RA, Wallace SE, Amemiya A, editors. GeneReviews(®). Seattle (WA): University of Washington, Seattle. Copyright © 1993–2025, University of Washington, Seattle. GeneReviews is a registered trademark of the University of Washington, Seattle. All rights reserved.; 1993.
36. Scherer SS, Kleopa KA. X-linked Charcot-Marie-tooth disease. J Peripher Nerv Syst. 2012;17 Suppl 3:9–13.
37. Abrams CK, Freidin M. GJB1-associated X-linked Charcot-Marie-tooth disease, a disorder affecting the central and peripheral nervous systems. Cell Tissue Res. 2015;360(3):659–73.
38. Saporta AS, Sottile SL, Miller LJ, Feely SM, Siskind CE, Shy ME. Charcot-Marie-tooth disease subtypes and genetic testing strategies. Ann Neurol. 2011;69(1):22–33.
39. Koutsis G, Karadima G, Floroskoufi P, Raftopoulou M, Panas M. Relapsing remitting multiple sclerosis in x-linked charcot-marie-tooth disease with central nervous system involvement. Case Rep Neurol Med. 2015;2015:841897.
40. Rosser T, Muir J, Panigrahy A, Baldwin EE, Boles RG. Transient leukoencephalopathy associated with X-linked Charcot-Marie-tooth disease. J Child Neurol. 2010;25(8):1013–6.
41. Kim GH, Kim KM, Suh SI, Ki CS, Eun BL. Charcot-Marie-tooth disease masquerading as acute demyelinating encephalomyelitis-like illness. Pediatrics. 2014;134(1):e270–3.
42. Segawa M. Hereditary progressive dystonia with marked diurnal fluctuation. Brain Dev. 2011;33(3):195–201.
43. Nygaard TG. Dopa-responsive dystonia. Curr Opin Neurol. 1995;8(4):310–3.
44. Salles PA, Teran-Jimenez M, Vidal-Santoro A, Chana-Cuevas P, Kauffman M, Espay AJ. Recognizing atypical dopa-responsive dystonia and its mimics. Neurol Clin Pract. 2021;11(6):e876–e84.
45. Yoshino H, Nishioka K, Li Y, Oji Y, Oyama G, Hatano T, et al. GCH1 mutations in dopa-responsive dystonia and Parkinson's disease. J Neurol. 2018;265(8):1860–70.
46. Tadic V, Kasten M, Bruggemann N, Stiller S, Hagenah J, Klein C. Dopa-responsive dystonia revisited: diagnostic delay, residual signs, and nonmotor signs. Arch Neurol. 2012;69(12):1558–62.
47. Wilder-Smith E, Tan EK, Law HY, Zhao Y, Ng I, Wong MC. Spinocerebellar ataxia type 3 presenting as an L-DOPA responsive dystonia phenotype in a Chinese family. J Neurol Sci. 2003;213(1–2):25–8.
48. Lee WW, Jeon B, Kim R. Expanding the spectrum of Dopa-Responsive Dystonia (DRD) and proposal for new definition: DRD, DRD-plus, and DRD look-alike. J Korean Med Sci. 2018;33(28):e184.

49. Teive HAG, Camargo CHF, Pereira ER, Coutinho L, Munhoz RP. Inherited metabolic diseases mimicking hereditary spastic paraplegia (HSP): a chance for treatment. Neurogenetics. 2022;23(3):167–77.
50. Furukawa Y. In: Adam MP, Feldman J, Mirzaa GM, Pagon RA, Wallace SE, Bean LJH, et al., editors. GTP cyclohydrolase 1-deficient dopa-responsive dystonia. Seattle (WA): GeneReviews((R)); 1993.
51. Opladen T, Lopez-Laso E, Cortes-Saladelafont E, Pearson TS, Sivri HS, Yildiz Y, et al. Consensus guideline for the diagnosis and treatment of tetrahydrobiopterin (BH(4)) deficiencies. Orphanet J Rare Dis. 2020;15(1):126.
52. Friedman J. In: Adam MP, Feldman J, Mirzaa GM, Pagon RA, Wallace SE, Bean LJH, et al., editors. Sepiapterin reductase deficiency. Seattle (WA): GeneReviews((R)); 1993.
53. Jen JC, Graves TD, Hess EJ, Hanna MG, Griggs RC, Baloh RW. Primary episodic ataxias: diagnosis, pathogenesis and treatment. Brain. 2007;130(Pt 10):2484–93.
54. Choi KD, Choi JH. Episodic ataxias: clinical and genetic features. J Mov Disord. 2016;9(3):129–35.
55. Muro García I, Toribio-Díaz ME, Quintas S. Episodic ataxia: a 20-year diagnostic delay. Neurologia (Engl Ed). 2020;35(7):500–1.
56. Hall DA, Birch RC, Anheim M, Jønch AE, Pintado E, O'Keefe J, et al. Emerging topics in FXTAS. J Neurodev Disord. 2014;6(1):31.
57. Jacquemont S, Leehey MA, Hagerman RJ, Beckett LA, Hagerman PJ. Size bias of fragile X premutation alleles in late-onset movement disorders. J Med Genet. 2006;43(10):804–9.
58. Rousseau F, Rouillard P, Morel ML, Khandjian EW, Morgan K. Prevalence of carriers of premutation-size alleles of the FMRI gene—and implications for the population genetics of the fragile X syndrome. Am J Hum Genet. 1995;57(5):1006–18.
59. Higuchi Y, Ando M, Yoshimura A, Hakotani S, Koba Y, Sakiyama Y, et al. Prevalence of fragile X-associated tremor/ataxia syndrome in patients with cerebellar ataxia in Japan. Cerebellum. 2022;21(5):851–60.
60. Orsucci D, Lorenzetti L, Baldinotti F, Rossi A, Vitolo E, Gheri FL, et al. Fragile X-Associated Tremor/Ataxia Syndrome (FXTAS): a gender perspective. J Clin Med. 2022;11(4)
61. Johnson K, Herring J, Richstein J. Fragile X Premutation Associated Conditions (FXPAC). Front Pediatr. 2020;8:266.
62. Leehey MA. Fragile X-associated tremor/ataxia syndrome: clinical phenotype, diagnosis, and treatment. J Investigat Med. 2009;57(8):830–6.
63. Abbasi DA, Nguyen TTA, Hall DA, Robertson-Dick E, Berry-Kravis E, Cologna SM. Characterization of the cerebrospinal fluid proteome in patients with fragile X-associated tremor/ataxia syndrome. Cerebellum. 2022;21(1):86–98.
64. Nagaraj AS, R. Fragile X Ataxia Syndrome misdiagnosed as multiple sclerosis 2020. Available from: https://theneurologyhub.com/article/fragile-x-ataxia-syndrome-misdiagnosed-as-multiple-sclerosis
65. Coffey SM, Cook K, Tartaglia N, Tassone F, Nguyen DV, Pan R, et al. Expanded clinical phenotype of women with the FMR1 premutation. Am J Med Genet A. 2008;146a(8):1009.
66. Hall DA, Berry-Kravis E, Jacquemont S, Rice CD, Cogswell J, Zhang L, et al. Initial diagnoses given to persons with the fragile X associated tremor/ataxia syndrome (FXTAS). Neurology. 2005;65(2):299–301.
67. Greco CM, Tassone F, Garcia-Arocena D, Tartaglia N, Coffey SM, Vartanian TK, et al. Clinical and neuropathologic findings in a woman with the FMR1 premutation and multiple sclerosis. Arch Neurol. 2008;65(8):1114–6.
68. Toko M, Ohshita T, Kurashige T, Morino H, Kume K, Yamashita H, et al. FXTAS is difficult to differentiate from neuronal intranuclear inclusion disease through skin biopsy: a case report. BMC Neurol. 2021;21(1):396.
69. Sone J, Mori K, Inagaki T, Katsumata R, Takagi S, Yokoi S, et al. Clinicopathological features of adult-onset neuronal intranuclear inclusion disease. Brain. 2016;139(Pt 12):3170–86.

70. Shribman S, Reid E, Crosby AH, Houlden H, Warner TT. Hereditary spastic paraplegia: from diagnosis to emerging therapeutic approaches. Lancet Neurol. 2019;18(12):1136–46.
71. Schule R, Wiethoff S, Martus P, Karle KN, Otto S, Klebe S, et al. Hereditary spastic paraplegia: clinicogenetic lessons from 608 patients. Ann Neurol. 2016;79(4):646–58.
72. Saputra L, Kumar KR. Challenges and controversies in the genetic diagnosis of hereditary spastic paraplegia. Curr Neurol Neurosci Rep. 2021;21(4):15.
73. Ebrahimi-Fakhari D, Saffari A, Pearl PL. Childhood-onset hereditary spastic paraplegia and its treatable mimics. Mol Genet Metab. 2022;137(4):436–44.
74. Murala S, Nagarajan E, Bollu PC. Hereditary spastic paraplegia. Neurol Sci. 2021;42(3):883–94.
75. Fink JK. Hereditary spastic paraplegia: clinico-pathologic features and emerging molecular mechanisms. Acta Neuropathol. 2013;126(3):307–28.
76. Ruano L, Melo C, Silva MC, Coutinho P. The global epidemiology of hereditary ataxia and spastic paraplegia: a systematic review of prevalence studies. Neuroepidemiology. 2014;42(3):174–83.
77. Pascual B, de Bot ST, Daniels MR, Franca MC Jr, Toro C, Riverol M, et al. "Ears of the Lynx" MRI sign is associated with SPG11 and SPG15 hereditary spastic paraplegia. AJNR Am J Neuroradiol. 2019;40(1):199–203.
78. da Graca FF, de Rezende TJR, Vasconcellos LFR, Pedroso JL, Barsottini OGP, Franca MC Jr. Neuroimaging in hereditary spastic paraplegias: current use and future perspectives. Front Neurol. 2018;9:1117.
79. Schrander-Stumpel C, Legius E, Fryns JP, Cassiman JJ. MASA syndrome: new clinical features and linkage analysis using DNA probes. J Med Genet. 1990;27(11):688–92.
80. Hewamadduma CA, Hoggard N, O'Malley R, Robinson MK, Beauchamp NJ, Segamogaite R, et al. Novel genotype-phenotype and MRI correlations in a large cohort of patients with SPG7 mutations. Neurol Genet. 2018;4(6):e279.
81. Hedera P, Eldevik OP, Maly P, Rainier S, Fink JK. Spinal cord magnetic resonance imaging in autosomal dominant hereditary spastic paraplegia. Neuroradiology. 2005;47(10):730–4.
82. Hobson GM, Garbern JY. Pelizaeus-Merzbacher disease, Pelizaeus-Merzbacher-like disease 1, and related hypomyelinating disorders. Semin Neurol. 2012;32(1):62–7.
83. Kjellin KG, Stibler H. Protein patterns of cerebrospinal fluid in hereditary ataxias and hereditary spastic paraplegia. J Neurol Sci. 1975;25(1):65–74.
84. de Freitas JL, Rezende Filho FM, Sallum JMF, Franca MC Jr, Pedroso JL, Barsottini OGP. Ophthalmological changes in hereditary spastic paraplegia and other genetic diseases with spastic paraplegia. J Neurol Sci. 2020;409:116620.
85. Martinuzzi A, Montanaro D, Vavla M, Paparella G, Bonanni P, Musumeci O, et al. Clinical and paraclinical indicators of motor system impairment in hereditary spastic paraplegia: a pilot study. PLoS One. 2016;11(4):e0153283.
86. Mereaux JL, Banneau G, Papin M, Coarelli G, Valter R, Raymond L, et al. Clinical and genetic spectra of 1550 index patients with hereditary spastic paraplegia. Brain. 2022;145(3):1029–37.
87. Romagnolo A, Masera S, Mattioda A, Superti G, Santorelli FM, Mongini T, et al. Atypical hereditary spastic paraplegia mimicking multiple sclerosis associated with a novel SPG11 mutation. Eur J Neurol. 2014;21(2):e14–5.
88. Mukai M, Koh K, Ohnuki Y, Nagata E, Takiyama Y, Takizawa S. Novel SPG11 mutations in a patient with symptoms mimicking multiple sclerosis. Intern Med. 2018;57(21):3183–6.
89. Giannoccaro MP, Matteo E, Bartiromo F, Tonon C, Santorelli FM, Liguori R, et al. Multiple sclerosis in patients with hereditary spastic paraplegia: a case report and systematic review. Neurol Sci. 2022;43(9):5501–11.
90. Macedo-Souza LI, Kok F, Santos S, Amorim SC, Starling A, Nishimura A, et al. Spastic paraplegia, optic atrophy, and neuropathy is linked to chromosome 11q13. Ann Neurol. 2005;57(5):730–7.
91. Bazvand F, Keramatipour M, Riazi-Esfahani H, Mahmoudi A. SPOAN syndrome: a novel mutation and new ocular findings; a case report. BMC Neurol. 2021;21(1):24.

92. Breza M, Koutsis G. Kennedy's disease (spinal and bulbar muscular atrophy): a clinically oriented review of a rare disease. J Neurol. 2019;266(3):565–73.
93. Malek EG, Salameh JS, Makki A. Kennedy's disease: an under-recognized motor neuron disorder. Acta Neurol Belg. 2020;120(6):1289–95.
94. La Spada A. In: Adam MP, Feldman J, Mirzaa GM, Pagon RA, Wallace SE, Amemiya A, editors. Spinal and bulbar muscular atrophy. Seattle (WA).: University of Washington, Seattle. Copyright © 1993–2025, University of Washington, Seattle. GeneReviews is a registered trademark of the University of Washington, Seattle. All rights reserved: GeneReviews(®); 1993.
95. Weisfeld-Adams JD, Katz Sand IB, Honce JM, Lublin FD. Differential diagnosis of Mendelian and mitochondrial disorders in patients with suspected multiple sclerosis. Brain. 2015;138(Pt 3):517–39.
96. Tschampa HJ, Greschus S, Vinahl M, Urbach H, Mueller MM, Gerding WM. MS-like presentation of Alexander disease with multifocal lesions and oligoclonal bands. J Neurol. 2011;258(5):935–7.
97. Balbi P, Salvini S, Fundarò C, Frazzitta G, Maestri R, Mosah D, et al. The clinical spectrum of late-onset Alexander disease: a systematic literature review. J Neurol. 2010;257(12):1955–62.
98. Farina L, Pareyson D, Minati L, Ceccherini I, Chiapparini L, Romano S, et al. Can MR imaging diagnose adult-onset Alexander disease? AJNR Am J Neuroradiol. 2008;29(6):1190–6.
99. Padiath QS, Saigoh K, Schiffmann R, Asahara H, Yamada T, Koeppen A, et al. Lamin B1 duplications cause autosomal dominant leukodystrophy. Nat Genet. 2006;38(10):1114–23.
100. Isohanni P, Linnankivi T, Buzkova J, Lönnqvist T, Pihko H, Valanne L, et al. DARS2 mutations in mitochondrial leucoencephalopathy and multiple sclerosis. J Med Genet. 2010;47(1):66–70.
101. Keegan BM, Kaufmann TJ, Weinshenker BG, Kantarci OH, Schmalstieg WF, Paz Soldan MM, et al. Progressive solitary sclerosis: gradual motor impairment from a single CNS demyelinating lesion. Neurology. 2016;87(16):1713–9.
102. Depienne C, Bugiani M, Dupuits C, Galanaud D, Touitou V, Postma N, et al. Brain white matter oedema due to ClC-2 chloride channel deficiency: an observational analytical study. Lancet Neurol. 2013;12(7):659–68.
103. Campion D, Dumanchin C, Hannequin D, Dubois B, Belliard S, Puel M, et al. Early-onset autosomal dominant Alzheimer disease: prevalence, genetic heterogeneity, and mutation spectrum. Am J Hum Genet. 1999;65(3):664–70.
104. Renvoize E, Hanson M, Dale M. Prevalence and causes of young onset dementia in an English health district. Int J Geriatr Psychiatry. 2011;26(1):106–7.
105. Mendez MF. Early-onset Alzheimer disease and its variants. Continuum (Minneap Minn). 2019;25(1):34–51.
106. Yang Y, Bagyinszky E, An SSA. Patient with PSEN1 Glu318Gly and other possible disease risk mutations, diagnosed with early onset Alzheimer's disease. Int J Mol Sci. 2023;24(20)
107. Chelban V, Breza M, Szaruga M, Vandrovcova J, Murphy D, Lee CJ, et al. Spastic paraplegia preceding PSEN1-related familial Alzheimer's disease. Alzheimers Dement (Amst). 2021;13(1):e12186.
108. Karlstrom H, Brooks WS, Kwok JB, Broe GA, Kril JJ, McCann H, et al. Variable phenotype of Alzheimer's disease with spastic paraparesis. J Neurochem. 2008;104(3):573–83.
109. Ringman JM, Dorrani N, Fernandez SG, Signer R, Martinez-Agosto J, Lee H, et al. Characterization of spastic paraplegia in a family with a novel PSEN1 mutation. Brain Commun. 2023;5(2):fcad030.
110. Yang Y, Bagyinszky E, An SSA. Presenilin-1 (PSEN1) mutations: clinical phenotypes beyond Alzheimer's disease. Int J Mol Sci. 2023;24(9)
111. Natelson Love M, Clark DG, Cochran JN, Den Beste KA, Geldmacher DS, Benzinger TL, et al. Clinical, imaging, pathological, and biochemical characterization of a novel presenilin 1 mutation (N135Y) causing Alzheimer's disease. Neurobiol Aging. 2017;49(216):e7–e13.
112. Appel-Cresswell S, Guella I, Lehman A, Foti D, Farrer MJ. PSEN1 p.Met233Val in a complex neurodegenerative movement and neuropsychiatric disorder. J Mov Disord. 2018;11(1):45–8.

113. Tiedt HO, Benjamin B, Niedeggen M, Lueschow A. Phenotypic variability in autosomal dominant familial Alzheimer disease due to the S170F mutation of Presenilin-1. Neurodegener Dis. 2018;18(2–3):57–68.
114. Lanoiselee HM, Nicolas G, Wallon D, Rovelet-Lecrux A, Lacour M, Rousseau S, et al. APP, PSEN1, and PSEN2 mutations in early-onset Alzheimer disease: a genetic screening study of familial and sporadic cases. PLoS Med. 2017;14(3):e1002270.
115. Verhaart IEC, Robertson A, Wilson IJ, Aartsma-Rus A, Cameron S, Jones CC, et al. Prevalence, incidence and carrier frequency of 5q-linked spinal muscular atrophy—a literature review. Orphanet J Rare Dis. 2017;12(1):124.
116. Mercuri E, Bertini E, Iannaccone ST. Childhood spinal muscular atrophy: controversies and challenges. Lancet Neurol. 2012;11(5):443–52.
117. Mugisha N, Oliveira-Carneiro A, Behlim T, Oskoui M. Brain magnetic resonance imaging (MRI) in spinal muscular atrophy: a scoping review. J Neuromuscul Dis. 2023;10(4):493–503.
118. Milella G, Introna A, D'Errico E, Fraddosio A, Scaglione G, Morea A, et al. Cerebrospinal fluid and clinical profiles in adult type 2-3 spinal muscular atrophy patients treated with nusinersen: An 18-month single-centre experience. Clin Drug Investig. 2021;41(9):775–84.
119. Hersheson J, Haworth A, Houlden H. The inherited ataxias: genetic heterogeneity, mutation databases, and future directions in research and clinical diagnostics. Hum Mutat. 2012;33(9):1324–32.
120. Sullivan R, Yau WY, O'Connor E, Houlden H. Spinocerebellar ataxia: an update. J Neurol. 2019;266(2):533–44.
121. Klockgether T, Mariotti C, Paulson HL. Spinocerebellar ataxia. Nat Rev Dis Primers. 2019;5(1):24.
122. Schmitz-Hübsch T, Coudert M, Bauer P, Giunti P, Globas C, Baliko L, et al. Spinocerebellar ataxia types 1, 2, 3, and 6: disease severity and nonataxia symptoms. Neurology. 2008;71(13):982–9.
123. Rossi M, Perez-Lloret S, Doldan L, Cerquetti D, Balej J, Millar Vernetti P, et al. Autosomal dominant cerebellar ataxias: a systematic review of clinical features. Eur J Neurol. 2014;21(4):607–15.
124. Kim DH, Kim R, Lee JY, Lee KM. Clinical, imaging, and laboratory markers of premanifest spinocerebellar ataxia 1, 2, 3, and 6: a systematic review. J Clin Neurol. 2021;17(2):187–99.
125. Jacobi H, Reetz K, du Montcel ST, Bauer P, Mariotti C, Nanetti L, et al. Biological and clinical characteristics of individuals at risk for spinocerebellar ataxia types 1, 2, 3, and 6 in the longitudinal RISCA study: analysis of baseline data. Lancet Neurol. 2013;12(7):650–8.
126. Yap KH, Abdul Manan H, Yahya N, Azmin S, Mohamed Mukari SA, Mohamed IN. Magnetic resonance imaging and its clinical correlation in spinocerebellar ataxia type 3: a systematic review. Front Neurosci. 2022;16:859651.
127. Kumar N, Miller GM. White matter hyperintense lesions in genetically proven spinocerebellar ataxia 8. Clin Neurol Neurosurg. 2008;110(1):65–8.
128. Nakayama T, Nakayama K, Takahashi Y, Ohkubo K, Tobe H, Soma M, et al. Case of spinocerebellar ataxia type 1 showing high intensity lesions in the frontal white matter on T2-weighted magnetic resonance images. Med Sci Monitor. 2001;7(2):299–303.
129. Trikamji B, Singh P, Mishra S. Spinocerebellar ataxia-10 with paranoid schizophrenia. Ann Indian Acad Neurol. 2015;18(1):93–5.
130. Saito N, Ishihara T, Kasuga K, Nishida M, Ishiguro T, Nozaki H, et al. Case report: a patient with spinocerebellar ataxia type 31 and sporadic Creutzfeldt-Jakob disease. Prion. 2018;12(2):147–9.
131. Alvarez G, Rey A, Sanchez-Dalmau FB, Muñoz E, Ríos J, Adán A. Optical coherence tomography findings in spinocerebellar ataxia-3. Eye (Lond). 2013;27(12):1376–81.
132. Linnemann C, Tezenas du Montcel S, Rakowicz M, Schmitz-Hübsch T, Szymanski S, Berciano J, et al. Peripheral neuropathy in spinocerebellar ataxia type 1, 2, 3, and 6. Cerebellum. 2016;15(2):165–73.

133. Vujosevic S, Parra MM, Hartnett ME, O'Toole L, Nuzzi A, Limoli C, et al. Optical coherence tomography as retinal imaging biomarker of neuroinflammation/neurodegeneration in systemic disorders in adults and children. Eye (Lond). 2023;37(2):203–19.
134. Galatolo D, Tessa A, Filla A, Santorelli FM. Clinical application of next generation sequencing in hereditary spinocerebellar ataxia: increasing the diagnostic yield and broadening the ataxia-spasticity spectrum. A retrospective analysis. Neurogenetics. 2018;19(1):1–8.
135. Neyal N, Keegan BM, Kantarci OH, Zeydan B. Coexistence of multiple sclerosis and spinocerebellar ataxia type-8. Mult Scler. 2023;29(9):1195–8.
136. Everest E, Gulec B, Uygunoglu U. A case of coexistent spinocerebellar ataxia type 2 and primary progressive multiple sclerosis-coincidental or associated? Cerebellum. 2023;23:1235.
137. Sundal C, Axelsson M, Wiklund L, Lindberg C, Andersen O. A SCA7 premutation may be a novel Mendelian modifier of MS course: a case report. Mult Scler Relat Disord. 2019;31:148–50.
138. Röhl JE, Lünemann JD, Zimmer C, Zschenderlein R, Valdueza JM. Multiple sclerosis coinciding with Machado-Joseph disease. Neurol Sci. 2005;26(2):135–6.
139. Han S, Bae DW, An JY. Neuromyelitis optica spectrum disorder in a patient with spinocerebellar ataxia type 6. Neurol Asia. 2019;24(4):377–9.
140. Takahashi Y, Manabe Y, Morihara R, Narai H, Yamashita T, Abe K. Neuromyelitis Optica Spectrum disorder coinciding with spinocerebellar ataxia type 31. Case Rep Neurol. 2017;9(2):127–30.

Neoplastic, Paraneoplastic, and Hematologic Disorders

9

9.1 Autoimmune Autonomic Ganglionopathy

9.1.1 Synonyms

- Subacute autonomic neuropathy; Autoimmune autonomic neuropathy, Idiopathic autonomic neuropathy.

9.1.2 Epidemiology

- Prevalence is unknown.
- Females are more commonly affected [1, 2].

9.1.3 Etiology and Definition

- Pathogenic autoantibodies to ganglionic nicotinic acetylcholine receptor (gnAChR) cause the failure of signal transmission through postganglionic autonomic nerve fibers, leading to postganglionic cholinergic failure. Therefore, this autoimmune disease affects the autonomic nervous system while relatively sparing motor and sensory nerves.
- The autoimmune autonomic ganglionopathy (AAG) is often associated with lung cancer, thymoma (paraneoplastic form), myasthenia gravis and other autoimmunities (idiopathic form) [1, 2].

T. Uher, *Mimics and Red Flags of Multiple Sclerosis*, https://doi.org/10.1007/978-3-031-98945-2_9

9.1.4 Clinical Features

- Focal neurological:
  - Paresthesia (50%).
  - Motor and other sensory deficits are absent or minimal.
- Parasympathetic failure:
  - Adie pupils (usually unilaterally mydriasis; decreased photoreaction; light sensitivity; blurry vision; difficulty reading).
  - Sicca syndrome (lacrimal and salivary secretomotor dysfunction).
  - Decreased heart rate response to deep breathing or Valsalva maneuver (e.g., fixed heart rate).
- Enteric failure:
  - Achalasia (neurogenic paralysis and dilatation of the esophagus associated with difficulty swallowing).
  - Gastroparesis, ileus, constipation.
  - Diarrhea, anorexia, early satiety, abdominal pain, vomiting after eating.
- Sympathetic failure:
  - Anhidrosis; Horner's syndrome; bradycardia; orthostatic hypotension.
- Parasympathetic and sympathetic failure in organs dually innervated by competing divisions of the autonomic nervous system:
  - Complex pupillary dysfunction.
  - Urinary dysfunction (urinary retention or incontinence).
  - Sexual dysfunction (erectile or ejaculatory dysfunction).
  - Pandysautonomia (widespread failure of the autonomic nervous system affecting all divisions simultaneously).
- Other less frequent features include psychiatric symptoms, coughing episodes, or endocrine dysfunction [2].

9.1.5 Disease Course

- Acute or subacute (days or weeks) onset of symptoms in middle age.
- Sometimes preceded by a viral illness (particularly in idiopathic form).
- The course is monophasic, with slow and incomplete recovery [2].

9.1.6 Brain Imaging

- Probably normal, but reliable data are lacking [3].
- The single case study reported a teenager with AAG and acute encephalitis with bilateral T2 lesions in basal ganglia, hippocampus, and insular cortex [4].

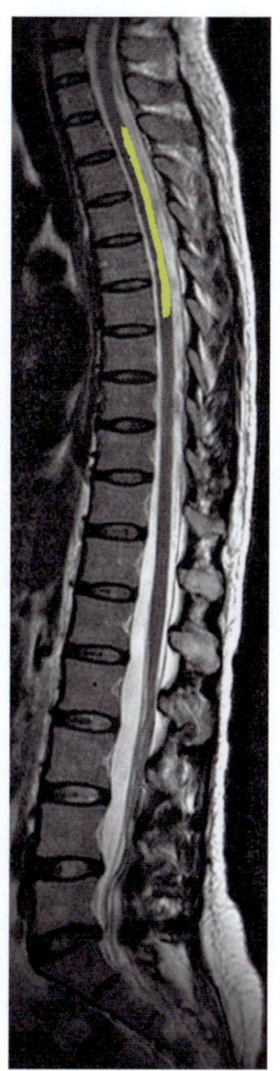

Fig. 9.1 Longitudinally extensive T2 hyperintensities in the dorsal columns in autoimmune autonomic ganglionopathy

9.1.7 Spinal Cord Imaging

- T2 hyperintensities in the dorsal columns, resulting from the degeneration of the central afferent tracts between the dorsal root ganglia and their synapse at the dorsal horn or even longitudinally extensive transverse myelitis (LETM) may be present [5, 6] (Fig. 9.1).

9.1.8 Blood Work

- Autoantibodies against the gnAChR can be detected only in acute stages of the disease and are present in only 50–70% of cases. Therefore, negative testing does not rule out the diagnosis [7, 8].
- Conversely, high levels of gnAChR correlate with disease severity.
- Some patients with positive gnAChR do not have AAG, due to a relatively high rate of false-positive results [7, 9].

9.1.9 Examination of CSF

- Data are lacking. A few case studies have shown normal findings or increased concentration of protein with or without pleocytosis. There are no data regarding the presence of cerebrospinal fluid (CSF)-restricted oligoclonal bands (OCB) [4, 7, 10].

9.1.10 Diagnosis

- Challenging to diagnose AAG owing to a lack of international consensus on diagnostic criteria and the absence of clear rules for interpreting of gnAChR levels [1].

9.1.11 Differential Diagnosis

- Diseases with dysautonomia that need to be distinguished from AAG include:
  - Neurodegenerative diseases such as multiple system atrophy.
  - Peripheral neuropathies (amyloidosis; diabetes; acute inflammatory demyelinating polyneuropathy [AIDP]).
  - Paraneoplastic syndrome (anti-Hu; anti-collapsin response-mediator protein-5 [CRMP-5]).
  - Rheumatologic diseases with autonomic manifestations (Sjögren's syndrome; systemic lupus erythematosus [SLE]; rheumatoid arthritis; ankylosing spondylitis; psoriatic arthritis; scleroderma).
  - Autoimmune neuromuscular conditions with prominent autonomic manifestations (Lambert–Eaton myasthenic syndrome; disorders with voltage-gated potassium channel [VGKC] complex antibodies).
  - Idiopathic gastrointestinal dysmotility.
  - Cholinergic neuropathy.
  - Idiopathic anhidrosis.
  - Acute sensory and autonomic neuronopathy (ASANN) is a rare, severe autoimmune condition typically preceded by a febrile illness. It is characterized by absence of motor deficit but damage to neurons in the dorsal root and autonomic ganglia, resulting in acute loss of all sensory modalities and autonomic failure with poor recovery and often fatal outcome [2, 3].

9.1.12 Treatment and Prognosis

- A few case studies reported benefits from intravenous immunoglobulins; plasmapheresis; mycophenolate mofetil; azathioprine; and anti-CD20 therapy.
- Spontaneous, usually incomplete recovery is observed in 30% of patients; severe cases may be life-threatening [2, 11].

9.2 Gliomas

9.2.1 Epidemiology

- Incidence of gliomas 5/100,000/year.
- Incidence of glioblastoma 3/100,000/year (most common subtype).
- Overall, demyelinating diseases are more prevalent than primary brain tumors.
- Females have a higher incidence of multiple sclerosis (MS) and tumefactive demyelination, but a lower incidence of brain tumors, with a female/male ratio of 1/1.6 [12–15].

9.2.2 Etiology and Definition

- Gliomas are neuroepithelial tumors arising from central nervous system (CNS) glial or supporting cells. They include 24% of all primary brain and CNS malignancies [15].

9.2.3 Clinical Features

- Depend on size and location of tumor and the amount of vasogenic edema.
- Focal neurological deficit.
- Headache, non-specific, often unilateral and progressive (50% of patients diagnosed with high-grade gliomas).
- Seizures (20–40%) [12, 14].
  - In MS are extremely rare at disease onset and not frequent through the disease course (1–3%) [16, 17].
- Increased intracranial pressure with positional headache, papilledema, encephalopathy or decreased consciousness.
- Commonly positive response to corticosteroids due to reduction of brain edema [12, 14].

9.2.4 Disease Course

- Gliomas can appear at any age, on average peak age is 20–30 years for grade 2 lesions, 40 years for grade 3, and 55–65 years for grade 4 (glioblastoma).
- Symptoms onset is typically subtle, subacute to chronic and progressive. However, high-grade tumors may present with more acute manifestations.
- Relapsing–remitting course is typical for MS, but uncommon in tumors [12–14].

9.2.5 Brain Imaging

- Lesions' location:
  - Most often occurs in the frontal and parietal lobes, less in temporal lobes.

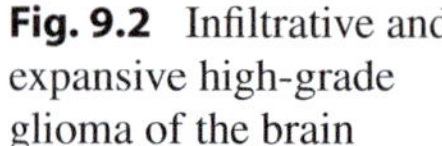

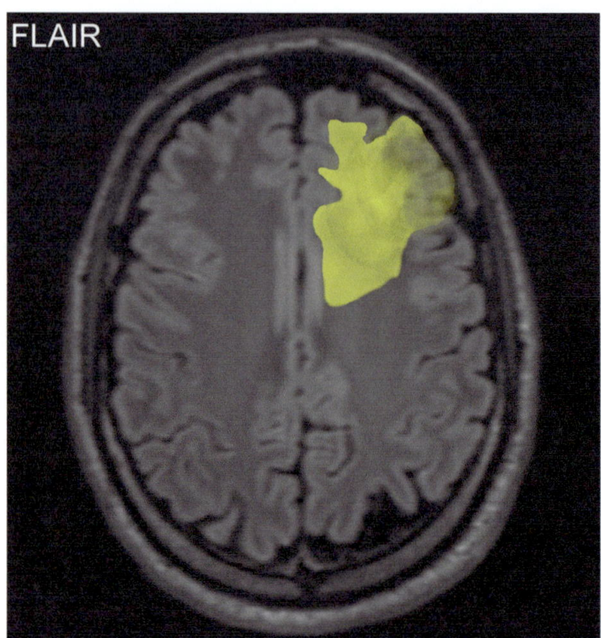

Fig. 9.2 Infiltrative and expansive high-grade glioma of the brain

 - Frequently subcortical white matter and deep gray matter but can expand to adjacent cortical gray matter or occur other brain locations such as brainstem or even spinal cord.
 - Gliomas never occur simultaneously in the brain and the spinal cord.
- Lesions' appearance:
 - Infiltrative, expansive, heterogeneous T2 hyperintense and T1 hypointense lesion (Fig. 9.2).
 - Cystic and hemorrhagic changes, or central necrosis may be seen in high-grade gliomas but not in MS.
 - MRI T2/fluid-attenuated inversion recovery (FLAIR) mismatch is typical for isocitrate dehydrogenase (*IDH*)-mutant gliomas, which is typical by hyperintense signal on T2-weighted sequence, but relative T2-weighted hypointense signal on FLAIR sequence, except for a hyperintense peripheral rim. This sign can distinguish *IDH*-mutant astrocytoma from other gliomas and non-malignant etiologies including demyelinating lesions.
 - Lesions do not show central vein sign (CVS); however, the usefulness of this marker is limited in patients with a single or very small number of lesions.
- Contrast enhancement:
 - Low-grade and often also grade 3 gliomas are non-enhancing initially.
 - Presence of enhancement with or without necrosis suggests a higher grade.
 - Grade 4 gliomas almost always show enhancement, which is variable, typically peripheral, and irregular with nodular components.

- Perilesional changes:
  - Edema and mass effect are more pronounced in high-grade gliomas.
  - In contrast to tumefactive demyelinating lesions, the mass effect of tumors is more pronounced relative to their size.
  - Tumefactive demyelinating lesions also often exhibit a perilesional edema (77%).
- Evolution over time:
  - Brain tumors typically increase in size and enhancement pattern over a short period of time (1–3 months). In contrast, acute MS lesions generally decrease in size following treatment. Over the long term (years), some MS lesions may show slow volume expansion, though this occurs at a significantly slower rate compared to brain tumors. Additionally, new distant lesions frequently develop in MS, which is atypical for brain neoplasms [18–20].
- Other imaging techniques
  - Diffusivity is usually unchanged, but the higher cellularity and grade of the tumor are associated with lower apparent diffusion coefficient (ADC) values due to decreased water diffusivity. However, simultaneously, ADC values may increase due to edema often seen in tumors.
  - Susceptibility weighted imaging (SWI) may show artifacts due to neoangiogenesis and microhemorrhage, whose presence indicates high-grade tumors (grade 4).
  - Magnetic resonance spectroscopy shows increased choline peak, decreased N-acetylaspartate (NAA) peak, and increased choline to creatinine ratio that may help to distinguish tumefactive MS lesions from high-grade gliomas, but not always from low-grade gliomas. However, its role in the differential diagnosis of gliomas has not yet been clearly established.
  - Dynamic-susceptibility contrast (DSC) MR perfusion imaging can evaluate for relative cerebral blood volume (rCBV), which reflect angiogenesis and can aid in differentiating low and high-grade gliomas and in differentiating of high-grade (not low-grade) gliomas showing increased rCBV from demyelinating lesions, which usually show decreased rCBV (only very rarely increased) due to absent neovascular proliferation [18, 21, 22].
  - Combination of DSC MR perfusion imaging with diffusion-tensor imaging (DTI) may also help to distinguish high-grade gliomas from demyelinating lesions [23].

9.2.6 Examination of Blood and CSF

- Routine testing typically yields normal results.
- Opening pressure can be elevated.
- Examination of CSF should be avoided in patients with large lesions, marked edema or with posterior fossa masses due to the risk of the brain herniation following the spinal tap [18].

9.2.7 Diagnosis

- Accurate diagnosis is essential to avoid unnecessary aggressive diagnostic and therapeutic procedures. Focusing on magnetic resonance imaging (MRI) only may lead to misdiagnosis.
- Biopsy of the lesion is required for diagnosis of neoplasm.
- Grading of tumors based on histological features and molecular abnormalities is important for estimating prognosis and guiding treatment [12–14, 19].

9.2.8 Differential Diagnosis

- Tumefactive lesions in MS may resemble gliomas, and conversely, early-stage gliomas may mimic MS lesions. In some patients, it may be difficult to differentiate between demyelinating lesions and brain neoplasms. In such cases, if surgery is feasible, a biopsy of the lesion is recommended. However, biopsy may be associated with complications, and their results may be uninformative or misleading. The patients undergoing biopsy are usually those without a pre-existing diagnosis of MS, with suspicious imaging findings, negative OCB, or from atypical populations (very old or young patients) [18, 24].
- Differentiating between low-grade glioma and tumefactive demyelination can be particularly challenging owing to their similar imaging features.
- There are no specific imaging markers to definitively distinguish gliomas from tumefactive demyelinating lesions in MS. Certain features, such as the following, tend to favor a diagnosis of tumefactive demyelination over glioma:
  - Well-circumscribed supratentorial lesions, rather than signs of diffuse and extensive demyelination. Lesion size is usually between 20 and 60 mm, but large lesions with a diameter >120 mm are also reported in rare cases.
  - Predilection for the frontal and parietal lobes, but lesions in corpus callosum, basal ganglia, infratentorial, and spinal cord may also occur.
  - More than 50% of lesions show contrast enhancement with any pattern (homogeneous, heterogeneous, nodular, punctate, closed-ring, or, less often, incomplete open-ring with the open portion toward the gray matter).
  - Less mass effect and perilesional edema relative to the size of the lesion.
  - Central necrosis may be observed rarely in severe MS cases and hemorrhagic leukoencephalopathy.
  - T2 hypointense rim.
  - Peripheral restricted diffusion in acute lesions.
  - Perivenular enhancement.
  - Presence of lesions in more than two distinct areas of the neuraxis, or additional lesions typical of MS.
  - Computed tomography (CT) hypodensity of MRI-enhanced regions (93% in demyelination vs. only 4% of cases with tumors).
  - Absence of blood or calcium in the center of a lesion favors a demyelination.
  - Some tumors (e.g., lymphoma) can appear hyperdense on CT.

  - 18-fludeoxyglucose positron emission tomography (FDG-PET) shows a lower degree of hypermetabolism (marginally above of normal cortex) in demyelinating lesions compared with that in tumors.
  - Presence of CSF-restricted OCB (>50% of cases with tumefactive demyelinating lesions) [24, 25].
- Not only demyelinating lesions but also neoplastic lesions such as high-grade gliomas or primary central nervous system (CNS) lymphomas often response to corticosteroids owing to an effect on brain edema. However, this prompt effect of corticosteroids is usually only temporary, and lesions rebound in a few weeks or months [24].
- Malignant brain tumors (especially in temporal lobe) can rarely present acutely with symptoms such as fever, encephalopathy, or bilateral abnormalities on MRI mimicking an inflammatory etiology (6%). Therefore, a brain neoplasm should always be considered as a potential diagnosis until a viral infection is confirmed. For example, patients with herpetic encephalitis may also have normal results of CSF examination [26, 27].
- Patients with MS probably do not have an increased risk of developing gliomas, but gliomas in MS have a worse prognosis. The co-occurrence of gliomas with MS, particularly in the early stages, often presents a diagnostic challenge. The average time between onset of MS and diagnosis of glioma is 12 years [25, 28].

9.2.9 Treatment and Prognosis

- Neurosurgery, radiotherapy, chemotherapy.
- Associated with high morbidity and mortality [12–15, 19].
- Radiotherapy for gliomas in patients with MS may accelerate the inflammatory disease activity of MS [28].

9.2.10 Gliomatosis Cerebri

- A rare growth pattern of diffuse gliomas involving the white matter of at least three brain lobes is often present as an extensive process on MRI, even at initial subclinical stages. Although radiotherapy can improve survival, the prognosis remains unfavorable [29].

9.3 Histiocytosis Disorders

9.3.1 Subtypes

A. Langerhans cell histiocytosis (LCH).
B. Erdheim–Chester disease (ECD).
C. Juvenile xanthogranuloma (JXG).
D. Rosai–Dorfman disease (RDD) (or Rosai–Dorfman–Destombes).
E. Haemophagocytic lymphohistiocytosis (HLH) [30].

9.3.2 Epidemiology

- Very rare conditions with a low incidence:

  A. LCH 0.26–0.89/100.000 children/year [30, 31].
  B. ECD not known; reported only hundreds of cases [30, 32].
  C. JXG 0.1/100.000 children/year [33].
  D. RDD not known; reported >1200 cases [34].
  E. HLH 0.13/100.000/year [35].

9.3.3 Etiology and Definition

- Characterized by inflammatory infiltrates of leukocytes with a macrophage and/or dendritic cell phenotype in different tissues.
- Subtypes A. to D. are associated with the accumulation of clonal mononuclear phagocytes and are considered as inflammatory myeloid neoplastic disorders.
- Only rarely progress to lymphoma-like malignancies, such as histiocytic sarcoma or malignant histiocytosis.
- HLH is characterized by activated CD8+ T cells that stimulate macrophage activation and extreme systemic inflammation and is considered a syndrome of immune dysregulation [30].

9.3.4 Clinical Features

- LCH
  - Primarily affects children (<10 years); rarely adults (3rd to 5th decade).
  - The manifestations vary widely and depend on the location and number of lesions, as well as the organ systems involved.
  - Lesions can occur in any organ system, with bones (especially skull lesions) and skin being the most affected.
  - Lesions in the pituitary gland may lead to diabetes insipidus and other endocrinopathies, whereas those in the CNS cause neurological deficits.
  - Progressive LCH-neurodegenerative disease can be diagnosed years after the disease was considered to be cured (around 10%) [30].
- ECD
  - Primarily affects adults.
  - Clinical manifestations resemble those of LCH but typically carry a worse prognosis.
  - Although ECD can affect any organ, skeletal system pathology is present in almost all patients, with bone pain being the most common symptom.
  - Systemic symptoms (fever or weight loss) may be present.
  - Often xanthelasma (yellowish deposits of the cholesterol beneath the eyes).

  - CNS involvement (30–50%) often leads to conditions such as diabetes insipidus, cerebellar syndromes, cranial neuropathy, seizures, hypophysitis with pan-hypopituitarism, or papilledema [30].
- JXG
  - Primarily affects young children (<4 years).
  - Single or multiple orange–red papules on the skin (xanthogranulomas), containing foamy macrophages (xanthoma cells) that usually resolve spontaneously.
  - Lesions may be in any organ system [30].
- RDD
  - Heterogeneous group of different conditions with a similar phenotype.
  - Primarily affects children (<10 years) but may occur in any age.
  - Occurs in isolation or conjunction with autoimmune, hereditary, and malignant diseases.
  - Painless enlargement of cervical lymph nodes, which may resolve spontaneously.
  - Lesions commonly occur in the orbit, nasal cavity, or parotid gland (22%), but are only rarely found in bones, subcutaneously, or in the brain [30].
- HLH
  - Affects primarily young children, but adults can be also affected.
  - Syndrome of extreme immune activation.
  - The primary, or genetic/familial, form is caused by mutations in genes responsible for cellular immunological functions.
  - Typically, progressive brain lesions alone or in association with recurrent fevers, splenomegaly, pancytopenia, hypertriglyceridemia, hypofibrinogenemia, and/or hyperferritinemia.
  - Dominant CNS involvement is rare.
  - The secondary form occurs in patients following a potent immunological stimulus, such as infection, malignancy (primarily leukemias and lymphomas, less commonly solid tumors), or autoimmune conditions. Therefore, all patients, especially adults, should undergo evaluation for the presence of malignancy or inflammation.
  - Can present with a relapsing–remitting course [30, 36].

9.3.5 Brain and Spinal Cord Imaging

- Several case studies have reported patients diagnosed with LHC and ECD exhibiting lesions in supra- and infra-tentorial regions of the brain and spinal cord, resembling MS.
- However, lesions linked to these histiocytoses frequently exhibit prolonged or chronic contrast enhancement, a feature atypical for MS [37–41].
- For example, ECD presents the following MRI patterns:
  - Multifocal brain lesions (nodules or tumefactive masses) (44%).

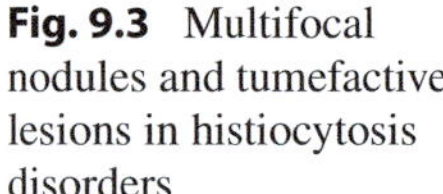

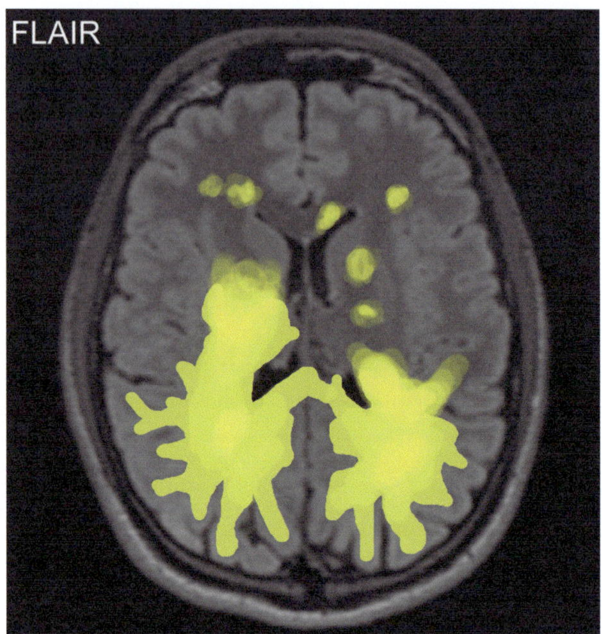

Fig. 9.3 Multifocal nodules and tumefactive lesions in histiocytosis disorders

- Meningioma-like tumors or nodular thickening of the dura mater (37%)
- Infiltrative and meningeal lesions (19%).
- Hence, ECD should also be considered in the differential diagnosis of gliomas and brain tumors [40, 41] (Fig. 9.3).

9.3.6 Blood Work

- Routine blood tests may appear normal or indicate systemic inflammation, characterized by increased levels of C-reactive protein and high erythrocyte sedimentation rate. Additionally, abnormalities such as elevated lactate dehydrogenase (LDH), anemia, leukocytopenia, or thrombocytopenia may be observed [30, 37, 38].

9.3.7 Examination of CSF

- Usually normal findings without CSF-restricted OCB.
- LCH: sometime slightly elevated concentration of protein [37].
- ECD: sometime mirror pattern (type IV) of OCB [38, 39].

9.3.8 Diagnosis

- The diagnosis is confirmed through a biopsy of the suspected lesion.
- In patients with CNS involvement, a brain biopsy is often necessary.
- The skeletal system is affected in 80% of LCH and 80–95% of ECD patients. However, in many patients, bone involvement is asymptomatic. Bone pathology can be visualized using X-ray, CT, MRI, scintigraphy, or FDG-PET [37–41].

9.3.9 Differential Diagnosis

- Neurological features only rarely precede systemic organ involvement, which can pose challenges in distinguishing them from MS [37].
- Histiocytoses may sometimes meet diagnostic MRI criteria for MS or present with a relapsing–remitting clinical course of CNS symptoms. Therefore, searching for red flags such as chronic contrast enhancement of CNS lesions, negative CSF-restricted OCB, bone lesions, endocrinopathy, skin lesions, or systemic symptoms such as fever or weight loss can help prevent misdiagnosis of MS [37, 38, 40–42].
- Many patients exhibit elevated concentrations of immunoglobulin G4 (IgG4), which can lead to misdiagnosis with IgG4-related disease [30, 37, 38].

9.3.10 Treatment and Prognosis

- The treatment approach varies depending on the disease subtype, but generally involves immunosuppressive (cytotoxic) therapies aimed at eliminating pathogenic clones of macrophages.
- Severe cases may require hematopoietic stem cell transplantation.
- The disease may progresses without therapy and can be potentially fatal [30].

9.4 Intramedullary Spinal Cord Tumors

9.4.1 Definition

- There are several subtypes of intradural intramedullar mass lesions, including:
  A. Primary intramedullary spinal cord neoplasms:
    - Ependymoma
    - Pilocytic astrocytoma
    - Diffuse midline glioma
    - Hemangioblastoma
    - Astrocytoma
    - Glioblastoma
    - Oligodendroglioma

- Primary central nervous system lymphoma
- Medulloblastoma
- Metastases to the intramedullary spinal cord
- Secondary central nervous system lymphoma

B. Benign tumors:
- Epidermoid cyst
- Dermoid cyst
- Lipoma
- Neuroenteric cyst [43]

9.4.2 Epidemiology

- The prevalence of ependymoma, the most common primary intramedullary spinal cord tumor is 0.21/100,000/year [44].

9.4.3 Clinical Features

- The outcome depends on the size and location of the pathology.
- Often subacute onset back pain, sensori-motor deficit, bowel/bladder dysfunction or radiculopathy [43].

9.4.4 Spinal Cord Imaging

- Lesions' location:
  - Mono- or multi-focal lesions in the spinal cord.
- Lesions' appearance:
  - The borders are typically well-defined, whereas in MS, signal changes are often less marginated compared to tumors.
  - Lesions are often longer compared to the shorter lesions seen in MS.
  - The signal intensity of the tumor may be heterogeneous and may contain cysts.
  - Small lesions or leptomeningeal pathology might be not evident on MRI.
  - Large tumors—such as ependymomas, astrocytomas, or metastases—can be longitudinal and mimick longitudinally extensive transverse myelitis (LETM) (Fig. 9.4).
- Contrast enhancement:
  - Enhancement is typically present, at least to some extent, and tends to persist (not only a few weeks as seen in MS).
  - In spinal cord metastases, a "flame sign" may be seen, which is an ill-defined triangular extension of ring contrast enhancement at the top and/or bottom of the cord lesion.

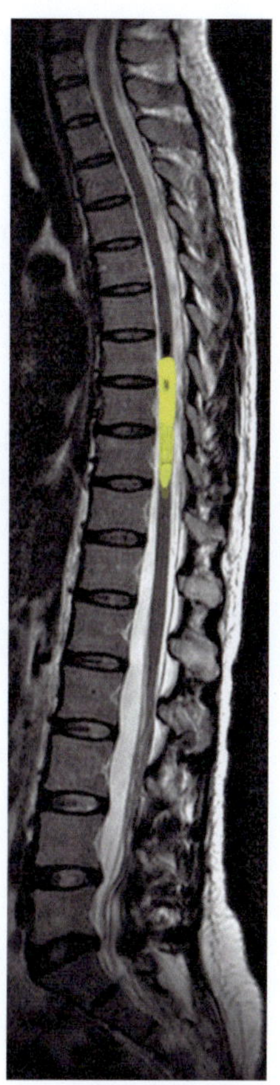

Fig. 9.4 Intramedullary spinal cord tumor mimicking longitudinally extensive transverse myelitis (LETM)

- Perilesional changes:
  - Varying degree of mass effect and edema, with marked spinal cord enlargement being more common compared to MS, where it is either absent or mild.
- Evolution over time:
  - Typically, a consistent increase in size over time, a characteristic not observed in MS lesions.
- Associated findings:
  - Typically no lesions present in the brain as seen in MS [43, 45].
- Since intramedullary spinal cord tumors and inflammatory demyelinating lesions share several MRI features, the differential diagnosis can be challenging [46].

9.4.5 Blood Work

- Normal

9.4.6 Examination of CSF

- Variable findings with often elevated (sometimes extremely) concentration of protein and low glucose level.
- Number of white blood cells is normal, or seen a mild pleocytosis [43].
- CSF-restricted OCB are rarely present (5.8%). The focal disruption of blood–brain barrier or destruction of CNS tissue associated with release of CNS antigens are hypothesized as possible mechanisms [47–49].
- Cytology of CSF may visualize neoplastic cells. However, the sensitivity is only around 60%. Repeated exams of CSF may increase sensitivity to 90% [50].
- Immunophenotyping and flow cytometry is indicated in patients with suspected hematologic malignancy [43].
- CSF analysis for cell surface markers and circulating tumor deoxyribonucleic acid (DNA) may improve the sensitivity of leptomeningeal tumor detection [51].
- Measuring opening pressure is essential to rule out elevated intracranial pressure, which may indicate leptomeningeal carcinomatosis [43].

9.4.7 Diagnosis

- Confirmed by biopsy, which is recommended in the majority of cases [43].

9.4.8 Differential Diagnosis

- Differential diagnosis is wide and includes the following disorders:
  - Myelopathies related to cancer treatment:
    Toxic myelopathy secondary to intrathecal chemotherapy (e.g., methotrexate, cytarabine).
    Immune checkpoint inhibitor-mediated myelitis.
    Radiation-induced myelopathy.
  - Vascular myelopathies.
  - Inflammatory infectious and autoimmune myelopathies.
  - Metabolic and toxic myelopathies.
  - Hereditary myelopathic syndromes [43, 52].
- MRI of the entire spine is required in all patients, regardless of the localization of neurologic deficits. Similarly, in all patients with leptomeningeal carcinomatosis performing the brain MRI with contrast agent is required. Evidence of asymptomatic lesions at other sites of CNS may help to clarify the diagnosis [43].
- Spinal cord tumors may mimic MS, there are several remarks helping to distinguish MS form spinal cord neoplasm such as:
  - Relapsing–remitting course in MS vs. steadily progression in tumors.
  - Presence of typical pattern of brain lesions in MS.
  - Presence of CSF-restricted OCB in MS and sometime also pleocytosis.
  - Temporal retinal nerve fiber layer (RNFL) thinning on optical coherence tomography (OCT) or increased P100 latencies on visual evoked potentials (VEP) in MS patients [47, 53–55].

- It's essential to consider that spinal cord tumors can rarely occur even in patients with a confirmed diagnosis of MS [56, 57].
- Absence of response to immunosuppressive therapy.
- Persistent contrast enhancement of lesion, marked mass effect, and edema [58].

9.4.9 Treatment and Prognosis

- Surgery, radiotherapy, and chemotherapy.
- The prognosis varies depending on the type and stage of the disease [43].

9.5 Paraneoplastic Neurologic Syndromes

9.5.1 Epidemiology

- Prevalence 1/300 in patients with cancer, but paraneoplastic neurologic syndromes/disorders (PNS) are probably underdiagnosed and underreported.
- The increasing use of immune checkpoint inhibitors for cancer treatment leads to an increased incidence of PNS [59, 60].

9.5.2 Etiology and Definition

- Heterogeneous group immune-mediated inflammatory disorders of the central and peripheral nervous system caused by cancer.
- Some antigens, which are released from lysed tumor cells, are expressed in the tumor and neural tissues. These antigens may escape immunotolerance, which cause production of neuronal autoantibodies directed against antigens expressed by neural tissue.
- Most high-risk antibodies target intracellular antigens. They are probably not directly pathogenic, but serve as biomarkers [61–63].
- There is a long list of paraneoplastic antibodies, which are stratified as high-risk, intermediate-risk, and low-risk based on their strength of association with underlying neoplasms (Table 9.1) [62–64].

9.5.3 Disease Course

- Subacute symptoms onset (few days to weeks).
- Cancer is diagnosed typically within 2, rarely 5 years of diagnosis of PNS [62, 65].
- The diagnosis of PNS usually precedes the diagnosis of cancer, but it can rarely present at the time of cancer diagnosis or even later [66].

Table 9.1 Overview of paraneoplastic antibodies (adapted and modified from Graus et al. 2021) [62]

Paraneoplastic antibody		Frequency of cancer	Associated tumors	Clinical phenotype
High risk		>70%		
ANNA1(Anti-Hu)	Antineuronal nuclear antibody 1	85%	SLCL, NSCL, other neuroendocrine tumors, neuroblastoma	Sensory neuronopathy, Chronic gastrointestinal pseudo-obstruction, Encephalomyelitis, and Limbic encephalitis
CRMP5 (CV2)	Collapsin response-mediator protein 5	>80%	SLCL, thymoma	Encephalomyelitis and Sensory neuronopathy
SOX1	SRY-Box Transcription Factor 1	80%	SLCL	LEMS with and without rapidly progressive cerebellar syndrome
PCA2 (also known as MAP1B)	Purkinje cell antibody 2 (microtubule-associated protein 1B)	80%	SCLC, NSCLC, breast cancer	Sensorimotor neuropathy, rapidly progressive cerebellar syndrome, and Encephalomyelitis
AMPH	Amphiphysin	80%	SCLC and breast cancer	Polyradiculoneuropathy, Sensorimotor neuropathy, Encephalomyelitis, stiff-person syndrome
ANNA2 (Anti-Ri)	Antineuronal nuclear antibody 2	70%	Breast, lung	Brainstem/cerebellar syndrome, Opsoclonus-myoclonus syndrome
PCA1 (Anti-Yo)	Purkinje cell antibody 1	>90%	Ovary and breast cancers	Rapidly progressive cerebellar syndrome
Ma2 and/or Ma		>75%	Testicular cancer and NSCLC	Limbic encephalitis, diencephalitis, and brainstem encephalitis
DNER (PCA-Tr)	Delta/notch-like epidermal growth factor-related receptor; Purkinje cell cytoplasmic antibody, type Tr	90%	Hodgkin lymphoma	Rapidly progressive cerebellar syndrome
KLHL11	Kelchlike protein 11	80%	Testicular cancer	Brainstem/cerebellar syndrome
LUZP4	Leucine zipper 4	Recently discovered autoantibodies with limited data		
TRIM46	Tripartite Motif Containing 46			
KCTD16	Potassium channel tetramerization domain containing 16			
ANNA3	Antineuronal nuclear antibody 3			

Intermediate risk		30–70%		
AMPAR	α-amino-3-hydroxy-5-methyl-4-isoxazolepropionic acid receptor	>50%	SCLC and malignant thymoma	Limbic encephalitis
GABA-B-R	Gamma-aminobutyric-acid B receptor	>50%	SCLC	Limbic encephalitis
mGluR5	Metabotropic glutamate receptor 5	50%	Hodgkin lymphoma	Encephalitis
P/Q VGCC	Voltage-gated calcium channel	>50%	SCLC	LEMS, rapidly progressive cerebellar syndrome
NMDAR	Anti-N-methyl-d-aspartate receptor	38%	Ovarian and extraovarian teratomas	Anti-NMDAR encephalitis
CASPR2	Contactin-associated protein-like 2	50%	Malignant thymoma	Morvan syndrome
Low risk		< 30%		
mGluR1	Metabotropic glutamate receptor	30%	Mostly hematologic	Cerebellar ataxia
GABA-A-R	Gamma-aminobutyric receptor	<30%	Malignant thymoma	Encephalitis
CASPR2	Contactin-associated protein-like 2	<30%	Malignant thymoma	Limbic encephalitis, acquired neuromyotonia, Morvan syndrome
GFAP	Glial fibrillary acidic protein	20%	Ovarian teratomas and adenocarcinomas	Meningoencephalitis
GAD65	Glutamic acid decarboxylase 65	<15%	SCLC, other neuroendocrine tumors, malignant thymoma	Limbic encephalitis, stiff-person syndrome, and cerebellar ataxia
LGI1	Leucine-rich glioma-inactivated 1	<10%	Malignant thymoma and Neuroendocrine tumors	Limbic encephalitis
DPPX	Dipeptidyl peptidase-like protein	<10%	B-cell neoplasms	Encephalitis with CNS hyperexcitability and PERM
GlyR	Glycine receptoracid-A	<10%	Malignant thymoma and Hodgkin lymphoma	Limbic encephalitis, PERM
AQP4	Aquaporin 4	<5%	Adenocarcinomas	NMOSD
MOG	Myelin oligodendrocyte glycoprotein	Rare cases	Mostly ovarian teratomas	MOG antibody-associated disease

Legend: *CNS* centran nervous system, *LEMS* Lambert–Eaton myasthenic syndrome, *NSCLC* non-small cell lung cancer, *PERM* progressive encephalomyelitis with rigidity and myoclonus, *SCLC* small cell lung cancer

9.5.4 Clinical and Imaging Features of High-Risk Phenotypes

- There is no pathognomonic neurologic presentations, but there are defined *"high-risk" phenotypes* (e.g., "classical" PNS) that are frequently associated with cancer. They include the following phenotypes [62, 64]:
- Limbic encephalitis
  - Rapidly progressing disease course (<3 months) with seizures, short-time memory loss, and psychiatric manifestations.
  - The etiology can be paraneoplastic or nonparaneoplastic. The most frequent types of limbic encephalitis are associated with cell surface antibodies such as LGI1 or CASPR2 antibodies, which are usually nonparaneoplastic.
  - However, limbic encephalitis can also be associated with onconeural antibodies against GABA-B-R, AMPAR, anti-Hu or anti-Ma2 which are often associated with paraneoplastic etiology [62, 64]. The detection of anti-Hu antibodies in children with limbic encephalitis is very rare and is usually not associated with cancer [67].
  - MRI shows inflammatory changes in the limbic system, including the hippocampus, amygdala, hypothalamus, and cingulate cortex, but other brain areas can also be affected. There is increased T2 signal and swelling in the mesial temporal lobes with or without contrast enhancement. Mass-like appearance or hypermetabolism on FDG-PET may be present.
  - Differential diagnosis includes mostly herpes simplex viral encephalitis (with cortical petechial hemorrhages, or rarely intracerebral hematomas); Wernicke encephalopathy (thiamine deficiency); drug intoxication; prion disease; neurosyphilis; Hashimoto encephalopathy; glioma or subclinical status epilepticus. In the cases with hypothalamic involvement should be excluded sarcoidosis or lymphocytic hypophysitis [68].
- Subacute cerebellar degeneration
  - Rapidly progressive (<3 months) severe bilateral cerebellar syndrome, which is initially not associated with a major cerebellar atrophy.
  - Rarely may be present hyperacute or unilateral onset. Conversely some patients may have slowly progressive phenotype mimicking neurodegenerative diseases.
  - Additional extracerebellar brainstem syndrome may be present.
  - The onconeural antibodies often associted with isolated cerebellar syndrome are PCA-1/Yo and DNER/PCA-Tr [62–64].
  - Brain MRI in the acute phase shows increaed T2 signal of the cerebellar hemispheres, therefore infectious or inflammatory cerebellitis need to be excluded.
  - In the chronic phase, T2 hyperintensities are less pronounced, but cerebellar atrophy and hypometabolism on FDG-PET are present [68].
- Opsoclonus-myoclonus
  - Present opsoclonus, action myoclonus (trunk, limbs, and head), cerebellar syndrome and encephalopathy (from confusion to coma).

  - Idiopathic form.
    Usually driven by an immune-mediated postinfectious process.
    More often in young patients; less frequently associated with encephalopathy; and has a better prognosis.
  - Paraneoplastic form
    In childred 50% of cases are associated with neuroblastoma.
    In adults is often associated with small cell lung cancer (SLCL) or breast cancer (often positive ANNA-2/anti-Ri antibodies).
    In young women can be associated with ovarian teratomas without neuronal autoantibodies.
    More often in older patients; more frequently associated with encephalopathy; and has a worse prognosis [62–64].
- Sensory neuronopathy
  - Caused by involvement of the sensory neurons of the dorsal root ganglia.
  - In addition to sensory deficit, some patients may also have motor deficit due to additional involvement of motor nerve roots or peripheral nerves.
  - The main differentials to consider are Sjogren's syndrome or platinum-based chemotherapy.
  - Paraneoplastic etiology should be suspected in patients with an inflammatory pattern of CSF and motor involvement.
  - The most frequent neural autoantibodies are ANNA-1/anti-Hu, CRMP5/anti-CV2 and AMPH [62–64].
- Encephalomyelitis
  - Can be diagnosed only in patients with clinical manifestations at multiple sites of the central but also PNS, including an involvement of dorsal root ganglia, nerve roots, or peripheral nerves.
  - Typically associates with SCLC with (ANNA-1/anti-Hu) or (CRMP5/anti-CV2) antibodies [62–64].
- Gastrointestinal pseudo-obstruction (enteric neuropathy)
  - Recurrent episodes of abdominal pain, distension, constipation, or vomiting, without evidence of mechanical obstruction caused by myenteric plexus dysfunction.
  - Abnormal gastric emptying or small bowel manometry can confirm the diagnosis.
  - Occasionally present other symptoms of autonomic dysfunction.
  - The positivity of anti-Hu antibodies suggests a paraneoplastic origin.
  - In contrast, antibodies against ganglionic acetylcholine receptor suggest a nonparaneoplastic origin [62, 63, 69].
- Lambert–Eaton myasthenic syndrome
  - Progressive proximal muscle weakness, often associated with autonomic dysfunction (dry mouth, erectile dysfunction, or constipation).
  - Decreased or absent muscle reflexes improve after repeat exercise or maximal voluntary contraction.
  - Diagnosis can be confirmed using electromyography (EMG).

- Around 90% of patients have positive antibodies against P/Q VGCCs, but they can be present also in non-paraneoplastic forms of the Lambert–Eaton syndrome (LEMS). Their presence is not required for the diagnosis.
- The positivity of SOX1 autoantibodies strongly suggest SLCL [62–64].

9.5.5 Clinical and Imaging Features of Intermediate-risk Phenotypes

- *"Intermediate-risk"* phenotypes (e.g., "non-classical" PNS) frequently occur in patients without cancer. Their presence should prompt consideration of a PNS, especially in unclear cases. Typically, these phenotypes also exhibit rapidly progressive onset of manifestations (<3 months) and inflammatory findings in the CSF or brain/spine MRI. They include the following phenotypes:
- Encephalitis (other than limbic)
  - May be associated with antibodies against mGluR5 or GABA-A-R [62–64].
  - Anti-NMDAR encephalitis can be associated with tumor, particularly in young women (40% have benign ovarian teratoma) [19].
  - Association with malignancy is commonly seen only in older adults [70].
- Brainstem encephalitis
  - Frequently oculomotor abnormalities and bulbar symptoms; sometimes also movement disorder or cerebellar syndrome.
  - Anti-Ma2 antibody positivity in patients with testicular tumors or non-small cell lung cancer (NSCLC) is often associated with limbic and brainstem encephalitis and sometime also diencephalic syndrome (with narcolepsy, hyperphagia, hyperthermia, and endocrine abnormalities).
  - Anti-Hu antibodies are often associated with bulbar syndrome and central hypoventilation.
  - Anti-Ri antibodies are often associated with opsoclonus-myoclonus syndrome and jaw dystonia.
  - Anti-KLHL11 antibodies in patients with testicular cancer or teratoma are often associated with sensorineural deafness [62–64].
  - Brain MRI can be normal, or in the acute phase are seen T2 hyperintensities and/or contrast enhancement in the cerebellum, cerebellar peduncles, or brainstem.
  - In the chronic phase may be present cerebellar and brainstem atrophy.
  - Similarly as in patients with multiple system atrophy may occur cruciform T2 hyperintensity in the pons ("hot cross bun sign") and T2 hyperintensity in the middle cerebellar peduncles secondary to Wallerian degeneration [68].
- Morvan syndrome
  - Co-occurrence of limbic encephalitis and neuromyotonia should not be considered as a synonym of Morvan syndrome.
  - Peripheral nerve hyperexcitability with encephalopathy (psychiatric syndromes, dysautonomia, and sleep disorders).
  - Malignant thymoma is sometimes associated with Morvan syndrome and myasthenia gravis.

  - Almost always associated with CASPR2, sometimes simultaneously with LGI1 and netrin 1 receptor antibodies [62–64].
- Stiff-person syndrome
  - Painful muscular spasms and stiffness due to co-activation of agonist and antagonist muscles.
  - Generalized or focal forms (affecting, for example, only lower limb)
  - The paraneoplastic forms are mostly associated with amphiphysin antibodies and breast cancer.
  - The nonparaneoplastic forms are often associated with GAD65 antibodies. However, in some patients, anti-GAD65 positivity may be associated with cancer.
  - There are also other non-paraneoplastic variants of Stiff-person syndrome with progressive encephalomyelitis, rigidity, and myoclonus associated with antibodies against GlyR antibodies [62–64].
- Myelopathy
  - Paraneoplastic myelitis is a rare but likely underreported condition.
  - May occur in isolation or together with brain involvement.
  - Disease onset is acute or insidious and progressive.
  - Often normal MRI (39%)
  - Most often symmetric longitudinally extensive transverse myelitis (LETM) (74% of those with abnormal MRI), can with contrast enhancement.
  - Affects predominantly tracts in the lateral columns and gray matter, therefore may mimic neuromyelitis optica spectrum disorders (NMOSD) or motor neuron disease.
  - Isolated bilateral lateral column involvement may occur. Tract-specific lateral column contrast enhancement is suggestive of a paraneoplastic myelopathy. (50%)
  - Central gray involvement is present in around 40–50%
  - Rarely presents as necrotizing myelopathy.
  - On the other hand, some patients may have normal MRI findings.
  - Often associated with breast and lung carcinomas, and with CV2/CRMP5 and amphiphysin antibodies.
  - Documented rare paraneoplastic AQP4 IgG seropositive NMOSD.
  - Some patients may not have neuronal antibodies; therefore, the paraneoplastic etiology should be considered also in patients with unclear myelopathies [62–64, 71].
- Paraneoplastic polyradiculoneuropathy
  - Sensorimotor deficit, pain, dysautonomia, often also CNS symptoms.
  - Distribution is symmetric or asymmetric.
  - Axonal pattern on nerve conduction studies.
  - The most frequently associated with CV2/CRMP5, amphiphysin, and PCA-2/MAP1B antibodies in patients with SCLC and breast cancer.
  - Peripheral neuropathies that fulfill the criteria of Guillain-Barre syndrome or chronic inflammatory demyelinating polyneuropathy (CIDP) in patients with cancer should not be considered paraneoplastic unless a high-risk antibody is identified [62–64].

- Nerve root contrast enhancement
  - Most common lumbar.
  - Clinically with acute or chronic polyradiculitis.
- Optic neuropathy
  - Present in 20% of patients with CRMP5-IgG-associated PNS.
  - Painless, subacute, bilateral, with optic disc edema and hemorrhages.
  - Sometime also nystagmus, diplopia, or opsoclonus.
  - Often accompanied by vitritis and/or retinopathy.
  - Owing to the presence of ocular inflammation, infectious causes of optic neuropathy must be excluded.
  - The most common malignancy is SCLC.
  - MRI does not show enhancement of the optic nerve.
  - Present inflammatory CSF with positive CRMP5 antibodies [72].
- Other less frequent "non-classical PNS" include cancer associated:
  - Retinopathy
  - Motor neuron disease
  - Movement disorders
  - Acute sensorimotor neuropathy
  - Acute pandysautonomia
  - Cranial neuropathy
  - Brachial neuritis [65, 68] (see Fig. 3.2 in the Sect. 3.2).

9.5.6 Examination of Blood and CSF

- Detection methods should include rodent brain tissue immunohistochemistry/immunofluorescence accompanied by confirmatory studies using immunoblot with recombinant proteins or cell-based assays. Although, commercial kits testing of multiple antibodies may be useful for the initial screening, the number of false-positive and false-negative results is relatively high.
- Testing for antibodies should include analysis of serum and CSF
- Only IgG antibodies have diagnostic significance [62]
- Common findings in the CSF
  - Inflammatory pattern (80–90%).
  - Elevated concentration of protein (70–80%).
  - Mild pleocytosis (ranging from 1 to 112 cells/mm^3) present in 30–50% of patients, with a higher frequency in acute than in chronic stages. In the acute stages is frequent pleocytosis without elevated protein.
  - Increased IgG index (60%).
  - CSF-restricted OCB (pattern II or III) (50%).
  - CSF-restricted OCB without inflammatory CSF pattern (10%).
  - A few patients may have normal CSF findings but positive neuronal antibodies. Conversely, some patients may exhibit an inflammatory pattern in the CSF but negative antibodies (seronegative PNS) [48, 65].

9.5.7 Diagnosis

- Established using the recent criteria (PNS-Care Score), distinguishing three levels of diagnostic certainty (possible, probable, and definite PNS) based on the type of clinical features, presence of neuronal antibodies, and presence of cancer [62].
- Cancer screening should be performed in patients with suspected PNS and guided by the neurological phenotype or antibody screening.
- Patients can have more than one tumor; thus, if the identified tumor is atypical for the clinical phenotype of PNS or antibody, additional studies for a second tumor should be considered [62].
- The tumors most often associated with PNS are SCLC, breast cancer, ovarian cancer, NSCLC, and lymphomas [61, 62].
- If the initial tumor screening is negative in patients with high-risk phenotypes and high-risk antibodies, it should be repeated every 4–6 months for at least 2 years, because a vast majority of tumours are diagnosed within 2 years after the onset of PNS [62].

9.5.8 Differential Diagnosis

- Diagnosis may be challenging because it requires distinguishing among involvement of the nervous system by cancer (metastasis or carcinomatous meningitis); systemic complications of cancer (coagulopathy, metabolic problems, or infections); treatment-related neurotoxicity or immune-mediated inflammatory PNS.
- Particularly, diagnosis of “non-classical PNS” can be easily missed, because clinical manifestations often mimic non-paraneoplastic diseases.
- Therefore, the diagnosis of PNS requires the exclusion of alternative causes.
- Establishing the direct link between a tumor and suspected PNS may be challenging in cases without positive neuronal antibodies because the presence of a tumor may be coincidental and not pathologically linked [61, 62, 65].
- However, PNS can also be diagnosed without evidence of positive neuronal antibody testing for example opsoclonus-myoclonus syndrome in children with neuroblastoma or Lambert–Eaton syndrome in patient with SCLC (seronegative PNS) [62].

9.5.9 Treatment and Prognosis

- Treatment of cancer together with early immunotherapy including high-dose corticosteroids, intravenous immunoglobulin, or plasmapheresis.
- Chronic therapy includes most often anti-CD20 therapy or cytostatics.
- Unfortunately, many PNS, particularly those targeting intra-neuronal antigens are treatment refractory [63, 64, 73].

- Immune checkpoint inhibitors enhance antitumor immunity by blocking immune checkpoint molecules, which increase long-term remissions of oncologic patients. However, they increase risk of immune-related adverse events including severe neurologic syndromes (in 1–3% of patients). The checkpoint inhibitor associated PNS predominantly affect the CNS and are associated with antibodies and cancer types, which are observed also in spontaneous PNS. Many patients are seronegative, and the detection of antibodies is not required for diagnosis in these cases [59, 60].

9.6 Primary CNS Lymphoma (PCNSL)

9.6.1 Epidemiology

- Incidence 0.45/100.000/years.
- Accounts for 2% of all brain tumors.
- Older age and immunosuppression are the main risk factors [74].

9.6.2 Etiology and Definition

- CNS lymphoma occurs in the CNS de novo (primary CNS lymphoma; PCNSL) or by the spreading of systemic disease (secondary CNS lymphoma).
- 90% of PCNSL cases are diffuse large B-cell primary lymphomas [75].

9.6.3 Clinical Features

- Depends on the site, size, and type of the PCNSL.
- The majority of patients have focal neurologic deficits, but around 40% of patients present with only nonspecific cognitive decline or behavioral changes.
- May be present cranial and peripheral neuropathy or radiculopathy due to leptomeningeal involvement or direct nerve invasion (neurolymphomatosis).
- Leptomeningeal involvement often causes increased intracranial pressure, which may be associated with headache, nausea, and vomiting.
- Ocular involvement is present in 25% of patients, but visual symptoms have only 4% of patients [75–77].

9.6.4 Disease Course

- Symptoms onset is typically subacute/insidious (over weeks to months) [75–77].
- Patients may present with a relapsing–remitting disease course [78] and often show rapid responses to corticosteroids, which can raise the risk of misdiagnosis with MS [79]. However, PCNSL primarily affects older patients, who typically

exhibit a primary or secondary progressive MS phenotype or generally experience a low number of relapses in the case of a relapsing–remitting phenotype. Hence, the manifestation of relapsing–remitting symptoms in older patients, particularly those with corticosteroid-resistant vision disorders (due to vitreoretinal involvement), should prompt suspicion of PCNSL [78].

9.6.5 Brain Imaging

- Lesions' location:
  - Single (70%) or multifocal lesions (30%) (multifocal lesions are more frequent in immunosuppressed patients).
  - Mostly supratentorial (70–80%), particularly in periventricular white matter, deep gray matter (basal ganglia or thalamus), and corpus callosum.
  - Typical subependymal extension and crossing of the corpus callosum.
  - Involvement of cortical gray matter or brainstem is less frequent.
  - Rarely isolated involvement of the leptomeninges or vitreoretinal space.
- Lesions' appearance:
  - Often large lesions mimicking tumefactive MS, NMOSD, MOGAD, other tumors, or infections.
  - T2 images show variable signal, most often iso or hypo-intense to gray matter, but can be also hyperintense, particularly if present necrosis.
  - T1 images show usually hypointense signal.
  - Diffusion-weighted imaging (DWI) typically shows intense restricted diffusion (increased DWI and decreased signal on ADC maps).
- Contrast enhancement:
  - Almost always present.
  - Homogeneous with well-defined borders, which is distinct from the open-ring enhancement commonly seen in MS or the heterogeneous/irregular enhancement with necrosis commonly observed in high-grade gliomas or metastases.
  - But immunocompromised patients might show only ring-like or no contrast enhancement and central necrosis.
  - May be present leptomeningeal enhancement (10–20%).
  - Even after successful treatment, small contrast–enhancing lesions may still be observed, but these do not necessarily indicate disease activity [75–77, 80–84].
- Perilesional changes:
  - Even large lesions may show relatively little mass effect and vasogenic edema (Fig. 9.5).
- Evolution over time:
  - Corticosteroids and cancer treatment may lead to substantial or even complete resolution of lesions and contrast enhancement. Despite of this, corticosteroid response is not diagnostic of CNS lymphoma because many other pathologies may improve following corticosteroids.

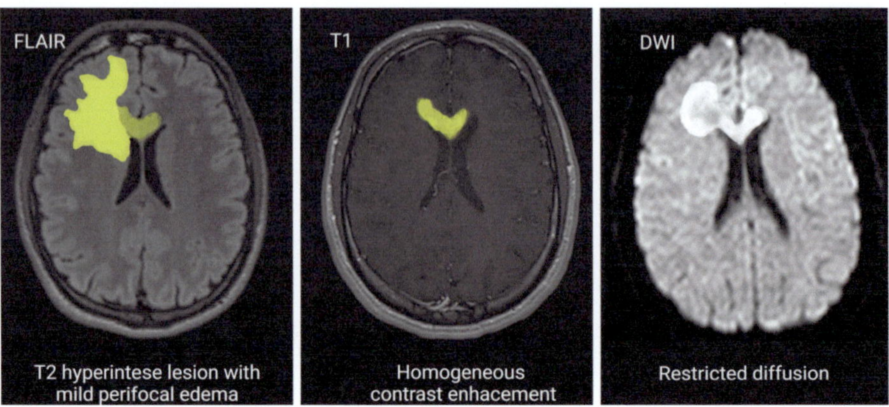

Fig. 9.5 MRI characteristics of primary CNS lymphoma (PCNSL)

  - Occasionally, corticosteroids induce sustained clinical and radiological improvement lasting 6–12 months; rarely up to 5 years.
- Associated findings:
  - Owing to high cellularity are lesions often hyperdense on CT.
  - Patients with isolated leptomeningeal or vitreoretinal involvement may show only enlarged and enhancing peripheral nerves or focal hypermetabolism on the FDG-PET [24, 75–77, 80–86].
  - Some patients may show inflammatory demyelinating brain lesions ("sentinel lesions") that occur months prior to the diagnosis of the primary CNS lymphoma. Histological assessment of the "sentinel lesion" suggest demyelination. It is hypothesized that "sentinel lesions" may represent the initial immunological response against a developing PCNSL, which may escape diagnosis in an inflammatory environment. There was also a hypothesized possibility of malignant transformation of tumefactive demyelination into B-cell lymphoma [78, 87].

9.6.6 Spinal Cord Imaging

- Isolated spinal involvement is uncommon (1.2–3.0%), but if present, it typically manifests as a solitary cord lesion, predominantly affecting cervical segments [81, 88, 89].

9.6.7 Blood Work

- Elevated concentration of lactate dehydrogenase (LDH), which is a marker of rapid cell turnover is associated with a worse prognosis. However, LDH is nonspecific marker and may be elevated in several other conditions such as liver failure, tissue ischemia, hemolysis, or infection [90].

9.6.8 Examination of CSF

- Low concentration of glucose. (10–54%)
- Elevated concentration of protein (34–70%) [90–93].
- Can be an elevated concentration of lactate.
- Elevated IgG index (20–30%).
- Positive OCB in CSF (60%).
- CSF-restricted OCB (17–27%) [79, 90, 94, 95].
- Pleocytosis
  - Present in the majority (40–70%), but not in all patients.
  - Positive cytomorphology of lymphoma cells (2–32%).
  - Sensitivity of detection of lymphoma cells on the first CSF sample, when combined cytomorphology and flow cytometry, is approximately 80%. Therefore, it is sometimes necessary to obtain multiple CSF samples.
  - Collecting of large volume of CSF (<30 mL) increases sensitivity of a detection of lymphoma cells.
  - Cytological analyses of CSF should be performed as soon as possible, because lymphocytes in native CSF break down rapidly. The time between CSF collection and assessment should be within 18–24 hours.
  - Rarely, a false-positive CSF result occurs if a CSF sample is contaminated by peripheral blood in patient with systemic lymphoma [79, 90–93].
- Combined elevation of LDH isozyme 5, ß2-microglobulin, and immunoglobulin heavy chain levels in CSF have a relatively high sensitivity (58–85%) and specificity (85%) for diagnosis of PCNSL. Furthermore, proteomics and microRNA analysis have high specificity in the diagnosis (95%) [90].
- Analysis of CSF is currently not as advanced enough to replace biopsy [92].

9.6.9 Diagnosis

- The clinical and imaging manifestations are not specific; therefore, definitive diagnosis requires cytologic proof of the PCNSL either by vitrectomy, CSF sampling, or brain biopsy (most frequently) [75, 77, 96].

9.6.10 Differential Diagnosis

- Differentiating between PCNSL and MS or other mimics can be challenging or sometimes impossible. As a result, the diagnosis of PCNSL is often delayed, and a biopsy of the lesion is typically required for a definitive diagnosis. However, sometimes, histopathological examination to distinguish PCNSL from its mimics can also be challenging, and repeated brain biopsies may be necessary [78, 85, 97, 98].
- Corticosteroids should be administered after evaluation for CNS lymphoma because they can mask imaging features and influence histological assessment.

- Patients with isolated leptomeningeal or vitreoretinal involvement may have normal MRI findings. Therefore, diagnosis requires examination of the CSF or, in the case of ocular involvement, ocular slit-lamp examination and vitrectomy [75].
- Intravascular lymphoma:
  - A rare variant with the proliferation of lymphoma cells only in the lumen of capillaries and postcapillary venules. Symptoms are caused by vessel occlusion (dementia, progressive strokes, or peripheral neuropathy). Patients often have skin lesions, night sweats, fever, weight loss, and increased markers of systemic inflammation such as C-reactive protein. The diagnosis is often made by biopsy of skin lesions [75].
- MS:
  - Red flags suggestive of PCNSL rather than MS include:
    Middle to older age.
    Rapidly deteriorating course.
    Corticosteroid dependence.
    Increased enhancement or lesion size over time.
    Intense restricted diffusion of lesions.
    Homogeneous contrast enhancement.
    Disproportionally low mass effect.
    Lack of spinal cord involvement.
    Abnormal cytology (clonal IgG gene rearrangement).
    Absence of CSF-restricted OCB [87].
  - Hyperacute MS lesions may also exhibit restricted diffusion, but they are typically detectable only for a few days/weeks, are less intense, and is usually located only in the periphery of the lesions, corresponding with a contrast-enhancing region. Additionally, lesions in MS are associated with a less marked decrease in the ADC map [75–77, 80–84].
- Acute ischemic stroke:
  - May also display restricted diffusion; however, in acute ischemic lesions typically do not exhibit round contrast enhancement, they are usually distributed within a vascular territory and present a wedge-shaped appearance with sharp borders. They often involve cortical gray matter, contrast enhancement is not as intense, and perfusion-weighted imaging typically reveals reduced cerebral blood flow. Additionally, the evolution of the lesions' characteristics over time often aids in differential diagnosis [99].

9.6.11 Treatment and Prognosis

- Disease progression can be rapid; therefore, treatment initiation should be initiated as soon as possible.
- Treatment protocol consists of induction and consolidation therapy.

- Although PCNSL is highly sensitive to chemotherapy and radiotherapy and tends to respond well to cancer treatment, relapses are common, and the prognosis is poor [75, 77, 96].
- MRI monitoring in remission should include imaging every 3 months for the first 2 years, then every 6 months for another 3 years, and then annually, because late relapses (>10 years) may occur [100].

9.7 Other Rare Hematologic Disorders

9.7.1 Crystal-Storing Histiocytosis

- Extremely rare disorder in patients expressing monoclonal immunoglobulins (such as multiple myeloma, monoclonal gammopathy of undetermined significance, lymphoma, or plasmacytoma) associated with the deposition of crystals within histiocytes.
- Isolated involvement of the CNS is very rare but may mimic MS. A case study reported an adult with a corticosteroid-responsive relapsing–remitting course of focal neurological symptoms, abnormal visual evoked potentials typical for MS, and MRI findings in the brain and spinal cord mimicking MS.
- Red flags against the diagnosis of MS include additional atypical clinical features (episodes of aphasia and confusion), absence of CSF-restricted OCB, persistent contrast enhancement, and progressive enlargement of T2 lesions.
- The diagnosis is established by brain biopsy showing macrophages containing intracellular kappa-light chain-restricted crystals [101, 102].

9.7.2 Monoclonal Gammopathy of Undetermined Significance (MGUS)

- MGUS is an asymptomatic, premalignant disorder that is often underdiagnosed. It is characterized by the presence of a monoclonal protein produced by an abnormal clone of plasma cells (with M-protein levels <30 g/L in serum and clonal bone marrow plasma cells <10%). The risk of progressing to multiple myeloma or other lymphoproliferative disorders is estimated at 1% per year. This condition affects approximately 3.2% of individuals over the age of 50.
- MGUS is generally considered benign and does not typically require treatment, as it is usually not associated with end-organ damage. It is often discovered incidentally. However, in some cases, MGUS can be associated with organ involvement, such as glomerulopathy.
- Around 5% of patients may experience peripheral neuropathy, chronic inflammatory demyelinating polyneuropathy, or, less commonly, myopathy.

- CNS involvement in MGUS is extremely rare, and its association with brain or spinal cord pathology remains a subject of ongoing discussion. Suggestions have been made that CNS involvement might present as focal asymptomatic or symptomatic brain lesions, cognitive deficits, or movement disorders.
- Case reports have documented instances where patients with MGUS also had MS, with M-protein detected in serum and CSF.
- There have also been reports of patients with MGUS experiencing longitudinally extensive transverse myelitis (LETM).
- Patients with MGUS and CNS involvement may present with multiple large demyelinating WM lesions, often with perifocal edema, mass effect, irregular "cloud-like" shapes, and ring-like contrast enhancement. These lesions might also show complete regression. In some cases, MRI features have been similar to those seen in acute disseminated encephalomyelitis (ADEM).
- Traditional immunomodulatory treatments for MS have shown limited effectiveness in these cases. However, corticosteroids, intravenous immunoglobulins, plasmapheresis, and therapies targeting B cells and plasmacytic cells have shown positive effects in some instances [103, 104].

References

1. Urriola N, Adelstein S. Autoimmune autonomic ganglionopathy: ganglionic acetylcholine receptor autoantibodies. Autoimmun Rev. 2022;21(2):102988.
2. Golden EP, Vernino S. Autoimmune autonomic neuropathies and ganglionopathies: epidemiology, pathophysiology, and therapeutic advances. Clin Auton Res. 2019;29(3):277–88.
3. Gutierrez J, Palma JA, Kaufmann H. Acute sensory and autonomic neuronopathy: a devastating disorder affecting sensory and autonomic ganglia. Semin Neurol. 2020;40(05):580–90.
4. Kuki I, Kawawaki H, Okazaki S, Hattori Y, Horino A, Higuchi O, et al. Autoimmune autonomic ganglionopathy in a pediatric patient presenting with acute encephalitis. Brain Dev. 2016;38(6):605–8.
5. Casseb RF, Martinez ARM, de Paiva JLR, França MC. Neuroimaging in sensory neuronopathy. J Neuroimaging. 2015;25(5):704–9.
6. Birnbaum J, Lalji A, Piccione EA, Izbudak I. Magnetic resonance imaging of the spinal cord in the evaluation of 3 patients with sensory neuronopathies: diagnostic assessment, indications of treatment response, and impact of autoimmunity: a case report. Medicine. 2017;96(49):e8483.
7. Vernino S, Low PA, Fealey RD, Stewart JD, Farrugia G, Lennon VA. Autoantibodies to ganglionic acetylcholine receptors in autoimmune autonomic neuropathies. New Engl J Med. 2000;343(12):847–55.
8. Vernino S, Lindstrom J, Hopkins S, Wang ZB, Low PA, Grp MS. Characterization of ganglionic acetylcholine receptor autoantibodies. J Neuroimmunol. 2008;197(1):63–9.
9. Li YB, Jammoul A, Mente K, Li JB, Shields RW, Vernino S, et al. Clinical experience of seropositive ganglionic acetylcholine receptor antibody in a tertiary neurology referral center. Muscle Nerve. 2015;52(3):386–91.
10. Suarez GA, Fealey RD, Camilleri M, Low PA. Idiopathic autonomic neuropathy – clinical, neurophysiologic, and follow-up-studies on 27 patients. Neurology. 1994;44(9):1675–82.
11. Bouxin M, Schvartz B, Mestrallet S, Debrumetz A, Hentzien M, Tabary T, et al. Rituximab treatment in seronegative autoimmune autonomic neuropathy and autoimmune autonomic ganglionopathy: case-report and literature review. J Neuroimmunol. 2019;326:28–32.
12. de la Fuente MI. Adult-type diffuse gliomas. Continuum (Minneap Minn). 2023;29(6):1662–79.

13. Ostrom QT, Price M, Neff C, Cioffi G, Waite KA, Kruchko C, et al. CBTRUS statistical report: primary brain and other central nervous system tumors diagnosed in the United States in 2015-2019. Neuro-Oncology. 2022;24(Suppl 5):v1–v95.
14. Omuro A, DeAngelis LM. Glioblastoma and other malignant gliomas: a clinical review. JAMA. 2013;310(17):1842–50.
15. Davis ME, editor. Epidemiology and overview of gliomas. Seminars in oncology nursing. Elsevier; 2018.
16. Mirmosayyeb O, Shaygannejad V, Nehzat N, Mohammadi A, Ghajarzadeh M. Prevalence of seizure/epilepsy in patients with multiple sclerosis: a systematic review and meta-analysis. Int J Prev Med. 2021;12:14.
17. Ooi S, Kalincik T, Perucca P, Monif M. The prevalence of epileptic seizures in multiple sclerosis in a large tertiary hospital in Australia. Mult Scler J Exp Transl Clin. 2021;7(1):2055217321989767.
18. Berkman JM, Nakhate V, Gonzalez Castro LN. Glioblastoma in patients with multiple sclerosis. Neurohospitalist. 2022;12(4):607–16.
19. Schaff LR, Mellinghoff IK. Glioblastoma and other primary brain malignancies in adults: a review. JAMA. 2023;329(7):574–87.
20. Ikeguchi R, Shimizu Y, Abe K, Shimizu S, Maruyama T, Nitta M, et al. Proton magnetic resonance spectroscopy differentiates tumefactive demyelinating lesions from gliomas. Mult Scler Relat Disord. 2018;26:77–84.
21. Cha S, Pierce S, Knopp EA, Johnson G, Yang C, Ton A, et al. Dynamic contrast-enhanced T2*-weighted MR imaging of tumefactive demyelinating lesions. AJNR Am J Neuroradiol. 2001;22(6):1109–16.
22. Blasel S, Pfeilschifter W, Jansen V, Mueller K, Zanella F, Hattingen E. Metabolism and regional cerebral blood volume in autoimmune inflammatory demyelinating lesions mimicking malignant gliomas. J Neurol. 2011;258(1):113–22.
23. Hiremath SB, Muraleedharan A, Kumar S, Nagesh C, Kesavadas C, Abraham M, et al. Combining diffusion tensor metrics and DSC perfusion imaging: can it improve the diagnostic accuracy in differentiating tumefactive demyelination from high-grade glioma? AJNR Am J Neuroradiol. 2017;38(4):685–90.
24. Abdoli M, Freedman MS. Neuro-oncology dilemma: tumour or tumefactive demyelinating lesion. Mult Scler Relat Disord. 2015;4(6):555–66.
25. Nafari A, Ghaffary EM, Shaygannejad V, Mirmosayyeb O. Concurrent glioma and multiple sclerosis: a systematic review of case reports. Mult Scler Relat Disord. 2024;84:105455.
26. Rees JH, Howard RS. High-grade glioma mimicking acute viral encephalitis—three case reports. Postgrad Med J. 1999;75(890):727–30.
27. Piper K, Foster H, Gabel B, Nabors B, Cobbs C. Glioblastoma mimicking viral encephalitis responds to acyclovir: a case series and literature review. Front Oncol. 2019;9:8.
28. Sahm K, Kessler T, Eisele P, Ratliff M, Sperk E, König L, et al. Concurrent gliomas in patients with multiple sclerosis. Commun Med. 2023;3(1):186.
29. Chen S, Tanaka S, Giannini C, Morris J, Yan ES, Buckner J, et al. Gliomatosis cerebri: clinical characteristics, management, and outcomes. J Neuro-Oncol. 2013;112(2):267–75.
30. McClain KL, Bigenwald C, Collin M, Haroche J, Marsh RA, Merad M, et al. Histiocytic disorders. Nat Rev Dis Primers. 2021;7(1):73.
31. Guyot-Goubin A, Donadieu J, Barkaoui M, Bellec S, Thomas C, Clavel J. Descriptive epidemiology of childhood Langerhans cell histiocytosis in France, 2000-2004. Pediatr Blood Cancer. 2008;51(1):71–5.
32. Tran TA, Fabre M, Pariente D, Craiu I, Haroche J, Charlotte F, et al. Erdheim-Chester disease in childhood: a challenging diagnosis and treatment. J Pediatr Hematol Oncol. 2009;31(10):782–6.
33. Janssen D, Harms D. Juvenile xanthogranuloma in childhood and adolescence: a clinicopathologic study of 129 patients from the Kiel pediatric tumor registry. Am J Surg Pathol. 2005;29(1):21–8.

34. Foucar E, Rosai J, Dorfman R. Sinus histiocytosis with massive lymphadenopathy (Rosai-Dorfman disease): review of the entity. Semin Diagn Pathol. 1990;7(1):19–73.
35. Ishii E, Ohga S, Imashuku S, Yasukawa M, Tsuda H, Miura I, et al. Nationwide survey of hemophagocytic lymphohistiocytosis in Japan. Int J Hematol. 2007;86(1):58–65.
36. Pastula DM, Burish M, Reis GF, Bollen A, Cha S, Ralph J, et al. Adult-onset central nervous system hemophagocytic lymphohistiocytosis: a case report. BMC Neurol. 2015;15:203.
37. Smith ME, Katz DA, Harris JO, Frank JA, Kufta CV, McFarlin DE. Systemic histiocytosis presenting as multiple sclerosis. Ann Neurol. 1993;33(5):549–54.
38. Sánchez-Villalobos JM, Jimeno-Almazán A, López-Peña C, Hernández-Hortelano E, Martínez-Francés A, Pérez-Vicente JA. Erdheim-Chester disease mimicking multiple sclerosis or a new association? Mult Scler Relat Disord. 2019;30:94–7.
39. Bohlega S, Alwatban J, Tulbah A, Bakheet SM, Powe J. Cerebral manifestation of Erdheim-Chester disease: clinical and radiologic findings. Neurology. 1997;49(6):1702–5.
40. Lachenal F, Cotton F, Desmurs-Clavel H, Haroche J, Taillia H, Magy N, et al. Neurological manifestations and neuroradiological presentation of Erdheim-Chester disease: report of 6 cases and systematic review of the literature. J Neurol. 2006;253(10):1267–77.
41. Haque A, Pérez CA, Reddy TA, Gupta RK. Erdheim-Chester disease with isolated CNS involvement: a systematic review of the literature. Neurol Int. 2022;14(3):716–26.
42. Gupta RK, Haque A, Reddy TA, Pérez CA. A patient with Erdheim-Chester disease limited to central nervous system. Neurol Int. 2022;14(3):678–82.
43. McFaline-Figueroa JR. Spinal cord neoplasms. Continuum (Minneap Minn). 2024;30(1):99–118.
44. Duong LM, McCarthy BJ, McLendon RE, Dolecek TA, Kruchko C, Douglas LL, et al. Descriptive epidemiology of malignant and nonmalignant primary spinal cord, spinal meninges, and cauda equina tumors, United States, 2004-2007. Cancer. 2012;118(17):4220–7.
45. Grossman RI, Yousem DM. Neuroradiology: the requisites. Mosby; 2003.
46. Zhuo Z, Zhang J, Duan Y, Qu L, Feng C, Huang X, et al. Automated classification of intramedullary spinal cord tumors and inflammatory demyelinating lesions using deep learning. Radiol Artif Intell. 2022;4(6):e210292.
47. Kageyama H, Suzuki T, Ohara Y. Intramedullary spinal cord germinoma clinically mimicking multiple sclerosis: a case report. Surg Neurol Int. 2019;10:201.
48. Psimaras D, Carpentier AF, Rossi C. Cerebrospinal fluid study in paraneoplastic syndromes. J Neurol Neurosurg Psychiatry. 2010;81(1):42–5.
49. Cohen O, Biran I, Steiner I. Cerebrospinal fluid oligoclonal IgG bands in patients with spinal arteriovenous malformation and structural central nervous system lesions. Arch Neurol. 2000;57(4):553–7.
50. Sener U, Kumthekar P, Boire A. Advances in the diagnosis, evaluation, and management of leptomeningeal disease. Neurooncol Adv. 2021;3(Suppl 5):v86–95.
51. Pajtler KW, Witt H, Sill M, Jones DT, Hovestadt V, Kratochwil F, et al. Molecular classification of ependymal tumors across all CNS compartments, histopathological grades, and age groups. Cancer Cell. 2015;27(5):728–43.
52. Shih RY, Koeller KK. Intramedullary Masses of the Spinal Cord: Radiologic-Pathologic Correlation. Radiographics. 2020;40(4):1125–45.
53. Braverman DL, Lachmann EA, Tunkel R, Nagler W. Multiple sclerosis presenting as a spinal cord tumor. Arch Phys Med Rehabil. 1997;78(11):1274–6.
54. Lammoglia FJ, Short SR, Sweet DE, Pay N, Abay EA 2nd. Multiple sclerosis presenting as an intramedullary cervical cord tumor. Kans Med. 1989;90(7):219–21, 28.
55. Selviaridis P, Zountsas B, Chatzisotiriou A, Zaraboukas T, Gerdemeli A. Demyelinating plaque imitates an intramedullary tumour. Clin Neurol Neurosurg. 2007;109(10):905–9.
56. Taricco MA, Machado A, Callegaro D, Marino R Jr. Spinal cord tumor in a patient with multiple sclerosis: case report. Arq Neuropsiquiatr. 2002;60(2-b):475–7.
57. Degirmenci E. Multiple sclerosis coexisting with spinal cord ependymoma: a case report. Ideggyogy Sz. 2012;65(9–10):342–4.

58. Safadi AL, Osborne B, Chitnis T, Graves JS, Newsome SD, Zamvil SS, et al. A 28-Year-Old Woman With Left-Sided Weakness and Atypical MRI Lesions: From the National Multiple Sclerosis Society Case Conference Proceedings. Neurol Neuroimmunol Neuroinflamm. 2023;10(6).
59. Graus F, Dalmau J. Paraneoplastic neurological syndromes in the era of immune-checkpoint inhibitors. Nat Rev Clin Oncol. 2019;16(9):535–48.
60. Farina A, Villagrán-García M, Vogrig A, Zekeridou A, Muñiz-Castrillo S, Velasco R, et al. Neurological adverse events of immune checkpoint inhibitors and the development of paraneoplastic neurological syndromes. Lancet Neurol. 2024;23(1):81–94.
61. Honnorat J, Antoine JC. Paraneoplastic neurological syndromes. Orphanet J Rare Dis. 2007;2:22.
62. Graus F, Vogrig A, Muñiz-Castrillo S, Antoine JG, Desestret V, Dubey D, et al. Updated diagnostic criteria for paraneoplastic neurologic syndromes. Neurol Neuroimmunol Neuroinflamm. 2021;8(4).
63. Ganaraja VH, Rezk M, Dubey D. Paraneoplastic neurological syndrome: growing spectrum and relevance. Neurol Sci. 2022;43(6):3583–94.
64. Abboud H, Probasco JC, Irani S, Ances B, Benavides DR, Bradshaw M, et al. Autoimmune encephalitis: proposed best practice recommendations for diagnosis and acute management. J Neurol Neurosurg Psychiatry. 2021;92(7):757–68.
65. Berger B, Bischler P, Dersch R, Hottenrott T, Rauer S, Stich O. "Non-classical" paraneoplastic neurological syndromes associated with well-characterized antineuronal antibodies as compared to "classical" syndromes – more frequent than expected. J Neurol Sci. 2015;352(1–2):58–61.
66. Giometto B, Grisold W, Vitaliani R, Graus F, Honnorat J, Bertolini G. Paraneoplastic neurologic syndrome in the PNS Euronetwork database: a European study from 20 centers. Arch Neurol. 2010;67(3):330–5.
67. Honnorat J, Didelot A, Karantoni E, Ville D, Ducray F, Lambert L, et al. Autoimmune limbic encephalopathy and anti-Hu antibodies in children without cancer. Neurology. 2013;80(24):2226–32.
68. Madhavan AA, Carr CM, Morris PP, Flanagan EP, Kotsenas AL, Hunt CH, et al. Imaging review of paraneoplastic neurologic syndromes. AJNR Am J Neuroradiol. 2020;41(12):2176–87.
69. Lee HR, Lennon VA, Camilleri M, Prather CM. Paraneoplastic gastrointestinal motor dysfunction: clinical and laboratory characteristics. Am J Gastroenterol. 2001;96(2):373–9.
70. Bost C, Chanson E, Picard G, Meyronet D, Mayeur ME, Ducray F, et al. Malignant tumors in autoimmune encephalitis with anti-NMDA receptor antibodies. J Neurol. 2018;265(10):2190–200.
71. Mustafa R, Zalewski NL, Flanagan EP, Kumar N. Challenging myelopathy cases. Semin Neurol. 2022;42(6):723–34.
72. Cross SA, Salomao DR, Parisi JE, Kryzer TJ, Bradley EA, Mines JA, et al. Paraneoplastic autoimmune optic neuritis with retinitis defined by CRMP-5-IgG. Ann Neurol. 2003;54(1):38–50.
73. Rojas I, Graus F, Keime-Guibert F, Reñé R, Delattre JY, Ramón JM, et al. Long-term clinical outcome of paraneoplastic cerebellar degeneration and anti-Yo antibodies. Neurology. 2000;55(5):713–5.
74. Ostrom QT, Cioffi G, Waite K, Kruchko C, Barnholtz-Sloan JS. CBTRUS statistical report: primary brain and other central nervous system tumors diagnosed in the United States in 2014-2018. Neuro-Oncology. 2021;23(12 Suppl 2):iii1–iii105.
75. Schaff L. Central nervous system lymphoma. Continuum (Minneap Minn). 2023;29(6):1710–26.
76. Bataille B, Delwail V, Menet E, Vandermarcq P, Ingrand P, Wager M, et al. Primary intracerebral malignant lymphoma: report of 248 cases. J Neurosurg. 2000;92(2):261–6.
77. Schlegel U. Primary CNS lymphoma. Ther Adv Neurol Disord. 2009;2(2):93–104.
78. Husseini L, Saleh A, Reifenberger G, Hartung HP, Kieseier BC. Inflammatory demyelinating brain lesions heralding primary CNS lymphoma. Can J Neurol Sci. 2012;39(1):6–10.

79. Hunt MA, Jahnke K, Murillo TP, Neuwelt EA. Distinguishing primary central nervous system lymphoma from other central nervous system diseases: a neurosurgical perspective on diagnostic dilemmas and approaches. Neurosurg Focus. 2006;21(5):E3.
80. Barajas RF, Politi LS, Anzalone N, Schöder H, Fox CP, Boxerman JL, et al. Consensus recommendations for MRI and PET imaging of primary central nervous system lymphoma: guideline statement from the International Primary CNS Lymphoma Collaborative Group (IPCG). Neuro-Oncology. 2021;23(7):1056–71.
81. Küker W, Nägele T, Korfel A, Heckl S, Thiel E, Bamberg M, et al. Primary central nervous system lymphomas (PCNSL): MRI features at presentation in 100 patients. J Neuro-Oncol. 2005;72(2):169–77.
82. Kalus S, Di Muzio B, Gaillard F. Demyelination preceding a diagnosis of central nervous system lymphoma. J Clin Neurosci. 2016;24:146–8.
83. Abrey LE, Batchelor TT, Ferreri AJ, Gospodarowicz M, Pulczynski EJ, Zucca E, et al. Report of an international workshop to standardize baseline evaluation and response criteria for primary CNS lymphoma. J Clin Oncol. 2005;23(22):5034–43.
84. Chiavazza C, Pellerino A, Ferrio F, Cistaro A, Soffietti R, Rudà R. Primary CNS lymphomas: challenges in diagnosis and monitoring. Biomed Res Int. 2018;2018:3606970.
85. Ohe Y, Hayashi T, Mishima K, Nishikawa R, Sasaki A, Matsuda H, et al. Central nervous system lymphoma initially diagnosed as tumefactive multiple sclerosis after brain biopsy. Intern Med. 2013;52(4):483–8.
86. Bromberg JE, Siemers MD, Taphoorn MJ. Is a "vanishing tumor" always a lymphoma? Neurology. 2002;59(5):762–4.
87. Kvarta MD, Sharma D, Castellani RJ, Morales RE, Reich SG, Kimball AS, et al. Demyelination as a harbinger of lymphoma: a case report and review of primary central nervous system lymphoma preceded by multifocal sentinel demyelination. BMC Neurol. 2016;16:72.
88. Carnevale J, Rubenstein JL. The challenge of primary central nervous system lymphoma. Hematol Oncol Clin North Am. 2016;30(6):1293–316.
89. Jiménez de la Peña MD, Vicente LG, Alonso RC, Cabero SF, Suárez AM, de Vega VM. The multiple faces of nervous system lymphoma. Atypical magnetic resonance imaging features and contribution of the advanced imaging. Curr Probl Diagn Radiol. 2017;46(2):136–45.
90. Scott BJ, Douglas VC, Tihan T, Rubenstein JL, Josephson SA. A systematic approach to the diagnosis of suspected central nervous system lymphoma. JAMA Neurol. 2013;70(3):311–9.
91. Fischer L, Jahnke K, Martus P, Weller M, Thiel E, Korfel A. The diagnostic value of cerebrospinal fluid pleocytosis and protein in the detection of lymphomatous meningitis in primary central nervous system lymphomas. Haematologica. 2006;91(3):429–30.
92. Nguyen-Them L, Alentorn A, Ahle G, Soussain C, Mathon B, Le Garff TM, et al. CSF biomarkers in primary CNS lymphoma. Rev Neurol. 2023;179(3):141–9.
93. Dux R, Kindler-Röhrborn A, Annas M, Faustmann P, Lennartz K, Zimmermann CW. A standardized protocol for flow cytometric analysis of cells isolated from cerebrospinal fluid. J Neurol Sci. 1994;121(1):74–8.
94. Bogdahn U, Bogdahn S, Mertens HG, Dommasch D, Wodarz R, Wünsch PH, et al. Primary non-Hodgkin's lymphomas of the CNS. Acta Neurol Scand. 1986;73(6):602–14.
95. Herrlinger U, Schabet M, Bitzer M, Petersen D, Krauseneck P. Primary central nervous system lymphoma: from clinical presentation to diagnosis. J Neuro-Oncol. 1999;43(3):219–26.
96. Schaff LR, Grommes C. Primary central nervous system lymphoma. Blood. 2022;140(9):971–9.
97. Naeem SB, Niazi F, Baig A, Sadiq H, Sattar M. Primary CNS lymphoma vs. tumefactive multiple sclerosis: a diagnostic challenge. J Coll Physicians Surg Pak. 2018;28(1):66–8.
98. Barrantes-Freer A, Engel AS, Rodríguez-Villagra OA, Winkler A, Bergmann M, Mawrin C, et al. Diagnostic red flags: steroid-treated malignant CNS lymphoma mimicking autoimmune inflammatory demyelination. Brain Pathol. 2018;28(2):225–33.
99. Adam G, Ferrier M, Patsoura S, Gramada R, Meluchova Z, Cazzola V, et al. Magnetic resonance imaging of arterial stroke mimics: a pictorial review. Insights Imaging. 2018;9(5):815–31.

100. Nabors LB, Portnow J, Ahluwalia M, Baehring J, Brem H, Brem S, et al. Central Nervous System Cancers, Version 3.2020, NCCN Clinical Practice Guidelines in Oncology. J Natl Compr Canc Netw. 2020;18(11):1537–70.
101. Costanzi C, Bourdette D, Parisi JE, Woltjer R, Rodriguez F, Steensma D, et al. Crystal-storing histiocytosis: an unusual relapsing inflammatory CNS disorder. Mult Scler Relat Disord. 2012;1(2):95–9.
102. Kaminsky IA, Wang AM, Olsen J, Schechter S, Wilson J, Olson R. Central nervous system crystal-storing histiocytosis: neuroimaging, neuropathology, and literature review. AJNR Am J Neuroradiol. 2011;32(2):E26–8.
103. Prakhova L, Lebedev V, Ilves A, Nazinkina Y. Monoclonal gammopathy of undetermined significance (MGUS) manifestation in CNS: a regular or chance occurrence? BMJ Case Rep. 2021;14(3).
104. Kaur J, Valisekka SS, Hameed M, Bandi PS, Varma S, Onwughalu CJ, et al. Monoclonal gammopathy of undetermined significance: a comprehensive review. Clin Lymphoma Myeloma Leuk. 2023;23(5):e195–212.

Primary Eye Diseases 10

10.1 Chronic Relapsing Inflammatory Optic Neuropathy (CRION)

10.1.1 Epidemiology

- A rare and underdiagnosed disorder with an unknown prevalence.
- Women are more commonly affected [1].
- A study of 214 patients with symptomatic optic neuritis found that 12 patients (5.6%) had CRION [2].

10.1.2 Etiology and Definition

- The exact pathogenesis of CRION is unclear, but it is considered to be at least partially immune-mediated.
- CRION is recognized as a distinct nosological entity separate from neuromyelitis optica spectrum disorders (NMOSD), myelin oligodendrocyte glycoprotein antibody-associated disease (MOGAD), or multiple sclerosis (MS) [1]. Some authors do not classify CRION as a distinct disease entity but rather as a clinical phenotype of any other aggressive systemic autoimmunity [3].

10.1.3 Clinical Features

- Visual loss is often severe. Approximately 28% of patients do not perceive light, compared to only 3.1% of those with MS [4].
- Another potential deficit may include constricted visual field (43%), altitudinal pattern of field loss (17%), central scotoma (17%), or uveitis (rare; 0–7%) [5].

T. Uher, *Mimics and Red Flags of Multiple Sclerosis*,
https://doi.org/10.1007/978-3-031-98945-2_10

- Periorbital pain is often severe, and may interfere with sleep, which is not typical for MS. The pain is often provoked by eye movement and worsens before or simultaneously with the reduction in vision. In rare cases, there is no pain.
- There is a prompt response to treatment with systemic corticosteroids. However, relapses often occur within days to months after tapering or withdrawing corticosteroids, resembling the pattern seen in granulomatous optic neuropathies or MOGAD.
- Almost all patients exhibit swollen or pale discs and positive relative afferent pupillary defect (RAPD) (in case of unilateral neuropathy) [1, 5].

10.1.4 Disease Course

- Relapsing-remitting subacute vision loss.
- Bilateral neuropathy is common (59%). Relapses typically occur sequentially (93%) rather than simultaneously (7%), with a latency period between involvement of both eyes ranging from weeks to several months.
- The mean age of symptoms onset is 35.7 years (range, 14–69) [1].

10.1.5 Brain and Spinal Cord Imaging

- Normal brain magnetic resonance imaging (MRI) (40%) [1].
- Unspecific focal T2 hyperintensities in brain (60%) [1, 6].
- Some patients might have MRI findings that fulfill criteria for dissemination in space, which can mimic MS [7].
- MRI of the affected optic nerve often reveals thickening, increased signal, or contrast enhancement (63%) [5].
- Advanced non-conventional imaging techniques have revealed microstructural changes in the optic chiasm and white matter of the brain [6].
- The spinal cord typically appears normal [1].

10.1.6 Blood Work

- There is no diagnostic blood biomarker [1].
- Patients do not exhibit increased concentrations of glial fibrillary acidic protein (GFAP) compared to patients with NMOSD, who almost always have elevated GFAP during relapses [8].
- Patients with relapsing inflammatory optic neuritis and corticosteroid dependency without the anti-aquaporin-4 (AQP4) immunoglobulin G (IgG) positivity should be tested for anti-MOG IgG [2, 10].

10.1.7 Examination of CSF

- Concentration of protein and cytology are usually normal.
- Cerebrospinal fluid (CSF)-restricted oligoclonal bands (OCB) are absent, but around 30% of patients have identical OCB in CSF and serum (pattern IV; mirror pattern) [5].

10.1.8 OCT

- On optical coherence tomography (OCT), the global, temporal, inferior, nasal, and superior quadrants of the retinal nerve fiber layer (RNFL) and ganglion cell layer (GCL) are significantly thinner in CRION patients compared to those with MS or NMOSD [2, 11].

10.1.9 Electrophysiology

- Visual evoked responses (VEP) demonstrate prolongation in latency without significant amplitude decrease or conduction block [5].

10.1.10 Diagnosis

- Many patients previously labeled as CRION (before anti-MOG-IgG testing became widely available) were later found to be anti-MOG-IgG positive. As a result, CRION is now considered a shrinking category, largely reserved for rare cases of seronegative relapsing optic neuritis. A diagnosis of CRION requires the exclusion of other neurological, ophthalmological, and systemic conditions, along with confirmation of the following five points:
    1. History of optic neuritis and ≥1 relapse.
    2. Objective clinical evidence of visual loss.
    3. Imaging: contrast enhancement of the optic nerve during the relapse.
    4. Laboratory: absence of anti-AQP4 IgG and anti-MOG IgG in blood.
    5. Response to immunosuppressive treatment and relapse upon withdrawal or dose reduction of this treatment [1].

10.1.11 Differential Diagnosis

- MS:
    - Compared with MS, CRION tends to result in more severe visual loss and pain. There is a clear dependence on corticosteroids, absence of CSF-restricted OCB, and MRI findings are often normal [5].
    - Recurrence of pain or deterioration in vision after reducing corticosteroids is a red flag for optic neuritis in MS. In these cases, alternative diagnoses such as NMOSD, MOGAD, sarcoidosis, or CRION should be suspected [1].

- SLE and Sarcoidosis:
  - In cases of suspected autoimmune etiology, it is recommended to examine antinuclear antibodies (ANA) titers. If positive, especially in young individuals, a more detailed laboratory work-up is necessary to rule out systemic autoimmune diseases, such as systemic lupus erythematosus (SLE) [1].
  - CRION-like presentations can be also observed in some other systemic autoimmune diseases. It cannot be ruled out that some patients presenting with CRION may eventually be diagnosed with a localized form of granulomatous disease, such as sarcoidosis, in the future [5].
- Ischemic and Hereditary Optic Neuropathies:
  - Conditions such as anterior ischemic optic neuropathy, posterior ischemic optic neuropathy, or giant cell arteritis can sometimes be difficult to distinguish from CRION. Additionally, primary ocular causes, such as posterior scleritis, maculopathies, and retinopathies must be excluded.
  - Suspecting a large list of hereditary optic atrophies, including the most frequent Leber hereditary optic neuropathy (LHON) and dominant optic atrophy, is particularly warranted when there is a positive family history [1].

10.1.12 Treatment and Prognosis

- Hyperacute corticosteroid treatment can prevent progression to severe visual loss during a relapse [12].
- Abrupt corticosteroid withdrawal may result in relapse and irreversible visual loss. Therefore, prolonged treatment with medium-dose corticosteroids is required in the majority of cases, and any reduction in dosage must be done very slowly, with close monitoring for evidence of relapsing activity [5].
- B-cell targeted treatments might be effective in CRION [2].
- Complete restoration of visual loss may occur even months after the onset.
- Outcome without treatment is likely to be very poor with a severe visual loss, but prognosis can vary widely [2, 5].
- Disease activity can settle over a decade [1].

10.2 Leber Hereditary Optic Atrophy (LHON)

10.2.1 Epidemiology

- Prevalence 2–3/100.000 (>30.000 patients in Europe) [13, 14].
- Female/male ratio 1/3.3 (owing to higher penetrance in males) [16].
- However, coexistence of LHON and MS is more frequent in females (66%) [15].

10.2.2 Etiology and Definition

- A maternally inherited mitochondrial disease [13] with an incomplete penetrance [16]. Three pathogenic mitochondrial deoxyribonucleic acid (mtDNA) variants account for 90–95% of cases.
- The retinal ganglion cells are preferentially affected. This leads to optic nerve degeneration [13, 16].
- The coexistence of LHON and MS (LHON-MS; "Harding's disease") occurs more frequently in patients with relapsing-remitting MS; (70%) than with primary progressive MS (30%). LHON-MS occurs 50 times more frequently than would be expected by chance [15, 17, 18].
- mtDNA mutations in LHON might not directly affect the risk of developing MS. However, they could potentially modify the course of MS through shared molecular pathways. The occurrence of mtDNA LHON mutations in individuals with MS might lead to atypical optic neuritis, characterized by increased severity, lack of pain, and irreversibility of visual loss. Conversely, the presence of MS might trigger LHON in individuals who would otherwise have remained asymptomatic, or it could be associated with greater severity of LHON [14].

10.2.3 Clinical Features

- Many patients with positive genetic testing for LHON are asymptomatic due to incomplete penetrance [16].
- Optic neuropathy
  - Typically bilateral.
  - Severe (often complete) visual loss.
  - Without or with only minimal and temporary recovery of visual loss.
  - There is no effect of corticosteroids [13, 18].
  - Sometime with loss of color vision and reduced contrast sensitivity resembling deficit in MS [19].
- May be present extra-ocular manifestations ("LHON plus syndromes"):
  - Cardiac arrhythmias; cardiomyopathy; tremor; ataxia; dementia; movement disorders; peripheral neuropathy; deformities of the vertebral column; seizures; or a MS-like presentations [13, 20].
- LHON-MS is characterized by:
  - More aggressive course with more frequent episodes of visual loss, a longer interval before the fellow eye becomes affected (on average 1.7 years), absence of eye pain, and a poorer visual outcome. This stands in contrast to patients with stand-alone LHON, who experience visual events less frequently, with both eyes being almost always affected within 6 months.
  - In contrast to MS, patients with LHON-MS typically experience little to no ocular pain (present in only 20%), a lack of visual recovery in most patients, and a poor visual outcome, often with blindness (50%) [18].

10.2.4 Disease Course

- The age of symptom onset is typically in early adulthood (<50 years)
- Begins with a subacute onset, followed by a plateau phase, and then transitions to a slowly progressive phase after 12 months [13, 14].

10.2.5 Brain and Spinal Cord Imaging

- Patients with a stand-alone LHON have often normal MRI findings, but some may have unspecific white matter lesions and/or a high signal or atrophy of the optic nerves.
- MRI in LHON-MS is similar as seen in patients with MS, but imaging of optic nerve usually does not show focal T2 lesions [21].
- If present spinal cord lesions, they are often atypical and may suggest comorbid MS [22].

10.2.6 Examination of Blood and CSF

- Some patients may have elevated concentrations of lactate and pyruvate in blood and CSF. The changes are more subtle compared with the other mitochondrial genetic disorders. Otherwise, the routine testing of blood and CSF findings in stand-alone LHON should be normal [13, 23].
- Occurrence of CSF-restricted OCB in the stand-alone LHON is unknown, but is expected to be negative. The frequency of CSF-restricted OCB in the LHON-MS copies findings in MS [15].

10.2.7 OCT

- Thinning of the retinal nerve fiber layer (RNFL), especially in the papillomacular bundle. The thinning may be masked in acute phase by the swelling. The RNFL thinning has a preferential loss of nerve fibers in the temporal (outer) quadrant of the optic nerve head but progress over time to all quadrants [24].

10.2.8 Electrophysiology

- VEP show abnormalities, often also in asymptomatic carriers [13, 25].

10.2.9 Diagnosis

- Genetic testing in clinically suspected cases [13]
- Screening of LHON in MS patients with atypical, severe or bilateral optic nerve involvement may identify LHON mutations in 1–15% of MS patients [15].

10.2.10 Treatment and Prognosis

- Idebenone may have some positive effect in early disease stages [26].
- LHON-MS is associated with a high likelihood of severe visual disability. In this respect, early disease-modifying therapy to prevent relapses is recommended despite the uncertainty relating to long-term benefits [18].
- Patients with a pre-excitation syndrome on electrocardiogram (ECG) should be referred to a cardiologist [13].

10.3 Neuroretinitis

10.3.1 Epidemiology

- A rare, likely underdiagnosed condition.

10.3.2 Etiology and Definition

- Caused by fluid leakage at the optic disc (not the macula) due to inflammation of unknown origin. This condition also involves fluid accumulation behind the macula, followed by its resorption, which leaves behind hard exudates in a star-shaped pattern [27–29].

10.3.3 Clinical Features

- Triad of:
  A. Subacute visual loss
     - Almost always unilateral
  B. Optic disc edema
  C. Macular star
     - Develops after 9–12 days (rarely up to 6 weeks)

10.3.4 Non-Infectious Subtypes

- Idiopathic
  - Typically occurs in young adults.
  - Often preceded by influenza-like illness (50%).
  - Visual loss is usually unilateral and painless.
  - Visual acuity ranges from 6/6 to perception of light.
  - Color vision may be impaired.
  - Typically results in central or centrocecal visual field loss.
  - Positive relative afferent pupillary defect (RAPD) (70%).
  - Most cases resolve spontaneously without treatment within 3 months.
  - Many authors recommend corticosteroids and antibiotics, at least until infectious causes have been ruled out.
  - Usually monophasic, only rarely recurrent.
  - Recurrent idiopathic neuroretinitis (RINR) has a relatively poor visual prognosis and long-term immunosuppression is required to prevent vision loss.
- Inflammatory
  - Probably underdiagnosed condition, which is often associated with the following inflammatory conditions:
    MOGAD
    Vogt–Koyanagi–Harada syndrome (bilateral granulomatous panuveitis)
    Polyarteritis nodosa
    Behçet's disease
    Sarcoidosis
    Inflammatory bowel disease
    Post-rabies vaccination
    Parry–Romberg syndrome (Progressive unilateral facial hemiatrophy of suspected autoimmune origin, which may represent a variant of localized scleroderma)
    Tubulointerstitial nephritis and uveitis
    Idiopathic retinal vasculitis, aneurysms, and neuroretinitis
      - Extremely rare
      - Raised intracranial pressure not responding to acetazolamide

10.3.5 Infectious Subtypes

- Cat scratch disease (Bartonella henselae) is the cause in most infectious cases (70%).
- Other common infections include syphilis, or tuberculosis.
- Other bacterial, viral, fungal, and parasitic organisms contribute to the wide spectrum of potential causative agents, including borrelia; leptospira; herpes simplex virus (HSV); varicella zoster virus (VZV); measles virus; Epstein-Barr virus (EBV); cytomegalovirus (CMV); hepatitis B virus (HBV); coxsackievirus B; or toxoplasma.

- Treatment typically includes antibiotics and corticosteroids.
- Compared to the idiopathic subtype, additional areas of focal chorioretinitis may be present [27–29].

10.3.6 Brain Imaging

- Often present contrast enhancement of the optic disc extending for a short segment of the optic nerve or enhancement of the optic nerve sheath [30, 31].
- MS-like brain lesions on MRI may possibly occur in some patients with neuroretinitis, particularly in those with hypertension [32].

10.3.7 OCT

- Subretinal fluid and thickening of the neurosensory retina and retinal exudates in the outer plexiform layer corresponding to the macular star [29].

10.3.8 Examination of Blood and CSF

- Routine blood tests in idiopathic subtype should be normal.
- In the case of infectious neuroretinitis may be elevated titers of antibodies against various infectious agents or elevated markers of systemic inflammation.

10.3.9 Diagnosis

- Ophthalmological examination, optic nerve MRI, OCT with angiography [27–29].

10.3.10 Differential Diagnosis

- Diagnosis can pose significant challenges for neurologists. Detecting the macular star necessitates detailed ocular examination, close monitoring, and collaboration with ophthalmologists.
- Neuroretinitis is often misdiagnosed as idiopathic demyelinating optic neuritis associated with MS and NMOSD or other optic neuropathies owing to:
  - Macular star formation typically occurs after 9–12 days (with a range extending up to 6 weeks), making it challenging to diagnose the condition during the initial days of disease onset.
  - Some macular stars may be imperfectly formed.
  - Similar ophthalmological findings may also be observed in other conditions, such as:

Hypertensive retinopathy
Papilledema (increased intracranial pressure; for example, in idiopathic intracranial hypertension)
Anterior ischemic optic neuropathy
Diabetic papillopathy
Local ophthalmic pathology (branch retinal vein occlusion, disc and juxtapapillary tumors, arteriovenous malformations, posterior vitreous traction)
Toxic etiologies (procarbazine, bis-chloroethylnitrosourea)

- Clinical red flags suggesting possible neuroretinitis
  - Pre-existing known inflammatory or infective disease
  - History of exposure to animals (especially cats), or overseas travel
  - History of preceding influenza-like illness or systemic symptoms
  - Lack of ocular pain in association with visual loss
  - Lack of RAPD in association with a central scotoma
- Eye red flags preceding development of macular star
  - Cells in the posterior vitreous (and possibly anterior chamber)
  - OCT may show subretinal fluid and inflammatory cells in vitreous, which are not seen in papilledema or ischemic optic neuropathy
  - Fluorescein angiography may show segmental disc involvement [27–29]
- Whether a neuroretinitis is associated with a higher risk for the future development of MS remains controversial [27, 33].
- However, neuroretinitis may coexist with MS, typically manifesting in later disease stages rather than as an initial presenting event. Speculations have arisen regarding whether treatment with interferons may act as a causative agent of neuroretinitis in some MS patients [34]. The causal relationship between neuroretinitis and MS remains unclear, and it is uncertain whether their occurrence is purely coincidental. Similarly, the question of whether an episode of neuroretinitis should be considered a demyelinating attack remains unanswered [33].

10.4 Non-arteritic Anterior Ischemic Optic Neuropathy (NAION)

10.4.1 Epidemiology

- Incidence 2.3–10.2/100.000/year (USA).
- The most common cause of optic neuropathy and optic nerve swelling in patients older than 50 years.
- Caucasians are more frequently affected [35].

10.4.2 Subtypes of Ischemic Optic Neuropathies

- Anterior ischemic neuropathy (pathology in the anterior portion of the optic nerve):
  - Non-arteritic (NAION).
  - Arteritic: associated with giant cell arteritis (also known as cranial arteritis; granulomatous arteritis; temporal arteritis or Horton's disease).
- Posterior ischemic neuropathy (pathology in the posterior portion of the optic nerve).
  - Non-arteritic (NPION) [36].

10.4.3 Etiology and Definition

- NAION is caused by restricted blood flow in the posterior ciliary arteries that supply blood to the optic nerve head (optic disc), resulting in an acute ischemic infarction of the axons in the optic nerve. It is primarily a hypotensive disorder and does not share mechanisms like those in stroke or thromboembolic disease in the vast majority of patients.
- Most frequently occurs in older patients and is often associated with vascular risk factors, such as hypertension, diabetes, sleep apnea, atherosclerosis, hypercoagulable states, migraine, prothrombotic state, and some medications (sildenafil, interferon-alpha, amiodarone, oral contraceptives, sumatriptan, anti-thrombotic agents, beta-blockers, statins, anti-hypertensives), infections (syphilis, rickettsia, hepatitis C virus [HCV], Borrelia burgdorferi, HSV, Chlamydia pneumoniae, severe acute respiratory syndrome coronavirus 2 [SARS-CoV-2]) and vaccinations.
- Generalized hypo-perfusion, nocturnal hypotension, vasospasm, impaired local blood flow autoregulation and congenital-variant anatomy of the optic nerve head are suggested as possible mechanisms. However, in most cases the cause remains unclear.
- Despite associated with several vascular risk factors, patients with NAION do not have increased risks of carotid stenosis, cardiac disease, or stroke [35–40].
- Although NAION has several genetic associations, including glycoprotein Ib platelet subunit alpha (GP1ab) polymorphisms, familial mitochondrial mutations, or *COL4A2* mutation, familial NAION is exceptionally rare [39, 41, 42].
- Arteritic anterior ischemic optic neuropathy (AAION) is associated with giant cell arteritis and typically causes more severe vision loss [39].

10.4.4 Clinical Features

- Visual loss:
  - Sudden unilateral.
  - Only rarely bilateral with sequential involvement of both eyes. The cumulative probability of the fellow eye developing NAION ranges between 15 and 25% within 3–5 years. Simultaneous bilateral onset is exceedingly rare and may occur in patients experiencing sudden and severe arterial hypotension, such as during shock.
  - Involves field defect and visual acuity loss.
  - Any pattern may occur, but altitudinal loss (usually inferior nasal), arcuate defect (55–80%) and central scotomas (20–25%) are most frequent.
  - Visual acuity varies from mild defects to no light perception, but very poor vision (hand motions or worse) is uncommon and should raise the suspicion for giant cell arteritis. In general, the visual loss tends to be worse compared to visual deficit in MS.
  - Often impaired color perception.
  - Photophobia might occur.
- Pain
  - Frequently absent, with only 8–15% of patients reporting discomfort or pain in or around the eye. This is unlike demyelinating optic neuritis, where pain with eye movements is typical and occurs in 94% of cases.
- Optic nerve edema
  - Occurs in all patients.
  - Sectorial or diffuse optic nerve head edema.
  - Persists for 4–6 weeks after onset.
  - In contrast, in demyelinating optic neuritis, optic nerve head edema is absent or only mild and usually without peripapillary hemorrhages (present in only 5% of patients).
  - Disc pallor starts to develop 2–3 weeks after the symptom's onset.
- Almost always present relative afferent pupillary defect (RAPD).
- There are no additional neurological manifestations.

10.4.5 Disease Course

- The mean age at symptom onset is 57–65 years; rarely occurs in young age.
- Acute onset of vision loss, not subacute or semi-acute as typically observed in optic neuritis.
- Symptoms firstly detected by patients often upon awakening (40–70%).
- The severity of symptoms either remains stable over time (65%) or worsens gradually over a period of days to 6–12 weeks, manifesting in either a steady or episodic manner before stabilizing.

- Nadir at disease onset or progress to peak visual loss over a week or more.
- Visual loss worsening can be usually attributed to a progression of NAION, rather than new episodes of NAION [36, 39, 40, 43–45].

10.4.6 Brain Imaging

- Usually normal, including MRI of the orbits [36, 40, 46].

10.4.7 Examination of Blood and CSF

- Routine testing is usually normal.

10.4.8 OCT

- In the acute stage, there is a thickening of the retinal nerve fiber layer (RNFL).
- "Disc at risk," cup to disc ratio of 0.2 or less in the fellow eye is almost always present (95%); if not the diagnosis of NAION should be questioned.
- The acute retinal swelling is followed by RNFL thinning in chronic stages [36].

10.4.9 Electrophysiology

- VEP show a reduction in amplitude, whereas in demyelinating optic neuritis is usually observed a reduction in the wave P100 latency [47].

10.4.10 Diagnosis

- Primarily based on clinical features, all patients must have optic nerve edema, and alternative etiologies must be excluded.
- Patients should undergo the following assessments:
  - Blood count, erythrocyte sedimentation rate (ESR), and C-reactive protein (CRP)
  - Evaluation of vascular risk factors (blood pressure, lipid profile, and glucose levels and others)
  - Screening for sleep apnea
  - Detailed medication history with a focus on drugs associated with nocturnal hypotension and phosphodiesterase (PDE) inhibitors
  - In younger patients (under age 50), assessment of homocysteine levels and hypercoagulable states [36, 40, 48]

10.4.11 Differential Diagnosis

- Posterior non-arteritic anterior ischemic optic neuropathy (NPION).
  - 9-times less common compared to NAION
  - Always a diagnosis of exclusion, because the typical funduscopic changes of anterior ischemic optic neuropathy are not seen, and a positive RAPD is nonspecific
- Giant cell arteritis
  - Mean age of symptoms onset around 70–75 years of age
  - Elevated inflammatory markers in blood (ESR; Leukocyte count; CRP)
  - Visual loss is usually more severe than in NAION
  - Visual loss is isolated (20%) or combined with other systemic manifestations (80%) such as:
    Headache/neck pain
    Jaw claudication
    Scalp/temporal tenderness
    Polymyalgia
    Fatigue/malaise
    Weight loss/anorexia
    Eye pain
    Diplopia
  - Temporal artery biopsy is the gold standard for diagnosis
- Demyelinating optic neuritis (MS, NMOSD, MOGAD).
  - Especially in patients under 50 years of age
  - Often associated with pain upon eye movements (94%)
  - Only rarely peripapillary hemorrhages (5%)
  - Often improving visual function. This stands in contrast to patients with NAION, where visual deficits tend to persist without major improvement.
  - Visual field loss tends to be central in optic neuritis rather than altitudinal as in NAION.
  - Only 35% of patients with acute optic neuritis exhibit mild to moderate disc swelling (less pronounced than in NAION). The remaining patients initially present with normal optic discs and are classified as retrobulbar neuritis. In NAION is marked disc swelling almost always present.
  - Disc swelling is usually vertically symmetric rather than segmental, as seen in NAION.
  - MRI may show contrast enhancement or lesional pathology of the optic nerves, which is typically absent in NAION.
  - MOGAD-associated optic neuritis is often associated with swollen optic nerve and hemorrhages but is associated with an improvement of visual loss and good prognosis as opposed to patients with NAION.

- Medication-associated NAION:
  - All patients should also be asked about their use of amiodarone; phosphodiesterase inhibitors, such as sildenafil; interferon-alpha; oral contraceptives; or prolonged and high-dose systemic corticosteroids. NAION may improve after discontinuation of these drugs.
- Compressive optic neuropathies (tumors, inflammatory conditions).
  - May be associated with swollen optic nerve, but typically is associated with an insidious onset, slowly progressive visual loss and optic atrophy.
- Retinal artery and vein occlusions.
  - Hyperacute onset, nadir of visual loss within minutes to hours, altitudinal or another visual field deficit. Patients usually have vascular risk factors.
  - The clinical manifestations are very similar to NAION, but funduscopic examination does not reveal severe optic disc swelling as seen in NAION.
  - Within hours from onset occurs superficial retinal edema with no optic disc swelling allowing distinguishing from NAION.
  - Unlike NAION, these conditions are frequently associated with atherosclerotic carotid disease and cardiogenic embolus, necessitating an evaluation similar to that for stroke.
- Diabetic papillopathy.
  - Diagnostic criteria require the presence of diabetes type 1 or 2 and other characteristic ophthalmological features, including unilateral or bilateral optic disc edema [36, 39, 40, 49].

10.4.12 Treatment and Prognosis

- There are no class I studies showing benefit from either medical or surgical treatments. Recommendations include optimizing vascular risk factors. The use of oral corticosteroids, intravitreal injections of corticosteroids, or anti-vascular endothelial growth factor agents remains a subject of controversy.
- Visual acuity typically remains stable in most patients after the acute event has resolved. However, spontaneous visual improvement may occur in some patients (41–43%), whereas others may experience worsening.
- NAION may lead to atrophy to the optic nerve and permanent blindness [36, 39, 50].

10.5 Retinal Vasculopathy with Cerebral Leukoencephalopathy and Systemic Manifestations (RVCL-S)

Synonyms: Historical descriptions have encompassed various terms, including: Cerebroretinal vasculopathy; Hereditary vascular retinopathy; Hereditary endotheliopathy, Retinopathy, nephropathy, and stroke; Hereditary systemic angiopathy; and Retinal vasculopathy with cerebral leukodystrophy.

10.5.1 Epidemiology

- Rare, underdiagnosed disease with unknown prevalence.
- Worldwide reported only dozens of families [51, 52].

10.5.2 Etiology and Definition

- Late-onset autosomal dominant microangiopathy with high penetrance attributed to mutations in the *TREX1* gene.
- Systemic small vessel endotheliopathy, which disrupts the vascular basal membrane and results in progressive diminishment of microvascular blood flow [51, 52].
- Other TREX1 mutations cause:
  - Aicardi-Goutiéres syndrome.
  - Autosomal dominant familial chilblain lupus.
  - SLE [51].

10.5.3 Clinical Features

- Visual symptoms due to vascular retinopathy (almost 100%):
  - Usually an initial clinical symptom.
  - Retinal micro-infarcts, sometime also hemorrhages.
  - Fundoscopy and fluorescein angiogram show telangiectasias, microaneurysms, cotton wool spots, later perifoveal capillary obliteration, and neovascularization [51, 53].
  - May be confused with diabetic, hypertensive or radiation retinopathy, branch retinal vein occlusion, infectious retinitis, sickle cell disease, and collagen vascular disease [54].
- Systemic Manifestations:
  - Anemia (74%), liver disease (70%), arterial hypertension (58%), nephropathy (49%), Raynaud syndrome (42%), subclinical hypothyroidism (37%), gastrointestinal bleeding (22%).
- Neurological Manifestations (26%):
  - Brain infarctions
  - Focal deficits (68%), migraine (53%), acute or progressive cognitive impairment (47%), psychiatric symptoms (39%), seizures (14%).
  - Tend to occur in later disease stages, as compared to visual and systemic manifestations. In contrast, migraine or Raynaud phenomenon may precede occurrence of visual symptoms and brain lesions up to 20 years [51, 53].
- The age of symptoms onset is between 35 and 50 years.
- Mutation carriers are seldom asymptomatic [51, 52].

10.5.4 Brain Imaging

- Small punctate to medium size white matter lesions (97%).
  - Mainly supratentorial.
  - Can be Dawson fingers and ovoid periventricular white matter lesions.
  - Spared subcortical U-fibers, corpus callosum, and gray matter.
  - Without or with temporary or permanent contrast enhancement.
  - May be restricted diffusion in center and the periphery of lesions.
  - Occurring of new lesions and sometime progression from small non-enhancing lesions to enhancing or tumor-like lesion.
- Tumor-like lesions (80–84%).
  - More frequent in advanced disease.
  - Often with ring-like or permanent contrast enhancement, edema, and mass effect mimicking tumefactive demyelination.
  - Can be leukodystrophy-like MRI pattern.
  - Associated with disability progression.
  - Effect of corticosteroids is usually present but often only partial (Fig. 10.1).
- Brain calcifications (50%).
  - In deep white matter sparing basal ganglia [51–53].

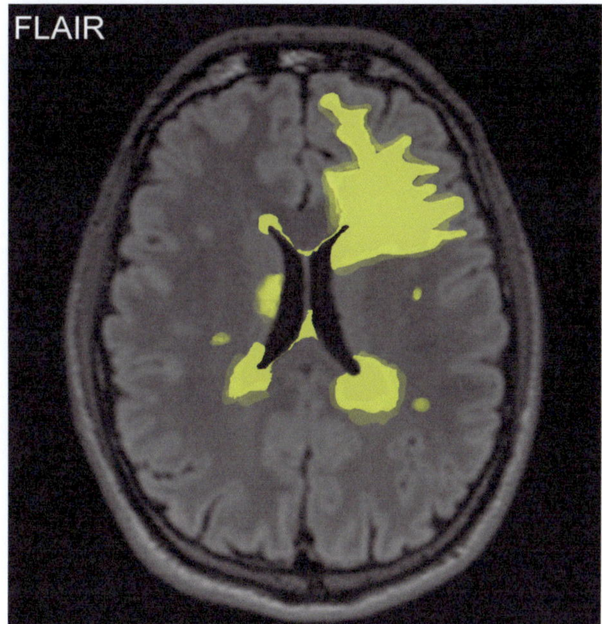

Fig. 10.1 Tumor-like lesions in retinal vasculopathy with cerebral leukoencephalopathy and systemic manifestations (RVCL-S)

10.5.5 Spinal Cord Imaging

- Usually normal.

10.5.6 Examination of Blood and CSF

- Routine blood testing is normal, but often positive CSF-restricted OCB [52, 53].

10.5.7 Diagnosis

- Genetic testing.
- Often misdiagnosed as brain tumor, MS, vasculitis, or organ disease of unknown origin, leading to unnecessary procedures and treatments.
- Red flags suggesting RVCL-S not MS include:
  - Persistent contrast enhancement of lesions.
  - Only partial effect of corticosteroids.
  - Brain calcifications.
  - Systemic manifestations.
  - Tumor-like brain lesions.
  - Spared the subcortical U-fibers and corpus callosum [51–53].

10.5.8 Treatment and Prognosis

- There is no effect of immunomodulatory treatments.
- Patients usually die between age 50 and 60 due to brain involvement [52, 53].

10.6 Trochleitis

10.6.1 Epidemiology

- Prevalence 12/100.000 (Spain).
- Higher incidence in women (87%).
- Often underdiagnosed.

10.6.2 Etiology and Definition

- Inflammation of the trochlea, a cartilaginous structure located in the superior and medial region of the orbit, which contains the tendon of the superior oblique muscle.

- The idiopathic (primary) form is the most common. It is hypothesized that stenosing tenosynovitis at the level of the superior oblique tendon sheath leads to chronic microtrauma of the tendon, resulting in local inflammation.
- The secondary form is rare and is associated with paranasal sinus inflammation, trauma, tumors, or systemic diseases such as rheumatoid arthritis, Behçet's disease, SLE, Still's disease, juvenile idiopathic arthritis, granulomatosis with polyangiitis, hidradenitis suppurativa, enteropathic arthropathy, sarcoidosis, or psoriasis.

10.6.3 Clinical Features

- Typically, trochleitis presents with a unilateral, sudden onset of hypersensitivity, tension, and sharp, pressure-like, or oppressive continuous pain of moderate to severe intensity in the trochlear region, which is considered pathognomonic.
- The pain is exacerbated by vertical eye movements.
- Palpation of the trochlear region is painful, but there is usually no local edema or erythema.
- Some patients may experience photophobia, blurred vision, asthenopia (convergence insufficiency), decreased or loss of depth perception, and even diplopia (due to motility impairment of the superior oblique muscle tendon).
- Bilateral trochleitis is rare (occurring in about 2% of cases), usually sequential, and is typically associated with secondary trochleitis.
- A high proportion of patients with trochleitis also report comorbid headaches or migraines, which may be caused or triggered by trochleitis.

10.6.4 Disease Course

- Mean age of symptoms onset is 43 ± 18 years.
- Typically, monophasic, but relapses may occur after months to years.

10.6.5 Brain and Spinal Imaging

- MRI or computed tomography (CT) may reveal thickening of the orbital pulley in about 20% of cases, especially in those with marked inflammation. However, due to the small size of the trochlea and the limited resolution of imaging, most cases show normal findings. Therefore, normal imaging cannot reliably rule out this condition.
- Orbital ultrasonography may show swelling of the peri-trochlear tissue and thickening of the superior oblique muscle, with low internal acoustic reflectivity in the trochlea.

10.6.6 Examination of Blood and CSF

- Routine testing is anticipated to yield normal results.

10.6.7 Diagnosis

- Based on clinical findings and imaging.
- In atypical cases, biopsy of the trochlear region may be required to confirm the diagnosis.

10.6.8 Differential Diagnosis

- Primary trochlear headache
- Orbital headaches with oculomotor cranial palsies
- Cavernous sinus thrombosis or fistula
- Horner syndrome
- Thyroid ophthalmopathy with superior oblique involvement
- Orbital myositis
- Tumors, and metastatic or inflammatory trochlear infiltration (sarcoidosis)
- Brown syndrome (usually painless congenital fibrosis and shortening of the superior oblique tendon resulting in decreased ocular motility; acquired secodary form can be painful).
- Talosa-Hunt syndrome

10.6.9 Treatment

- Systemic or locally injected corticosteroids may be used.
- Oral, topical, or systemic nonsteroidal anti-inflammatory drugs (NSAIDs) may be helpful in some cases, but there is no scientific evidence to support their routine use.
- In patients with secondary trochleitis, treatment should focus on addressing the underlying condition.
- Trochleectomy may be considered in severe and resistant cases.

10.6.10 Prognosis

- Most patients experience rapid and complete improvement, usually within 2 days and almost always within a few weeks [55–58].

10.7 Uveitis

10.7.1 Definition

- Inflammation of uveal tract (choroid, ciliary body, and iris) and/or the adjacent ocular tissues (retina, vitreous, and optic nerve).

10.7.2 Epidemiology

- Uveitis is a major cause of visual impairment and blindness (10% in USA) [59].
- Incidence 17.4–52.4/100.000/year.
- Prevalence 69.0–114.5/100.000.
- Prevalence of uveitis in patients with MS 0.53–1.34% (tenfold higher than in general population).
- The prevalence of MS in patients with uveitis ranges from 0.52 to 3.2%.
- Uveitis is more often associated with relapsing-remitting than primary progressive MS [60–62].

10.7.3 Anatomic Subtypes

- Anterior
  - Affects the ciliary body and iris.
- Intermediate uveitis
  - Affects the vitreous.
  - 10–20% of all uveitis cases.
  - Most often etiology: Idiopathic (pars planitis); MS; and sarcoidosis.
- Posterior uveitis
  - Affects the retina and/or choroid.
- Panuveitis
  - Refers to combined anterior, intermediate, and posterior uveitis [60, 63].

10.7.4 Etiology Subtypes

- Idiopathic
  - This subtype includes MS-related uveitis.
- Traumatic
- Inflammatory
  - Sarcoidosis, Behçet's disease, ankylosing spondylitis, etc.
- Infectious
- Neoplastic [61, 64]

10.7.5 Etiology

- MS-related uveitis is most often intermediate (61–80%), less often panuveitis (33–50%).
- Although, MS and uveitis share similar genetic risk factors and immunologic effector pathways, it is still unclear whether uveitis should be considered a distinct autoimmune disorder or an extension of the MS.
- The pathophysiology of MS-related uveitis is not fully understood. Given that retinal neurons are unmyelinated, intermediate uveitis is not a consequence of demyelination.
- However, it is hypothesized concept of epitope spreading between myelin and non-myelin antigens, which may result in similar T-cell responses and a predisposition to uveitis in MS patients [60, 61, 65].

10.7.6 Clinical Features

- Most frequently bilateral (50–94%).
- Typically, blurred vision, floaters, pain, red eye and photophobia.
- Often mild, in some cases asymptomatic.
- Ophthalmological exam may reveal diffuse vitreous cells, inflammatory aggregates and exudate, retinal periphlebitis, and uncommon vitreous hemorrhages or optic disc edema [60].
- The prevalence of periphlebitis and other vasculitic changes in the retina is higher in patients with MS-related uveitis compared to those with uveitis unrelated to MS. Nevertheless, their clinical significance remains uncertain [65].
- It is not clear, whether there is association between the severity of uveitis and the severity of MS [60, 65]; but there is association between a presence of retinal periphlebitis (perivenular inflammation; analogy of periventricular Dawson fingers) and clinical and radiological disease activity of MS [66].

10.7.7 Disease Course

- The onset of MS-associated uveitis is usually in middle age.
- Monophasic or relapsing-remitting course [65].
- MS-associated uveitis occurs most frequently before the diagnosis of MS and may precede neurological manifestations of MS by years [67].

10.7.8 Brain and Spinal Imaging

- If uveitis is not linked to MS, imaging studies are expected to yield normal findings.

10.7.9 Examination of Blood and CSF

- Routine testing is anticipated to yield normal results.

10.7.10 Retinal Fluorescein Angiography

- May detect the retinal periphlebitis [60].

10.7.11 Diagnosis

- The diagnosis of intermediate uveitis is based on clinical (floaters, blurred vision) and ophthalmoscopic (vitreous cells, snowballs, snowbanks, and retinal periphlebitis) findings [60, 65].
- The uveitis is not currently considered an inflammatory relapse of MS, and uveitis is treated separately with local and systemic corticosteroids [67, 68].

10.7.12 Differential Diagnosis

- Given that uveitis is often associated with systemic diseases, an etiology of the uveitis should always be investigated. For example, infectious and neoplastic etiologies must be excluded [60].
- Brain MRI is recommended for uveitis patients exhibiting the following: neurological manifestations; retinal vasculitis; age over 40 years; intermediate uveitis; and posterior uveitis or panuveitis to rule out the presence of an oculocerebral lymphoma [65, 69].
- Optic neuritis can be distinguished from uveitis by the following features:
  - Usually improve spontaneously over a few weeks. In contrast, untreated visual symptoms in uveitis typically persist over time.
  - Uveitis typically does not result in a relative afferent pupillary defect (RAPD), unless it is rarely complicated by optic disc edema.
  - Uveitis typically does not present with neurological manifestations and abnormal MRI findings, as optic neuritis often does [65].

10.7.13 Treatment

- Systemic or local corticosteroids (such as periocular corticosteroid injections or intravitreal injections of corticosteroid implants) are employed in the treatment of acute relapses of uveitis, including cases associated with MS.
- Frequent or chronic local or systemic corticosteroids may cause complications, such as cataract, glaucoma, or central serous chorioretinopathy.

- Uveitis patients with sight-threatening or corticosteroid-resistant disease may require additional immunomodulatory therapies.
- In untreated MS patients who develop uveitis, initiating disease-modifying treatment is not indicated. Management should instead be tailored to address the uveitis. For MS patients already on disease-modifying treatment who develop uveitis, local therapies such as intravitreal dexamethasone implants should be considered.
- Some immunomodulatory treatments for MS, such glatiramer acetate, mycophenolate mofetil, teriflunomide, natalizumab, alemtuzumab, and anti-CD20 therapies may target uveitis and MS [65, 67].

10.7.14 Prognosis

- Treated uveitis typically results in relatively favorable visual outcomes in most cases [60, 65].

References

1. Petzold A, Plant GT. Chronic relapsing inflammatory optic neuropathy: a systematic review of 122 cases reported. J Neurol. 2014;261(1):17–26.
2. Lee HJ, Kim B, Waters P, Woodhall M, Irani S, Ahn S, et al. Chronic relapsing inflammatory optic neuropathy (CRION): a manifestation of myelin oligodendrocyte glycoprotein antibodies. J Neuroinflammation. 2018;15(1):302.
3. Navarro CE, Arango GJ, Cubides MF. Chronic relapsing inflammatory optic neuropathy in a patient with triple antiphospholipid antibody positivity. Neurol Sci. 2021;42(8):3439–43.
4. The clinical profile of optic neuritis. Experience of the Optic Neuritis Treatment Trial. Optic Neuritis Study Group. Arch Ophthalmol. 1991;109(12):1673–8.
5. Kidd D, Burton B, Plant GT, Graham EM. Chronic relapsing inflammatory optic neuropathy (CRION). Brain. 2003;126(Pt 2):276–84.
6. Colpak AI, Kurne AT, Oguz KK, Has AC, Dolgun A, Kansu T. White matter involvement beyond the optic nerves in CRION as assessed by diffusion tensor imaging. Int J Neurosci. 2015;125(1):10–7.
7. Sharma A, Khurana D, Kesav P. MRI findings in chronic relapsing inflammatory optic neuropathy. BMJ Case Rep. 2013;2013.
8. Storoni M, Verbeek MM, Illes Z, Marignier R, Teunissen CE, Grabowska M, et al. Serum GFAP levels in optic neuropathies. J Neurol Sci. 2012;317(1–2):117–22.
9. Petzold A, Woodhall M, Khaleeli Z, Tobin WO, Pittock SJ, Weinshenker BG, et al. Aquaporin-4 and myelin oligodendrocyte glycoprotein antibodies in immune-mediated optic neuritis at long-term follow-up. J Neurol Neurosurg Psychiatry. 2019;90(9):1021–6.
10. Liu H, Zhou H, Wang J, Xu Q, Wei S. Antibodies to myelin oligodendrocyte glycoprotein in chronic relapsing inflammatory optic neuropathy. Br J Ophthalmol. 2019;103(10):1423–8.
11. Eslami M, Lichtman-Mikol S, Razmjou S, Bernitsas E. Optical coherence tomography in chronic relapsing inflammatory optic neuropathy, neuromyelitis optica and multiple sclerosis: a comparative study. Brain Sci. 2022;12(9):1140.
12. Plant GT, Sibtain NA, Thomas D. Hyperacute corticosteroid treatment of optic neuritis at the onset of pain may prevent visual loss: a case series. Mult Scler Int. 2011;2011:815068.
13. Yu-Wai-Man P, Chinnery PF. Leber Hereditary Optic Neuropathy. In: Adam MP, Feldman J, Mirzaa GM, Pagon RA, Wallace SE, Bean LJH, et al., editors. GeneReviews(®). Seattle

(WA): University of Washington, Seattle. Copyright © 1993–2023, University of Washington, Seattle. GeneReviews is a registered trademark of the University of Washington, Seattle. All rights reserved.; 1993.

14. Bargiela D, Chinnery PF. Mitochondria in neuroinflammation – Multiple sclerosis (MS), Leber hereditary optic neuropathy (LHON) and LHON-MS. Neurosci Lett. 2019;710:132932.
15. Palace J. Multiple sclerosis associated with Leber's Hereditary Optic Neuropathy. J Neurol Sci. 2009;286(1–2):24–7.
16. Yu-Wai-Man P, Griffiths PG, Brown DT, Howell N, Turnbull DM, Chinnery PF. The epidemiology of Leber hereditary optic neuropathy in the North East of England. Am J Hum Genet. 2003;72(2):333–9.
17. Harding AE, Riordan-Eva P, Govan GG. Mitochondrial DNA diseases: genotype and phenotype in Leber's hereditary optic neuropathy. Muscle Nerve Suppl. 1995;3:S82–4.
18. Pfeffer G, Burke A, Yu-Wai-Man P, Compston DA, Chinnery PF. Clinical features of MS associated with Leber hereditary optic neuropathy mtDNA mutations. Neurology. 2013;81(24):2073–81.
19. Sadun AA, Salomao SR, Berezovsky A, Sadun F, Denegri AM, Quiros PA, et al. Subclinical carriers and conversions in Leber hereditary optic neuropathy: a prospective psychophysical study. Trans Am Ophthalmol Soc. 2006;104:51–61.
20. Nikoskelainen EK, Marttila RJ, Huoponen K, Juvonen V, Lamminen T, Sonninen P, et al. Leber's "plus": neurological abnormalities in patients with Leber's hereditary optic neuropathy. J Neurol Neurosurg Psychiatry. 1995;59(2):160–4.
21. Matthews L, Enzinger C, Fazekas F, Rovira A, Ciccarelli O, Dotti MT, et al. MRI in Leber's hereditary optic neuropathy: the relationship to multiple sclerosis. J Neurol Neurosurg Psychiatry. 2015;86(5):537–42.
22. Bursle C, Riney K, Stringer J, Moore D, Gole G, Kearns LS, et al. Leber hereditary optic neuropathy and longitudinally extensive transverse myelitis. JIMD Rep. 2018;42:53–60.
23. Ninomiya T, Yamazaki H, Munakata S, Yoshino H, Sato T. A case of Leber's hereditary optic neuropathy with elevated blood levels of lactate and pyruvate. Br J Ophthalmol. 1997;81(5):422.
24. Hedges TR, Gobuty M, Manfready RA, Erlich-Malona N, Monaco C, Mendoza-Santiesteban CE. The optical coherence tomographic profile of Leber hereditary optic neuropathy. Neuro-Ophthalmology (Aeolus Press). 2016;40(3):107–12.
25. Salomao SR, Carelli V, Sacai PY, Berezovsky A, Andrade RE, Chicani CF, et al. Pattern-reversal Visually Evoked Potential (VEP) in asymptomatic carriers from an extensive Brazilian pedigree with 11778 Leber's Hereditary Optic Neuropathy (LHON). Invest Ophthalmol Vis Sci. 2003;44(13):936.
26. Carelli V, Carbonelli M, de Coo IF, Kawasaki A, Klopstock T, Lagrèze WA, et al. International consensus statement on the clinical and therapeutic management of Leber hereditary optic neuropathy. J Neuroophthalmol. 2017;37(4):371–81.
27. Purvin V, Sundaram S, Kawasaki A. Neuroretinitis: review of the literature and new observations. J Neuroophthalmol. 2011;31(1):58–68.
28. Lueck CJ. Neuroretinitis: a tricky mimic. Pract Neurol. 2020;20(6):430–2.
29. Abdelhakim A, Rasool N. Neuroretinitis: a review. Curr Opin Ophthalmol. 2018;29(6):514–9.
30. Schmalfuss IM, Dean CW, Sistrom C, Bhatti MT. Optic neuropathy secondary to cat scratch disease: distinguishing MR imaging features from other types of optic neuropathies. AJNR Am J Neuroradiol. 2005;26(6):1310–6.
31. Wals KT, Ansari H, Kiss S, Langton K, Silver AJ, Odel JG. Simultaneous occurrence of neuroretinitis and optic perineuritis in a single eye. J Neuroophthalmol. 2003;23(1):24–7.
32. Kasundra GM, Sood I, Prakash S, Mehta DP. Neuroretinitis with abnormal brain imaging in Ask-Upmark kidney: a novel case report. J Pediatr Neurosci. 2014;9(2):172–4.
33. Miller NR, Johnson LN, Bakaeva T, Van Stavern GP, Lee AG. Is neuroretinitis associated with multiple sclerosis? J Neuroophthalmol. 2022;42(1):126–30.
34. Williams KE, Johnson LN. Neuroretinitis in patients with multiple sclerosis. Ophthalmology. 2004;111(2):335–40; discussion 40–1.

35. Hattenhauer MG, Leavitt JA, Hodge DO, Grill R, Gray DT. Incidence of nonarteritic anterior ischemic optic neuropathy. Am J Ophthalmol. 1997;123(1):103–7.
36. Raizada K, Margolin E. Non-arteritic anterior ischemic optic neuropathy. Treasure Island (FL) ineligible companies: StatPearls; 2024. Disclosure: Edward Margolin declares no relevant financial relationships with ineligible companies.
37. Archer EL, Pepin S. Obstructive sleep apnea and nonarteritic anterior ischemic optic neuropathy: evidence for an association. J Clin Sleep Med. 2013;9(6):613–8.
38. Sharma RA, Newman NJ, Biousse V. New concepts on acute ocular ischemia. Curr Opin Neurol. 2019;32(1):19–24.
39. Hayreh SS. Ischemic optic neuropathy. Prog Retin Eye Res. 2009;28(1):34–62.
40. Morrow MJ. Ischemic optic neuropathy. Continuum (Minneap Minn). 2019;25(5):1215–35.
41. Fingert JH, Grassi MA, Janutka JC, East JS, Howard JG, Sheffield VC, et al. Mitochondrial variant G4132A is associated with familial non-arteritic anterior ischemic optic neuropathy in one large pedigree. Ophthalmic Genet. 2007;28(1):1–7.
42. Qureshi K, Farooq MU, Deol A, Glisson C, Gorelick PB. Bilateral non-arteritic anterior ischaemic optic neuropathy in a patient with a COL4A2 mutation. Neuro-Ophthalmology (Aeolus Press). 2022;46(3):190–3.
43. Hayreh SS, Podhajsky PA, Zimmerman B. Nonarteritic anterior ischemic optic neuropathy: time of onset of visual loss. Am J Ophthalmol. 1997;124(5):641–7.
44. Hayreh SS, Zimmerman MB. Nonarteritic anterior ischemic optic neuropathy: natural history of visual outcome. Ophthalmology. 2008;115(2):298–305.e2.
45. Characteristics of patients with nonarteritic anterior ischemic optic neuropathy eligible for the ischemic optic neuropathy decompression trial. Arch Ophthalmol. 1996;114(11):1366–74.
46. Rizzo JF 3rd, Andreoli CM, Rabinov JD. Use of magnetic resonance imaging to differentiate optic neuritis and nonarteritic anterior ischemic optic neuropathy. Ophthalmology. 2002;109(9):1679–84.
47. Arnold AC, Hepler RS. Natural history of nonarteritic anterior ischemic optic neuropathy. J Neuroophthalmol. 1994;14(2):66–9.
48. Hayreh SS. Anterior ischaemic optic neuropathy III. Treatment, prophylaxis, and differential diagnosis. Br J Ophthalmol. 1974;58(12):981–9.
49. González-Gay MA, Blanco R, Rodríguez-Valverde V, Martínez-Taboada VM, Delgado-Rodriguez M, Figueroa M, et al. Permanent visual loss and cerebrovascular accidents in giant cell arteritis: predictors and response to treatment. Arthritis Rheum. 1998;41(8):1497–504.
50. Ischemic Optic Neuropathy Decompression Trial: twenty-four-month update. Arch Ophthalmol. 2000;118(6):793–8.
51. Stam AH, Kothari PH, Shaikh A, Gschwendter A, Jen JC, Hodgkinson S, et al. Retinal vasculopathy with cerebral leukoencephalopathy and systemic manifestations. Brain. 2016;139(11):2909–22.
52. Ayrignac X, Carra-Dallière C, Marelli C, Taïeb G, Labauge P. Adult-onset genetic central nervous system disorders masquerading as acquired neuroinflammatory disorders: a review. JAMA Neurol. 2022;79(10):1069–78.
53. de Boer I, Pelzer N, Terwindt G. Retinal vasculopathy with cerebral leukoencephalopathy and systemic manifestations. In: Adam MP, Feldman J, Mirzaa GM, Pagon RA, Wallace SE, Bean LJH, et al., editors. GeneReviews(®). Seattle (WA): University of Washington, Seattle. Copyright © 1993–2024, University of Washington, Seattle. GeneReviews is a registered trademark of the University of Washington, Seattle. All rights reserved.; 1993.
54. Gass JD, Blodi BA. Idiopathic juxtafoveolar retinal telangiectasis. Update of classification and follow-up study. Ophthalmology. 1993;100(10):1536–46.
55. Collado Sánchez L, Munuera I, Rodrigo Sanjuán MJ, Garcia-Martin E. Orbital trochleitis: Literature review. Arch Soc Esp Oftalmol (Engl Ed). 2024;99(10):436–49.
56. Al-Zubidi N, Braga Soares AF, Bindiganavile SH, Yen MT, Al Belushi F, Silkiss RZ, et al. Trochleitis: EyeWiki; Accessed January 2025 [Available from: https://eyewiki.org/Trochleitis.
57. Jarrín E, García-García Á, Hurtado-Ceña FJ, Rodríguez-Sánchez JM. Clinical characteristics, treatment, and outcome of trochleitis. Strabismus. 2017;25(1):1–4.

58. Fonseca P, Manno RL, Miller NR. Bilateral sequential trochleitis as the presenting feature of systemic lupus erythematosus. J Neuroophthalmol. 2013;33(1):74–6.
59. Thorne JE, Suhler E, Skup M, Tari S, Macaulay D, Chao J, et al. Prevalence of noninfectious uveitis in the United States: a claims-based analysis. JAMA Ophthalmol. 2016;134(11):1237–45.
60. Casselman P, Cassiman C, Casteels I, Schauwvlieghe PP. Insights into multiple sclerosis-associated uveitis: a scoping review. Acta Ophthalmol. 2021;99(6):592–603.
61. Tsirouki T, Dastiridou A, Symeonidis C, Tounakaki O, Brazitikou I, Kalogeropoulos C, et al. A focus on the epidemiology of uveitis. Ocul Immunol Inflamm. 2018;26(1):2–16.
62. Olsen TG, Frederiksen J. The association between multiple sclerosis and uveitis. Surv Ophthalmol. 2017;62(1):89–95.
63. Jakob E, Reuland MS, Mackensen F, Harsch N, Fleckenstein M, Lorenz HM, et al. Uveitis subtypes in a german interdisciplinary uveitis center—analysis of 1916 patients. J Rheumatol. 2009;36(1):127–36.
64. Duplechain A, Conrady CD, Patel BC, Baker S. Uveitis. Treasure Island (FL) ineligible companies: StatPearls; 2024. Disclosure: Christopher Conrady declares no relevant financial relationships with ineligible companies. Disclosure: Bhupendra Patel declares no relevant financial relationships with ineligible companies. Disclosure: Stephen Baker declares no relevant financial relationships with ineligible companies.
65. Abraham A, Nicholson L, Dick A, Rice C, Atan D. Intermediate uveitis associated with MS: diagnosis, clinical features, pathogenic mechanisms, and recommendations for management. Neurol Neuroimmunol Neuroinflamm. 2021;8(1):e909.
66. Sepulcre J, Murie-Fernandez M, Salinas-Alaman A, García-Layana A, Bejarano B, Villoslada P. Diagnostic accuracy of retinal abnormalities in predicting disease activity in MS. Neurology. 2007;68(18):1488–94.
67. Fitoussi R, Gascon P, Denis D, Mathis T, Tieulé N, Schneider-Rouhaud C, et al. Epidemiological, clinical, and therapeutic profile of uveitis in multiple sclerosis: a multicenter study. Ocul Immunol Inflamm. 2024:1–5.
68. Jouve L, Benrabah R, Héron E, Bodaghi B, Le Hoang P, Touitou V. Multiple sclerosis-related Uveitis: does MS treatment affect uveitis course? Ocul Immunol Inflamm. 2017;25(3):302–7.
69. Chirpaz NM, Kerever SMP, Gavoille AM, Kodjikian LMP, Bernier RM, Gerfaud-Valentin MM, et al. Relevance of brain MRI in patients with uveitis: retrospective cohort on 402 patients. Ocul Immunol Inflamm. 2022;30(5):1109–15.

Vascular Non-inflammatory Diseases 11

11.1 Cerebral Amyloid Angiopathy (CAA)

11.1.1 Epidemiology, Definition, and Subtypes

- A small vessel disease associated with aging.
- CAA presents in three variants:
- Sporadic.
  - Very common, around 23% of the older people from general population (mean age 84.9 years) exhibit CAA in brain biopsy [1].
- Hereditary
  - Rare genetically determined variant (Dutch, Icelandic, Finnish and other subtypes) [2, 3].
- Inflammatory (synonyms: CAA-related inflammation (CAA-ri); amyloid beta-related angiitis).
  - Rare, underdiagnosed variant with prevalence 0.13/100.000 [4].

11.1.2 Etiology

- CCA is caused by deposition of amyloid beta in the walls of small arteries, arterioles, and capillaries of the leptomeninges, cerebral and cerebellar cortex.
- The disease progresses through the following stages:
  1. Presymptomatic cerebrovascular amyloid deposition.
  2. Presymptomatic impairment of cerebrovascular reactivity that can be measured by transcranial Doppler or functional magnetic resonance imaging (MRI).
  3. Non-hemorrhagic brain tissue pathology including focal tissue damage and microstructural brain changes. This stage begins 10–15 years before the occurrence of the first symptomatic brain hemorrhage.

T. Uher, *Mimics and Red Flags of Multiple Sclerosis*,
https://doi.org/10.1007/978-3-031-98945-2_11

4. Brain hemorrhage. Overall, it stands as one of the primary causes (15–20%) of spontaneous brain intracerebral hemorrhages in older people over 60 years of age. In certain cases, it may also cause subarachnoid hemorrhage [5].

- The rare inflammatory variant CAA-ri is caused by inflammatory response to increased amyloid beta deposition in the brain [6].

11.1.3 Clinical Features

- Recurrent hemorrhagic strokes.
- Often cognitive impairment, which is driven not only by hemorrhages but also by microinfarcts and other microstructural brain changes [2, 5, 7].
- Often comorbid with Alzheimer's disease [8].
- Manifestistations of CAA-ri are different and include:
  - Subacute cognitive decline (48%), acute or subacute focal neurological deficit, headache (33%), encephalopathy, behavioral changes (27%), or seizures.
  - It occurs mostly in younger patients (>40 years old) [2, 9–12]

11.1.4 Brain Imaging

- Non-hemorrhagic brain tissue pathology (3. stage) includes:
  - Lobar lacunes (resorbed necrotic tissue of a small infarct).
  - Cortical microinfarcts.
  - T2 hyperintensities in white matter (posterior predominant, asymmetric, patchy, or confluent lesions).
  - Enlarged perivascular spaces.
  - Brain atrophy.
- Hemorrhagic brain tissue pathology (4. stage) includes:
  - Macrobleeds

    Usually are larger than 1 cm in diameter.

    Cortical-subcortical regions (often occipital and temporal lobe).

    Typically, multiple lobar macrobleeds of different age.

    Recurrence: 9% per year.
  - Strictly lobar microbleeds

    "Black dots" on susceptibility weighted images (SWI).

    May be clinically silent.

    Multiple strictly lobar microbleeds represent one of the most significant biomarkers for the diagnosis of CAA and exhibit a high positive predictive value for CAA (Fig. 11.1).
  - Microbleeds or multifocal small hemorrhages may present also in patients with other brain diseases such as state after cardiac bypass for surgery; cavernous malformations; chronic hypertensive encephalopathy; brain trauma with diffuse axonal injury; Fabry disease; cerebral autosomal dominant arteriopathy with subcortical infarcts and leukoencephalopathy (CADASIL); COL4A1 brain small vessel disease; acute hepatic encephalopathy; cerebral hyperperfusion

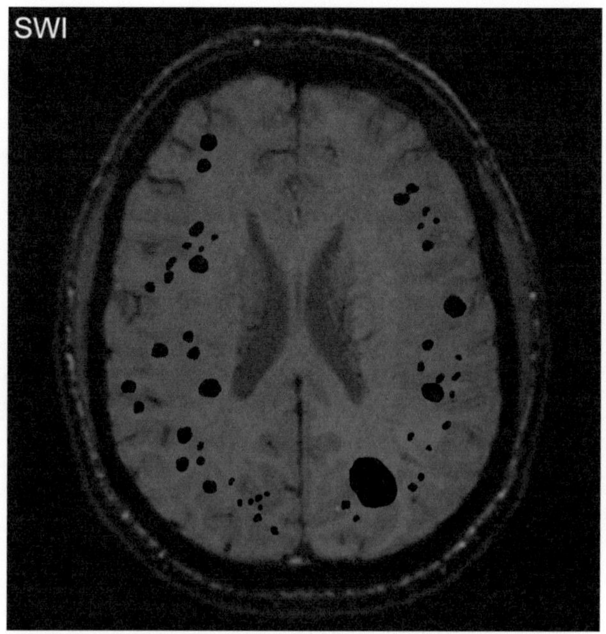

Fig. 11.1 Multiple strictly lobar microbleeds and multifocal small hemorrhages in cerebral amyloid angiopathy (CAA)

syndrome; cerebral vasculitis; cerebral small vessel disease (CSVD); intracranial embolism; brain infections; intravascular lymphoma; moyamoya disease; sarcoidosis; posterior reversible encephalopathy syndrome (PRES); radiation-induced cerebral vasculopathy (unilateral gyral thickening and contrast enhancement with mild mass effect with or without diffusion restriction); Sneddon syndrome; thrombotic microangiopathies and others [5, 7, 13, 14].

- Inflammatory CAA-ri:
  - Brain macrobleeds are usually not present, but frequently microhemorrhages and T2 lesions in white matter.
  - Vasogenic edema (often frontal and temporal subcortical white matter).
  - May be parenchymal or leptomeningeal contrast enhancement [7, 10–12, 15, 16].

11.1.5 Spinal Cord Imaging

- Usually only age-related changes.
- Rarely may histopathology reveal deposits of amyloid beta protein in the spinal leptomeningeal vessels [17].

11.1.6 Blood Work

- Routine blood tests are normal.

11.1.7 Examination of CSF

- May be elevated concentration of protein.
- Cytology is normal.
- Decreased levels of amyloid beta 40 and 42 peptides.
- Concentrations of total and phosphorylated tau proteins are only mildly elevated compared to controls, but significantly lower than those observed in Alzheimer's disease [2, 18, 19].
- During acute phase of CAA-ri can be found:
  - Increased levels of anti-amyloid beta autoantibodies
  - Increased concentration of protein (80%) and pleocytosis (44%) without cerebrospinal fluid (CSF)-restricted oligoclonal bands (OCB) [9, 11, 12, 20].

11.1.8 Diagnosis

- Established through the presence of typical imaging findings or genetic testing in cases of rare hereditary forms of CAA [2].
- For definite diagnosis of CAA-ri is required pathological confirmation [10, 11].
- Used the Boston criteria version 2.0 [21].
- There is a rare case study of patient diagnosed with hereditary form of CAA and MS [3].

11.1.9 Treatment and Prognosis

- The treatment is only symptomatic, as in any other spontaneous brain hemorrhage [7, 22].
- In patients with atrial fibrillation and a history of brain hemorrhage due to CAA, the use of non-vitamin K antagonist oral anticoagulants (NOACs) or acetylsalicylic acid may be considered, although the evidence supporting this is limited [2].
- CAA-ri is treated with corticosteroids and immunosuppression to achieve remission and prevent relapses [12].

11.2 Cerebral Autosomal Dominant Arteriopathy with Subcortical Infarcts and Leukoencephalopathy (CADASIL)

11.2.1 Epidemiology

- Prevalence 2–5/100.000 (probably underestimated).
- Most frequent monogenic cerebral small vessel disease [23, 24].

11.2.2 Etiology and Definition

- Autosomal dominant genetic disorder.
- Only rarely occurs sporadically due to a de novo mutation [25].
- Mutations in the causative *NOTCH3* gene (comprising over 200 subtypes) result in alterations to the NOTCH3 receptor protein, which is expressed by vascular smooth muscle cells and pericytes. These mutations lead to small vessel disease characterized by impaired cerebrovascular autoregulation, hypoperfusion, and ischemia. Cerebral vessels exhibit narrowing, along with intimal thickening and degeneration of vascular smooth muscle cells, accompanied by deposition of granular osmiophilic material [24].
- Cerebral Autosomal Recessive Arteriopathy with Subcortical Infarcts and Leukoencephalopathy (CARASIL) is similar but rarer disease with recessive inheritance [26].

11.2.3 Clinical Features

- A broad spectrum of clinical manifestations:
- Migraine (55–75%) [24].
  - Complicated with aura (84%) [27].
  - Often first clinical symptoms of CADASIL (41%) [28].
  - Occurs typically around 30 years of age [29].
  - Migraine with aura might be the only symptoms of CADASIL (12.1%).
  - Often present atypical aura features including prolonged visual auras, gastrointestinal symptoms, dysarthria, confusion, focal neurological deficits, or aura occurring without migraine headaches (60%) [28].
- Recurrent subcortical ischemic events (transient ischemic attack [TIA] or stroke) (85%) [30].
  - Mean age 45–50 years, though the range vary widely (30–80) [24, 31].
  - Occlusions of small penetrating arteries (lacunar subcortical infarctions) or large cerebral arteries (large territorial strokes).
  - Subcortical hemorrhages rarely occur, particularly in patients on anticoagulation [24].
- Acute encephalopathy (10%)
  - Mean age 42 years [32].
  - Evolves from migraine relapse and progress to confusion, seizures, and cortical signs. This is followed by spontaneous remission [24, 33].
- Psychiatric symptoms
  - Apathy, depression, and other psychiatric disturbances.
  - Cognitive impairment is progressive, primarily affecting information processing speed and executive functions. Episodic memory typically becomes impaired only in later stages. Cognitive decline can manifest in isolation, without accompanying neurological symptoms [24, 34].

- Other less frequent manifestations include:
  - Ischemic damage of the optic nerve [35] or retina [36].
  - Myopathy and peripheral neuropathy [24].
  - Epilepsy [37].
  - Isolated ataxia (dominant truncal ataxia rather than limb ataxia) [38].
  - CARASIL has some additional symptoms including early-onset cognitive impairment, gait disturbance, early-onset spondylosis with low back pain and early-onset alopecia [26].

11.2.4 Brain Imaging

- Lesions' location:
  - Typical locations (may not always be involved):
    A. Confluent bilateral anterior temporal lobe T2 hyperintensities (90% sensitivity and specificity for CADASIL; but less often in Asian populations).
    B. External capsule (90% sensitivity, but specificity only 50% because it also occurs very often in sporadic small vessel disease).
    C. Superior frontal gyrus (Fig. 11.2).
  - Other locations:
    Periventricular (96%) and deep white matter (85%).
    Less frequent subcortical white matter (25%).
    Basal ganglia (60%).
    Brainstem (45%).
    Thalamus.
    Corpus callosum; rare but may mimic MS [24, 39–42].
  - Relative sparing of:
    Occipital and orbitofrontal white matter.

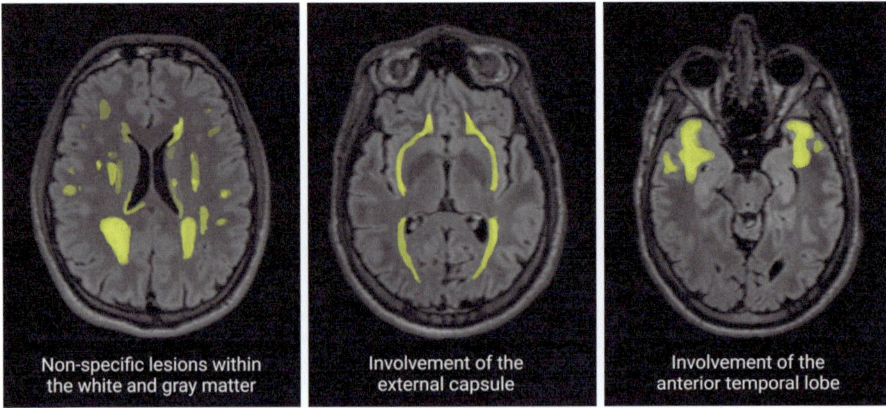

Fig. 11.2 MRI characteristics of cerebral autosomal dominant arteriopathy with subcortical infarcts and leukoencephalopathy (CADASIL)

Subcortical U-fibers.

Cerebral cortex (although lesions seen on 7-Tesla MRI) [40, 43].

- Lesions' appearance:
  - Large, sometime confluent, symmetrical T2 hyperintense lesions.
  - Lacunes (fluid isointense signal of CSF).
  - T1 hypointense lesions (62%).
  - Diffusion-weighted imaging (DWI) with restricted diffusion in sub/acute ischemic lesions [24, 39–41].
- Contrast enhancement:
  - Rare [44–46]
- Evolution over time:
  - Lesions may already be present in young individuals (20–30 years old) who are presymptomatic carriers of the CADASIL mutation [47]. Conversely, patients in the early stages of the disease may exhibit normal MRI findings [38].
- Associated findings:
  - Brain atrophy.
  - Cerebral microbleeds (25–70%; more frequent in older patients with vascular risk factors).
  - Intracerebral hemorrhages are rare [24, 48].

11.2.5 Spinal Cord Imaging

- Cord lesions are rare. The nature of these lesions, whether ischemic or inflammatory demyelinating, remains unknown. However, the majority of previous studies have interpreted the lesions as ischemic [49, 50].

11.2.6 Blood Work

- Routine testing is normal.
- A small sample size study demonstrated decreased Aβ42 levels compared to controls, akin to Alzheimer's disease patients. However, it also showed normal levels of total tau (t-tau) and phosphorylated tau (p-tau), distinguishing CADASIL patients from those with vascular dementia and Alzheimer's disease, who typically exhibit elevated tau and p-tau levels [51].

11.2.7 Examination of CSF

- Routine CSF testing is usually normal.
- However, a few case studies have reported abnormal CSF findings resembling those seen in MS, such as mildly elevated protein concentration, mild pleocytosis, and CSF-restricted OCB. It remains unclear whether these patients have comorbid MS and CADASIL or if they present with an inflammatory-like manifestation of CADASIL [44, 45, 52–54].

11.2.8 OCT

- On OCT (optical coherence tomography), retinal nerve fiber layer (RNFL) thinning might be evident even in the absence of subjective visual deficits and is often prominent in the temporal quadrant, akin to findings in MS [36].

11.2.9 Diagnosis

- *NOTCH3* sequencing of encoding exons is used to confirm the diagnosis.
- Skin biopsy is recommended only for patients with suspected CADASIL, but absence of *NOTCH3* mutation or unclassified variant in *NOTCH3* and should include NOTCH3 immunohistochemistry and electron microscopy.
- Genetic counseling should be offered to all patients and should precede genetic testing of patient and family members [24].

11.2.10 Differential Diagnosis

- The disorder is often overlooked and misdiagnosed.
- Although corpus callosum lesions can be in CADASIL (not frequently) and MS; most patients with CADASIL do not have spinal cord or optic nerve lesions, nor abnormal CSF. In contrast, in CADASIL are very often temporo-polar lesions not usually seen in MS [24].
- Additionally, acute onset, normal CSF, and lack of response to corticosteroids may help with differential diagnosis from MS [44, 45, 55].
- However, a few case studies described CADASIL patients with isolated optic neuritis with CSF-restricted OCB and positive response to high-dose corticosteroids. These cases reflect possible an inflammatory process associated with CADASIL or two separate diseases occurring in the same patient. Therefore, immunomodulatory treatments, including corticosteroids, could be considered for these patients because there are no effective therapeutic options available for CADASIL [44, 45, 52, 54].
- CADASIL-associated encephalopathy is often misdiagnosed as encephalitis, especially in cases where encephalopathy is the initial symptom [24, 33].
- Differential diagnosis of CADASIL also includes CARASIL; mitochondrial encephalomyopathy, lactic acidosis and stroke-like episodes (MELAS); Krabbe and Fabry disease; cathepsin A-related arteriopathy with strokes and leukoencephalopathy (CARASAL); adult-onset leukoencephalopathy with axonal spheroids and pigmented glia (ALSP); and other rare monogenic forms of small vessel disease [24].
- CARASAL is exceptionally rare (only few cases documented). It represents a monogenic cause of cerebral small vessel disease. Although its phenotype shares similarities with CADASIL, CARASAL is distinguished by its notable involvement of the brainstem, characterized by symptoms such as hearing loss, tinnitus, vertigo, and dysphagia. It is also associated with alopecia. Brain MRI typically reveals prominent thalamic and brainstem abnormalities [56].

- Pontine autosomal dominant microangiopathy and leukoencephalopathy (PADMAL) is genetic disorder sharing similarities with conditions such as CADASIL, CARASIL, and CARASAL, leading to multiple lacunar infarcts and microbleeds primarily affecting the deep white matter, pons, cerebellum, corpus callosum, and occasionally the cervical spinal cord. Unlike CARASAL, thalamic involvement is not a typical feature in PADMAL [57, 58].
- Fabry disease can also have confluent symmetrical white matter lesions and microbleeds. The pulvinar sign (hyperintense on T1 but not on T2 images) is likely of limited clinical value [59, 60].

11.2.11 Treatment and Prognosis

- Only vascular risk prevention (antiplatelet drugs) because causal and effective treatment is not available [24].
- Reduced life expectancy (men 64.6 and women 70.7 years) [31].

11.3 Cerebral Small Vessel Disease (CSVD)

11.3.1 Alternative Terms

- Leukoaraiosis; Leukoencephalopathy; or White matter disease should not be used [61].

11.3.2 Epidemiology

- Very common neurological disease; 5–15% of general middle-aged population have at least one T2 hyperintensity in white matter.
- This proportion increases to over 90% in people of age 80 years or older and to 100% in people over 90 years of age.
- Cerebral microbleeds are present in 6.5% of people aged 50 years, but in 10–28% of people aged 70 years and 36% for people aged 80–89 years.
- CSVD in middle-aged individuals is more prevalent in those with vascular risk factors including arterial hypertension, diabetes mellitus, smoking, obstructive sleep apnea, or chronic kidney disease.
- There are no significant sex differences, but males are more likely to present with moderate to severe CSVD and acute strokes [62–67].

11.3.3 Etiology and Definition

- A disorder of cerebral microvessels (arterioles, venules, and capillaries) leading to focal white matter hyperintensities and other abnormalities observed on brain imaging. These imaging abnormalities are usually associated with permanent WM damage due to demyelination and axon loss.

- CSVD is a group of imaging features predominantly in brain locations with poor collateral vascularization (e.g., watershed areas, fronto-subcortical regions).
- Pathology is characterized by loss of smooth muscle cells from the tunica media, lipohyalinosis, the development of microatheroma, and segmental arterial disorganization leading to imaging changes associated with CSVD.
- Other abnormalities associated with CSVD include cerebral microvessel endothelial dysfunction, including blood–brain barrier dysfunction, impaired vasodilation, vessel stiffening, dysfunctional blood flow and interstitial fluid drainage, white matter rarefaction, ischemia, inflammation, myelin damage, and secondary neurodegeneration.
- It remains unclear which vascular dysfunctions are most crucial in the pathogenesis, which abnormalities are reversible, and why there is such variability in lesion progression and symptomatology.
- CSVD causes about 25% of all ischemic strokes, most intracerebral hemorrhages in older people (85%), and 45% of dementia [61, 67–69].
- There is wide variability in the previous research regarding terminology. The recent Standards for Reporting Vascular Changes on Neuroimaging 1 (STRIVE-1) involves the following MRI features related to CSVD:
  A. Recent small subcortical infarct
  B. Lacune
  C. White matter hyperintensity
  D. Perivascular space
  E. Cerebral microbleed
  F. Cortical superficial siderosis
  G. Cortical cerebral microinfarct
  H. Spontaneous intracerebral hemorrhages presumed due to CSVD
  I. Incidental DWI-positive lesion
  J. Brain atrophy
- The subtypes of CSVD based on different pathological characteristics include:
  - Atherosclerosis
  - Cerebral amyloid angiopathy
  - Hereditary vascular diseases (CADASIL, Fabry disease, MELAS, retinal vasculopathy with cerebral leukoencephalopathy, COL4A1 brain small vessel disease, etc.)
  - Inflammatory vascular diseases (primary angiitis of the central nervous system [CNS], Susac's syndrome, etc.)
  - Venous collagenosis

    Associated with periventricular white matter hyperintensities; common in older age; and associated with cognitive and motor decline. Collagen deposition in veins is associated with enlargement of the periventricular space. The etiology remains unknown.
  - Other types of small vessel diseases (post-radiation angiopathy, non-amyloid microvessel degeneration in Alzheimer's disease, etc.) [62, 70, 71].

11.3.4 Clinical Features

- CSVD is associated with asymptomatic brain infarcts and/or symptomatic small vessel ischemic strokes.
- In many cases, CSVD is asymptomatic. However, over time, cumulative, repeated small vessel ischemic events in most cases lead to a gradually progressive sensory-motor deficit, abnormal gait, and cognitive decline culminating in vascular dementia.
- Relationships between lesion burden and clinical manifestations are highly variable and poorly understood [61–63, 68].

11.3.5 Brain Imaging

A. Recent small subcortical infarct ("acute lacunar infarct")
   - Most common acute clinical manifestation of CSVD.
   - 20–30% of all ischemic stroke cases.
   - Imaging evidence of a recent small infarction in the territory of one perforating arteriole with clinical symptoms consistent with a lesion occurring within the previous 3 weeks.
   - Does not include asymptomatic lesions and lesions associated with atypical neurobehavioral manifestations or gradual neurological deterioration.
   - Lesions' location:
     - Territory of perforating arterioles in the subcortical white matter, deep gray matter (basal ganglia, internal capsule, thalamus) or infratentorial region (often pons).
   - Lesions' appearance:
     - Small (axial diameter < 20 mm).
     - Hyperintense on fluid-attenuated inversion recovery (FLAIR) and T2 images; hypointense on T1 images; in the acute stage with restricted diffusion.
     - Large variability in residual appearances of recent small subcortical infarcts, including disappearance; lacunes with or without a hemosiderin (T2*-hypointense) rim; or a small hemosiderin spot. The cause of variability in residual appearance is unclear, but it is probably influenced by factors such as the initial lesion size, tissue injury, inflammation, comorbidities, location, microcirculatory variations, and individual vulnerabilities.
     - White matter tract degeneration around the recent small subcortical infarcts may lead to new T2 hyperintensities in adjacent white matter.
   - Origin:
     - Not all recent small subcortical infarcts are due to intrinsic perforating arterial disease (primary pathology within the small blood vessels). Some infarcts are caused by large artery disease or non-intrinsic factors, where small vessel pathology is secondary to another underlying condition, such as hypertension, diabetes, or autoimmune disorders [69, 72].

B. Lacune (of presumed vascular origin)
   - Location:
     - Subcortical white matter.
     - Deep gray matter (basal ganglia and thalamus).
     - Infratentorial region.
   - Appearance
     - A small (axial 3–15 mm), round or ovoid, fluid-filled (CSF-like), sharply defined cavity with a tissue loss.
     - Hypointense on FLAIR and T1 images; hyperintense on T2 images; often surrounded by a hyperintense rim on T2 images.
     - There is a subtype of lacunes that is not cavitated yet and may represent an intermediate stage between white matter hyperintensities and a fully cavitated lacune.
     - Some perivascular spaces may have diameter greater than 3 mm and their distinguishing from lacunes may be challenging.
   - Origin:
     - Incident lacunes in the subcortical white matter have often a different pathogenesis than those in the deep GM and infratentorial region.
   1. End-stage cavitation in a white matter hyperintensity.
      - This subtype of lacunes is more often seen in subcortical white matter. Penetrating vessels supplying the subcortical white matter lack collateral networks (watershed areas) are susceptible to ischemia. Therefore, lacunes in subcortical white matter often develop slowly within in an area of preexistent white matter hyperintensity with compromised perfusion and are often surrounded by significant new white matter hyperintensity.
   2. From an occlusion of a single small deep perforating artery (thalamoperforant, lenticulostriate, or pontine paramedian arteriole).
      - This subtype of lacunes is more often seen in deep gray matter and infratentorial region. They usually occur with only few surrounding white matter hyperintensities in locations that appeared normal at baseline indicating a more acute development.
      - Their direct origin from large arteries might make these arterioles more prone to acute occlusion.
   3. End tissue damage from a recent small subcortical infarct (by definition, a lacune should not be associated with an infarct unless it results from a small subcortical infarct).
   4. From a small subcortical hemorrhage.
   5. From an incidental DWI-positive lesion.
   - Clinical significance:
     - Associated with major neurological disability or asymptomatic.
     - Their presence increases the risk of future stroke and worse outcome following the stroke [69, 72].

C. White matter hyperintensity (of presumed vascular origin)
   - The term ischemic white matter hyperintensity should be avoided.
   - The most studied feature of CSVD.

- Location:
  - Mainly periventricular and deep subcortical white matter.
  - Lesions in the deep gray matter or brainstem are not included into this category unless explicitly stated (deep gray matter hyperintensities; brainstem hyperintensities; or subcortical hyperintensities).
- Appearance:
  - Typically, symmetrical.
  - Hyperintense on FLAIR and T2 images; slightly hypointense or isointense on T1 images; without restricted diffusion.
  - May decrease in size over time due to resolution of excess interstitial fluid before permanent damage occur.
  - May become confluent.
  - Without contrast enhancement or mass effect.
  - Although occurrences of new lesions over time are common, regression of white matter lesion volume might also take place in considerable proportion of patients (30%).
- Origin:
  - Their prevalence increases with age and varies considerably across different age groups in the general population.
  - Subtle diffuse ischemia/hypoxia or incomplete infarction (not complete infarction leading to lacune).
  - Associated with impaired cerebrovascular reactivity, increased blood-brain barrier permeability; increased vascular pulsatility; venous collagenosis; and reduced resting cerebral blood flow.
  - Quantitative MRI often detects additional areas of tissue damage in the normal-appearing brain tissue surrounding the lesion, which are not identified by conventional MRI methods.
- Clinical significance:
  - Associated with future risk of stroke, stroke severity, cognitive decline, death, dependency, or impaired gait.
- The following findings may sometimes occur:
  - Periventricular cap: A smooth T2-hyperintense area around the lateral ventricles, particularly the frontal and posterior horns, likely reflecting increased interstitial water content due to dysfunctional transependymal transportation rather than ischemic-gliotic changes. Quantifying the water content in these lesions may help determine their origin.
  - Periventricular rim: A segmental or complete, sharply defined continuous rim of thin hyperintensity in the periventricular white matter.
  - Periventricular halo: A more widespread, and less well-defined area of T2 hyperintense signal in the white matter surrounding the ventricles. Often seen in hydrocephalus, advanced demyelinating diseases and chronic small vessel ischemic changes.
  - Periventricular caps, rims, and halos might originate from different causes, such as demyelination, gliosis, ischemic changes, edema, or hydrocephalus.

  - These mild periventricular hyperintensities are often seen in healthy individuals, and their frequency increases with age. However, if they are extensive, it is usually pathological, though often a nonspecific finding [69, 72–75].
- Evolution over time:
  - Initially, periventricular lesions typically manifest at the apex of the lateral ventricles (capping). Subsequently, these lesions spread around the ventricles, typically originating in the frontal lobes and later extending to the parieto-occipital region. Lesions in the brainstem and basal ganglia typically occur in more advanced stages of the disease.
  - Over time can progress from punctate to clustered to confluent hyperintensities [61, 73–77].

D. Perivascular (Virchow-Robin) spaces
- Location:
  - Most prominent in the basal ganglia and centrum semiovale.
- Appearance:
  - Small (<2 mm diameter when imaged perpendicular to the course of the vessel), fluid-filled round, ovoid, or linear spaces that follow the course of small perforating vessels (predominantly periarteriolar) through white matter and deep gray matter.
  - Signal like CSF (hypo or isointense on FLAIR, hyperintense on T2 images; hypointense on T1 images; without restricted diffusion; without T2-hyperintense rim).
- Origin:
  - May reflect impaired clearance of interstitial fluid and waste from the brain, potentially occurring during sleep and preceding the occurrence of lacunes, cerebral microbleeds, or white matter lesions.
- Clinical significance:
  - The presence of a few perivascular spaces can be considered physiological across a wide age range. However, a significant burden of perivascular spaces is frequently linked to neurological conditions such as stroke, cerebral amyloid angiopathy, or Alzheimer's disease.
  - The prevalence rises with age and vascular risk factors and exhibits a high heritability.
  - A high burden of perivascular spaces in the centrum semiovale combined with a single strictly lobar hemorrhagic feature (such as intracerebral hemorrhage, cerebral microbleed, or cortical superficial siderosis) suggests probable cerebral amyloid angiopathy [69, 76, 77].

E. Cerebral microhemorrhages
- Location:
  - Cortical gray matter and juxtacortical white matter or strictly lobar microbleeds in older patients are typical for cerebral amyloid angiopathy.
  - Deep gray matter, subcortical white matter and brainstem or mixed deep-lobar microbleeds are typical for arteriolosclerosis; but regions and pathologies overlap.

- Appearance:
  - Small (2–5 mm diameter; sometime 10 mm) ovoid hypointensities on T2* or susceptibility-weighted sequences due to the paramagnetic properties of the blood breakdown product hemosiderin.
- Origin:
  - Caused by small parenchymal hemorrhages due to damage of the small cerebral arteries.
- Clinical significance:
  - Predict risks of intracerebral hemorrhages and ischemic stroke during antithrombotic therapy. However, their presence should not limit the use of antiplatelet or anticoagulant drugs for prevention of ischemic stroke [69, 76, 77] (Fig. 11.3).

F. Cortical superficial siderosis
- Location and appearance:
  - Defined by the presence of chronic blood products within or covering the superficial cortex.
  - T2*-weighted gradient-echo or other blood-sensitive sequences show cortical superficial siderosis as a linear hypointensity over the cortex.
- Origin:
  - Convexity subarachnoid hemorrhage, superficial cortical bleeding from vascular malformations, hemorrhagic transformation of infarcts, or trauma. The most cases in older population may be attributed to subarachnoid hemorrhage from advanced leptomeningeal vessel cerebral amyloid angiopathy, sometimes with secondary cortical ischemic injury.
- Clinical significance:
  - Diagnostic marker of advanced cerebral amyloid angiopathy.
  - Its presence predicts risk of future intracerebral hemorrhages, functional decline, and post-intracerebral hemorrhage dementia [69, 76, 77].

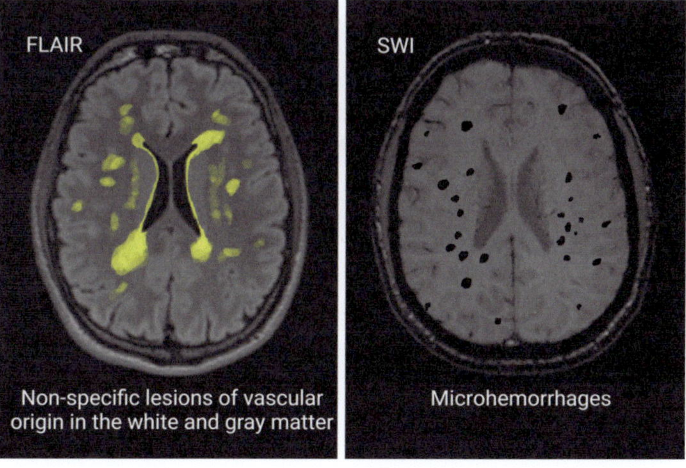

Fig. 11.3 Selected MRI characteristics of cerebral small vessel disease (CSVD)

G. Cortical cerebral microinfarcts
  - Location and appearance:
    - Small (<4 mm) strictly cortical lesions (T1 hypointense; T2 hyperintense; T2*isointense; restricted diffusion in acute stage).
    - Larger microinfarcts (0.5–4.0 mm) can be detected using conventional MRI, but even 7 Tesla MRI detects only a small proportion of the lesions observed on neuropathology.
  - Clinical significance:
    - The most widespread form of infarction in the ageing brain. They are present in 16–42% of individuals who had died of natural or age-related conditions at autopsy.
    - Not typical for CSVD, because also occur because of microembolism from cardiac or arterial sources.

Associated with cognitive decline [69, 76, 77].

H. Intracerebral hemorrhage presumed due to CSVD
  - Around 85% of all intracerebral hemorrhages are caused by CSVD.
  - Either through arteriolosclerotic vasculopathy of perforating arteries or via cerebral amyloid angiopathy associated with lobar intracerebral hemorrhages.

I. Incidental DWI-positive lesion
  - Small (<20 mm) subcortical or cortical location.
  - Caused by CSVD, embolism or altered hemodynamics.
  - Most common in severe CSVD.
  - May disappear or evolve into a white matter hyperintensity, lacune, or old cortical cerebral microinfarct.
  - They overlap with recent small subcortical infarcts or cortical cerebral microinfarcts when occurring within the previous few weeks.

J. Brain atrophy
  - Unspecific marker of CSVD.
  - Frequently present subcortical (with increased ventricular volume) and cortical (with thinning and sulcal widening) atrophy [69, 76, 77].

11.3.6 Scores to Quantify the Amount of WM T2 Hyperintense Lesions Attributed to CSVD

- Summary small vessel disease score [69].
- Fazekas scale
  - Periventricular white matter lesions (0 = absent; 1 = "caps" or pencil-thin lining; 2 = smooth "halo"; 3 = irregular periventricular signal extending into the deep white matter).
  - Deep white matter lesions (0 = absent; 1 = punctate foci; 2 = beginning confluence; 3 = large confluent areas) [78].

11.3.7 Examination of Blood and CSF

- Routine testing should yield normal results.

11.3.8 Diagnosis

- Based on imaging findings.

11.3.9 Differential Diagnosis

- MS
  A. Recent small subcortical infarct
    - Acute ischemic lesions (almost always) and MS lesions (rarely) may show restricted diffusion. The etiology of the early restricted diffusion in the MS lesions is unknown. However, most acute demyelinating lesions in MS with restricted diffusion also exhibit contrast enhancement, which helps distinguish them from ischemic lesions. Importantly, in a small proportion of patients with MS, restricted diffusion may precede contrast enhancement. The rare, restricted diffusion in hyperacute MS lesions usually lasts only a few days to about 2–3 weeks and is in the periphery of the lesions.

  B. Lacune
    - Not associated with MS but with vascular comorbidities in MS patients. Their occurrence (19.6%) in MS patients increases with age [79].

  C. White matter hyperintensity
    - MRI features may resemble demyelinating lesions in MS, making the differential diagnosis challenging, especially in patients with atypical phenotypes.
    - Often symmetric involvement of both hemispheres, which is atypical for MS.
    - Periventricular white matter lesions in MS are often perpendicular to the lateral ventricle ("Dawson fingers").
    - Infratentorial region is usually not affected in early stages of CSVD, which is not the true for MS.
    - Locations of lesions atypical for CSVD but typical for MS include:
      - Corpus callosum, because of redundant blood supply.
      - Juxtacortical/subcortical U-fibers because of rich blood supply.
      - Temporal lobe.
    - Central vein sign is not present in majority of CSVD lesions.
    - Lesions might sometime disappear, which is extremely rare in MS.
    - Lesions in CSVD do not increase in size over time, unlike some chronic active lesions in MS, which typically do.
    - Lesions in CSVD do not show contrast enhancement [80–83].

D. Perivascular space
    - Although enlarged perivascular spaces are more common in MS patients compared to healthy controls, it is typically of a mild extent. The hypothesized contribution of neuroinflammatory or degenerative pathology in MS may underlie this observation. However, there is insufficient evidence to support their use for diagnostic and/or prognostic purposes in MS [84].
E. Cerebral microbleed
    - Probably not associated with MS but with vascular comorbidities in MS patients. Their occurrence in MS (19.8%) increases with age and disability and predict progression of disability [85].
F. Cortical superficial siderosis;
G. Cortical cerebral microinfarct;
H. Spontaneous intracerebral hemorrhages presumed due to CSVD.
I. Incidental DWI-positive lesion are not associated with MS.
J. Brain atrophy is nonspecific marker occurring in CSVD and MS [86].

- Binswanger disease (subcortical vascular dementia)
    - A progressive type of CSVD overlapping with other vascular cognitive impairment and neurodegenerative conditions. It is associated with extensive confluent subcortical white matter ischemic changes with or without lacunar strokes. The white matter injury is related to endothelial dysfunction with secondary inflammatory response and breakdown of the neurovascular unit. Patients suffer from cognitive impairment, gait problems, pyramidal signs, and pseudobulbar syndrome [71].

11.3.10 Treatment and Prognosis

- Treatment is focused on addressing vascular risk factors, tailored based on the underlying etiology.
- The rate of progression of CSVD remains unknown. Studies have demonstrated a high variability in the proportion of patients experiencing new lesion accrual per year, ranging from 5% to 50% [87].
- CSVD is associated with increased risk of ischemic and hemorrhagic stroke, dementia, and death [66].

11.4 COL4A1-Related Disorders

11.4.1 Epidemiology

- Prevalence is unknown and this condition is likely underdiagnosed [88].

11.4.2 Etiology, Subtypes, and Definition

- Group of inherited autosomal dominant diseases characterized by mutations in a *COL4A1* gene encoding type IV collagen. These mutations lead to a pathology in the basement membrane of vascular endothelium in many tissues. This is associated with "fragile" small blood vessels and increased susceptibility to stress-induced arterial and arteriolar rupture. These disorders cause cerebrovascular diseases.

- Can occur as de novo mutations (>27%) [88, 89].
- *COL4A1*-related disorders have similar phenotypes and include:
  - COL4A1 brain small vessel disease.
  - COL4A2-related porencephaly and intracerebral hemorrhages.
  - Pontine autosomal dominant microangiopathy with leukoencephalopathy (PADMAL).
  - Familial porencephaly (Porencephaly type 1, Hereditary porencephaly).
  - Hereditary angiopathy with nephropathy, aneurysms, and muscle cramps syndrome [88, 90].

11.4.3 Clinical Features

- Can manifest already prenatally (as a severe or fatal intraparenchymal hemorrhage) or in the early childhood (severe developmental delay, mental retardation, microcephaly, and motor pyramidal and extrapyramidal abnormalities).
- Some patients may exhibit a late adult-onset phenotype, characterized by small vessel disease or have an asymptomatic course.
- Manifestations in the adult-onset phenotype mainly include:
  - Recurrent strokes and silent microhemorrhages (mean age at stroke 30–40 years; hemorrhagic strokes are twice as often as ischemic strokes).
  - Epilepsy.
  - Migraine.
  - Cognitive impairment.
  - Congenital cataract or tortuosity of retinal arteries.
  - Other manifestations include: other abnormalities of eyes (cataracts, glaucoma, microphthalmia, etc.); renal cysts; nephrosis; micro-albuminuria; cardiac arrhythmia; skeletal muscles dystrophic changes; myoglobinuria; creatine kinase elevation; muscle cramps; Raynaud's phenomenon; or hemolytic anemia [88, 91–93].

11.4.4 Brain Imaging

- Micro- or macrohemorrhages.
- Lacunar infarcts and multifocal areas with restricted diffusion (recent infarction)
- Dilated perivascular spaces and brain atrophy.
- Leukoencephalopathy with diffuse relatively symmetrical T2 hyperintensities in periventricular and deep white matter (sparing subcortical white matter) and basal ganglia.
- Angiography may show aneurysmal dilatation or stenosis of cerebral arteries.
- Other findings may include congenital porencephaly (CSF-filled cavities), hydrocephalus, focal cortical dysplasia, Dandy Walker malformation, dysplastic brain stem, or schizencephaly [91–93] (Fig. 11.4).

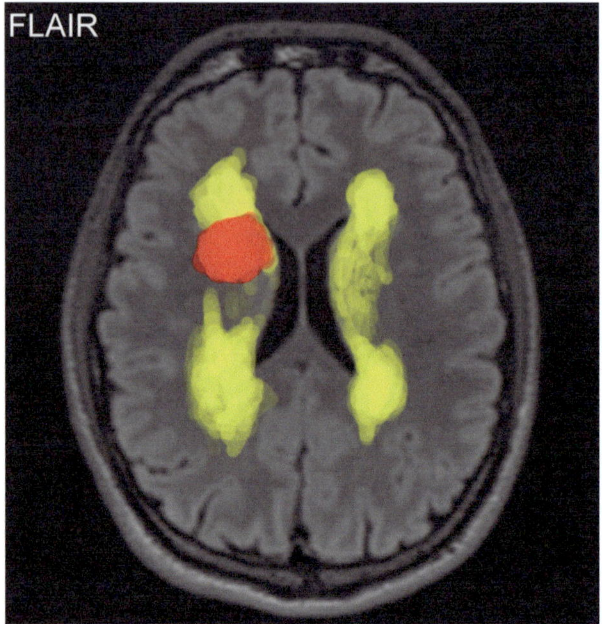

Fig. 11.4 Leukoencephalopathy and micro- or macrohemorrhages in COL4A1-related disorders

11.4.5 Spinal Cord Imaging

- Normal findings.

11.4.6 Examination of CSF

- Normal or shows elevated concentration of protein [92].

11.4.7 Diagnosis

- Extensive leukoencephalopathy with microhemorrhages, coupled with the absence of cardiovascular risk factors, a history of congenital cataracts or glaucoma, and a positive family history in young adults, should raise suspicion for this rare group of disorders.
- Genetic testing (*COL4A1* sequencing) is recommended for suspected patients, particularly those with a positive family history [89, 91–93].

11.4.8 Differential Diagnosis

- Reported cases of patients initially misdiagnosed with MS.
- The differential diagnosis should also include acute disseminated hemorrhagic encephalomyelitis, inflammatory leukoencephalopathy, or inflammatory amyloidosis [89, 91–93].

11.4.9 Treatment and Prognosis

- Only preventive measures, including avoidance of strenuous physical activity, intravenous thrombolysis, and antiplatelet and anticoagulant treatments.
- The fetus should be delivered via Cesarean section [90].
- If misdiagnosed with an autoimmune disorder, administration of corticosteroids may be associated with disease worsening [88, 92].
- The prognosis varies widely [88].

11.5 Ischemic Stroke

11.5.1 Epidemiology

- Incidence in women 178/100.000/year.
- Incidence in men 117/100.000/year [94].
- Increased prevalence in patients with MS [95].

11.5.2 Clinical Features

- Hyperacute symptoms onset (seconds-minutes) is atypical for MS, where symptoms onset usually evolves over hours-days.
- No specific clinical signs and/or symptoms; neurological manifestations vary depending on the location and extent of the ischemic territory [94].

11.5.3 Brain Imaging

- Early hyperacute (within minutes of arterial occlusion).
  - DWI: increased signal; apparent diffusion coefficient (ADC): reduced signal; T1 and T2 signals are normal
  - A minority of cases have normal DWI.
  - Occlusion in MR angiography.

- Late hyperacute (after 6 hours)
  - T2 hyperintensity; initially better seen on FLAIR.
  - T1 hypointensity seen after 16 hours.
  - Sulcal effacement (local mass effect that pushes adjacent gyri together and displaces the CSF from the sulci).
  - DWI shows restricted diffusion.
- Acute (during the first week)
  - Remains high DWI signal and low ADC signal.
  - T2 hyperintensity (signal increases during the first 4 days).
  - T1 hypointensity.
  - After 5 days, present the cortical contrast enhancement.
  - Less common arterial contrast enhancement after 3 days (50%), or uncommon leptomeningeal enhancement after 2–6 days.
  - Increase of edema, mass effect, gyral swelling, and sulcal effacement with nadir after 3–4 days (mass effect decreases after 7 days).
  - Might occur hemorrhagic transformation (5%) due to petechial hemorrhages (89%) or less frequent hematomas (11%).
- Subacute (after 10–15 days)
  - Decreased ADC values continue to rise (they normalize), but DWI signal remains increased due to persistent high T2 signal (T2 shine through).
  - May occur temporary loss of visibility of an infarct called "T2 fogging" (50%), which may cause underestimation of true infarct size.
  - T1 hypointensity.
  - Often present cortical contrast enhancement.
- Chronic
  - ADC signal is high; DWI signal is variable but decreases over time.
  - T2 hyperintensity.
  - T1 signal remains low.
  - Cortical contrast enhancement usually persists for 2 to 4 months. But if parenchymal enhancement persists for >12 weeks the presence of alternative pathology should be suspected.
  - Focal brain atrophy [96, 97] (Fig. 11.5).

11.5.4 Other Imaging Features of Ischemic Lesions

- Often single lesion (in MS are usually multiple).
- Located in the territory of a specific artery or in watershed territory (different distribution than in MS).
- Watershed (border zone) infarcts at the borders between cerebral vascular territories have atypical shapes and locations, as compared with MS lesions.
  - Cortical border zones infarcts: wedge-shaped or gyriform.
  - Deep border zones infarcts: ≥3 lesions, each ≥3 mm in diameter, in a linear fashion (string of pearls) parallel to the lateral ventricles in the deep white matter; sometimes become confluent (band-like).

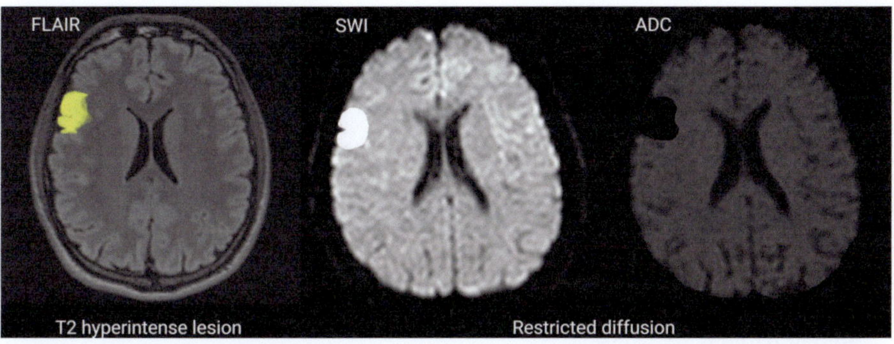

Fig. 11.5 MRI characteristics of ischemic stroke

- Shows restricted diffusion but not contrast enhancement (hyperacute MS lesions shows simultaneous contrast enhancement and sometime also mostly peripheral restricted diffusion over days to 2–3 weeks; restricted diffusion may precede contrast enhancement in some active MS lesions).
- Perfusion imaging may show hypoperfusion (active MS lesions exhibit increased blood flow due to inflammation).
- Loss of gray-white differentiation in ischemic lesions and sulcal effacement (do not occur in MS).
- Central vein sign (CVS) is negative in vast majority of lesions (majority of MS lesions has CVS) [80–83, 97, 98].

11.5.5 Examination of Blood and CSF

- Routine blood tests are usually normal.
- Often slightly elevated concentration of protein in CSF (40–50%) [99].
- Very mild pleocytosis (<15 cells in mm^3) is rare (12.7%), but can occur. However, marked pleocytosis following ischemic stroke is uncommon and should prompt further investigations [100, 101].

11.5.6 Diagnosis

- Based on clinical manifestations and imaging
- Brain imaging, particularly MRI with DWI, is most reliable imaging method to confirm the presence of acute ischemic stroke [94, 97].

11.5.7 Treatment

- Thrombolysis, thrombectomy, secondary ischemic stroke prevention [94].

11.6 Migraine

11.6.1 Epidemiology

- The global prevalence is estimated to be 14–15% of the population [102, 103].
- More common in the young age.
- Female/male ratio 2–3/1 [102, 103].
- Patients with MS have higher prevalence of migraine (21–36%) [104]. Female sex, young age, early disease stage, relapsing-remitting phenotype, and treatment with interferons are all associated with a higher frequency of migraine among patients with MS [105].

11.6.2 Etiology and Definition

- The precise etiology of this chronic neurovascular disorder remains unclear. It is hypothesized that a combination of environmental and genetic factors contributes to dysfunction of brainstem nuclei, leading to cortical excitatory-inhibitory imbalance, vascular dysfunction, and abnormalities in the synthesis of neurotransmitters and neuromodulators [106, 107]

11.6.3 Clinical Features

- Headache:
  - Typical migraine headaches manifest as frontal, unilateral, throbbing, and pulsating pain exacerbated by physical activity, accompanied by autonomic symptoms such as nausea, vomiting, photophobia, phonophobia, eyelid/facial swelling, conjunctival redness, tearing, and nasal congestion. The duration typically ranges from 4 to 72 hours, with a median duration of 24 hours.
  - Prodromal symptoms may precede the headache and include mood and behavioral changes, fatigue, yawning, pallor, blurred vision, decreased concentration, neck stiffness, photophobia, and phonophobia, occurring 24–48 hours before the onset of the headache.
  - Postdromal symptoms, experienced hours to days after the headache, may include decreased concentration, neck stiffness, and fatigue [108, 109].
- Aura:
  - Aura is most commonly visual (90%) and typically develops gradually over 5–60 minutes, with the duration usually within 1 hour. Polysymptomatic aura can persist for up to 3 hours, whereas motor aura can rarely last for 72 hours or longer.
  - A typical migraine headache should develop during or within 60 minutes after the onset of aura.
  - Visual aura affects one hemifield (not just one eye) and typically presents with positive symptoms such as scintillations, flashing lights, wavy lines, dots, distorted, or tunnel vision. However, sometimes only scotoma is present.

- Sensory aura is the second most common subtype. Sensory symptoms can migrate and include positive sensations such as tingling dysesthesia, pins, or needles. Negative symptoms such as numbness are also common and can occur without any accompanying positive symptoms.
- Motor and speech disorders, such as aphasia, are less common.
- When aura symptoms are multiple, they typically occur successively, starting with visual symptoms, followed by sensory symptoms, and then aphasia. However, variations in this sequence, including the reverse order and other patterns, have also been observed.
- Motor aura often follows sensory symptoms in its presentation [108–110].

11.6.4 Subtypes of Migraine and Diagnostic Criteria

- Migraine without aura.
  A. ≥5 attacks fulfilling criteria B, C, and D
  B. Headache attacks lasting 4–72 hours (when untreated or unsuccessfully treated)
  C. Headache has ≥2 of the following four characteristics:
    1. unilateral location
    2. pulsating quality
    3. moderate or severe pain intensity
    4. aggravation by or causing avoidance of routine physical activity (e.g. walking or climbing stairs)
  D. During headache ≥1 of the following:
    1. nausea and/or vomiting
    2. photophobia and phonophobia
  E. Not better accounted for by another diagnosis.

- Migraine with aura (30%):
  A. ≥2 migraine attacks fulfilling criteria B and C
  B. ≥1 of the following fully reversible aura symptoms (visual, sensory, speech and/or language, motor, brainstem, retinal)
  C. ≥3 of the following six characteristics
    1. ≥1 aura symptom spreads gradually over ≥5 minutes
    2. ≥2 aura symptoms occur in succession
    3. each individual aura symptom lasts 5–60 minutes (It is not rare for aura to last >1 hour, but in most such cases, patients have at least two of the other characteristics)
    4. ≥1 aura symptom is unilateral
    5. ≥1 aura symptom is positive
    6. The aura is accompanied, or followed within 60 minutes, by headache with or without migraine characteristics. Aura is sometimes associated

with a headache not fulfilling criteria for migraine, but this is still considered as a migraine headache because of its relation to the aura.

- Aura without headache (5%)
  - No headache accompanies or follows the aura within 60 minutes.
- Migraine with brainstem aura
  - Migraine with brainstem symptoms has almost always additional typical aura symptoms. When the aura includes motor weakness, it should be diagnosed as hemiplegic migraine.
- Hemiplegic migraine
  - Separate subtype with genetic and pathophysiological differences.
  - Typically associated with paresis rather than plegia and typically lasts less than 72 hours. However, in rare cases, it may persist for weeks.
  - Familial hemiplegic migraine frequently manifests with brainstem symptoms alongside typical aura symptoms, with headache being nearly always present. Occasionally, during relapses, disturbances of consciousness (including coma), confusion, fever, and CSF pleocytosis may occur. It can be misinterpreted as epilepsy. In half of these families, chronic progressive cerebellar ataxia develops, progressing independently of migraine attacks.
- Retinal migraine
  - Repeated monocular visual disturbance including scintillations, scotomata, or blindness, and associated with migraine headache. It should spread gradually over ≥5 minutes and last 5–60 minutes.
  - Extremely rare cause of transient monocular visual loss.
- Vestibular migraine
  - Episodic vertigo lasting from 5 minutes to 72 hours is common. At least half of these episodes are associated with typical migraine headache, photophobia or phonophobia, or visual aura.
- Complications of migraine
  - Status migrainosus (debilitating migraine attack lasting >72 hours).
  - Migrainous infarction occurs mainly in the posterior circulation and predominantly affects young women.
  - Persistent aura without infarction is characterized by the persistence of aura symptoms for at least one week without evidence of infarction on MRI. These symptoms are often bilateral and can persist for months.
  - Migraine aura-triggered seizure refers to a seizure that occurs either during or within 1 hour after an attack of migraine with aura.
  - Other complications: abdominal migraine, cyclic vomiting syndrome, recurring gastrointestinal disturbance, benign paroxysmal vertigo, benign paroxysmal torticollis [108, 109].

11.6.5 Brain Imaging

- Lesions' location:
  - Microstructural alterations in normal-appearing gray and white matter.

  - Focal T2 lesions (30–70%) in migraine patients without any vascular risks.
  - Patients experiencing aura and more severe migraines typically have a higher lesion burden [104, 111].
  - Typically located in deep white matter, with periventricular and juxtacortical lesions being less common. The presence of at least three typical periventricular lesions is associated with a higher probability of a MS.
  - Frontal and parietal lobes are most affected, whereas the temporal lobe is only rarely involved. Conversely, in MS, the temporal lobe is often affected.
  - Although, patients with migraines exhibit global structural changes in gray matter, cortical lesions are not typically present. If cortical lesions are detected, this should raise suspicion for a possible diagnosis of MS [112, 113].
  - Higher prevalence of T2 stroke-like lesions in the vascular border zone of the cerebellum (5.4% in migraine vs. 0.7% in controls). This frequency is increased in patients with often migraine attacks [114, 115].
  - Sometime T2 lesions in the brainstem (often in pons) (4–5%) [114]
  - The corpus callosum is typically unaffected [104, 116–118]
- Lesions' appearance:
  - Lesions in migraine are typically smaller compared to those in MS (median 2.5 mm versus usually >5.0 mm in MS).
  - Often punctate or round shape, rather than being ovoid and perpendicular to the lateral ventricle as seen in MS.
  - Lesions usually lack the central vein sign [119] and do not exhibit restricted diffusion on DWI [104, 116–118] (Fig. 11.6).
- Contrast enhancement and perilesional changes:
  - Absent [104, 116–118].
- Evolution over time:
  - The size and number of lesions remain relatively stable over time [104].

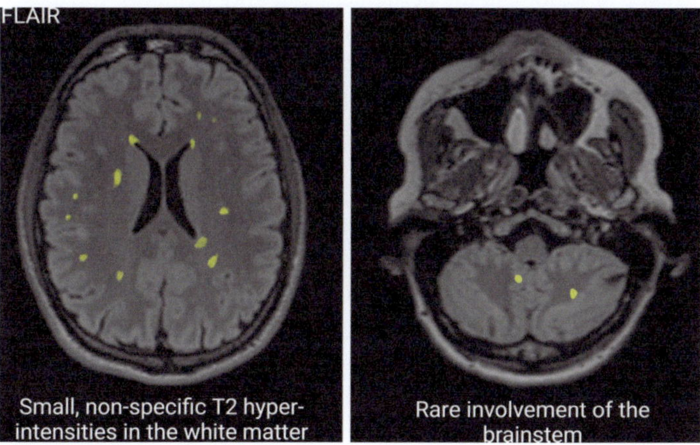

Fig. 11.6 MRI characteristics of migraine

11.6.6 Spinal Cord Imaging

- Normal [120].

11.6.7 Examination of Blood and CSF

- Normal [107, 121].

11.6.8 Electrophysiology

- Patients with migraine with visual aura might have rarely (5%) slightly prolonged latencies on visual evoked potentials (VEP) [122, 123].

11.6.9 Diagnosis

- See "Subtypes of migraine and diagnostic criteria."

11.6.10 Differential Diagnosis

- MS:
  - High proportion of patients with migraine fulfill MRI criteria for dissemination in space of MS [116] and migraine is one of the most common sources of false-positive diagnosis of MS [124].
  - In contrast, migraine is often comorbid with MS and occurs during prodromal phase of MS [125]. Patients with comorbid MS and migraine exhibit a higher occurrence of lesions in the periaqueductal gray matter of the mesencephalon [126]. Additionally, they experience an increase frequency of contrast-enhancing lesions [127] and possibly also cortical microbleeds, which are otherwise extremely rare in MS [85].
  - Distinguishing a demyelinating event (relapse) from a prolonged aura without headache in patients with MS is only rarely challenging [104], because relapses in MS:

    Usually not accompanied with headache.

    Develop and progress slowly over hours-days (not minutes).

    Duration of the relapse is longer (days-weeks, not minutes).

    Retrobulbar neuritis in MS typically impacts only one eye due to prechiasmatic involvement (not a hemifield). Symptoms are characterised mainly by negative features, such as blurred vision, scotoma, mild pain, and a relative afferent pupillary defect (RAPD) [128].

- Cerebrovascular events:
  - When suspected aura with or without headache occurs first after 40 years of age, when symptoms are only negative or when aura is prolonged or very short, other causes, particularly transient ischemic attacks, should be ruled out [109].

11.6.11 Treatment

- Symptomatic relief to stop headaches as well as chronic treatments aimed at preventing migraine recurrence [106].
- Some studies suggest the pathogenetic role of patent foramen ovale (PFO) in generating symptoms and white matter lesions in migraine patients, especially those with visual aura and occipital lesions [129]. However, further research is necessary to determine whether the occlusion of PFO, which is more prevalent in migraine patients, may have any positive effects [130].

11.7 Moyamoya Disease and Syndrome

11.7.1 Epidemiology

- Incidence 0.09/100,000/year (USA).
- In Asia, the incidence is tenfold higher compared to the rest of the world.
- The incidence exhibits two peaks: in children around the age of 5 years, and in adults between 40 and 50 years of age.
- Female/male ratio 2/1 [131–134].

11.7.2 Etiology and Definition

- Moyamoya disease and syndrome (MM) represent progressive non-inflammatory vasculopathies characterized by bilateral stenosis of the intracranial segments of the internal carotid arteries and their proximal branches, leading to strokes or subclinical brain infarcts.
- In this condition, the occlusion of vessels results from a combination of smooth muscle cell hyperplasia and luminal thrombosis.
- Genetic factors play a significant role in the pathogenesis of MM. Most familial cases involve polygenic inheritance or an autosomal dominant pattern, where abnormal regulation of specific proteins leads to the Moyamoya phenotype in susceptible individuals when certain environmental triggers are present. However, the exact etiology and pathogenesis of MM remain unknown.

- Stenosis of the large vessels leads to the development of compensatory collateral vasculature, comprising dilated perforating small arteries. These arteries, a combination of preexisting and newly formed vessels, emerge near the apex of the carotid, on the cortical surface, within the leptomeninges, and from branches of the external carotid artery, which supply the dura and the base of the skull. Vertebrobasilar (posterior) circulation is affected rarely.

11.7.3 Subtypes

- Idiopathic (Moyamoya disease).
- Associated with the following conditions (Moyamoya syndrome):
  - Sickle cell disease; neurofibromatosis type I; state after therapeutic cranial radiotherapy; congenital cardiac anomaly; renal-artery stenosis; giant cervicofacial hemangiomas; Down syndrome; and a wide spectrum of other disorders [131].

11.7.4 Clinical Features

- Cerebrovascular events (i.e., ischemic, or hemorrhagic stroke, transient ischemic attacks) is the most common manifestation. Therefore, clinical symptoms occur usually acutely/paroxysmally not like in MS, when relapses develop usually subacutely over hours or days.
- Headache is usually migraine-like (63%).
- An enlargement of the optic disk with concomitant retinovascular anomalies is relatively typical.
- Rarely seizures, movement disorders (mainly chorea due to dilated collaterals in the basal ganglia), cognitive and psychiatric manifestations [131].

11.7.5 Brain Imaging

- Lesions' location:
  - Often in the cortex, subcortical regions, and deep gray matter (atypical for MS)
  - Less frequently in periventricular and juxtacortical white matter, resembling those seen in MS. Infratentorial involvement is usually absent.
  - Involvement may be asymmetric. If it is unilateral, progression to bilateral involvement occurs in 40% of patients [135] (Fig. 11.7).
- Lesions' appearance:
  - Acute infarcts with restricted diffusion and old post-ischemic lesions.
- Contrast enhancement:
  - Prominent leptomeningeal collaterals exhibit high signal intensity on FLAIR images due to slow flow and contrast enhancement on post-contrast T1 images. This pattern manifests as linear leptomeningeal hyperintensities following a sulcal pattern, giving the appearance of the brain being covered with ivy ("ivy sign").

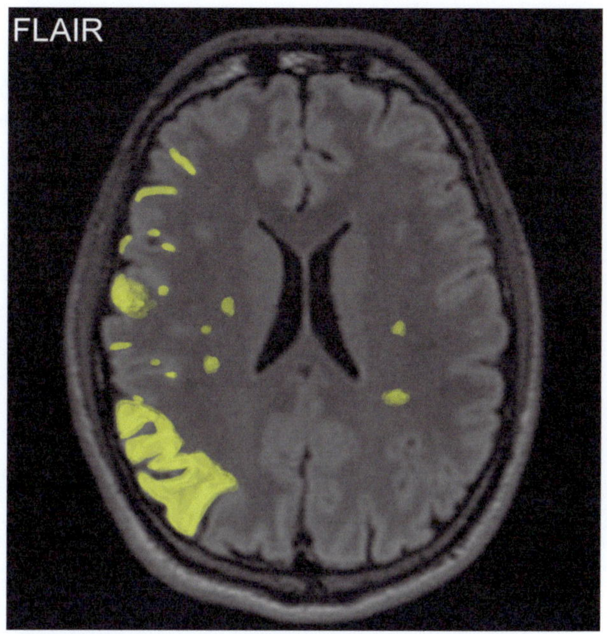

Fig. 11.7 Initially asymmetric involvement predominantly affecting the cortex, subcortical regions, and deep gray matter in Moyamoya disease and syndrome

- Evolution over time:
  - The occurrence of new cerebrovascular pathology over time.
- Associated Findings:
  - Frequently cerebral microhemorrhages (more in males and older patients).
  - MRI angiographic findings suggestive of MM are present in only 50–75% of patients and may reveal decreased flow voids in the main cerebral arteries, but increased flow voids can be observed through the basal ganglia and thalamus due to compensatory collateral vessels.
  - The network of abnormally dilated compensatory vasculature of small vessels can be visualized using the gold standard examination digital subtraction angiography (DSA), which resembles a "puff of cigarette smoke" (translated in Japanese as "moyamoya").
  - Cortical atrophy [135–140]

11.7.6 Spinal Cord Imaging

- Normal [135–139].

11.7.7 Examination of Blood and CSF

- Routine tests are normal, including negative OCB [135, 137].

11.7.8 Diagnosis

- Imaging is most important for definite diagnosis. Early diagnosis can prompt timely intervention and help prevent stroke-related disability [135–140].

11.7.9 Differential Diagnosis

- MS:
  - MM can mimic MS and is often misdiagnosed due to its rarity and sometimes asymptomatic or atypical presentation. More than 3% of patients with MM were initially diagnosed with MS [141].
  - The presence of transient focal neurological deficits, cortical symptoms such as aphasia, the absence of typical MS brain MRI findings, the lack of spinal cord and infratentorial lesions, and normal CSF should raise suspicion of MM [135–138].
  - In contrast, very rare case studies describe patients with coexisting MM disease and MS. The presence of typical MS lesions, involvement of the spinal cord, and positive OCB should arise suspicion of a comorbid diagnosis of MS [142].
- Stroke:
  - MM should be considered in children and young adults presenting with cerebrovascular events or ischemic changes on brain imaging.
  - Screening for MM should be considered in suspected patients with high-risk disorders such as neurofibromatosis type 1, Down syndrome, sickle cell disease, or following therapeutic cranial radiation [131].

11.7.10 Treatment and Prognosis

- Moyamoya can progress slowly or rapidly, leading to rapid neurological decline.
- Antiplatelet therapy does not halt disease progression. Therefore, surgery is often necessary to provide a new source of blood flow by bypassing a branch of the external carotid artery with a cortical artery. Other surgical approaches are also utilized [131].

11.8 Posterior Reversible Encephalopathy Syndrome (PRES)

11.8.1 Synonym

- Posterior leukoencephalopathy syndrome (PLES).

11.8.2 Epidemiology

- Prevalence
  - 0.8% of patients with end-stage renal disease.
  - 0.7% of patients with systemic lupus erythematosus (SLE).
  - 20–98% of women with preeclampsia or eclampsia [143].

11.8.3 Etiology and Definition

- Usually associated with other medical conditions such as hypertensive crisis, renal failure, (pre)-eclampsia, severe hypercalcemia, thrombocytopenic syndromes, Henoch–Schönlein purpura, hemolytic uremic syndrome, amyloid angiopathy, SLE, sepsis, anaphylaxis, alcohol withdrawal or medications (especially immunosuppressive, immunomodulatory, chemotherapeutic, and cytotoxic agents) [143–147].
- Hypertensive encephalopathy, which may or may not be associated with PRES, is the most common cause of PRES [148].
- Case studies reported PRES associated with using of disease-modifying drugs for treatment of MS such as fingolimod, anti-CD20, natalizumab or interferon-beta [149–152].
- Although the exact pathophysiology remains unclear, dysfunction in cerebral autoregulation, endothelial dysfunction, and impairment of the blood-brain barrier likely contribute to the extravasation of fluid and the development of cortical or subcortical vasogenic edema [144, 145, 147].
- Vasogenic edema may progress to cytotoxic edema if left untreated [153].

11.8.4 Clinical Features

- The onset is acute or subacute.
- Variable symptoms including the headache (50%); encephalopathy with mild confusion or coma (94%); focal or generalized seizures (75%); visual disturbances (20–39%); or also other focal neurological deficits such as ophthalmoplegia, dysarthria, hemianopia, or ataxia [143, 144, 146, 147].
- Some patients have residual irreversible neurological symptoms [150].
- High blood pressure is not always present in PRES [154].

11.8.5 Brain Imaging

- Lesions' location:
  - PRES tends to favor the posterior circulation, likely due to a relative lack of sympathetic innervation in the arterioles, which protects the brain from

increases in intravascular pressure. Hence, cortical gray matter and subcortical white matter in the parieto-occipital regions are typically affected (70–90%).
  - Other, less frequently affected regions include the posterior frontal cortical region, temporal lobe, brainstem, cerebellum, and deep gray matter structures such as the basal ganglia.
  - Involvement is usually bilateral and symmetric; however, approximately 3–5% of patients present with asymmetrical or unilateral pathology (Fig. 11.8).
- Lesions' appearance:
  - T2 hyperintense and T1 hypointense signal in affected regions.
  - Vasogenic edema (with increased signal on DWI); but restricted diffusion (with decreased signal on the ADC map) is not frequent (17–26%).
  - SWI may show subarachnoid or rarely parenchymal micro- or macrohemorrhages (11–65%).
- Contrast enhancement:
  - Patchy leptomeningeal or gyriform/cortical (33–37%).
- Perilesional changes:
  - Typically, no mass effect, but rare case studies reported unilateral tumefactive PRES [145, 147, 150, 155, 156].
- Evolution over time:
  - MRI findings may improve significantly already 72 hours after the discontinuation of causing mechanism or medication [149, 150].

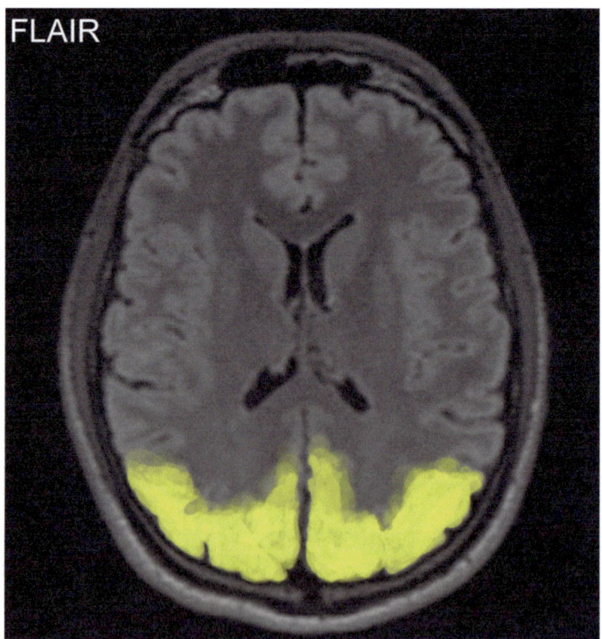

Fig. 11.8 Posterior reversible encephalopathy syndrome (PRES) with bilateral and symmetric involvement of the cortical gray matter and subcortical white matter in the parieto-occipital regions

11.8.6 Spinal Cord Imaging

- Typically normal, but a few case studies reported patients with isolated involvement of the spinal cord ("posterior reversible encephalopathy syndrome with spinal cord involvement; PRES-SCI") with cervical, confluent, centrally located longitudinally extensive transverse myelitis (LETM) originating from cervicomedullary junction.
- These cord lesions completely resolve on follow-up MRI in most cases.
- Brain MRI can be normal in these patients [157, 158].

11.8.7 Blood Work

- Normal.

11.8.8 Examination of CSF

- May be elevated concentration of protein.
- Rare presence of CSF-restricted OCB is usually related to the underlying condition, such as autoimmune disease [149, 157, 159].

11.8.9 Diagnosis

- It is not a single disease entity but rather a clinico-radiologic syndrome with various underlying causes.
- The clinical manifestations are often atypical; therefore, a combination of clinical history and MRI features, which are often typical for PRES, is important for diagnosis. In some atypical cases, diagnosis might be challenging, and follow-up MRI may be needed [145, 147, 150].

11.8.10 Differential Diagnosis

- Includes stroke, cerebral venous thrombosis, encephalitis, neoplasm, acute hepatic encephalopathy, reversible cerebral vasoconstriction syndrome, osmotic demyelination syndrome, rhombencephalitis, and other inflammatory or infectious leukoencephalopathies or demyelinating disorders [145, 147, 155].
- In patients on certain immunomodulatory treatments, such as natalizumab may PRES mimic progressive multifocal leukoencephalopathy [151].

11.8.11 Treatment and Prognosis

- A rapid normalization of elevated blood pressure if present, anti-epileptic therapy if needed and withdrawal of the causing medication or treatment of underlying condition.
- Treated patients have generally a good outcome [143, 147], but PRES associated with hypertensive encephalopathy may progress to coma and death if left untreated [148].

11.9 Superficial Siderosis of CNS

11.9.1 Epidemiology

- Prevalence 100/100.000 [160].

11.9.2 Etiology and Definition

- Linear hemosiderin depositions in the leptomeninges and on the surface of the cerebral and cerebellar cortex, brainstem, or spinal cord. The neurotoxic iron within the hemosiderin leads to demyelination and axonal loss [160–162].
- The sources of iron depositions include:
  - Type 1 (classical): Chronic or repeated low-volume bleeding into the subarachnoid space in patients with spinal dural abnormalities (dural tears in the upper thoracic spinal cord), cerebral amyloid angiopathy, CNS tumors, arteriovenous malformations, spontaneous intracranial hypotension, CNS trauma, traumatic nerve root avulsion, or after craniospinal surgery.
  - Type 2 (secondary; less common): Monophasic bleeding into the subarachnoid space due to subarachnoid hemorrhage, arteriovenous malformation, vasculitis, cerebral venous thrombosis, or trauma [160, 162, 163].

11.9.3 Clinical Features (Type 1)

- The early asymptomatic stage is followed by insidious onset and slow progression of the following symptoms:
  - Cerebellar syndrome often manifesting with dominant gait ataxia, primarily due to the preferential involvement of the cerebellar vermis.
  - Sensorineural hearing loss, typically one of the initial symptoms.
  - Hyposmia (the olfactory and vestibulocochlear nerves are most frequently affected because these are pure glial nerves and have close contact with the CSF).
  - Less frequent spinal cord symptoms including spasticity, anterior horn signs, sensory symptoms, radicular pain, or sphincter symptoms.
  - Some patients may experience cognitive decline.

11.9.4 Clinical Features (Type 2)

- Clinical symptoms are more closely associated with the underlying pathological process rather than the focal superficial siderosis [160–163].

11.9.5 Brain Imaging

- SWI sequences show signal loss (dark rims) on the surface of the brain indicating the presence of blood breakdown products.
  - Type 1 (infratentorial; classical): symmetrical involvement of posterior fossa structures is common, but it can often also extend to cortical sulci.
  - Type 2 (infratentorial; secondary): asymmetric depositions in the infratentorial structures around the source of the bleeding [161, 162].
  - Cortical type of superficial siderosis: hemosiderin deposits are limited to a supratentorial cortex. This subtype is primarily associated with cerebral amyloid angiopathy, although it can also occur in traumatic brain injury, subarachnoid bleeding, reversible cerebral vasoconstriction syndrome, hemorrhagic transformation of an infarct, dural fistulae, or cortical vein thrombosis (Fig. 11.9).

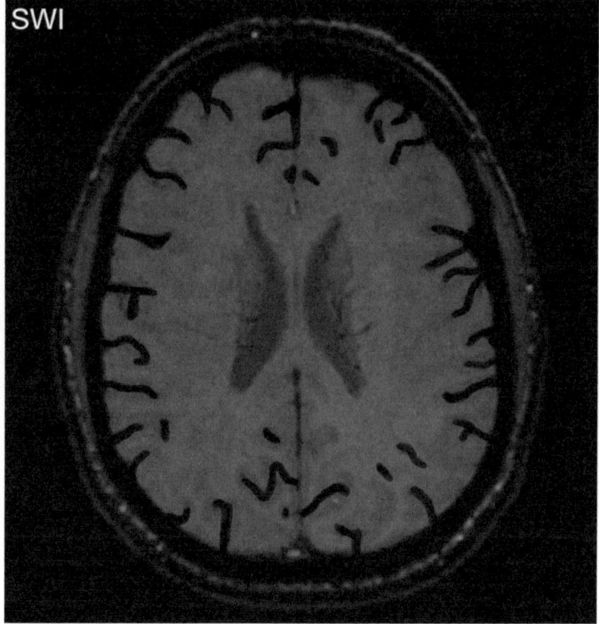

Fig. 11.9 Cortical type of superficial siderosis characterized by hemosiderin deposits limited to the supratentorial cortex

11.9.6 Spinal Cord Imaging

- Linear hemosiderin depositions on the surface of the spinal cord, and sharp delineations of hemosiderin deposits in the cranial nerves and spinal nerve roots at the transition zone between central glial cells and peripheral Schwann cells may be present [160, 162, 164, 165].

11.9.7 Blood Work

- Normal.

11.9.8 Examination of CSF

- Red cells indicating recent bleeding and/or blood breakdown products such as hemosiderin or ferritin indicating older bleeding may be present (still present in the CSF months after bleeding) [160–163].

11.9.9 Diagnosis

- Based on clinical symptoms and MRI showing iron deposits.
- The brain and whole spine imaging, including SWI sequences (or other paramagnetic-sensitive sequence) is required to define the pattern of siderosis and search for a potential source of bleeding.
- CT, MR and DSA are often not helpful because larger vascular lesions visible on angiography would usually not cause chronic low-volume subarachnoid bleeding [160, 162, 163].

11.9.10 Treatment and Prognosis

- Identification and treatment a source of subarachnoid bleeding (for example surgical repair of the dural defect) and reduction of an adverse effect of neurotoxic iron by iron-chelating agents, such as deferiprone.
- Although some patients might be stable, many untreated patients have progressive irreversible neurological deficit [160, 162, 163].

11.10 Vascular Myelopathies

11.10.1 Epidemiology

- Spinal cord infarction

- Incidence 3.1/100.000/year (75% periprocedural; 25% spontaneous)
- 1% of all strokes in the CNS and 5–8% of all acute myelopaties [166, 167]
- Older patients with vascular risk factors are most commonly affected, but young people may also be affected due to fibrocartilaginous embolism or vertebral dissection [168].

• Arteriovenous (AV) fistulas
  - Incidence 0.5–1/100.000/year.
  - Female/male ratio 1/4.
  - Usually in adults between 40 and 80 years of age [169, 170].

11.10.2 Etiology and Definition

• There are many different vascular mechanisms responsible for vascular myelopathies:
• Arterial ischemia
  - Periprocedural spinal cord infarction
    Thoracic aortic aneurysm surgery is responsible for half of the cases. Other cases include cardiac surgery, spinal decompression, epidural injection, angiography, nerve block, embolization, as well as other vascular or thoracic surgeries [171].
  - Spontaneous spinal cord infarction and TIA
    Dissection (aortic, vertebral, or subclavian artery).
    Mechanical (fibrocartilaginous embolism, surfer's myelopathy, arterial compression by disk or fascial compression).
    Embolic.
    Vasculitis (rare; primary angiitis of the CNS; other systemic autoimmune, infectious, or paraneoplastic [e.g., Hodgkin lymphoma]).
    Low blood pressure.
    Hypercoagulability (SLE, disseminated intravascular coagulation, malignancy, dehydration).
    Pharmacologic (sildenafil, oral contraceptives, phentermine, cocaine, cannabis).
    Arterial vasospasm.
    Some patients report physical maneuver at or before onset of deficit such as lifting, back hyperextension, neck movement, or Valsalva suggesting potential mechanism such as arterial dissection, fibrocartilaginous embolism, or radicular artery compression from disc).
    In many cases, the mechanism remains unclear.
• Venous congestion/ischemia.
  - Spinal dural arteriovenous fistulas (70% of the spinal AV malformations)
    AV shunt consisting of a connection between a radiculo-meningeal artery and single radicular vein, typically in the neural foramen. This connection

leads to arterialization of the vein, venous hypertension, spinal cord congestion, and venous ischemia [172].

In many patients, an association with previous cervical and thoracic spinal cord surgeries or trauma (typically within <2 years after the event) is observed, which may contribute to the development of an AV fistula [170, 173].

- Spinal epidural and pial arteriovenous fistula

  Less frequent mechanism resulting from a connection between paraspinal or paravertebral arteries and the epidural venous plexus [168, 174].

- Miscellaneous causes of venous ischemic myelopathy.

  Various conditions associated with decreased venous outflow from the intrinsic veins of the spinal cord such as:

  - Vasculitis in Behçet's disease affecting venous system.
  - Inferior vena cava thrombosis or obstruction.
  - Overshunting-associated myelopathy can occur in patients with ventriculo-peritoneal shunt causing decreased CSF pressure.
  - Epidural infections and others [168].

- Hematomyelia (Intraparenchymal spinal cord hemorrhage).
  - A highly uncommon condition caused by trauma; spinal cord cavernous and AV malformations; neoplasm or other rare causes.
- Extraparenchymal hemorrhage.
  - Subarachnoid or subdural hemorrhage.
  - Epidural hematoma.

    Most commonly caused by trauma, surgery, epidural catheterization, or lumbar puncture [168].

11.10.3 Clinical Features

- Arterial ischemia
  - Periprocedural spinal cord infarction.

    Approximately 80% of patients awaken from the procedure with maximum deficits. In the remaining 20% of cases, deficits may manifest hours to days after the procedure or progress gradually over days or hours following the procedure.

    Flaccid paraplegia (70%).

    Mild or less severe deficit (30%).

    Only a small proportion of patients (15%) experience pain, a frequency lower than that observed in cases of spontaneous spinal cord infarction [171].

  - Spontaneous spinal cord infarction

    The acute bilateral neurological deficit depends upon the topography of the ischemic lesion.

    Unilateral manifestations are rare.

    Onset to nadir of severe deficit is usually within 12 hours.

The faster and more severe the deficits, the easier to diagnose spinal cord infarction.

Infarction in the anterior spinal artery territory has bilateral corticospinal (motor weakness) and spino-thalamic (pain/temperature loss) tract involvement.

Less frequently are infarctions localized in the posterior spinal artery territory causing dorsal column dysfunction with dominating sensory loss [168].

Rare cases of Brown-Séquard syndrome, central cord syndrome, and complete cord syndrome were also described [175].

Premorbid conditions such as peripheral neuropathy can often confound clinical picture [168].

Intense acute pain in the back, chest, neck, or limbs occurring at or prior to onset is a common feature (60–70%) and characteristic symptom of spinal cord infarction. This symptom is atypical for myelitis and can aid in the differential diagnosis [176].

  - Spinal cord TIA

    Rare condition, which is often difficult to prove. Usually painless with a short duration of symptoms (seconds to minutes).

    In a minority of cases recurrent spinal TIA may precede spinal cord infarction (3%) [168, 177].

- Venous congestion/ischemia
  - Spinal dural arteriovenous fistula

    Insidious onset with (often stepwise) progressive thoracic myelopathy.

    Motor weakness and sensory loss on lower limbs, bowel/bladder dysfunction, conus syndrome or radicular symptoms.

    Back or radicular pain is frequent [173].

    Acute paraplegia (2–5%) or stepwise progression (11–32%) [168].

    Combined upper and lower motor findings (70%) [178].

    Sensory level (18–37%; mostly at L1 level) [179].

    Often dramatic worsening of deficit during activities associated with elevating venous pressure, such as exertion, Valsalva, or lumbar puncture [180].

    A significant exacerbation of deficits after corticosteroids, attributed to venous hypertension (50%), which may serve as a diagnostic indicator for the presence of an AV fistula [181, 182].

    In contrast, there are case reports of patients showing improvement after undergoing plasmapheresis [183].

    Rarely is AV fistula asymptomatic incidental finding [184].

  - Spinal epidural and pial arteriovenous fistula

    Slowly progressive myelopathy with venous distension that may compress the spinal cord or nerve roots [168, 174].

- Hematomyelia (Intraparenchymal spinal cord hemorrhage)
  - The clinical presentation closely resembles that of spinal cord infarction, characterized by intense back pain at onset followed by rapid and severe myelopathy. However, in contrast to the typical rapid progression observed in

spinal cord infarction over hours, the progression in this condition may be slower, extending over days [168].

- Extraparenchymal hemorrhage
  - The clinical manifestations vary depending on the extent and location of the hemorrhage [168].

11.10.4 Spinal Cord Imaging

- Arterial ischemia
  - Acute stage:

    MRI may appear normal (50–70%) [176].

    Otherwise, T2 hyperintensities typically occur in the antero-medial part of the spinal cord.

    May be seen bilaterally symmetric circular/ovoid T2 hyperintensity in the anterior horns ("Owl-eyes" or "snake-eyes" sign) or bilateral T2 lesions showing U or V-shape on transversal planes.

    In severe cases may be affected all gray matter of the spinal cord.

    Residual cystic myelomalacia with bright T2 hyperintensity and T1 hypointensity indicates matrix destruction and axonal loss.

    Sagittal plane may show non-contiguous anterior pencil-like T2 hyperintensity ("pencil sign").

    Although marked edema is uncommon, it can occur in severe cases.

    Contrast enhancement is uncommon in the acute stage [168, 176].
  - Subacute stage (after days).

    The spectrum of MRI patterns can vary widely.

    Ischemic lesions are often large and do not respect vascular territories.

    If present restricted diffusion, it should be confirmed on ADC map, because of technical difficulties in DWI of the spinal cord.

    Contrast enhancement may occur (40%).
    - Usually, a linear craniocaudal strip.
    - Sometime present in adjacent nerve roots (non-nodular).
    - Typically resolves within months.

    Vertebral body infarction (10–20% of cases) should not be misinterpreted with vertebral body hemangiomas and degenerative changes.

    Hyperintense T2 signal in the anterior spinal artery may suggest slow flow or thrombus.

    Sometime seen adjacent arterial dissection, which detection may be challenging (T1-weighted fat saturation sequence).

    MR angiography of the spinal canal has limited value and can usually show only a rare acute presentation of spinal dural arteriovenous fistula/arteriovenous malformation.

    DSA is usually not used, unless suspected alternative vascular pathology such as spinal dural arteriovenous fistula or vasculitis.

Red flags indicating alternative diagnoses other than spinal cord ischemia include:
  - Large lesion with mild clinical deficits.
  - Lesion extending the entire length of the cord.
  - Separate well-defined lesions (although noncontiguous lesions are common in spinal cord ischemia).
  - A small lesion with severe edema [168, 171, 176].
- Chronic stage (after weeks-months).

  At this stage differentiating the spinal cord infarction from other myelopathies is more difficult.

  Can be found spinal cord atrophy, or residual T2 hyperintensity respecting a vascular territory [168] (Fig. 11.10).

- Spinal dural arteriovenous, epidural, and pial arteriovenous fistulas.
  - Almost all patients have T2 hyperintense lesions (95%).
  - Often longitudinally extensive transverse myelitis (LETM) extending to the conus (90%) with edema.
  - Contrast enhancement is seen in majority of cases (see Fig. 15.3 in Sect. 15.22.6).
  - Flow voids (enlarged perimedullary veins), which are located on the dorsal more than the ventral surface of the cord (seen best on post-contrast T1 but may be visible also on T2 images) (80%) [168, 185].
  - Therefore, high-quality MRI of the entire spine without evidence of T2-hyperintense signal or flow voids usually reliably excludes spinal dural AV fistulas [186, 187].
  - However, flow voids can also be seen with tumors and or AV malformations, and mild prominence of nontortuous vasculature in the lower thoracolumbar cord is normal finding.
  - Although, DSA is the gold standard for diagnosis, the spinal MR angiography can detect 80–95% of the fistulas and can be considered as an initial step to localize the fistula level [188].
  - DSA is highly sensitive, but may show false-negative findings, especially if performed by a non-experienced angiographer [189].
  - Visualization of the AV fistula may be compromised by atherosclerosis of segmental arteries or thrombosis of veins of the fistula [190].
  - In negative cases, suspected cervical AV fistulas should be considered intracranial four-vessel DSA.
  - Postcontrast MRI may show abrupt segments without contrast-enhancement, called the "missing-piece sign" [168, 174, 191, 192].
- Intraparenchymal (hematomyelia) and extra-parenchymal spinal cord hemorrhage:
  - MRI shows blood products within or around the spinal cord [168].

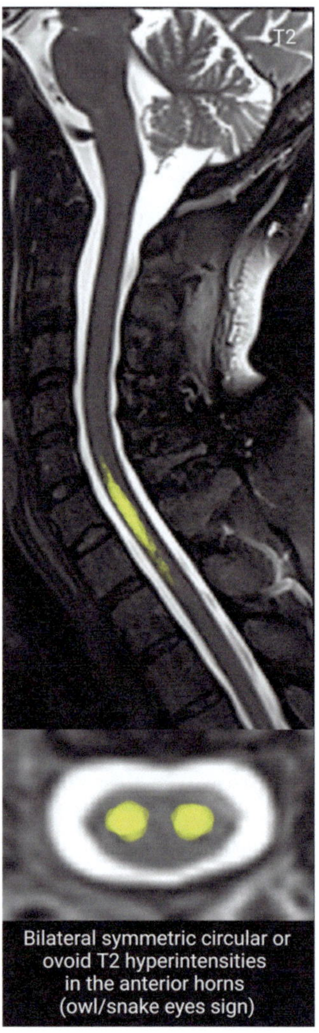

Fig. 11.10 Selected MRI characteristics of spinal cord infarction

11.10.5 Electrophysiology

- Some patients with spinal dural AV fistulas may show signs of polyradiculopathy on conduction studies due to involvement of lower motor neurons [193].

11.10.6 Blood Work

- Normal.

11.10.7 Examination of CSF

- Periprocedural and spontaneous spinal cord infarctions:
  - Often mildly to moderately elevated concentration of protein
  - Mild pleocytosis (<10%)
  - Marked pleocytosis (>25 cells/mm^3) is atypical for spinal cord ischemia
  - IgG index is normal, and CSF-restricted OCB are negative [168, 176]
- Spinal dural AV fistulas:
  - Lumbar puncture should be avoided [168, 180]
  - If a CSF analysis is conducted, it typically does not exhibit an inflammatory pattern. However, cases displaying an inflammatory pattern with marked pleocytosis have also been described [194], including rare instances of patients with positive CSF-restricted OCB [195].

11.10.8 Diagnosis

- Vascular myelopathies are rare and frequently underrecognized disorders. Although some clinical features may suggest vascular myelopathy, accurate interpretation of MRI findings is key factor for correct diagnosis [168].

11.10.9 Differential Diagnosis

- Vascular myelopathies are often misdiagnosed. Around 15% of patients with a diagnosis of idiopathic acute transverse myelitis have vascular myelopathy [196].
- Many patients with spontaneous spinal cord infarction are initially suspected to have Guillain–Barré syndrome due to spinal shock with hyporeflexia [168, 177].
- Spinal dural AV fistula is frequently misdiagnosed as a peripheral neurological disorder, such as cauda equina syndrome, primarily due to the absence of upper motor neuron signs and the presence of progressive lower motor neuron signs at the level of the conus or roots. LETM in the thoracic spinal cord, especially in elderly patients, should always raise suspicion of a spinal dural AV fistula [168, 170].
- "Owl-eyes" or "snake-eyes" sign can be observed also in other diagnoses such as amyotrophic lateral sclerosis (ALS), compressive myelopathy, Hopkins syndrome, myelin oligodendrocyte glycoprotein antibody-associated disease (MOGAD), neuromyelitis optica spectrum disorders (NMOSD), neuroinfections (poliovirus, West Nile virus, enterovirus), or spinal muscular atrophy [197].
- Cobb syndrome (Spinal arteriovenous metameric syndrome) is a rare disorder characterized by a port-wine-colored vascular skin nevus and an angioma within the spinal canal, which can potentially lead to vascular myelopathy [198].

11.10.10 Treatment and Prognosis

- Delay in diagnosis of vascular myelopathies can be associated with worse outcome [199].
- Anti-inflammatory treatment (such as corticosteroids) used in patients with misdiagnosed vascular myelopathies can worsen symptoms and outcomes of patients [182].
- Arterial ischemia.
  - Periprocedural spinal cord infarction
    An increase of the spinal cord perfusion pressure through collaterals by CSF drainage and/or arterial blood pressure augmentation.
    Many patients have substantial improvements despite significant initial deficits [171].
  - Spontaneous spinal cord infarction
    Although, there is only limited evidence, intravenous recombinant tissue plasminogen activator (rtPA) within the first 4.5 hours after onset could be considered.
    Alternatively, arterial pressure augmentation with or without lumbar drainage can have a positive effect.
    Secondary stroke prevention of ischemic vascular events is recommended [168].
    Despite often severe deficits at onset, 50% of patients are able to walk without the need for a gait aid after they recover [176].
- Spinal dural fistulas
  - Embolization of the fistula or surgical disconnection of the draining vein [168] lead to stabilization or improvement of neurological deficit (>30–40%) and improvement or resolution of the spinal cord lesions (80%) [200].

References

1. Jäkel L, De Kort AM, Klijn CJM, Schreuder F, Verbeek MM. Prevalence of cerebral amyloid angiopathy: a systematic review and meta-analysis. Alzheimers Dement. 2022;18(1):10–28.
2. Banerjee G, Carare R, Cordonnier C, Greenberg SM, Schneider JA, Smith EE, et al. The increasing impact of cerebral amyloid angiopathy: essential new insights for clinical practice. J Neurol Neurosurg Psychiatry. 2017;88(11):982–94.
3. Kobylarek D, Iwanowski P, Masolak D, Limphaibool N, Chou JT, Kozubski W. A case report: co-occurrence of cerebral amyloid angiopathy and multiple sclerosis. Mult Scler Relat Disord. 2020;46:102517.
4. Sakai K, Ueda M, Fukushima W, Tamaoka A, Shoji M, Ando Y, et al. Nationwide survey on cerebral amyloid angiopathy in Japan. Eur J Neurol. 2019;26(12):1487–93.
5. Koemans EA, Chhatwal JP, van Veluw SJ, van Etten ES, van Osch MJP, van Walderveen MAA, et al. Progression of cerebral amyloid angiopathy: a pathophysiological framework. Lancet Neurol. 2023;22(7):632–42.
6. Kinnecom C, Lev MH, Wendell L, Smith EE, Rosand J, Frosch MP, et al. Course of cerebral amyloid angiopathy-related inflammation. Neurology. 2007;68(17):1411–6.
7. Charidimou A, Boulouis G, Gurol ME, Ayata C, Bacskai BJ, Frosch MP, et al. Emerging concepts in sporadic cerebral amyloid angiopathy. Brain. 2017;140(7):1829–50.

8. Boyle PA, Yu L, Nag S, Leurgans S, Wilson RS, Bennett DA, et al. Cerebral amyloid angiopathy and cognitive outcomes in community-based older persons. Neurology. 2015;85(22):1930–6.
9. Corovic A, Kelly S, Markus HS. Cerebral amyloid angiopathy associated with inflammation: a systematic review of clinical and imaging features and outcome. Int J Stroke. 2018;13(3):257–67.
10. Kang P, Bucelli RC, Ferguson CJ, Corbo JC, Kim AH, Day GS. Teaching NeuroImages: cerebral amyloid angiopathy-related inflammation presenting with isolated leptomeningitis. Neurology. 2017;89(6):e66–e7.
11. Berry-Noronha A, Bonavia L, Smith T, Sahathevan R. Cerebral amyloid angiopathy related inflammation: an under recognized but treatable complication of cerebral amyloid angiopathy. Radiol Case Rep. 2023;18(7):2362–5.
12. Regenhardt RW, Thon JM, Das AS, Thon OR, Charidimou A, Viswanathan A, et al. Association between immunosuppressive treatment and outcomes of cerebral amyloid angiopathy-related inflammation. JAMA Neurol. 2020;77(10):1261–9.
13. Poon MT, Fonville AF, Al-Shahi SR. Long-term prognosis after intracerebral haemorrhage: systematic review and meta-analysis. J Neurol Neurosurg Psychiatry. 2014;85(6):660–7.
14. Blitstein MK, Tung GA. MRI of cerebral microhemorrhages. AJR Am J Roentgenol. 2007;189(3):720–5.
15. Renard D, Tatu L, Collombier L, Wacongne A, Ayrignac X, Charif M, et al. Cerebral amyloid angiopathy and cerebral amyloid angiopathy-related inflammation: comparison of hemorrhagic and DWI MRI features. J Alzheimer's Dis. 2018;64(4):1113–21.
16. Coulette S, Renard D, Lehmann S, Raposo N, Arquizan C, Charif M, et al. A clinico-radiological study of cerebral amyloid angiopathy-related inflammation. Cerebrovasc Dis. 2019;48(1–2):38–44.
17. Tokuda T, Ikeda S, Maruyama K, Yanagisawa N, Ito N. Spinal cord vascular and leptomeningeal amyloid beta-protein deposition in a case with cerebral amyloid angiopathy. Acta Neuropathol. 1992;84(2):207–10.
18. Verbeek MM, Kremer BP, Rikkert MO, Van Domburg PH, Skehan ME, Greenberg SM. Cerebrospinal fluid amyloid beta(40) is decreased in cerebral amyloid angiopathy. Ann Neurol. 2009;66(2):245–9.
19. Charidimou A, Friedrich JO, Greenberg SM, Viswanathan A. Core cerebrospinal fluid biomarker profile in cerebral amyloid angiopathy: a meta-analysis. Neurology. 2018;90(9):e754–e62.
20. Piazza F, Greenberg SM, Savoiardo M, Gardinetti M, Chiapparini L, Raicher I, et al. Anti-amyloid β autoantibodies in cerebral amyloid angiopathy-related inflammation: implications for amyloid-modifying therapies. Ann Neurol. 2013;73(4):449–58.
21. Charidimou A, Boulouis G, Frosch MP, Baron JC, Pasi M, Albucher JF, et al. The Boston criteria version 2.0 for cerebral amyloid angiopathy: a multicentre, retrospective, MRI-neuropathology diagnostic accuracy study. Lancet Neurol. 2022;21(8):714–25.
22. Kozberg MG, Perosa V, Gurol ME, van Veluw SJ. A practical approach to the management of cerebral amyloid angiopathy. Int J Stroke. 2021;16(4):356–69.
23. Razvi SS, Davidson R, Bone I, Muir KW. The prevalence of cerebral autosomal dominant arteriopathy with subcortical infarcts and leucoencephalopathy (CADASIL) in the west of Scotland. J Neurol Neurosurg Psychiatry. 2005;76(5):739–41.
24. Di Donato I, Bianchi S, De Stefano N, Dichgans M, Dotti MT, Duering M, et al. Cerebral Autosomal Dominant Arteriopathy with Subcortical Infarcts and Leukoencephalopathy (CADASIL) as a model of small vessel disease: update on clinical, diagnostic, and management aspects. BMC Med. 2017;15(1):41.
25. Coto E, Menendez M, Navarro R, Garcia-Castro M, Alvarez V. A new de novo Notch3 mutation causing CADASIL. Eur J Neurol. 2006;13(6):628–31.
26. Tikka S, Baumann M, Siitonen M, Pasanen P, Poyhonen M, Myllykangas L, et al. CADASIL and CARASIL. Brain Pathol. 2014;24(5):525–44.
27. Guey S, Mawet J, Herve D, Duering M, Godin O, Jouvent E, et al. Prevalence and characteristics of migraine in CADASIL. Cephalalgia. 2016;36(11):1038–47.

28. Eikermann-Haerter K, Yuzawa I, Dilekoz E, Joutel A, Moskowitz MA, Ayata C. Cerebral autosomal dominant arteriopathy with subcortical infarcts and leukoencephalopathy syndrome mutations increase susceptibility to spreading depression. Ann Neurol. 2011;69(2):413–8.
29. Tan RY, Markus HS. CADASIL: migraine, encephalopathy, stroke and their inter-relationships. PLoS One. 2016;11(6):e0157613.
30. Dichgans M, Mayer M, Uttner I, Bruning R, Muller-Hocker J, Rungger G, et al. The phenotypic spectrum of CADASIL: clinical findings in 102 cases. Ann Neurol. 1998;44(5):731–9.
31. Opherk C, Peters N, Herzog J, Luedtke R, Dichgans M. Long-term prognosis and causes of death in CADASIL: a retrospective study in 411 patients. Brain. 2004;127(Pt 11):2533–9.
32. Adib-Samii P, Brice G, Martin RJ, Markus HS. Clinical spectrum of CADASIL and the effect of cardiovascular risk factors on phenotype: study in 200 consecutively recruited individuals. Stroke. 2010;41(4):630–4.
33. Schon F, Martin RJ, Prevett M, Clough C, Enevoldson TP, Markus HS. "CADASIL coma": an underdiagnosed acute encephalopathy. J Neurol Neurosurg Psychiatry. 2003;74(2):249–52.
34. Peters N, Opherk C, Danek A, Ballard C, Herzog J, Dichgans M. The pattern of cognitive performance in CADASIL: a monogenic condition leading to subcortical ischemic vascular dementia. Am J Psychiatry. 2005;162(11):2078–85.
35. Rufa A, De Stefano N, Dotti MT, Bianchi S, Sicurelli F, Stromillo ML, et al. Acute unilateral visual loss as the first symptom of cerebral autosomal dominant arteriopathy with subcortical infarcts and leukoencephalopathy. Arch Neurol. 2004;61(4):577–80.
36. Rufa A, Pretegiani E, Frezzotti P, De Stefano N, Cevenini G, Dotti MT, et al. Retinal nerve fiber layer thinning in CADASIL: an optical coherence tomography and MRI study. Cerebrovasc Dis. 2011;31(1):77–82.
37. Haddad N, Ikard C, Hiatt K, Shanmugam V, Schmidley J. Recurrent status epilepticus as the primary neurological manifestation of CADASIL: a case report. Epilepsy Behav Case Rep. 2015;3:26–9.
38. Park DG, Min JH, Sohn SH, Sohn YB, Yoon JH. Ataxia associated with CADASIL: a pathology-confirmed case report and literature review. Cerebellum. 2020;19(6):907–10.
39. Singhal S, Rich P, Markus HS. The spatial distribution of MR imaging abnormalities in cerebral autosomal dominant arteriopathy with subcortical infarcts and leukoencephalopathy and their relationship to age and clinical features. AJNR Am J Neuroradiol. 2005;26(10):2481–7.
40. Auer DP, Putz B, Gossl C, Elbel G, Gasser T, Dichgans M. Differential lesion patterns in CADASIL and sporadic subcortical arteriosclerotic encephalopathy: MR imaging study with statistical parametric group comparison. Radiology. 2001;218(2):443–51.
41. O'Sullivan M, Jarosz JM, Martin RJ, Deasy N, Powell JF, Markus HS. MRI hyperintensities of the temporal lobe and external capsule in patients with CADASIL. Neurology. 2001;56(5):628–34.
42. Chabriat H, Levy C, Taillia H, Iba-Zizen MT, Vahedi K, Joutel A, et al. Patterns of MRI lesions in CADASIL. Neurology. 1998;51(2):452–7.
43. De Guio F, Reyes S, Vignaud A, Duering M, Ropele S, Duchesnay E, et al. In vivo high-resolution 7 Tesla MRI shows early and diffuse cortical alterations in CADASIL. PLoS One. 2014;9(8):e106311.
44. Schiess N, Huether K, Szolics M, Agarwal G, El-Hattab AW, Sathe S. Multiple sclerosis or "inflammatory CADASIL?": case report and review of the literature. Clin Neurol Neurosurg. 2018;173:196–9.
45. Collongues N, Derache N, Blanc F, Labauge P, de Seze J, Defer G. Inflammatory-like presentation of CADASIL: a diagnostic challenge. BMC Neurol. 2012;12:78.
46. Chabriat H, Vahedi K, Iba-Zizen MT, Joutel A, Nibbio A, Nagy TG, et al. Clinical spectrum of CADASIL: a study of 7 families. Cerebral autosomal dominant arteriopathy with subcortical infarcts and leukoencephalopathy. Lancet. 1995;346(8980):934–9.
47. Stromillo ML, Dotti MT, Battaglini M, Mortilla M, Bianchi S, Plewnia K, et al. Structural and metabolic brain abnormalities in preclinical cerebral autosomal dominant arteriopathy with subcortical infarcts and leucoencephalopathy. J Neurol Neurosurg Psychiatry. 2009;80(1):41–7.

48. Lesnik Oberstein SA, van den Boom R, van Buchem MA, van Houwelingen HC, Bakker E, Vollebregt E, et al. Cerebral microbleeds in CADASIL. Neurology. 2001;57(6):1066–70.
49. Jing XZ, Jiang W, Gan L, Zhu WA, Dong M, Yu P, et al. CADASIL with spinal cord involvement: a case report and literature review. J Neurol. 2019;266(9):2330–3.
50. Hinze S, Goonasekera M, Nannucci S, Quaghebeur G, Briley D, Markus HS, et al. Longitudinally extensive spinal cord infarction in CADASIL. Pract Neurol. 2015;15(1):60–2.
51. Formichi P, Parnetti L, Radi E, Cevenini G, Dotti MT, Federico A. CSF biomarkers profile in CADASIL-A model of pure vascular dementia: usefulness in differential diagnosis in the dementia disorder. Int J Alzheimer's Dis. 2010;2010:959257.
52. Moura J, Mendes Pinto C, Pinto P, Santos E. Inflammatory optic neuropathy as a presenting feature of cerebral autosomal dominant arteriopathy with subcortical infarcts and leukoencephalopathy. Neurohospitalist. 2023;13(2):183–7.
53. Dichgans M, Wick M, Gasser T. Cerebrospinal fluid findings in CADASIL. Neurology. 1999;53(1):233.
54. Lee HJ, Shin KJ, Kang Y, Oh SI. Multiple sclerosis in a patient with neurogenic locus notch homolog protein 3 mutation. J Clin Neurol. 2023;19(2):201–3.
55. Bentley P, Wang T, Malik O, Nicholas R, Ban M, Sawcer S, et al. CADASIL with cord involvement associated with a novel and atypical NOTCH3 mutation. J Neurol Neurosurg Psychiatry. 2011;82(8):855–60.
56. Budhdeo S, de Paiva ARB, Wade C, Lopes LCG, Della-Ripa B, Davagnanam I, et al. A rare cause of monogenic cerebral small vessel disease and stroke: Cathepsin A-related arteriopathy with strokes and leukoencephalopathy (CARASAL). J Neurol. 2022;269(12):6673–7.
57. Li Q, Wang C, Li W, Zhang Z, Wang S, Wupuer A, et al. A novel mutation in COL4A1 gene in a Chinese family with pontine autosomal dominant microangiopathy and leukoencephalopathy. Transl Stroke Res. 2022;13(2):238–44.
58. Ding XQ, Hagel C, Ringelstein EB, Buchheit S, Zeumer H, Kuhlenbaumer G, et al. MRI features of pontine autosomal dominant microangiopathy and leukoencephalopathy (PADMAL). J Neuroimaging. 2010;20(2):134–40.
59. Germain DP. Fabry disease. Orphanet J Rare Dis. 2010;5:30.
60. Cocozza S, Russo C, Pisani A, Olivo G, Riccio E, Cervo A, et al. Redefining the pulvinar sign in fabry disease. AJNR Am J Neuroradiol. 2017;38(12):2264–9.
61. Sharrief A. Diagnosis and management of cerebral small vessel disease. Continuum (Minneap Minn). 2023;29(2):501–18.
62. Pantoni L. Cerebral small vessel disease: from pathogenesis and clinical characteristics to therapeutic challenges. Lancet Neurol. 2010;9(7):689–701.
63. Prins ND, Scheltens P. White matter hyperintensities, cognitive impairment and dementia: an update. Nat Rev Neurol. 2015;11(3):157–65.
64. Sachdev P, Chen X, Wen W. White matter hyperintensities in mid-adult life. Curr Opin Psychiatry. 2008;21(3):268–74.
65. Brown R, Low A, Markus HS. Rate of, and risk factors for, white matter hyperintensity growth: a systematic review and meta-analysis with implications for clinical trial design. J Neurol Neurosurg Psychiatry. 2021;92(12):1271–7.
66. Debette S, Schilling S, Duperron MG, Larsson SC, Markus HS. Clinical significance of magnetic resonance imaging markers of vascular brain injury: a systematic review and meta-analysis. JAMA Neurol. 2019;76(1):81–94.
67. Cannistraro RJ, Badi M, Eidelman BH, Dickson DW, Middlebrooks EH, Meschia JF. CNS small vessel disease: a clinical review. Neurology. 2019;92(24):1146–56.
68. Wardlaw JM, Smith C, Dichgans M. Small vessel disease: mechanisms and clinical implications. Lancet Neurol. 2019;18(7):684–96.
69. Duering M, Biessels GJ, Brodtmann A, Chen C, Cordonnier C, de Leeuw FE, et al. Neuroimaging standards for research into small vessel disease-advances since 2013. Lancet Neurol. 2023;22(7):602–18.

70. Wang B, Li X, Li H, Xiao L, Zhou Z, Chen K, et al. Clinical, radiological and pathological characteristics between cerebral small vessel disease and multiple sclerosis: a review. Front Neurol. 2022;13:841521.
71. Huisa BN, Rosenberg GA. Binswanger's disease: toward a diagnosis agreement and therapeutic approach. Expert Rev Neurother. 2014;14(10):1203–13.
72. Gouw AA, van der Flier WM, Pantoni L, Inzitari D, Erkinjuntti T, Wahlund LO, et al. On the etiology of incident brain lacunes: longitudinal observations from the LADIS study. Stroke. 2008;39(11):3083–5.
73. Sichtermann T, Furtmann JK, Dekeyzer S, Gilmour G, Oros-Peusquens AM, Bach JP, et al. Increased water content in periventricular caps in patients without acute hydrocephalus. AJNR Am J Neuroradiol. 2019;40(5):784–7.
74. Zimmerman RD, Fleming CA, Lee BC, Saint-Louis LA, Deck MD. Periventricular hyperintensity as seen by magnetic resonance: prevalence and significance. AJR Am J Roentgenol. 1986;146(3):443–50.
75. Jochems ACC, Arteaga C, Chappell F, Ritakari T, Hooley M, Doubal F, et al. Longitudinal changes of white matter hyperintensities in sporadic small vessel disease: a systematic review and meta-analysis. Neurology. 2022;99(22):e2454–e63.
76. Wardlaw JM, Smith EE, Biessels GJ, Cordonnier C, Fazekas F, Frayne R, et al. Neuroimaging standards for research into small vessel disease and its contribution to ageing and neurodegeneration. Lancet Neurol. 2013;12(8):822–38.
77. Duering M, Adam R, Wollenweber FA, Bayer-Karpinska A, Baykara E, Cubillos-Pinilla LY, et al. Within-lesion heterogeneity of subcortical DWI lesion evolution, and stroke outcome: a voxel-based analysis. J Cereb Blood Flow Metab. 2020;40(7):1482–91.
78. Fazekas F, Chawluk JB, Alavi A, Hurtig HI, Zimmerman RA. MR signal abnormalities at 1.5 T in Alzheimer's dementia and normal aging. AJR Am J Roentgenol. 1987;149(2):351–6.
79. Zhang L, Yu X, Zheng Y, Lin A, Zhang Z, Li S, et al. Lacunes are associated with late-stage multiple sclerosis comorbidities. Front Neurol. 2023;14:1224748.
80. Hyland M, Bermel RA, Cohen JA. Restricted diffusion preceding gadolinium enhancement in large or tumefactive demyelinating lesions. Neurol Clin Pract. 2013;3(1):15–21.
81. Balashov KE, Lindzen E. Acute demyelinating lesions with restricted diffusion in multiple sclerosis. Mult Scler. 2012;18(12):1745–53.
82. Abou Zeid N, Pirko I, Erickson B, Weigand SD, Thomsen KM, Scheithauer B, et al. Diffusion-weighted imaging characteristics of biopsy-proven demyelinating brain lesions. Neurology. 2012;78(21):1655–62.
83. Filippi M, Preziosa P, Banwell BL, Barkhof F, Ciccarelli O, De Stefano N, et al. Assessment of lesions on magnetic resonance imaging in multiple sclerosis: practical guidelines. Brain. 2019;142(7):1858–75.
84. Granberg T, Moridi T, Brand JS, Neumann S, Hlavica M, Piehl F, et al. Enlarged perivascular spaces in multiple sclerosis on magnetic resonance imaging: a systematic review and meta-analysis. J Neurol. 2020;267(11):3199–212.
85. Zivadinov R, Ramasamy DP, Benedict RR, Polak P, Hagemeier J, Magnano C, et al. Cerebral microbleeds in multiple sclerosis evaluated on susceptibility-weighted images and quantitative susceptibility maps: a case-control study. Radiology. 2016;281(3):884–95.
86. Uher T, Krasensky J, Malpas C, Bergsland N, Dwyer MG, Kubala Havrdova E, et al. Evolution of brain volume loss rates in early stages of multiple sclerosis. Neurol Neuroimmunol Neuroinflamm. 2021;8(3):e979.
87. Shaaban CE, Jorgensen DR, Gianaros PJ, Mettenburg J, Rosano C. Cerebrovascular disease: neuroimaging of cerebral small vessel disease. Prog Mol Biol Transl Sci. 2019;165:225–55.
88. Plaisier E, Ronco P. COL4A1-related disorders. In: Adam MP, Feldman J, Mirzaa GM, Pagon RA, Wallace SE, Bean LJH, et al., editors. GeneReviews((R)). Seattle (WA); 1993.
89. Zagaglia S, Selch C, Nisevic JR, Mei D, Michalak Z, Hernandez-Hernandez L, et al. Neurologic phenotypes associated with COL4A1/2 mutations: expanding the spectrum of disease. Neurology. 2018;91(22):e2078–e88.

90. Mancuso M, Arnold M, Bersano A, Burlina A, Chabriat H, Debette S, et al. Monogenic cerebral small-vessel diseases: diagnosis and therapy. Consensus recommendations of the European Academy of Neurology. Eur J Neurol. 2020;27(6):909–27.
91. Shah S, Kumar Y, McLean B, Churchill A, Stoodley N, Rankin J, et al. A dominantly inherited mutation in collagen IV A1 (COL4A1) causing childhood onset stroke without porencephaly. Eur J Paediatr Neurol. 2010;14(2):182–7.
92. Plancher JM, Hufnagel RB, Vagal A, Peariso K, Saal HM, Broderick JP. Case of small vessel disease associated with COL4A1 mutations following trauma. Case Rep Neurol. 2015;7(2):142–7.
93. Meuwissen ME, Halley DJ, Smit LS, Lequin MH, Cobben JM, de Coo R, et al. The expanding phenotype of COL4A1 and COL4A2 mutations: clinical data on 13 newly identified families and a review of the literature. Genet Med. 2015;17(11):843–53.
94. Campbell BCV, De Silva DA, Macleod MR, Coutts SB, Schwamm LH, Davis SM, et al. Ischaemic stroke Nat Rev Dis Primers. 2019;5(1):70.
95. Hong Y, Tang HR, Ma M, Chen N, Xie X, He L. Multiple sclerosis and stroke: a systematic review and meta-analysis. BMC Neurol. 2019;19(1):139.
96. Allen LM, Hasso AN, Handwerker J, Farid H. Sequence-specific MR imaging findings that are useful in dating ischemic stroke. Radiographics. 2012;32(5):1285–97. discussion 97-9
97. Boulter DJ, Schaefer PW. Stroke and stroke mimics: a pattern-based approach. Semin Roentgenol. 2014;49(1):22–38.
98. Derdeyn CP, Khosla A, Videen TO, Fritsch SM, Carpenter DL, Grubb RL Jr, et al. Severe hemodynamic impairment and border zone – region infarction. Radiology. 2001;220(1):195–201.
99. Koenig M, Aldrich EM. Chapter 25 – Cerebrovascular disorders. In: Irani DN, editor. Cerebrospinal fluid in clinical practice. Philadelphia: W.B. Saunders; 2009. p. 225–31.
100. Rundblad LIS, Iversen HK, West AS. Pleocytosis in cerebrospinal fluid attributed to ischemic stroke: a review of the literature. J Neurol Sci. 2023;449:120664.
101. Ramirez-Lassepas M, Patrick BK. Cerebrospinal fluid cellular response in uncomplicated acute ischemic stroke. J Stroke Cerebrovasc Dis. 1992;2(3):168–72.
102. Steiner TJ, Stovner LJ. Global epidemiology of migraine and its implications for public health and health policy. Nat Rev Neurol. 2023;19(2):109–17.
103. Allais G, Chiarle G, Sinigaglia S, Airola G, Schiapparelli P, Benedetto C. Gender-related differences in migraine. Neurol Sci. 2020;41(Suppl 2):429–36.
104. Mrabet S, Wafa M, Giovannoni G. Multiple sclerosis and migraine: links, management and implications. Mult Scler Relat Disord. 2022;68:104152.
105. Moisset X, Ouchchane L, Guy N, Bayle DJ, Dallel R, Clavelou P. Migraine headaches and pain with neuropathic characteristics: comorbid conditions in patients with multiple sclerosis. Pain. 2013;154(12):2691–9.
106. Goadsby PJ, Lipton RB, Ferrari MD. Migraine – current understanding and treatment. N Engl J Med. 2002;346(4):257–70.
107. Onderwater GLJ, van Dongen RM, Harms AC, Zielman R, van Oosterhout WPJ, van Klinken JB, et al. Cerebrospinal fluid and plasma amine profiles in interictal migraine. Ann Neurol. 2022;93:715.
108. Headache Classification Committee of the International Headache Society (IHS). The International Classification of Headache Disorders, 3rd edition (beta version). Cephalalgia. 2013;33(9):629–808.
109. Headache Classification Committee of the International Headache Society (IHS). The International Classification of Headache Disorders, 3rd edition. Cephalalgia. 2018;38(1):1–211.
110. Fraser CL, Hepschke JL, Jenkins B, Prasad S. Migraine Aura: pathophysiology, mimics, and treatment options. Semin Neurol. 2019;39(6):739–48.
111. Bashir A, Lipton RB, Ashina S, Ashina M. Migraine and structural changes in the brain: a systematic review and meta-analysis. Neurology. 2013;81(14):1260–8.
112. Absinta M, Rocca MA, Colombo B, Copetti M, De Feo D, Falini A, et al. Patients with migraine do not have MRI-visible cortical lesions. J Neurol. 2012;259(12):2695–8.

113. Rocca MA, Ceccarelli A, Falini A, Colombo B, Tortorella P, Bernasconi L, et al. Brain gray matter changes in migraine patients with T2-visible lesions: a 3-T MRI study. Stroke. 2006;37(7):1765–70.
114. Kruit MC, van Buchem MA, Launer LJ, Terwindt GM, Ferrari MD. Migraine is associated with an increased risk of deep white matter lesions, subclinical posterior circulation infarcts and brain iron accumulation: the population-based MRI CAMERA study. Cephalalgia. 2010;30(2):129–36.
115. Kruit MC, van Buchem MA, Hofman PA, Bakkers JT, Terwindt GM, Ferrari MD, et al. Migraine as a risk factor for subclinical brain lesions. JAMA. 2004;291(4):427–34.
116. Liu S, Kullnat J, Bourdette D, Simon J, Kraemer DF, Murchison C, et al. Prevalence of brain magnetic resonance imaging meeting Barkhof and McDonald criteria for dissemination in space among headache patients. Mult Scler. 2013;19(8):1101–5.
117. Lapucci C, Saitta L, Bommarito G, Sormani MP, Pardini M, Bonzano L, et al. How much do periventricular lesions assist in distinguishing migraine with aura from CIS? Neurology. 2019;92(15):e1739–e44.
118. Maggi P, Absinta M, Sati P, Perrotta G, Massacesi L, Dachy B, et al. The "central vein sign" in patients with diagnostic "red flags" for multiple sclerosis: a prospective multicenter 3T study. Mult Scler. 2020;26(4):421–32.
119. Solomon AJ, Watts R, Ontaneda D, Absinta M, Sati P, Reich DS. Diagnostic performance of central vein sign for multiple sclerosis with a simplified three-lesion algorithm. Mult Scler. 2018;24(6):750–7.
120. Rovaris M, Bozzali M, Rocca MA, Colombo B, Filippi M. An MR study of tissue damage in the cervical cord of patients with migraine. J Neurol Sci. 2001;183(1):43–6.
121. Pannewitz-Makaj K, Wurster U, Jendretzky KF, Gingele S, Suhs KW, Stangel M, et al. Evidence of oligoclonal bands does not exclude non-inflammatory neurological diseases. Diagnostics (Basel). 2020;11(1):37.
122. Khalil NM, Legg NJ, Anderson DJ. Long term decline of P100 amplitude in migraine with aura. J Neurol Neurosurg Psychiatry. 2000;69(4):507–11.
123. Boylu E, Domac FM, Kocer A, Unal Z, Tanridag T, Us O. Visual evoked potential abnormalities in migraine patients. Electromyogr Clin Neurophysiol. 2010;50(6):303–8.
124. Solomon AJ, Bourdette DN, Cross AH, Applebee A, Skidd PM, Howard DB, et al. The contemporary spectrum of multiple sclerosis misdiagnosis: a multicenter study. Neurology. 2016;87(13):1393–9.
125. Yusuf FLA, Ng BC, Wijnands JMA, Kingwell E, Marrie RA, Tremlett H. A systematic review of morbidities suggestive of the multiple sclerosis prodrome. Expert Rev Neurother. 2020;20(8):799–819.
126. Gee JR, Chang J, Dublin AB, Vijayan N. The association of brainstem lesions with migraine-like headache: an imaging study of multiple sclerosis. Headache. 2005;45(6):670–7.
127. Graziano E, Hagemeier J, Weinstock-Guttman B, Ramasamy DP, Zivadinov R. Increased contrast enhancing lesion activity in relapsing-remitting multiple sclerosis migraine patients. Neuroimage Clin. 2015;9:110–6.
128. Thompson AJ, Banwell BL, Barkhof F, Carroll WM, Coetzee T, Comi G, et al. Diagnosis of multiple sclerosis: 2017 revisions of the McDonald criteria. Lancet Neurol. 2018;17(2):162–73.
129. Signoriello E, Cirillo M, Puoti G, Signoriello G, Negro A, Koci E, et al. Migraine as possible red flag of PFO presence in suspected demyelinating disease. J Neurol Sci. 2018;390:222–6.
130. Lip PZ, Lip GY. Patent foramen ovale and migraine attacks: a systematic review. Am J Med. 2014;127(5):411–20.
131. Scott RM, Smith ER. Moyamoya disease and moyamoya syndrome. N Engl J Med. 2009;360(12):1226–37.
132. Yonekawa Y, Ogata N, Kaku Y, Taub E, Imhof HG. Moyamoya disease in Europe, past and present status. Clin Neurol Neurosurg. 1997;99(Suppl 2):S58–60.
133. Baba T, Houkin K, Kuroda S. Novel epidemiological features of moyamoya disease. J Neurol Neurosurg Psychiatry. 2008;79(8):900–4.

134. Uchino K, Johnston SC, Becker KJ, Tirschwell DL. Moyamoya disease in Washington State and California. Neurology. 2005;65(6):956–8.
135. Preziosa P, Martinelli V, Ferre L, Guaschino C, Simionato F, Moiola L, et al. Moyamoya disease mimicking the first attack of multiple sclerosis. J Neurol. 2017;264(5):1005–7.
136. Dorfman LJ, Fischbein NJ, Woodard JI, Choudhri O, Bell-Stephens TE, Steinberg GK. Moyamoya disease can masquerade as multiple sclerosis. Neurologist. 2012;18(6):398–403.
137. Zaheer F, Berger JR. Moyamoya: another multiple sclerosis mimic. Mult Scler Relat Dis. 2012;1(2):100–3.
138. Spanou I, Evangelopoulos ME, Velonakis G, Logiotatos N, Chatziioannou A, Potagas C, et al. Moyamoya disease may mimic multiple sclerosis? Case Rep Neurol Med. 2019;2019:1.
139. Wolf B. Why screen newborns for profound and partial biotinidase deficiency? Mol Genet Metab. 2015;114(3):382–7.
140. Kelly ME, Bell-Stephens TE, Marks MP, Do HM, Steinberg GK. Progression of unilateral moyamoya disease: a clinical series. Cerebrovasc Dis. 2006;22(2–3):109–15.
141. Das S, Ray BK, Pandit A, Kumar S, Dubey S. Multiple sclerosis and Moyamoya angiopathy: mimic and misdiagnosis. Mult Scler Relat Disord. 2022;66:104036.
142. Si XL, Li LF, Fang YJ, Yan YP, Pu JL. A patient with multiple sclerosis and coexisting Moyamoya disease: why and how. Front Neurol. 2020;11:516587.
143. Geocadin RG. Posterior reversible encephalopathy syndrome. N Engl J Med. 2023;388(23):2171–8.
144. Lee VH, Wijdicks EF, Manno EM, Rabinstein AA. Clinical spectrum of reversible posterior leukoencephalopathy syndrome. Arch Neurol. 2008;65(2):205–10.
145. McKinney AM, Short J, Truwit CL, McKinney ZJ, Kozak OS, SantaCruz KS, et al. Posterior reversible encephalopathy syndrome: incidence of atypical regions of involvement and imaging findings. AJR Am J Roentgenol. 2007;189(4):904–12.
146. Hinchey J, Chaves C, Appignani B, Breen J, Pao L, Wang A, et al. A reversible posterior leukoencephalopathy syndrome. N Engl J Med. 1996;334(8):494–500.
147. Lamy C, Oppenheim C, Mas JL. Posterior reversible encephalopathy syndrome. Handb Clin Neurol. 2014;121:1687–701.
148. Price RS, Kasner SE. Hypertension and hypertensive encephalopathy. Handb Clin Neurol. 2014;119:161–7.
149. Dietz N, Mufti Z, Yousaf M, Brown R, Counts C, Bjurström MF, et al. Acute posterior reversible encephalopathy syndrome (PRES) in setting of interferon-beta use: case presentation with reduction of edema in 72 h after cessation of interferon-beta therapy with sub-clinical inflammation. BMC Neurol. 2021;21(1):445.
150. Lindå H, von Heijne A. A case of posterior reversible encephalopathy syndrome associated with gilenya(®) (fingolimod) treatment for multiple sclerosis. Front Neurol. 2015;6:39.
151. Décard BF, Haghikia A, Tönnes C, Thöne J, Lukas C, Chan A, et al. Natalizumab-associated reversible encephalopathy syndrome mimicking progressive multifocal leukoencephalopathy. Mult Scler. 2013;19(2):249–51.
152. Sánchez-Carteyron A, Alarcia R, Ara JR, Martín J. Posterior reversible encephalopathy syndrome after rituximab infusion in neuromyelitis optica. Neurology. 2010;74(18):1471–3.
153. Ito T, Sakai T, Inagawa S, Utsu M, Bun T. MR angiography of cerebral vasospasm in preeclampsia. AJNR Am J Neuroradiol. 1995;16(6):1344–6.
154. Ay H, Buonanno FS, Schaefer PW, Le DA, Wang B, Gonzalez RG, et al. Posterior leukoencephalopathy without severe hypertension: utility of diffusion-weighted MRI. Neurology. 1998;51(5):1369–76.
155. Rykken JB, McKinney AM. Posterior reversible encephalopathy syndrome. Semin Ultrasound CT MR. 2014;35(2):118–35.
156. Gao B, Yu BX, Li RS, Zhang G, Xie HZ, Liu FL, et al. Cytotoxic edema in posterior reversible encephalopathy syndrome: correlation of MRI features with serum albumin levels. AJNR Am J Neuroradiol. 2015;36(10):1884–9.

157. Liu L, Dai D, Cao F, Zhang L, Wang X. Posterior reversible encephalopathy syndrome with spinal cord involvement but without hemisphere lesions: a case report. Medicine (Baltimore). 2019;98(2):e13649.
158. de Havenon A, Joos Z, Longenecker L, Shah L, Ansari S, Digre K. Posterior reversible encephalopathy syndrome with spinal cord involvement. Neurology. 2014;83(22):2002–6.
159. Nelke C, Schulte-Mecklenbeck A, Pawlitzki M, Rolfes L, Räuber S, Gross CC, et al. The innate immune response characterizes posterior reversible encephalopathy syndrome. J Clin Immunol. 2021;41(6):1229–40.
160. Kharytaniuk N, Cowley P, Sayal P, Eleftheriou P, Farmer SF, Chan E, et al. Classical infratentorial superficial siderosis of the central nervous system: pathophysiology, clinical features and management. Pract Neurol. 2022;22:274.
161. Fearnley JM, Stevens JM, Rudge P. Superficial siderosis of the central nervous system. Brain. 1995;118(Pt 4):1051–66.
162. Weidauer S, Neuhaus E, Hattingen E. Cerebral superficial siderosis : etiology, neuroradiological features and clinical findings. Clin Neuroradiol. 2023;33(2):293–306.
163. Kumar N. Superficial siderosis: a clinical review. Ann Neurol. 2021;89(6):1068–79.
164. Charidimou A, Boulouis G, Fotiadis P, Xiong L, Ayres AM, Schwab KM, et al. Acute convexity subarachnoid haemorrhage and cortical superficial siderosis in probable cerebral amyloid angiopathy without lobar haemorrhage. J Neurol Neurosurg Psychiatry. 2018;89(4):397–403.
165. Charidimou A, Linn J, Vernooij MW, Opherk C, Akoudad S, Baron JC, et al. Cortical superficial siderosis: detection and clinical significance in cerebral amyloid angiopathy and related conditions. Brain. 2015;138(Pt 8):2126–39.
166. Sandson TA, Friedman JH. Spinal cord infarction. Report of 8 cases and review of the literature. Medicine (Baltimore). 1989;68(5):282–92.
167. Rabinstein AA. Vascular myelopathies. Continuum (Minneap Minn). 2015;21(1 Spinal Cord Disorders):67–83.
168. Zalewski NL. Vascular myelopathies. Continuum (Minneap Minn). 2021;27(1):30–61.
169. Bradac GB, Daniele D, Riva A, Bracchi M, Stura G, Riccio A, et al. Spinal dural arteriovenous fistulas: an underestimated cause of myelopathy. Eur Neurol. 1994;34(2):87–94.
170. Jellema K, Tijssen CC, van Gijn J. Spinal dural arteriovenous fistulas: a congestive myelopathy that initially mimics a peripheral nerve disorder. Brain. 2006;129(Pt 12):3150–64.
171. Zalewski NL, Rabinstein AA, Krecke KN, Brown RD, Wijdicks EFM, Weinshenker BG, et al. Spinal cord infarction: clinical and imaging insights from the periprocedural setting. J Neurol Sci. 2018;388:162–7.
172. Hurst RW, Kenyon LC, Lavi E, Raps EC, Marcotte P. Spinal dural arteriovenous fistula: the pathology of venous hypertensive myelopathy. Neurology. 1995;45(7):1309–13.
173. Fugate JE, Lanzino G, Rabinstein AA. Clinical presentation and prognostic factors of spinal dural arteriovenous fistulas: an overview. Neurosurg Focus. 2012;32(5):E17.
174. Brinjikji W, Yin R, Nasr DM, Lanzino G. Spinal epidural arteriovenous fistulas. J Neurointerventional Surg. 2016;8(12):1305–10.
175. Kramer CL. Vascular disorders of the spinal cord. Continuum (Minneap Minn). 2018;24(2, Spinal Cord Disorders):407–26.
176. Zalewski NL, Rabinstein AA, Krecke KN, Brown RD Jr, Wijdicks EFM, Weinshenker BG, et al. Characteristics of spontaneous spinal cord infarction and proposed diagnostic criteria. JAMA Neurol. 2019;76(1):56–63.
177. English SW, Rabinstein AA, Flanagan EP, Zalewski NL. Spinal cord transient ischemic attack: insights from a series of spontaneous spinal cord infarction. Neurol Clin Pract. 2020;10(6):480–3.
178. Lee J, Lim YM, Suh DC, Rhim SC, Kim SJ, Kim KK. Clinical presentation, imaging findings, and prognosis of spinal dural arteriovenous fistula. J Clin Neurosci. 2016;26:105–9.
179. Jellema K, Canta LR, Tijssen CC, van Rooij WJ, Koudstaal PJ, van Gijn J. Spinal dural arteriovenous fistulas: clinical features in 80 patients. J Neurol Neurosurg Psychiatry. 2003;74(10):1438–40.

180. Koerts G, Vanthuyne V, Delavallee M, Rooijakkers H, Raftopoulos C. Spinal dural arteriovenous fistula presenting with paraplegia following lumbar puncture. J Neurosurg Spine. 2013;19(1):57–60.
181. Lee CS, Pyun HW, Chae EY, Kim KK, Rhim SC, Suh DC. Reversible aggravation of neurological deficits after steroid medication in patients with venous congestive myelopathy caused by spinal arteriovenous malformation. Interv Neuroradiol. 2009;15(3):325–9.
182. Nasr DM, Brinjikji W, Rabinstein AA, Lanzino G. Clinical outcomes following corticosteroid administration in patients with delayed diagnosis of spinal arteriovenous fistulas. J Neurointerv Surg. 2017;9(6):607–10.
183. McKeon A, Lindell EP, Atkinson JL, Weinshenker BG, Piepgras DG, Pittock SJ. Pearls & oy-sters: clues for spinal dural arteriovenous fistulae. Neurology. 2011;76(3):e10–2.
184. Shimizu K, Takeda M, Mitsuhara T, Tanaka S, Nagano Y, Yamahata H, et al. Asymptomatic spinal dural arteriovenous fistula: case series and systematic review. J Neurosurg Spine. 2019;1-9:733.
185. Muralidharan R, Saladino A, Lanzino G, Atkinson JL, Rabinstein AA. The clinical and radiological presentation of spinal dural arteriovenous fistula. Spine. 2011;36(25):E1641–7.
186. Toossi S, Josephson SA, Hetts SW, Chin CT, Kralik S, Jun P, et al. Utility of MRI in spinal arteriovenous fistula. Neurology. 2012;79(1):25–30.
187. Gilbertson JR, Miller GM, Goldman MS, Marsh WR. Spinal dural arteriovenous fistulas: MR and myelographic findings. AJNR Am J Neuroradiol. 1995;16(10):2049–57.
188. Luetmer PH, Lane JI, Gilbertson JR, Bernstein MA, Huston J 3rd, Atkinson JL. Preangiographic evaluation of spinal dural arteriovenous fistulas with elliptic centric contrast-enhanced MR angiography and effect on radiation dose and volume of iodinated contrast material. AJNR Am J Neuroradiol. 2005;26(4):711–8.
189. Zalewski NL, Rabinstein AA, Brinjikji W, Kaufmann TJ, Nasr D, Ruff MW, et al. Unique gadolinium enhancement pattern in spinal dural arteriovenous fistulas. JAMA Neurol. 2018;75(12):1542–5.
190. Rodriguez FJ, Crum BA, Krauss WE, Scheithauer BW, Giannini C. Venous congestive myelopathy: a mimic of neoplasia. Mod Pathol. 2005;18(5):710–8.
191. Kalamangalam GP, Bhattacharya J, Teasdale E, Thomas M. Myelopathy from intracranial dural arteriovenous fistula. J Neurol Neurosurg Psychiatry. 2002;72(6):816–8.
192. Wrobel CJ, Oldfield EH, Di Chiro G, Tarlov EC, Baker RA, Doppman JL. Myelopathy due to intracranial dural arteriovenous fistulas draining intrathecally into spinal medullary veins. Report of three cases. J Neurosurg. 1988;69(6):934–9.
193. Shin MJ, Kim W, Baik SK, Kim SY, Kim SN. Cauda equina syndrome caused by spinal dural arteriovenous fistula. Ann Rehabil Med. 2011;35(6):928–33.
194. Manners J, Jadhav AP, Xia Z. Mystery case: a 61-year-old woman with lower extremity paralysis and sensory loss. Neurology. 2017;89(22):e257–e63.
195. Cohen O, Biran I, Steiner I. Cerebrospinal fluid oligoclonal IgG bands in patients with spinal arteriovenous malformation and structural central nervous system lesions. Arch Neurol. 2000;57(4):553–7.
196. Zalewski NL, Flanagan EP, Keegan BM. Evaluation of idiopathic transverse myelitis revealing specific myelopathy diagnoses. Neurology. 2018;90(2):e96–e102.
197. Mariano R, Flanagan EP, Weinshenker BG, Palace J. A practical approach to the diagnosis of spinal cord lesions. Pract Neurol. 2018;18(3):187–200.
198. Clark MT, Brooks EL, Chong W, Pappas C, Fahey M. Cobb syndrome: a case report and systematic review of the literature. Pediatr Neurol. 2008;39(6):423–5.
199. Brinjikji W, Nasr DM, Morris JM, Rabinstein AA, Lanzino G. Clinical outcomes of patients with delayed diagnosis of spinal dural arteriovenous fistulas. AJNR Am J Neuroradiol. 2016;37(2):380–6.
200. Muralidharan R, Mandrekar J, Lanzino G, Atkinson JL, Rabinstein AA. Prognostic value of clinical and radiological signs in the postoperative outcome of spinal dural arteriovenous fistula. Spine. 2013;38(14):1188–93.

12 Miscellaneous Diseases and Normal Findings

12.1 Amyotrophic Lateral Sclerosis (ALS)

12.1.1 Epidemiology

- Incidence 1–2.6/100.000/years.
- Prevalence 6/100.000 [1].

12.1.2 Etiology and Definition

- A fatal neurodegenerative disease of central nervous system (CNS).
- Most cases are sporadic (90–95%); only 5–10% is hereditary.
- Sporadic ALS is suspected to involve genetic susceptibility to unknown environmental risk factors [1, 2].

12.1.3 Clinical Features

- Combination of upper and lower motor neuron pathology but may occur as a pure upper or lower motor neuron phenotype [2].
- Multiple phenotypes, but bulbar- and spinal-onset are the most common [2].
- Multiple sclerosis (MS) is primarily associated with pathology affecting upper motor neurons, but lesions causing damage to lower motor neurons can also occur. This typically happens when demyelination occurs in the ventral root exit zone or similarly in the brainstem [3].
- Unexplained weight loss, pseudobulbar affect, or respiratory dysfunction is typical for ALS but usually not seen in early stages of MS.

T. Uher, *Mimics and Red Flags of Multiple Sclerosis*,
https://doi.org/10.1007/978-3-031-98945-2_12

- In contrast, ALS patients do not experience sensory symptoms, optic neuritis, internuclear opthalmopparesis, or extraocular muscles disorders, which are typical for MS [2, 4, 5].
- Although bowel and bladder disorders were once considered rare in ALS, approximately 30% of patients report urgency, frequency, and urge incontinence and 60% of them experience hesitancy, a sensation of incomplete emptying, post-micturition dribble, and straining during voiding due to neurogenic bladder or pelvic floor spasticity [6].
- Cognitive and behavioral changes occur in 35–50% of ALS patients already in the early disease stages, and 15% of patients meet the criteria for fronto-temporal dementia [7]. Although, cognitive or behavioral changes occur also in MS, their severity is generally milder [8].

12.1.4 Disease Course

- Slowly progressive (not relapsing-remitting) phenotype and disease onset is insidious [2] not acute or subacute as observed in relapsing-remitting MS [9].
- The average age of symptom onset is 58–60 years, which is higher than in MS [1].

12.1.5 Brain and Spinal Cord Imaging

- Magnetic resonance imaging (MRI) shows T2 hyperintensities in the corticospinal tracts. They can be seen for example in capsula interna (best seen on coronal plane) or in the spinal cord. This sign has specificity <70% and sensitivity <40% [10] (Fig. 12.1).
- "Motor band sign" from iron deposition in the motor cortex (particularly precentral gyrus) might be present on susceptibility weighted imaging (SWI) sequences [11].
- Both features are nonspecific and may occasionally be observed in the general population.

12.1.6 Blood Work

- Except for elevated creatine phosphokinase concentrations in some patients, routine blood testing is normal [2].

12.1.7 Examination of CSF

- Glucose level and leukocyte count is usually normal.
- Commonly elevated concentration of protein and albumin quotient indicating blood–brain barrier damage [12].
- Extremely increased markers of neuroaxonal damage, such as neurofilaments light chain (correlate with worse prognosis) [13].

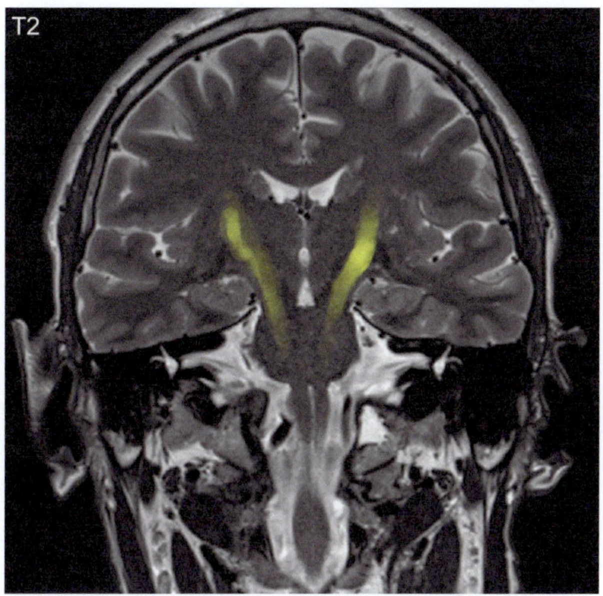

Fig. 12.1 Increased T2 signal in the corticospinal tracts in amyotrophic lateral sclerosis (ALS)

- The occasional presence of cerebrospinal fluid (CSF)-restricted oligoclonal (OCB) is probably not related to ALS pathophysiology:
  - OCB (pattern II; oligoclonal IgG bands only in CSF) (2%).
  - OCB (pattern III; oligoclonal bands in CSF and serum with additional bands in CSF) (8%).
  - OCB (pattern IV; identical oligoclonal bands in CSF and serum; caused by disruption of blood-brain barrier; mirror pattern) (60%).
  - OCB (pattern V; monoclonal bands in CSF and serum) (2%) [14].

12.1.8 OCT

- Optical coherence tomography (OCT) may sometime show peripapillary retinal nerve fiber layer (RNFL) thinning in the superior and inferior quadrants [15].

12.1.9 Electrophysiology

- Similar to MS, nerve conduction studies typically do not reveal sensory nerve involvement or motor nerve conduction block. Repetitive stimulation of a nerve does not show decrements or increments of the muscle action potential. Needle electromyography (EMG) can confirm lower motor neuron involvement (denervation findings), a feature usually absent in MS [2, 16].

12.1.10 Diagnosis

- Diagnosing ALS early can be challenging due to its heterogeneous phenotypes and the overlap of disease manifestations with other disorders [2].
- The most commonly used diagnostic criteria are revised El Escorial criteria to subclassify ALS as possible, probable, probable laboratory supported, and definite ALS, depending on clinical presentation and EMG findings [17].

12.1.11 Differential Diagnosis

- Primary progressive MS (see above).
- Primary lateral sclerosis (PLS) and progressive muscular atrophy (PMA) are often regarded as spectra of ALS. However, they could also be considered as separate clinical entities [2].
- PLS manifests with an insidious onset of symmetric, slowly progressing spastic paresis, which progresses slower than ALS. Clinically, signs of upper motor neuron involvement are predominant, although EMG often reveals concomitant lower motor neuron involvement. Spasticity is a common early sign in PLS patients, unlike ALS, and limb atrophy is rare. Unlike ALS, PLS is not usually fatal for most patients. Histologically, PLS is characterized by degeneration of the lateral medullary tracts, anterior horn cells of the spinal cord, and the premotor region of the motor cortex. The unilateral variant of PLS is referred to as Mills' syndrome [18].
- PMA affects only the lower motor neurons, is less common than ALS, progress slower and paresis occurs firstly in the hands. Around 20% of patients who are diagnosed with PMA over time develop upper motor neuron symptoms and are re-diagnosed with ALS [19].
- Other, most often, conditions mimicking ALS include: multifocal motor neuropathy with conduction block; axonal motor predominant chronic inflammatory demyelinating polyneuropathy; spinobulbar muscular atrophy; inclusion body myositis; hereditary spastic paraparesis; hyper-parathyroidism; hexosaminidase A deficiency (Tay-Sachs disease) or simultaneous cervical nerve root and spinal cord compression by mass lesions [2, 20].
- There is a case study of a patient with neuro-Behçet's disease and ALS presenting with longitudinally extensive (LETM) spinal cord lesion [21].

12.1.12 Treatment and Prognosis

- Symptomatic treatment [2].
- Glutamate antagonist Riluzole, the antioxidant Edaravone, Tofersen (for approximately 2% of patients with familial ALS associated with an superoxide dismutase 1 [*SOD1*] gene mutation) and the Sodium phenylbutyrate/Taurursodiol may slow down disease progression, prolong autonomy and increase survival by a few months [22].
- The average survival from onset to death is 3–4 years [1].

12.2 Bell's Palsy

12.2.1 Epidemiology

- Incidence 20–30/100.000/year (lowest in children; increases in adulthood; and peaks at around the age of 70).
- Female/male ratio 1/1 [23, 24].
- Accounts for 70% of peripheral facial palsies.
- Although, brain stem involvement in MS is common, isolated cranial mononeuropaties including peripheral facial palsies are rare (1.6% of MS patients) [25].

12.2.2 Etiology and Definition

- Idiopathic isolated unilateral peripheral facial palsy [26].
- The exact cause is unknown, but inflammation of the facial nerve due to herpes virus infection is suggested as a possible etiological factor [27].

12.2.3 Clinical Features

- Acute or subacute unilateral facial palsy involving the lower and the upper half of the face (central facial palsy affects only the lower half of the face).
- The nadir of symptoms typically occurs within 72 h. Other causes of peripheral facial palsy usually develop more slowly.
- Some patients also experience hyperacusis, hypolacrimation, hyposalivation, and unilateral loss of taste (on the anterior two-thirds of the tongue).
- The traditional clinical definition of central and peripheral facial palsy has limitations. It should be kept in mind that clinically peripheral facial palsy might be caused by lesions located in the CNS [24].

12.2.4 Brain Imaging

- Normal or may show contrast enhancement of the distal intracanalicular and labyrinthine segments of the facial nerve, geniculate ganglion, distal tympanic, and mastoid portions of the facial nerve [28].
- Among MS patients with clinically peripheral facial palsy, only around 60–70% of them have focal lesions in the brainstem explaining the clinical presentation, (data from a 1.5 Tesla MRI scanner) [25, 29].
- Although routine brain MRI in patients with typical Bell's palsy is generally not recommended, some authors recommend performing a brain MRI to exclude alternative diagnoses. Misdiagnosis of MS-related facial palsy may delay treatment of MS and increase risk of disability progression in the future [29–31].

12.2.5 Spinal Cord Imaging

- Normal.

12.2.6 Blood Work

- Normal.

12.2.7 Examination of CSF

- Abnormal findings (10–25%).
- Mildly elevated concentrations of protein and/or mild mononuclear pleocytosis may sometimes be present.
- CSF-restricted OCB are almost always absent.
- If the CSF analysis does show any clear pathological findings, a search for an alternative diagnosis should be initiated.
- CSF analysis is not mandatory in typical cases [32].

12.2.8 Diagnosis

- Based on clinical features and exclusion of alternative diagnoses.

12.2.9 Differential Diagnosis

- Rarely, isolated facial palsy may be caused by a small pontine lesion, but typically these patients also exhibit additional neurological features. In these cases may be facial palsy misdiagnosed as Bell's palsy [24, 29, 30].
- In MS patients, facial palsy is often associated with other neurological signs and symptoms, such as hearing loss or vestibular syndrome.
- Isolated peripheral facial palsy may be rarely the first presentation of the MS and can be misdiagnosed as Bell's palsy, especially when is associated with some typical clinical features of Bell's palsy, such as pain around the ear or ipsilateral loss of taste which can be also present in MS-related facial palsy.
- MS-related facial palsy and Bell's palsy typically respond to corticosteroids. Therefore, treatment response may not help with the diagnosis of MS [29, 30].
- In MS patients with a newly occurring peripheral facial palsy, it is important to distinguish between MS relapse, Bell's palsy, or infectious facial palsy.
- Bell's palsy rarely recurs; therefore, recurrent or bilateral facial palsy should prompt consideration of alternative diagnosis, such as myasthenia gravis, lymphoma, sarcoidosis, Lyme disease, or the Guillain–Barré syndrome or MS [24, 33].

- The Ramsay Hunt syndrome (Varicella-zoster virus [VZV] herpetic infection in older adults causing peripheral facial palsy along with a maculopapular, vesicular rash affecting the ear or mouth) is typically unilateral and monophasic [24].
- Peripheral facial palsy may be confused with hemifacial spasm, in which the corner of the mouth is drawn up and the eye is partially or completely closed due to involuntary contraction of the risorius and orbicularis oculi muscles [24].
- Other rare causes of peripheral facial palsy include diabetes, human immunodeficiency virus (HIV) infection, boreliosis, sarcoidosis, Sjögren's syndrome, parotid gland tumors, eclampsia, amyloidosis, recent infection or vaccination [24].

12.2.10 Treatment and Prognosis

- Corticosteroids shorten the time to complete recovery, but antivirotic treatment did not show any effect in majority of studies [27].
- Complete recovery within 6 months in 70% of cases. The remaining 30% of patients have residual paresis, contractures, or synkinesis [23].
- The risk factors associated with incomplete recovery include hypertension, older age, impairment of taste, pain other than in the ear, and severe palsy [24].
- Also, the absence of excitability on nerve conduction studies between the fourth and tenth day from disease onset predicts a poorer recovery [34].
- Aberrant regeneration of the parasympathetic fibers of the facial nerve may occur, leading to lacrimation after a salivary stimulus, a condition known as the syndrome of crocodile tears [24].

12.3 Chemoradiation-Induced Demyelination

12.3.1 Epidemilogy

- Clinically significant brain injury occurs in 5–10% of patients, while mild cognitive symptoms are more common.

12.3.2 Etiology and Definition

- Chemotherapy and radiation in cancer patients induce neurotoxicity by disrupting neural precursor cells, particularly oligodendrocytes, and causing chronic neuroinflammation through persistent microglial activation. Radiotherapy can also lead to necrosis of white matter tracts, axonal degeneration, and vascular injury. Early demyelination after radiotherapy is dose-dependent, while late progressive diffuse demyelination may occur beyond 4–6 months following treatment.

12.3.3 Classification of Clinical Post-Radiation Side Effects

- A. Acute stage (days to weeks): transient fatigue, headache, nausea, and lethargy with or without corticosteroids; associated with endothelial damage and disruption of the blood–brain barrier.
- B. Early delayed stage (1–6 months): somnolence, worsening of pre-existing symptoms, temporary cognitive impairment, and new focal deficits; associated with transient demyelination of the CNS.
- C. Late delayed stage (>6 months to years after radiotherapy): usually associated with moderate to severe permanent cognitive impairment.

12.3.4 Brain and Spinal Imaging

- Radiation-induced demyelination typically occurs in healthy brain parenchyma adjacent to the tumor.
- A. Acute Stage: Normal findings or diffuse brain vasogenic edema.
- B. Early Delayed Stage: MRI findings range from discrete non-enhancing T2 hyperintensities in deep white matter to diffuse, confluent, or necrotic lesions with thick, irregular, contrast-enhancing borders, and vasogenic brain edema.
- C. Late Delayed Stage: Necrosis of white matter tracts, axonal degeneration, leukoencephalopathy, vascular injury, accelerated brain atrophy, and in some patients, cystic porencephaly.
- Occasionally, the MRI pattern may resemble findings seen in patients with MS.

12.3.5 Examination of Blood and CSF

- CSF-restricted OCB are rarely present in cancer patients (6%).

12.3.6 Diagnosis

- History of (chemo) radiation and MRI findings.

12.3.7 Differential Diagnosis

- It has been observed that patients with MS have a higher risk of chemoradiation-induced neurotoxicity, likely due to the negative impact of chemoradiation on oligodendrocytes and the disruption of the blood-brain barrier. This may possibly also apply to patients with myelin oligodendrocyte glycoprotein antibody-associated disease (MOGAD) and neuromyelitis optica spectrum disorders (NMOSD).
- Although there is no clear association between radiotherapy and a higher risk of developing MS (with only a few case reports), radiotherapy may increase the risk of relapses in MS patients.

- In some cases, differentiating between Radiologically Isolated Syndrome (RIS) and MS-like late-delayed demyelination secondary to chemoradiation therapy in previously predisposed patients can be challenging.

12.3.8 Treatment

- Corticosteroids may be used for managing of acute adverse effects [35–37].

12.4 Fibromyalgia

12.4.1 Epidemiology

- Prevalence 2.000–5.000/100.000 [38, 39].
- More prevalent among: Women; Patients with other central sensitivity syndromes such as irritable bowel syndrome; Patients with immune-mediated diseases such as MS, systemic lupus erythematosus (SLE), rheumatoid arthritis, psoriatic arthritis, or patients with Hashimoto's thyroiditis [38, 40, 41].
- MS is associated with a twofold higher prevalence compared to the general population [42].

12.4.2 Etiology and Definition

- The etiology is unclear, but it is believed that genetic and environmental factors (psychosocial stressors and physical trauma), likely play a role.
- Has been suggested that fibromyalgia has a neurogenic origin associated with abnormal processing of painful stimuli in the CNS (central sensitivity syndrome) due to diminished activation of pain inhibitory systems and a "central amplification"of pain perception [39, 40, 43]. In this context, some authors suggest that could arise because of MS in some patients [42].
- Whether fibromyalgia might be an autoimmune disease is discussed [44].

12.4.3 Clinical Features

- Fibromyalgia is a form of chronic widespread diffuse musculoskeletal pain.
- AAPT (by American Pain Society) diagnostic criteria (2019):
  - Presence of pain in multiple sites: Pain must be present in six or more pain sites from a total of nine possible sites, which include the head, left arm, right arm, chest, abdomen, upper back and spine, lower back and spine, including buttocks, left leg, and right leg.
  - Pain causing moderate to severe sleep problems or fatigue.

  - The pain associated with sleep problems or fatigue must persist for at least 3 months [39].
- ACR (American College of Rheumatology) diagnostic criteria (2016):
  - Bilateral pain above and below the waist lasting at least 3 months and
  - Pain on palpation in at least 11 of 18 specific body sites [45].
- The pain is often associated with emotional distress and/or functional disability, affective disorders, and cognitive complaints.
- The symptoms cannot be explained better with other comorbid diagnosis.
- Patients have increased sensitivity to pressure, but also to several other sensory stimuli, including heat, cold, auditory, and electrical stimuli.
- The pain is predominantly nociplastic caused by altered nociceptive processing (central hypersensitivity). This contrasts with nociceptive pain, which is caused by a nociceptive stimulus, or neuropathic pain, which is caused by pathology of the nervous system [39, 43].

12.4.4 Brain and Spinal Cord Imaging

- Conventional imaging studies reveal normal or age-related findings.
- Diffusion-tensor imaging (DTI) and voxel-based morphometry MRI have demonstrated changes in the microstructure of brain areas linked to core pain sensation [46].

12.4.5 Examination of Blood and CSF

- Routine testing is normal.
- Occasionally positive for antinuclear antibodies (ANA), often displaying the speckled pattern [47].
- Neurotransmitters associated with increasing ascending sensory inputs, such as: substance P; nerve growth factor; brain-derived neurotrophic factor, and glutamate (an excitatory amino acid), are often increased.
- Nevertheless, activity in descending anti-nociceptive pathways is decreased, as evidenced by decreased concentrations of serotonin, norepinephrine, and dopamine.
- Although opioid levels are increased, opioid receptor binding is decreased, which can explain the lower effectiveness of opioids in fibromyalgia [43].

12.4.6 Diagnosis

- See Sect. 12.4.3.

12.4.7 Treatment and Prognosis

- Symptomatic management, which may include tricyclic antidepressants, antiepileptic drugs, selective serotonin reuptake inhibitors, norepinephrine/ serotonin reuptake inhibitors, and physiotherapy [48].
- Patients have decreased quality of life [39, 43].

12.5 Functional Neurological Disorders

12.5.1 Epidemiology

- Prevalence 50/100.000.
- Women are more frequently affected (60–75%) [49].

12.5.2 Etiology and Definition

- The exact cause of Functional neurological disorders (FND) is not fully understood. However, it is suggested that the pathophysiology involves overactivity of the limbic system, the development of an internal symptom model within a predictive coding framework, and dysfunction of brain networks that contribute to the sense of voluntariness in movement. Although psychological stressors are common risk factors, they are often absent [50].

12.5.3 Clinical Features

- Motor manifestations
  - General features:
    - Sudden onset.
    - Disappearance with distraction and increase with attention.
    - Excessive slowness, fatigue, and demonstration of effort.
    - Inconsistency in performance with high variability of severity over time and discordant performance between assessments.
    - Incongruency with clinical features not compatible with organically determined patterns.
    - Giveaway weakness with inability to rotate the head toward the paralyzed limb.
  - Arm weakness:
    - Upper arm weakness with drift without pronation.
    - Finger abduction sign (weakness of fingers abduction that resolves with contralateral finger abduction against resistance).
    - Able to remove objects from bag or put on clothes inconsistent with upper limb examination.

- Leg weakness:
  - Hoover sign (involuntary extension of the affected leg when flexing the contralateral leg against resistance).
  - Hip abductor sign (weakness of hip abduction in a paretic leg that resolves with contralateral hip abduction against resistance).
  - Able to stand on toes or ankles despite weak plantar flexion or dorsiflexion on bed.
- Parkinsonism:
  - Lack of speed or amplitude decrement on repetitive tapping.
  - Variable resistance during passive manipulation (Gegenhalten).
- Tremor
  - Variability in frequency.
  - Response to externally cued rhythmic movements (positive tremor entrainment test), in which occurs synchronization or cessation of tremor to externally cued rhythmic movement.
  - Tonic coactivation of antagonistic muscles at tremor onset.
  - Pause during contralateral ballistic movements.
  - Whack-a-mole sign (appearance or worsening of an involuntary movement in a separate body part when the initially affected body part is suppressed by someone holding it down).
- Myoclonus
  - Entrainment or full suppressibility.
  - Variability in duration, distribution or latency of jerks (if stimulus sensitive).
  - Predominance of axial or facial jerks.
- Dystonia
  - Fixed dystonia at onset.
  - Variable resistance to passive manipulation.
  - Lack of sensory trick and overflow.
  - Face: tonic pulling of the lips or jaw to 1 side; closed eyelids resist retraction by examiner.
- Tics
  - Not fully stereotypical.
  - Interference with speech or voluntary actions.
  - Lack of premonitory urge.
  - Inability to voluntarily suppress.
- Gait and balance
  - Excessive gait slowness or a gait similar to walking on ice.
  - Excessive demonstration of effort (huffing and puffing sign).
  - Astasia-abasia.
  - Knee buckling (knees gives out or feel weak; not specific for FND).
  - Dragging gait with forefoot in contact with ground.
  - No or controlled falls despite excessive swaying when walking.
  - Swaying and imbalance lessened with dual tasks.

    - Persistent perceptual postural dizziness involves a persistent sense of disequilibrium or nonspinning dizziness triggered by changes in position, motion, or exposure to moving visual stimuli or complex visual patterns. Initially, it is often associated with acute dizziness related to conditions like vestibular neuronitis or panic attacks. Symptoms persist due to the failure of vestibular and brain readaptation. It commonly leads to the development of anxiety and functional gait disorders.
  - Posture
    - Variability of positions over time.
    - Inconsistent, uneconomic postures.
    - Myoclonic jerks affecting the trunk (often diagnosed as propriospinal myoclonus) or fixed forward–flexion of the thoracolumbar spine (camptocormia).
- Speech manifestations
  - Effortful speech.
  - Sudden onset of dysphonia, stuttering, or dysprosody.
  - Dysfluency similar to stuttering and articulation deficits.
  - Prosodic abnormalities (including foreign accent).
- Sensory and visual manifestations
  - Less reliable than motor manifestations.
  - Atypical sensory loss, which either takes the form of a circle or does not have typical root or nerve distribution (for example precise midline splitting of vibration sense on the forehead or sternum; or sharply demarcated hypoesthesia at the groin or shoulder).
  - Visual field testing may show a tubular or missing half defect (an ipsilateral hemianopia on testing the "affected" eye, normal vision in the other eye, and a complete hemianopia toward the affected side on testing with both eyes open).
  - Pain syndromes are not classified as FND but often coexist with them.
- Paroxysmal manifestations (including seizures/attacks)
  - Paroxysmal akinesia (typical positive features include long-duration attacks with closed eyes).
  - Paroxysmal hyperkinesias (e.g., tremor, dystonia, and jerks).
  - Psychogenic nonepileptic seizure can be distinguished from epileptic seizures by the long duration of shaking episodes (>3 min), fluctuating course of seizures, asynchronous limb movements, pelvic movements, side to-side head movements, closed eyes, ictal crying, and recall of ictal events.
- Functional cognitive symptoms
  - Subjective memory deficit and decreased ability to concentrate [50–54].

12.5.4 Brain and Spinal Cord Imaging

- Comprehensive data are lacking, but imaging studies are expected to be normal.

12.5.5 Examination of Blood and CSF

- Although, comprehensive data are lacking and routine blood and CSF testing are expected to yield normal results. A recent study on 26 patients and 26 controls showed mildly increased leukocyte count in considerable proportion of patients with FND (65% vs. 15% in controls) [55].

12.5.6 Diagnosis

- The diagnosis necessitates not only the exclusion of other diseases but also the presence of positive signs, as listed above, during the neurological examination. Therefore, FND should not be approached as a diagnosis of exclusion [51, 56].
- In general, patients with FND exhibit positive signs such as internal inconsistency (changing patterns of clinical features over time with susceptibility to distraction) and incongruency (clinical features are not compatible with organically determined patterns). These signs are both required for the diagnosis of FND [50–54].

12.5.7 Differential Diagnosis

- FND and MS do not have highly specific biomarkers and can present with similar neurological symptoms, therefore differential diagnosis may be challenging and relies on a skilled clinical assessment.
- Around 0.1–0.4% of MS patients are misdiagnosed with FND. The proportion of patients with FND who are misdiagnosed with MS is likely even higher [51].
- Misinterpretation of nonspecific and temporary symptoms that do not clearly indicate involvement of the CNS, along with nonspecific MRI findings, are responsible for misdiagnosing MS in many patients with FND [57].
- Conversely, placing too much emphasis on a history of psychiatric comorbidity or adverse experiences, as well as focusing on "bizarre" clinical presentations, can often lead to an incorrect diagnosis of FND [58].
- Misdiagnosing a patient with FND as having MS or vice versa, causes harm to patients because of delay to diagnosis and treatment [51, 59].
- FND can coexist with MS, and several hypotheses have been suggested to interpret this association [51, 59–61]. Given the potential comorbidity of FND with MS, it is necessary to establish whether new symptoms are attributable to a new relapse, progression independent of relapsing activity, or FND, and vice versa. Especially in cases of atypical and refractory symptoms in MS patients, it is important to consider FND in the differential diagnosis [59].

12.5.8 Treatment and Prognosis

- Multidisciplinary management including explaining the diagnosis, psychological interventions, rehabilitation, and physical treatment, is recommended. FNDs are potentially reversible with treatment. However, due to their under-recognition and a lack of experienced therapists, the prognosis remains poor [50, 52–54].

12.6 Headache and Neurological Deficits with Cerebrospinal Fluid Lymphocytosis (HaNDL)

12.6.1 Epidemiology

- Very rare condition, slightly more prevalent in men.
- Most frequently occurs in the third to fourth decades of life, though it is occasionally seen in children.

12.6.2 Etiology and Definition

- One hypothesis suggests that infections could play a role in its pathogenesis, as some patients exhibit flu-like symptoms and test positive for human herpesvirus (HHV)-7, borrelia, or Epstein–Barr Virus (EBV).
- Another theory proposes the involvement of vasospasms and transient reductions in cerebral perfusion. In some cases, a cortical spreading depression pattern, similar to that seen in migraines, is observed.
- Additionally, it is speculated that an autoimmune process may contribute to the condition's development.
- The exact pathophysiology remains uncertain and is likely multifactorial.
- Notably, 15% of patients with HaNDL have a history of migraines.

12.6.3 Clinical Features

- Episodes of headache:
  - Typically lasting over 4 h.
  - Migraine-like in nature
  - Often unilateral, commonly on the left side
  - A pulsating or throbbing quality
  - Generally severe, though occasionally of moderate intensity
  - Precedes or accompanies the onset of neurological deficits.
  - Frequently associated with vegetative symptoms, such as nausea and vomiting (occurring in over 50% of cases).

- Transient neurological deficit:
  - Includes at least one of the following key features: hemiparesthesia (60%), aphasia (47%), or hemiparesis (55%).
  - Other possible manifestations may include confusion (33%), papilledema (16%), visual disturbances (rare), dysarthria (11%), abducens nerve palsy or other cranial nerve deficits, agraphia, nystagmus, ataxia, and various other sensorimotor signs and symptoms.
  - Unlike migraine, visual symptoms are uncommon.

12.6.4 Disease Course

- Relapsing remitting
- Relapses typically occur within 1–3 months.
- Monophasic course is rare (4%).

12.6.5 Brain and Spinal Cord Imaging

- Typically, normal (75%)
  - A few patients may exhibit:
  - Leptomeningeal enhancement (7.5%)
  - Nonspecific white matter lesions (10%)
  - Corpus callosum lesions (5.1%)
  - Restricted diffusion (2.2%)
  - Gray matter swelling and enhancement in the temporal and occipital sulci.

12.6.6 Examination of Blood and CSF

- Glucose concentration is normal, but most patients exhibit elevated concentration of protein, albumin quotient, and CSF opening pressure.
- Lymphocytic pleocytosis is present in the CSF (average 147.5 cells/mL); a minimum of 15 cells/mL is required for diagnosis.
- Improvement or worsening of headaches and neurological deficits often corresponds with changes in CSF pleocytosis.
- Pleocytosis may persist after symptom resolution and, in rare cases, may appear a few days after a headache episode.
- CSF-restricted or corresponding OCB are very rare (2.2%).
- CSF abnormalities typically resolve spontaneously within several months; but after 99 days (range 56–196), nearly all patients still show CSF pleocytosis.

12.6.7 Electrophysiology

- Nearly half of the cases (46%) exhibit diffuse or focal slowing on electroencephalography (EEG).

12.6.8 Diagnosis

- HaNDL syndrome is a diagnosis of exclusion.
- Diagnosis relies on a combination of transient headache episodes, neurological deficits, and CSF pleocytosis, with alternative diagnoses ruled out (i.e., no better explanation exists for the symptoms).

12.6.9 Differential Diagnosis

- Infectious encephalitis or meningitis, Syphilis, Lyme's disease, neoplastic (carcinomatous) meningitis, CNS vasculitis, migraine with aura, epilepsy, stroke, autoimmune and paraneoplastic encephalitis, tumors and other structural lesions in the CNS.

12.6.10 Treatment and Prognosis

- HaNDL syndrome is benign and self-limiting, typically involving 1–12 episodes; thus, treatment focuses on symptoms relief.
- If preventive treatment is necessary, options may include flunarizine, acetazolamide, propranolol, valproic acid, nimodipine, or corticosteroids [62–65].

12.7 Spondylotic and Other Structural Myelopathies

12.7.1 Epidemiology

- Prevalence of surgically treated or hospitalization required cases of cervical spondylotic myelopathy: 1.6–4.0/100.000/years [66].
- Degenerative thoracic myelopathy is less frequent [67].

12.7.2 Etiology and Definition

- Compression of the spinal cord occurs due to osteoarthritic changes in the spine, including disk degeneration and migration, loss of disk height, altered biomechanics of the cervical spine, hypertrophy of the ligamentum flavum, laxity of facet joints, strain and hypertrophy of spinal joints, or less common conditions such as spondylolisthesis and ossification of the posterior longitudinal ligament.

- Chronic spinal cord compression leads to the prolonged stretching of the spinal cord and a decrease in intraparenchymal spinal cord blood flow, resulting in ischemic injury to the spinal cord and aseptic neuroinflammation [68].

12.7.3 Clinical Features

- Neck pain:
  - Moderate or severe (60%); mild (20%); without pain (20%).
  - The neck pain is attributed to abnormalities of the structures surrounding the spinal cord rather than dysfunction of the cord itself [69].
  - Radiculopathy with radicular pain is present in only 40% of patients, and its absence often correlates with delayed diagnosis and treatment.
- Neurological deficit:
  - Decreased dexterity or weakness of the hands may be present.
  - Upper extremities are affected symmetrically or asymmetrically.
  - Lower extremities are typically affected symmetrically, and often display motor weakness, dorsal column syndrome and gait instability.
  - A dominant upper motor neuron syndrome is typically observed, with lower motor neuron syndrome occasionally present to a lesser extent.
  - Sensory manifestations, including Lhermitte's sign, are common.
  - Bowel/bladder dysfunction is frequent but usually not dominant [70].
- The manifestations of spondylotic myelopathy are often confounded by arthritis, degenerative lumbar spine disorders, peripheral neuropathies, or other CNS disorders such as stroke, Parkinson's disease, or MS [71].

12.7.4 Disease Course

- Insidious symptoms onset over months to years and chronic stepwise progression.
- Acute onset is atypical, unless preceded by trauma or long-lasting hyperflexion or hyper-extension of the spine [71].

12.7.5 Spinal Cord Imaging

- Spinal canal stenosis (<10 mm diameter) with completely effaced subarachnoid space at the level of compression.
- T2 hyperintesity in a compressed segment of the spinal cord is not present in all clinically symptomatic patients (58–85%).
- Some patients have asymptomatic T2 lesions, or only transient reversible increase of T2 signal in the spinal cord.
- Although the presence of T2 signal changes has not prognostic value, multiple hyperintensities across several spinal segments and decreased signal on T1 images indicate poorer outcomes [72–74].

- Contrast enhancement.
  - Rare (7%), but may persist for months to 2 years, even after successful decompressive surgery.
  - Often pancake-like enhancement pattern ("pancake sign") with:
    - A. Transverse band appearance, greater in transverse than vertical extent on sagittal images;
    - B. Location just below the site of maximum stenosis at the center of the spindle-shaped T2 hyperintensity, and
    - C. Uni- or bilateral circumferential enhancement sparing gray matter on axial images ("croissant sign") [75] (Fig. 12.2; also see Figs. 15.2, 15.3, and 15.4 in Sect. 15.22.6)
- X-rays should be performed because can highlight the presence of spondylolisthesis, stress fractures facet arthropathy, or scoliosis.
- Computed tomography (CT) myelography is an alternative in patients with contraindicated MRI [71].
- In some patients dynamic cervical spine MRI in extension can show spinal cord compression from spondylosis hidden in the neutral position [76].

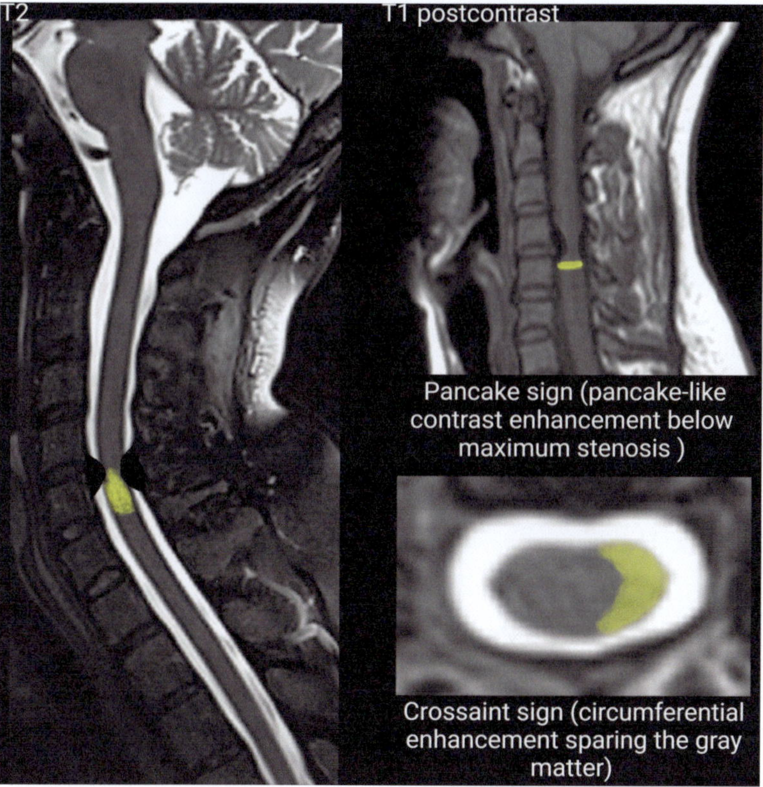

Fig. 12.2 MRI characteristics of spondylotic myelopathy

12.7.6 Blood Work

- Normal.

12.7.7 Examination of CSF

- Occasionally mildly elevated concentration of protein [77].
- CSF-restricted OCB is extremely rare [78].

12.7.8 Electrophysiology

- Motor evoked potentials (MEP) is the most sensitive test for detecting myelopathy, and they correlate with its severity [79].
- The amplitude of MEP and the frequency of F waves evoked by peripheral nerve stimulation could aid in differentiating cervical myelopathy from mimics such as ALS [80].

12.7.9 Diagnosis

- Based on clinical manifestation and spinal cord MRI [71].

12.7.10 Differential Diagnosis

- ALS may mimic spondylotic myelopathy; however, it is not associated with sensory symptoms and often presents with abnormal EMG findings.
- Hereditary spastic paraplegia (HSP) may resemble spondylotic myelopathy, but patients with HSP often display early spasticity despite preserved motor strength. This presentation is atypical for spondylotic myelopathy, where spasticity and paresis typically develop simultaneously.
- Multifocal motor neuropathy and peripheral neuropathies are characterized by diminished reflexes and typical findings on nerve conduction studies and EMG [71].

12.7.11 Treatment and Prognosis

- Treatment options include either conservative measures such as waiting, wearing a cervical collar, bed rest, medication, and physical therapy, or surgical intervention [71].
- Surgery is not recommended for patients with compression of the cervical cord in the absence of clinical myelopathic symptoms. However, patients require

monitoring due to the risk of clinical worsening over time (23% develop myelopathic symptoms within 4 years).
- No clear evidence to support the indication of prophylactic surgery in patients with spinal canal stenosis to prevent cord injury from minor trauma [81].
- In MS patients with coexisting symptomatic cervical myelopathy, surgery is recommended to improve the quality of life [82].

12.7.12 Other Causes of Structural Myelopathy

12.7.12.1 Chiari Malformation
- The cerebellar tonsils extend into the spinal canal below the foramen magnum and into the upper cervical spinal canal. A half of the patients are asymptomatic, the rest experience myelopathy, headache, or cerebellar syndrome [71].

12.7.12.2 Hirayama Disease
- Abnormal forward shifting of the posterior dura matter during neck flexion, which compress the spinal cord. This causes juvenile painless weakness and amyotrophy of hand and forearm muscles.
- MRI shows asymmetric focal spinal cord flattening and atrophy (mostly at the cervical vertebrae C4-C7), loss of attachment between the posterior dural sac and subjacent lamina, and noncompressive intramedullary T2 hyperintensity.
- Treatment of this rare disorder is conservative or surgical [71, 83].

12.7.12.3 Idiopathic Spinal Cord Herniation
- In this rare disorder of unclear etiology, the thoracic spinal cord herniates through a small dural defect [71, 84].

12.7.12.4 Spinal Arachnoid Cysts
- Symptoms mimic degenerative thoracic myelopathy.
- Typically located extramedullary (extra- or intra-duraly) on the dorsal aspect of the thoracic spine. The cyst is non-enhancing and has the same signal as CSF, thus visualization is indirect through the displacement of the spinal cord.
- Treatment is surgical (fenestration, decompression, or shunting) [71, 85].

12.7.12.5 Syringomyelia
- Abnormal, CSF-filled cavity within the adult spinal cord
- Origin is either idiopathic or caused by Chiari malformation, tumors, trauma, adhesions, and arachnoid webs.
- Asymptomatic or have clinical manifestations including dissociated sensory loss, atrophy of the hands, hyperreflexia and spasticity, or Horner syndrome.
- Surgery is performed in only some patients depending on etiology. For example, patients with a syrinx and Chiari malformations are usually recommended for surgery [71, 86].

12.8 Traumatic Axonal Injury

12.8.1 Synonyms

- Diffuse axonal injury.

12.8.2 Epidemiology

- The incidence is unknown, but around 10% of all patients with brain injury admitted to the hospital have some degree of traumatic axonal injury (TAI) [87].

12.8.3 Etiology and Definition

- TAI is defined as brain trauma followed by a prolonged (>6 h) loss of consciousness without a visible mass lesion or increased intracranial pressure, but with diffuse traumatic pathological findings, especially in white matter tracts.
- The combination of sudden translational and angular acceleration, along with rotational acceleration, has been proposed as the most important mechanisms. TAI can also be caused by trauma involving low rates of acceleration. Severe or even deadly TAI can occur even if the initial impact force is not strong enough to cause skull fracturing or evident macroscopic brain pathology.
- Primary (mechanical stretch and tearing of axons due to traumatic acceleration or deceleration) and secondary (driven mostly by hydroxylation of proteins of microtubules due to an inflammatory and apoptotic cascade) axotomy are pathological substrates of TAI [88, 89].

12.8.4 Clinical Features

- Typically, loss of consciousness at the time and after the brain trauma. TAI is considered in patients with a Glasgow Coma Scale (GCS) of <8 for >6 h.
- The diagnosis is initially often not suspected until later when patients fail to recover neurologically as expected and remain in a persistent vegetative state.
- The mild TAI has signs and symptoms corresponding to a brain concussion or contusion (headache, dizziness, nausea, vomiting, and fatigue) [88, 90].

12.8.5 Brain Imaging

- Lesions' location:
  - A brain CT scan may appear normal.
  - Although normal MRI findings may not rule out TAI, MRI typically reveals multiple lesions predominantly in white matter tracts located in the midline of

the brain. These lesions are especially noticeable in the gray-white matter junction of the cerebral cortex, the corpus callosum, and in more severe cases, in the brainstem.
  - Other locations include the internal capsule or cerebral peduncles.
- Lesions' appearance:
  - Multiple small hemorrhagic and/or non-hemorrhagic T2 hyperintense lesions with surrounding edema.
  - T1 signal is decreased in the case of non-hemorrhagic lesions and increased in the case of the hemorrhagic component of the lesion.
  - Paramagnetic-sensitive sequences such as SWI or and gradient-echo (GRE) can detect small hemorrhagic lesions (multiple "dark spots") in the subacute or chronic phases (less in the acute phase) and aid in the differential diagnosis of TAI (Fig. 12.3).
  - The majority of lesions show restricted diffusion, reflecting cytotoxic edema and indicating disruption of normal cellular processes. In the subacute to chronic phase, lesions may exhibit increased apparent diffusion coefficient (ADC) values compared to normal brain tissue, which reflects the resolution of cytotoxic edema and the presence of vasogenic edema [88, 89, 91].

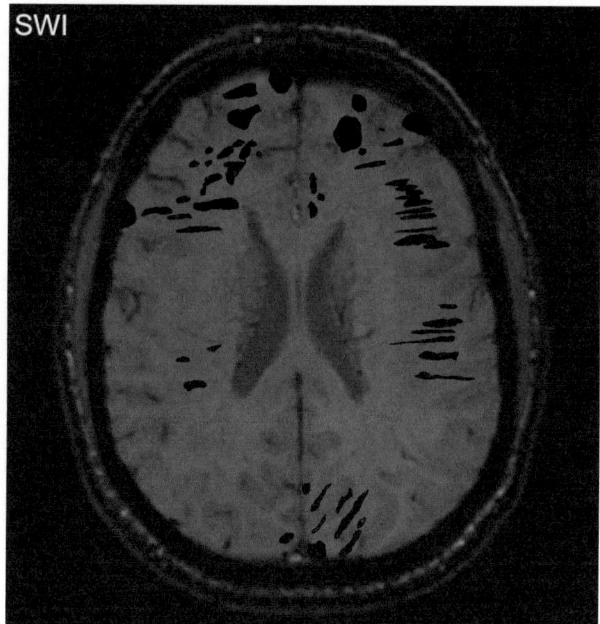

Fig. 12.3 Microhemorrhages in traumatic axonal injury

12.8.6 Spinal Cord Imaging

- TAI in the spinal cord has been described in babies [92].

12.8.7 Examination of Blood and CSF

- Elevated concentrations of markers of neuronal injury in blood, such as neurofilament licht chain (NfL), glial fibrillary acidic protein (GFAP), ubiquitin C-terminal hydrolase L1 (UCH-L1), S100 beta protein, or Neuron-specific enolase (NSE). Their levels may have prognostic value [88, 93].

12.8.8 Diagnosis

- Based on history of traumatic event, clinical manifestations, and MRI.
- There are no established criteria for diagnosing TAI [88, 89, 91].
- The history of brain trauma, the clinical presentation, and the presence of hemorrhagic lesions can help distinguish TAI from MS.
- Although brain injury has not been conclusively identified as a risk factor for MS, several case studies from the literature, as well as clinical experience show rare coincidences of brain injury and the clinical symptoms onset of MS [94, 95].

12.8.9 Treatment and Prognosis

- Same management as in severe traumatic brain injury.
- The calcium channel blocker nimodipine may decrease a secondary axotomy.
- The prognosis of patients with severe TAI is poor [87–89].

12.9 Normal Findings in the General Population

12.9.1 Brain Imaging

- Brain aging is associated with accumulation of non-specific small T2 hyperintensities in the white matter.
  - Usually absent in adults younger than 30 years
  - Occasionally present in adults over 40 years of age
  - Present in vast majority (>90%) of adults over 60–65 years of age.

The etiology of these hyperintensities heterogeneous, mostly attributed to the chronic ischemia caused by CSVD [96, 97, 98].

12.9.2 Spinal Cord Imaging

- Normal, except for cases of degenerative cervical myelopathy, which occurs in 0.19% of the population, with a peak prevalence of 0.42% at 50–54 years of age [99].

12.9.3 Examination of Cerebrospinal Fluid

- Positive CSF-restricted OCB is very rare in healthy individuals (>4%; although this prevalence may be overestimated) but relatively common in healthy siblings of patients with MS (19%) [100].
- A mildly increased CSF cell count may rarely be seen in healthy people, and is often attributed to automated cell counting, which may overestimate low CSF cell counts [101].

References

1. Talbott EO, Malek AM, Lacomis D. The epidemiology of amyotrophic lateral sclerosis. Handb Clin Neurol. 2016;138:225–38.
2. Feldman EL, Goutman SA, Petri S, Mazzini L, Savelieff MG, Shaw PJ, et al. Amyotrophic lateral sclerosis. Lancet. 2022;400(10360):1363–80.
3. Shefner JM, Mackin GA, Dawson DM. Lower motor neuron dysfunction in patients with multiple sclerosis. Muscle Nerve. 1992;15(11):1265–70.
4. Solomon AJ, Hills W, Chen Z, Rosenbaum J, Bourdette D, Whitham R. Autoantibodies and Sjogren's syndrome in multiple sclerosis, a reappraisal. PLoS One. 2013;8(6):e65385.
5. Solomon AJ, Arrambide G, Brownlee WJ, Flanagan EP, Amato MP, Amezcua L, et al. Differential diagnosis of suspected multiple sclerosis: an updated consensus approach. Lancet Neurol. 2023;22(8):750–68.
6. Lopes de Carvalho ML, Motta R, Battaglia MA, Brichetto G. Urinary disorders in amyotrophic lateral sclerosis subjects. Amyotroph Lateral Scler. 2011;12(5):352–5.
7. Ringholz GM, Appel SH, Bradshaw M, Cooke NA, Mosnik DM, Schulz PE. Prevalence and patterns of cognitive impairment in sporadic ALS. Neurology. 2005;65(4):586–90.
8. Uher T, Krasensky J, Sobisek L, Blahova Dusankova J, Seidl Z, Kubala Havrdova E, et al. Cognitive clinico-radiological paradox in early stages of multiple sclerosis. Ann Clin Transl Neurol. 2018;5(1):81–91.
9. Lublin FD, Reingold SC, Cohen JA, Cutter GR, Sorensen PS, Thompson AJ, et al. Defining the clinical course of multiple sclerosis: the 2013 revisions. Neurology. 2014;83(3):278–86.
10. Simon NG, Turner MR, Vucic S, Al-Chalabi A, Shefner J, Lomen-Hoerth C, et al. Quantifying disease progression in amyotrophic lateral sclerosis. Ann Neurol. 2014;76(5):643–57.
11. Chakraborty S, Gupta A, Nguyen T, Bourque P. The "Motor Band Sign": susceptibility-weighted imaging in amyotrophic lateral sclerosis. Can J Neurol Sci. 2015;42(4):260–3.
12. Leonardi A, Abbruzzese G, Arata L, Cocito L, Vische M. Cerebrospinal fluid (CSF) findings in amyotrophic lateral sclerosis. J Neurol. 1984;231(2):75–8.
13. Brousse M, Delaby C, De La Cruz E, Kuhle J, Benkert P, Mondesert E, et al. Serum neurofilament light chain cut-off definition for clinical diagnosis and prognosis of amyotrophic lateral sclerosis. Eur J Neurol. 2023;30(7):1919–27.

14. Klose V, Jesse S, Lewerenz J, Kassubek J, Dorst J, Tumani H, et al. CSF oligoclonal IgG bands are not associated with ALS progression and prognosis. Front Neurol. 2023;14:1170360.
15. Rojas P, de Hoz R, Ramírez AI, Ferreras A, Salobrar-Garcia E, Muñoz-Blanco JL, et al. Changes in retinal OCT and their correlations with neurological disability in early ALS patients, a follow-up study. Brain Sci. 2019;9(12)
16. Grana EA, Kraft GH. Electrodiagnostic abnormalities in patients with multiple sclerosis. Arch Phys Med Rehabil. 1994;75(7):778–82.
17. Brooks BR, Miller RG, Swash M, Munsat TL, World Federation of Neurology Research Group on Motor Neuron D. El Escorial revisited: revised criteria for the diagnosis of amyotrophic lateral sclerosis. Amyotroph Lateral Scler Other Motor Neuron Disord. 2000;1(5):293–9.
18. Tartaglia MC, Rowe A, Findlater K, Orange JB, Grace G, Strong MJ. Differentiation between primary lateral sclerosis and amyotrophic lateral sclerosis: examination of symptoms and signs at disease onset and during follow-up. Arch Neurol. 2007;64(2):232–6.
19. Liewluck T, Saperstein DS. Progressive muscular atrophy. Neurol Clin. 2015;33(4):761–73.
20. Goutman SA. Diagnosis and clinical management of amyotrophic lateral sclerosis and other motor neuron disorders. Continuum (Minneap Minn). 2017;23(5, Peripheral Nerve and Motor Neuron Disorders):1332–59.
21. Sato T, Ouchi H, Shimbo J, Sato A, Yamazaki M, Hashidate H, et al. Coexistence of amyotrophic lateral sclerosis with neuro-Behcet's disease presenting as a longitudinally extensive spinal cord lesion: clinicopathologic features of an autopsied patient. Neuropathology. 2014;34(2):185–9.
22. Masrori P, Van Damme P. Amyotrophic lateral sclerosis: a clinical review. Eur J Neurol. 2020;27(10):1918–29.
23. Peitersen E. Bell's palsy: the spontaneous course of 2,500 peripheral facial nerve palsies of different etiologies. Acta Otolaryngol Suppl. 2002;549:4–30.
24. Gilden DH. Clinical practice. Bell's Palsy N Engl J Med. 2004;351(13):1323–31.
25. Zadro I, Barun B, Habek M, Brinar VV. Isolated cranial nerve palsies in multiple sclerosis. Clin Neurol Neurosurg. 2008;110(9):886–8.
26. May M, Hughes GB. Facial nerve disorders: update 1987. Am J Otol. 1987;8(2):167–80.
27. Engström M, Berg T, Stjernquist-Desatnik A, Axelsson S, Pitkäranta A, Hultcrantz M, et al. Prednisolone and valaciclovir in Bell's palsy: a randomised, double-blind, placebo-controlled, multicentre trial. Lancet Neurol. 2008;7(11):993–1000.
28. Sartoretti-Schefer S, Wichmann W, Valavanis A. Idiopathic, herpetic, and HIV-associated facial nerve palsies: abnormal MR enhancement patterns. AJNR Am J Neuroradiol. 1994;15(3):479–85.
29. Di Stadio A, Dipietro L, Ralli M, Greco A, Ricci G, Messineo D, et al. Clinical and radiological findings of facial paralysis in multiple sclerosis. Mult Scler Relat Disord. 2020;37:101456.
30. Fukazawa T, Moriwaka F, Hamada K, Hamada T, Tashiro K. Facial palsy in multiple sclerosis. J Neurol. 1997;244(10):631–3.
31. Uher T, Adzima A, Srpova B, Noskova L, Marechal B, Maceski AM, et al. Diagnostic delay of multiple sclerosis: prevalence, determinants and consequences. Mult Scler. 2023;29(11–12):1437–51.
32. Kohler A, Chofflon M, Sztajzel R, Magistris MR. Cerebrospinal fluid in acute peripheral facial palsy. J Neurol. 1999;246(3):165–9.
33. Ivanković M, Demarin V. From recurrent peripheral facial palsy to multiple sclerosis. Acta Clin Croat. 2011;50(3):419–21.
34. Campbell ED, Hickey RP, Nixon KH, Richardson AT. Value of nerve-excitability measurements in prognosis of facial palsy. Br Med J. 1962;2(5296):7–10.
35. Borges A, Garcez D, Pedro C, Passos J. Chemoradiation induced multiple sclerosis-like demyelination. eNeurologicalSci. 2021;22:100315.

36. Guillemin F, Biau J, Conde S, Clavelou P, Dupic G. Multiple sclerosis as differential diagnosis of radionecrosis for post-irradiation brain lesions: a case report. Clin Transl Radiat Oncol. 2020;21:44–8.
37. Sterpi AE, Triantafyllou AS, Tzanetakos D, Ampantzi E, Kitsos D, Theodorou A, et al. Multiple sclerosis-like lesions induced by radiation: a case report and systematic review of the literature. J Clin Med. 2024;13(24)
38. Branco JC, Bannwarth B, Failde I, Abello Carbonell J, Blotman F, Spaeth M, et al. Prevalence of fibromyalgia: a survey in five European countries. Semin Arthritis Rheum. 2010;39(6):448–53.
39. Arnold LM, Bennett RM, Crofford LJ, Dean LE, Clauw DJ, Goldenberg DL, et al. AAPT diagnostic criteria for fibromyalgia. J Pain. 2019;20(6):611–28.
40. Yunus MB. The prevalence of fibromyalgia in other chronic pain conditions. Pain Res Treat. 2012;2012:584573.
41. Applbaum E, Lichtbroun A. Novel Sjögren's autoantibodies found in fibromyalgia patients with sicca and/or xerostomia. Autoimmun Rev. 2019;18(2):199–202.
42. Marrie RA, Yu BN, Leung S, Elliott L, Warren S, Wolfson C, et al. The incidence and prevalence of fibromyalgia are higher in multiple sclerosis than the general population: a population-based study. Mult Scler Relat Disord. 2012;1(4):162–7.
43. Clauw DJ, Arnold LM, McCarberg BH. The science of fibromyalgia. Mayo Clin Proc. 2011;86(9):907–11.
44. Clauw D, Sarzi-Puttini P, Pellegrino G, Shoenfeld Y. Is fibromyalgia an autoimmune disorder? Autoimmun Rev. 2023:103424.
45. Wolfe F, Clauw DJ, Fitzcharles MA, Goldenberg DL, Häuser W, Katz RL, et al. 2016 revisions to the 2010/2011 fibromyalgia diagnostic criteria. Semin Arthritis Rheum. 2016;46(3):319–29.
46. Lutz J, Jäger L, de Quervain D, Krauseneck T, Padberg F, Wichnalek M, et al. White and gray matter abnormalities in the brain of patients with fibromyalgia: a diffusion-tensor and volumetric imaging study. Arthritis Rheum. 2008;58(12):3960–9.
47. Smart PA, Waylonis GW, Hackshaw KV. Immunologic profile of patients with fibromyalgia. Am J Phys Med Rehabil. 1997;76(3):231.
48. Chinn S, Caldwell W, Gritsenko K. Fibromyalgia pathogenesis and treatment options update. Curr Pain Headache Rep. 2016;20(4):25.
49. Carson A, Lehn A. Epidemiology. Handb Clin Neurol. 2016;139:47–60.
50. Hallett M, Aybek S, Dworetzky BA, McWhirter L, Staab JP, Stone J. Functional neurological disorder: new subtypes and shared mechanisms. Lancet Neurol. 2022;21(6):537–50.
51. Walzl D, Solomon AJ, Stone J. Functional neurological disorder and multiple sclerosis: a systematic review of misdiagnosis and clinical overlap. J Neurol. 2022;269(2):654–63.
52. Espay AJ, Aybek S, Carson A, Edwards MJ, Goldstein LH, Hallett M, et al. Current concepts in diagnosis and treatment of functional neurological disorders. JAMA Neurol. 2018;75(9):1132–41.
53. Bennett K, Diamond C, Hoeritzauer I, Gardiner P, McWhirter L, Carson A, et al. A practical review of functional neurological disorder (FND) for the general physician. Clin Med (Lond). 2021;21(1):28–36.
54. Serranová T, Di Vico I, Tinazzi M. Functional movement disorder: assessment and treatment. Neurol Clin. 2023;41(4):583–603.
55. Serranova T, Slovak M, Forejtova Z, Sieger T, Dusek P, Srpova B, et al. Abnormal cerebrospinal fluid cytology in functional movement disorders. Psychosom Med. 2024;86(6):555–60.
56. Diagnostic and statistical manual of mental disorders: DSM-5™, 5th ed. Arlington, VA, US: American Psychiatric Publishing, Inc.; 2013. xliv, 947-xliv, p.
57. Solomon AJ, Pettigrew R, Naismith RT, Chahin S, Krieger S, Weinshenker B. Challenges in multiple sclerosis diagnosis: misunderstanding and misapplication of the McDonald criteria. Mult Scler. 2021;27(2):250–8.

58. Stone J, Reuber M, Carson A. Functional symptoms in neurology: mimics and chameleons. Pract Neurol. 2013;13(2):104–13.
59. Aybek S, Chan A. The borderland of multiple sclerosis and functional neurological disorder: a call for clinical research and vigilance. Eur J Neurol. 2023;30(1):3–8.
60. Caplan LR, Nadelson T. Multiple sclerosis and hysteria. Lessons learned from their association. JAMA. 1980;243(23):2418–21.
61. Stone J, Carson A, Duncan R, Roberts R, Coleman R, Warlow C, et al. Which neurological diseases are most likely to be associated with "symptoms unexplained by organic disease". J Neurol. 2012;259(1):33–8.
62. Al-Chalabi M, Hegde P, Asghar F, Aladamat N, Delcimmuto N, Gharaibeh K, et al. Transient headache and neurological deficits with cerebrospinal fluid lymphocytosis syndrome: a comprehensive systematic review of 93 patients from 57 studies. Cephalalgia. 2023;43(4):3331024231157694.
63. Fiamingo G, Canavero I, Gastaldi M, Coloberti E, Buongarzone G, Ghiotto N, et al. HaNDL syndrome: a reversible cerebral vasoconstriction triggered by an infection? A case report and a case-based review. Eur J Med Res. 2022;27(1):196.
64. Gómez-Aranda F, Cañadillas F, Martí-Massó JF, Díez-Tejedor E, Serrano PJ, Leira R, et al. Pseudomigraine with temporary neurological symptoms and lymphocytic pleocytosis. A report of 50 cases. Brain. 1997;120(Pt 7):1105–13.
65. Mulroy E, Yap J, Danesh-Meyer H, Anderson N. Symptomatic intracranial hypertension during recovery from the syndrome of headache with neurologic deficits and cerebrospinal fluid lymphocytosis (HANDL). Pract Neurol. 2017;17(2):145–8.
66. Boogaarts HD, Bartels RH. Prevalence of cervical spondylotic myelopathy. Eur Spine J. 2015;24(Suppl 2):139–41.
67. Aizawa T, Sato T, Tanaka Y, Ozawa H, Hoshikawa T, Ishii Y, et al. Thoracic myelopathy in Japan: epidemiological retrospective study in Miyagi prefecture during 15 years. Tohoku J Exp Med. 2006;210(3):199–208.
68. Karadimas SK, Erwin WM, Ely CG, Dettori JR, Fehlings MG. Pathophysiology and natural history of cervical spondylotic myelopathy. Spine. 2013;38(22 Suppl 1):S21–36.
69. Schneider MM, Badhiwala JH, Alvi MA, Tetreault LA, Kalsi P, Idler RK, et al. Prevalence of neck pain in patients with degenerative cervical myelopathy and short-term response after operative treatment: a cohort study of 664 patients from 26 global sites. Global Spine J. 2022;14:21925682221124098.
70. Lavelle WF, Bell GR. Cervical myelopathy: history and physical examination. Semin Spine Surg. 2007;19(1):6–11.
71. Onofrei LV. Structural myelopathies. Continuum (Minneap Minn). 2024;30(1):73–98.
72. Tetreault LA, Dettori JR, Wilson JR, Singh A, Nouri A, Fehlings MG, et al. Systematic review of magnetic resonance imaging characteristics that affect treatment decision making and predict clinical outcome in patients with cervical spondylotic myelopathy. Spine. 2013;38(22 Suppl 1):S89–110.
73. Takahashi M, Yamashita Y, Sakamoto Y, Kojima R. Chronic cervical cord compression: clinical significance of increased signal intensity on MR images. Radiology. 1989;173(1):219–24.
74. Nouri A, Martin AR, Mikulis D, Fehlings MG. Magnetic resonance imaging assessment of degenerative cervical myelopathy: a review of structural changes and measurement techniques. Neurosurg Focus. 2016;40(6):E5.
75. Flanagan EP, Krecke KN, Marsh RW, Giannini C, Keegan BM, Weinshenker BG. Specific pattern of gadolinium enhancement in spondylotic myelopathy. Ann Neurol. 2014;76(1):54–65.
76. Mustafa R, Zalewski NL, Flanagan EP, Kumar N. Challenging myelopathy cases. Semin Neurol. 2022;42(6):723–34.
77. Kheram N, Pfender N, Boraschi A, Farshad M, Kurtcuoglu V, Curt A, et al. Cerebrospinal fluid pressure dynamics reveal signs of effective spinal canal narrowing in ambiguous spine conditions. Front Neurol. 2022;13:951018.

78. Cohen O, Biran I, Steiner I. Cerebrospinal fluid oligoclonal IgG bands in patients with spinal arteriovenous malformation and structural central nervous system lesions. Arch Neurol. 2000;57(4):553–7.
79. Lyu RK, Tang LM, Chen CJ, Chen CM, Chang HS, Wu YR. The use of evoked potentials for clinical correlation and surgical outcome in cervical spondylotic myelopathy with intramedullary high signal intensity on MRI. J Neurol Neurosurg Psychiatry. 2004;75(2):256–61.
80. Kamei N, Nakamae T, Maruyama T, Nakao K, Farid F, Adachi N. Differentiating neurodegenerative disease from compressive cervical myelopathy using motor evoked potentials. Spine. 2023;49:726.
81. Fehlings MG, Tetreault LA, Riew KD, Middleton JW, Aarabi B, Arnold PM, et al. A clinical practice guideline for the Management of Patients with Degenerative Cervical Myelopathy: recommendations for patients with mild, moderate, and severe disease and Nonmyelopathic patients with evidence of cord compression. Glob Spine J. 2017;7(3 Suppl):70s–83s.
82. Owiti W, Peev N, Arif S, Brady Z, AbdelHafiz T. Is surgery beneficial for patients with concurrent multiple sclerosis and degenerative cervical myelopathy? A review of literature. Brain Spine. 2022;2:100870.
83. Wang H, Tian Y, Wu J, Luo S, Zheng C, Sun C, et al. Update on the pathogenesis, clinical diagnosis, and treatment of Hirayama disease. Front Neurol. 2021;12:811943.
84. Sharma P, Soin P, Elbanan M, Kochar PS. Understanding idiopathic spinal cord herniation – a comprehensive review of imaging and literature. J Clin Imaging Sci. 2019;9:22.
85. Sadek AR, Nader-Sepahi A. Spinal arachnoid cysts: presentation, management and pathophysiology. Clin Neurol Neurosurg. 2019;180:87–96.
86. Flint G. Syringomyelia: diagnosis and management. Pract Neurol. 2021;21(5):403–11.
87. Vieira RC, Paiva WS, de Oliveira DV, Teixeira MJ, de Andrade AF, de Sousa RM. Diffuse axonal injury: epidemiology, outcome and associated risk factors. Front Neurol. 2016;7:178.
88. Lampros M, Vlachos N, Tsitsopoulos PP, Zikou AK, Argyropoulou MI, Voulgaris S, et al. The role of novel imaging and biofluid biomarkers in traumatic axonal injury: an updated review. Biomedicines. 2023;11(8)
89. Bruggeman GF, Haitsma IK, Dirven CMF, Volovici V. Traumatic axonal injury (TAI): definitions, pathophysiology and imaging-a narrative review. Acta Neurochir. 2021;163(1):31–44.
90. Adams JH, Mitchell DE, Graham DI, Doyle D. Diffuse brain damage of immediate impact type: its relationship to ‘primary brain-stem damage’ in head injury. Brain. 1977;100(3):489–502.
91. Huisman TAGM, Sorensen AG, Hergan K, Gonzalez RG, Schaefer PW. Diffusion-weighted imaging for the evaluation of diffuse axonal injury in closed head injury. J Comput Assist Tomogr. 2003;27(1)
92. Shannon P, Smith CR, Deck J, Ang LC, Ho M, Becker L. Axonal injury and the neuropathology of shaken baby syndrome. Acta Neuropathol. 1998;95(6):625–31.
93. Korley FK, Jain S, Sun X, Puccio AM, Yue JK, Gardner RC, et al. Prognostic value of day-of-injury plasma GFAP and UCH-L1 concentrations for predicting functional recovery after traumatic brain injury in patients from the US TRACK-TBI cohort: an observational cohort study. Lancet Neurol. 2022;21(9):803–13.
94. Pfleger CC, Koch-Henriksen N, Stenager E, Flachs EM, Johansen C. Head injury is not a risk factor for multiple sclerosis: a prospective cohort study. Mult Scler. 2009;15(3):294–8.
95. Goldacre MJ, Abisgold JD, Yeates DG, Seagroatt V. Risk of multiple sclerosis after head injury: record linkage study. J Neurol Neurosurg Psychiatry. 2006;77(3):351–3.
96. Garnier-Crussard A, Bougacha S, Wirth M, André C, Delarue M, Landeau B, et al. White matter hyperintensities across the adult lifespan: relation to age, Aβ load, and cognition. Alzheimers Res Ther. 2020;12(1):127.
97. Longstreth WT Jr, Manolio TA, Arnold A, Burke GL, Bryan N, Jungreis CA, et al. Clinical correlates of white matter findings on cranial magnetic resonance imaging of 3301 elderly people. The Cardiovascular Health Study. Stroke. 1996;27(8):1274–82.
98. Habes M, Erus G, Toledo JB, Zhang T, Bryan N, Launer LJ, et al. White matter hyperintensities and imaging patterns of brain ageing in the general population. Brain. 2016;139(Pt 4):1164–79.

99. Grodzinski B, Stubbs DJ, Davies BM. Most degenerative cervical myelopathy remains undiagnosed, particularly amongst the elderly: modelling the prevalence of degenerative cervical myelopathy in the United Kingdom. J Neurol. 2023;270(1):311–9.
100. Haghighi S, Andersen O, Rosengren L, Bergström T, Wahlström J, Nilsson S. Incidence of CSF abnormalities in siblings of multiple sclerosis patients and unrelated controls. J Neurol. 2000;247(8):616–22.
101. Kleine TO, Nebe CT, Löwer C, Lehmitz R, Geilenkeuser WJ, Kruse R, et al. Evaluation of cell counting and leukocyte differentiation in cerebrospinal fluid controls using hematology analyzers by the German Society for Clinical Chemistry and Laboratory Medicine. Clin Chem Lab Med. 2010;48(6):839–48.

13 Clinical Red Flags and Key Features in the Differential Diagnosis of Multiple Sclerosis

13.1 Bilateral Visual Loss

- Bilateral simultaneous or sequential optic neuritis in patients with multiple sclerosis (MS) is very rare and is considered a red flag for the diagnosis of MS [1–3].
- Bilater visual loss is observed in the following conditions that may mimic MS:
  - Acute disseminated encephalomyeliti (ADEM)
  - Autoimmune glial fibrillary acidic protein (GFAP) astrocytopathy
  - Behçet's disease
  - Biotinidase deficiency
  - Cobalamin and folate deficiency
  - Cooper deficiency and zinc overload
  - Chronic relapsing inflammatory optic neuropathy (CRION)
  - Churg-strauss syndrom (Wegener granulomatosis)
  - Graves' disease (hyperthyroidism) associated with dysthyroid optic neuropathy, which occurs due to compression of the optic nerves caused by the enlargement of the extraocular muscles.
  - Infections (rare)
    - Viral (A viral prodrome in children, herpes simplex virus [HSV], varicella-zoster virus [VZV], Epstein–Barr virus [EBV], cytomegalovirus [CMV], measles, mumps, influenza, human immunodeficiency virus [HIV])
    - Bacterial (syphilis, tuberculosis, Lyme disease, leptospirosis, cat scratch disease)
    - Parasitic (toxoplasmosis, cryptococcosis) or fungal (aspergillosis, candidiasis)
  - Mitochondrial disorders such as Leber hereditary optic atrophy (LHON), Dominant optic atrophy (DOA), but also other subtypes
  - Marburg disease
  - Myelin oligodendrocyte glycoprotein antibody-associated disease (MOGAD)
  - Non-arteritic anterior ischemic optic neuropathy (NAION) (rare)

T. Uher, *Mimics and Red Flags of Multiple Sclerosis*,
https://doi.org/10.1007/978-3-031-98945-2_13

  - Neuromyelitis optica spectrum disorders (NMOSD)
  - Paraneoplastic optic neuropathy (CRMP-5) and infiltrative or compressive neoplasms such as glioma, lymphoma, leukemia, or metastases affecting the optic nerves or chiasm
  - Retinal vasculopathy with cerebral leukoencephalopathy and systemic manifestations (RVCL-S)
  - Sarcoidosis
  - Sjogren's syndrome
  - Susac's syndrome
  - Systemic lupus erythematosus (SLE)
  - Uveitis
  - Vogt–Koyanagi–Harada disease
- Other disorders that are usually not considered in the differential diagnosis of MS include for example methanol poisoning and other toxic optic neuripathies, giant cell arteritis, infiltrative/compressive neoplasms (glioma, lymphoma, leukemia, metastases) or primary eye diseases.

13.2 Cardiovascular Involvement

- It is not associated with MS [4, 5] but occurs in the following conditions that may mimic MS:
  - Anti-phospholipid syndrome
    - Valve abnormalities, coronary artery disease, myocardial dysfunction, pulmonary hypertension, intracardiac thrombi
  - Autoimmune autonomic ganglionopathy
    - Bradycardia, orthostatic hypotension
  - Autosomal recessive cerebelar ataxias (ARCA), such as Friedreich ataxia (FRDA) or Refsum disease
  - Autoimmune/inflammatory arteritis (giant cell arteritis, Takayasu arteritis, polyarteritis nodosa)
  - Churg-strauss syndrom
  - Cerebrotendinous xanthomatosis (CTX)
  - Cogan's syndrome
    - Aortitis with aortic vasculitis; aortic aneurysm, dissection or insufficiency
  - COL4A1-related disorders
  - Fabry disease
    - Left ventricular hypertrophy, arrhythmias
  - Homocystinuria
  - Infections (brucellosis; coxsackievirus B; cytomegalovirus [CMV]; dengue fever; enteroviruses; hepatitis C virus [HCV]; hepatitis E virus [HEV]; human immunodeficiency virus [HIV]; Chagas disease; Lyme boreliosis; Mycoplasma pneumonia; syphilis; toxocarosis; varicella-zoster virus [VZV] associated vasculopathy)
  - Mitochondrial disorders
    - Hypertrophic cardiomyopathy; atrial fibrillation; conduction abnormalities; hypertension; and pre-excitation syndrome in Leber hereditary optic atrophy (LHON)

- Moyamoya syndrome
  - Congenital cardiac anomaly
- Pompe disease
- Presenilin-1 related familial Alzheimer's disease
- Rheumatoid arthritis
  - Pericarditis; pericardial effusion; valvular heart disease; conduction defects; myocardial infarction; heart failure; peripheral vascular disease; hypertension
- Sarcoidosis
  - Arrhythmias; heart failure; pericardial disease; pulmonary hypertension; sudden cardiac death; aneurysm; small fiber neuropathy related cardiovascular dysautonomia
- Sjogren's syndrome
  - Pericarditis and heart valve disorders
- Systemic lupus erythematosus (SLE)
  - Pericardial effusion and acute pericarditis
- Vitamin E deficiency
  - Left ventricular hypertrophy, mild dilated cardiomyopathy, and congestive heart failure
- Wernicke encephalopathy
  - Hypotension and tachycardia

13.3 Cerebellar Ataxia

- Cerebellar syndrome is commonly observed in patients with MS but can also result from any brain disease affecting the cerebellum and its connections, such as tumors, strokes, or demyelinating lesions. The following conditions that may mimic MS are more frequently associated with cerebellar syndrome:
  - Alexander's disease
  - Anti-GQ1b antibody syndromes including Bickerstaff's brainstem encephalitis and Miller–Fischer syndrome (but it is not clear here, whether ataxia does not have purely peripheral origin)
  - Autoimmune and paraneoplastic encephalitis (Hu, Ri, Yo, Tr, CASPR2, KLHL11, NIF, mGluR1, GAD65, VGCC, DNER/PCA-T) and primary cerebellar or brainstem tumours
  - Autoimmune glial fibrillary acidic protein (GFAP) astrocytopathy
  - Autosomal recessive cerebellar ataxias (ARCA)
  - Behçet's disease (but also other systemic autoimmune diseases, when affecting cerebellum and its connections)
  - Celiac disease
  - Cerebellar ataxia with neuropathy and vestibular areflexia syndrome (CANVAS)
  - Cerebrotendinous xanthomatosis (CTX)
  - Charcot-Marie-Tooth Neuropathy
  - Coenzyme Q10 Deficiency

- Cytotoxic T lymphocyte antigen 4 (CTLA-4) haploinsufficiency
- Dopa-responsive dystonia
- Episodic ataxias
- Fragile X-Associated Tremor/Ataxia Syndrome (FXTAS)
- Glut1 deficiency syndrome
- Hashimoto's encephalopathy also known as Steroid-responsive encephalopathy associated with autoimmune thyroiditis (SREAT)
- Hereditary spastic paraplegia (HSP) (for example SPG 4 or 7)
- Chiari malformation
- Chronic lymphocytic inflammation with pontine perivascular enhancement responsive to steroids (CLIPPERS)
- Heavy metal toxicity
- Infections (Sporadic Creutzfeldt–Jakob disease; human T-cell lymphotropic virus type 1 [HTLV-1]; human immunodeficiency virus [HIV]; Listeria rhombencephalitis; Lyme boreliosis; progressive multifocal leukoencephalopathy [PML] and John Cunningham virus [JCV]-associated granule cell neuronopathy; syphilis; tuberculosis; Whipple's disease)
- Mitochondrial disorders
- Multiple system atrophy (MSA), type C
- Nonmetabolic inherited leukodystrophies and leukoencephalopathies (Adult-onset Alexander disease, ClC-2 chloride channel deficiency leukoencephalopathy, Autosomal dominant leukodystrophy, or Adult-onset neuronal intranuclear inclusion disease and others)
- Opsoclonus myoclonus ataxia syndrome
- Postinfectious cerebellitis
- Spinocerebellar ataxias (SCA)
- Superficial siderosis of CNS
- Vascular causes such as cerebellar infarction, hemorrhage, or venous sinus thrombosis
- Vitamin deficiencies (B12, folate, and cooper deficiency; neuroferritinopathy; vitamin E deficiency; Wilson's disease) and toxic causes (alcohol, phenytoin, lithium, metronidazol, chemotherapy agents etc.)
- Wernicke encephalopathy
- Wide range of inherited metabolic disorders such as glutamate and urea cycle disorders, X-linked adrenoleukodystrophy, Pelizaeus-Merzbacher disease, Fabry disease (often transient due to vertebrobasilar ischemic attacks) etc.

13.4 Constitutional Symptoms

- Fever and flu-like symptoms are not associated with MS [4, 5] but may occur in the following conditions that mimic MS:
- Acute disseminated encephalomyelitis (ADEM) and myelin oligodendrocyte glycoprotein antibody-associated disease (MOGAD), especially in children.
  - Some patients have prodromal symptoms (malaise, headache, mild fever).

- Anti-GQ1b antibody syndromes (Bickerstaff's brainstem encephalitis, Miller–Fischer syndrome and Guillain–Barré syndrome)
  - Commonly preceded by an infection with fever.
- Autoimmune glial fibrillary acidic protein (GFAP) astrocytopathy
  - The onset of disease is often preceded by flu-like symptoms including rhinorrhea, sore throat, fever, and cough (30-40%).
- Baló concentric sclerosis
  - Sometime prodromal symptoms (malaise, headache, mild fever).
- Behçet's disease
  - Relapses in are typically associated with systemic flare-ups, often accompanied by systemic symptoms such as fatigue, malaise, subfebrile fever, ulcers, or uveitis and elevated inflammatory markers.
- Brain tumors
  - Malignant tumors, especially in temporal lobe can rarely present acutely with symptoms such as fever, encephalopathy, or bilateral abnormalities on magnetic resonance imaging (MRI) mimicking inflammatory etiology.
- Churg–Strauss syndrom
  - Prodromal phase and eosinophilic phase may be associated with fever and other systemic symptoms.
- Cogan's syndrome
  - Systemic vasculitis may be associated with fever, headaches, polyarthralgia, arthritis, myalgia, spleno-megaly, lymphadenopathy.
- Combined central and peripheral demyelination
- Fabry disease
  - Some patients experience episodes of unexplained high fever.
- Familial hemiplegic migraine
  - Occasionally, during relapses, disturbances of consciousness (including coma), confusion, fever, and cerebrospinal fluid (CSF) pleocytosis may occur.
- Hematologic malignancies including intravascular lymphoma
  - May occur night sweats, fever, weight loss and increased markers of systemic inflammation.
- Histiocytosis disorders (e.g., Erdheim–Chester disease)
  - Commonly systemic symptoms, including fever or weight loss.
- Sarcoidosis
  - Can occur systemic symptoms including mild fever.
  - Rare Heerfordt syndrome is associated with facial palsy, parotitis, anterior uveitis, and fever.
- Schilder's disease
  - Some patients have prodromal symptoms (malaise, headache, mild fever).
- Sjogren's syndrome
  - Extra-glandular systemic features may include fever.
  - Aseptic meningoencephalitis is commonly associated with flu-like symptoms.
- Systemic lupus erythematosus (SLE)
  - Commonly associated with systemic features including fever.
- Systemic vasculitis of different etiologies

  - However, in primary angitis of the central nervous system (CNS) are systemic symptoms uncommon.
- Wide spectrum of infections and intoxications

13.5 Cognitive Impairment

- Majority of brain disorders can be associated with some degree of cognitive impairment, either acutely (as in acute encephalitis, meningoencephalitis, or encephalopathy) or chronically.
- Cognitive impairment can be present in some patients with MS even in the very early stages of the disease, but its prevalence significantly increases, affecting up to 50% of patients as the disease progresses. However, dementia syndrome is observed in only a very small proportion of patients with MS [6–8].
- Cognitive impairment without motor or sensory deficits, severe encephalopathy, and significant cognitive deficits in the early stages of the disease, rapid cognitive decline, and pronounced neuropsychiatric symptoms are all red flags when diagnosing MS [1, 2, 8].
- Insidious cognitive decline may be prominent in the following conditions that mimic MS:
  - Amyotrophic lateral sclerosis (ALS)
  - Anti-phospholipid syndrome
  - Autoimmune and inflammatory multisystem diseases such as Behçet's disease, Hashimoto's encephalopathy, sarcoidosis, relapsing polychondritis, systemic sclerosis and localized scleroderma, celiac disease, Sjogren's syndrome, systemic lupus erythematosus (SLE)
  - Autoimmune and paraneoplastic encephalitis
  - Autosomal recessive cerebellar ataxias
  - Brain tumors including lymphoma
  - Cerebral amyloid angiopathy
  - Cerebral autosomal dominant arteriopathy with subcortical infarcts and leukoencephalopathy (CADASIL)
  - Cerebral small vessel disease (CSVD) (especially in advanced stages) and Binswanger's disease
  - Cerebrotendinous xanthomatosis (CTX)
  - Cobalamin and folate deficiency, nitrous oxide-induced myeloneuropathy or intoxications (alcohol, haevy metals, carbon monoxide etc.)
  - COL4A1-related disorders
  - Fragile X-Associated Tremor/Ataxia Syndrome (FXTAS)
  - Hereditary spastic paraplegia (HSP) (some complicated subtypes)
  - Homocysteine remethylation disorders
  - Hyperornithinemia–hyperammonemia-homocitrullinuria (HHH) syndrome and other disorders of glutamate and urea cycle metabolism
  - Lysosomal storage and peroxisomal function disorders including Fabry disease, X-linked adrenoleukodystrophy, Krabbe disease, metachromatic leukodystrophy, Niemann-Pick disease type C, Tay-Sachs disease, or Pompe disease
  - Mitochondrial disorders

  - Moyamoya disease and syndrome (advanced stages)
  - Neuroinfections such as cryptococcal infection, human immunodeficiency virus (HIV) encephalopathy or progressive multifocal leukoencephalopathy (PML), prion diseases, syphilis, tuberculosis, Whipple's disease
  - Nonmetabolic inherited leukodystrophies and leukoencephalopathies
  - Presenilin-1 related familial Alzheimer's disease and other neurodegenerative dementias
  - Primary angitis of the CNS (PACNS)
  - Retinal vasculopathy with cerebral leukoencephalopathy and systemic manifestations (RVCL-S)
  - Spinocerebellar ataxias (SCA) (some subtypes)
  - Superficial siderosis of CNS (not frequently)
  - Susac's syndrome
  - Wilson's disease
- Although encephalopathy is also associated with cognitive impairment, it is typically more acute and severe, often accompanied by a wide range of other manifestations, including but not limited to changes in consciousness, behavior, motor functions, or seizures. Many brain disorders can involve both insidious cognitive decline and episodes of acute or subacute encephalopathy, making it challenging to classify some conditions as one or the other. Below is a list of MS mimics that may present with encephalopathy:
  - ADEM
  - Acute hemorrhagic leukoencephalitis (AHLE)
  - Autoimmune and inflammatory multisystem diseases such as Behçet's disease, sarcoidosis, relapsing polychondritis, systemic sclerosis and localized scleroderma, celiac disease, Sjogren's syndrome, SLE
  - Autoimmune and paraneoplastic encephalitis
  - Baló concentric sclerosis
  - Bickerstaff's brainstem encephalitis
  - Brain tumors including lymphoma
  - Central pontine myelinolisis
  - Cerebral amyloid angiopathy related inflammation
  - MOGAD
  - Cogan's syndrome encephalitis
  - Encephalitis in NMOSD (rare)
  - Hashimoto's encephalopathy
  - Ig4-related hypertrophic pachymeningitis
  - Marburg's variant of MS
  - Marchiafava–Bignami disease
  - Neuroinfections
  - Posterior reversible encephalopathy syndrome (PRES)
  - Schilder's disease
  - Susac's syndrome
  - Traumatic axonal injury
  - Tumefactive MS
  - Wernicke encephalopathy

13.6 Cough and Respiratory Manifestations

- Cough may occur in various neurological disorders affecting the respiratory muscles, such as myasthenia gravis or acute inflammatory demyelinating polyneuropathy (AIDP), as well as in diseases involving the brainstem due to impaired swallowing and aspiration. However, only certain conditions are typically associated with cough and other respiratory manifestations. MS is not associated with cough or other respiratory symptoms [4, 5], but these may be present in several conditions that can mimic MS:
  - Autoimmune autonomic ganglionopathy
    - May occur infrequent coughing episodes.
  - Cerebellar ataxia, neuropathy, and vestibular areflexia syndrome (CANVAS)
    - Chronic dry spasmodic cough (65%).
    - May occur up to 30 years before the onset of the neurological symptoms.
  - Chiari malformation
    - From compression of the brainstem.
  - Churg-Strauss syndrome
    - The prodromal phase often includes asthma bronchiale and rhino-sinusitis, allergic rhinitis, and recurrent or chronic sinusitis.
    - Eosinophilic phase is associated with peripheral eosinophilia and organ involvement including lungs (60–70%).
  - Histiocytosis disorders
  - Infections
  - Lymphoma
  - Rheumatoid arthritis
  - Sarcoidosis
  - Schistosomiasis
    - Sympotomatic acute phase may include a skin rash, headache, fever, dry cough, abdominal and muscle pain, bloody diarrhea, hepatosplenomegaly and eosinophilia, sometime also myocarditis, pericarditis, septic meningitis, or interstitial pneumonitis.
  - Systemic vasculitis
  - Systemic lupus erythematosus (SLE)
  - Toxocarosis
    - Productive cough, bronchospasm, recurrent pneumonia, hepatomegaly, diarrhea, nausea, vomiting, angioedema, pruritic rash, cardiac conduction, and muscle abnormalities.

13.7 Epileptic Seizures

- Seizures are relatively rare in patients with MS (1–2%), and in most cases, they occur after the diagnosis of MS, typically in the context of advanced disease [9, 10]. Epileptic seizures, occurring with varying frequency, are more commonly seen in the following MS mimickers:
  - Acute disseminated encephalomyelitis (ADEM)

- Acute intermittent porphyria
- Adult-onset Alexander disease (children)
- Adult-onset leukoencephalopathy with axonal spheroids and pigmented glia (ALSP)
- Alpha-methylacyl-coA racemase deficiency
- Anti-phospholipid syndrome
- Arginase 1 deficiency
- Autoimmune and paraneoplastic encephalitis
- Autoimmune glial fibrillary acidic protein (GFAP) astrocytopathy
- Baló concentric sclerosis
- Behçet's disease (2.0–2.5%), less common than in SLE
- Brain tumors
- Celiac disease
- Central pontine myelinolisis
- Cerebral amyloid angiopathy related inflammation
- Cerebral autosomal dominant arteriopathy with subcortical infarcts and leukoencephalopathy (CADASIL)
- Myelin oligodendrocyte glycoprotein antibody-associated disease (MOGAD)
- Coenzyme Q10 Deficiency
- Cogan's syndrome
- COL4A1-related disorders
- Cytotoxic T lymphocyte antigen 4 (CTLA-4) haploinsufficiency
- Delta-1-pyrroline-5-carboxylase synthetase deficiency
- Episodic ataxias
- Fragile X Syndrome (FXS; in children)
- Functional neurological disorders (non-epileptic seizures)
- Glut1 deficiency syndrome
- Hashimoto's encephalopathy
- Hereditary spastic parapaplegia (HSP) (for example SPG11)
- Histiocytosis disorders (Erdheim–Chester disease)
- IgG4-related hypertrophic pachymeningitis
- Inflammatory bowel disease
- Inherited metabolic diseases
  - Homocysteine remethylation disorders (children)
  - Biotinidase deficiency (infancy)
  - Cerebrotendinous xanthomatosis (33%)
  - Glutamate and urea cycle metabolism disorders
  - Niemann-Pick disease type C (gelastic cataplexy)
- Leukoencephalopathy with brainstem and spinal cord involvement and lactate elevation
- Marburg's variant of MS
- Marchiafava-Bignami disease
- Mitochondrial disorders (children or adult-onset)
- Moyamoya disease and syndrome (rare) and other vascular causes such as cerebral cavernous malformations, venous sinus thrombosis or arteriovenous malformations

- Neuroinfections (Herpes simplex virus [HSV], varicella-zoster virus [VZV], West Nile, or enteroviruses encephalitis; neurocysticercosis etc.)
- Posterior reversible encephalopathy syndrome (PRES)
- Presenilin-1 related familial Alzheimer's disease and some other neurodegenerative or prion diseases
- Primary angitis of the CNS (PACNS) (not frequent)
- Rasmussen's encephalitis
- Relapsing polychondritis
- Retinal vasculopathy with cerebral leukoencephalopathy and systemic manifestations (RVCL-S)
- Sarcoidosis
- Schilder's disease
- Sjogren's syndrome
- Spinocerebellar ataxia (e.g., SCA 10, 19/22, ATN1)
- Susac syndrome (rare)
- Systemic lupus erythematosus (SLE; in 7–20%)
- Systemic sclerosis and localized scleroderma
- Tumefactive MS
- Wernicke encephalopathy

13.8 Extrapyramidal Movement Disorders

- They are atypical for patients with MS [4, 5] but occur with variable frequency in several conditions that may mimic MS:
  - Adult-onset neuronal intranuclear inclusion disease
  - Anti-phospholipid syndrome
  - Autoimmune encephalitis with antibodies against neuronal surface
  - Autoimmune glial fibrillary acidic protein (GFAP) astrocytopathy
  - Autosomal recessive cerebellar ataxias (ARCA)
  - Behçet's disease
  - Cerebrotendinous xanthomatosis
  - COL4A1-related disorders
  - Dopa-responsive dystonia
  - Fragile X-Associated Tremor/Ataxia Syndrome (FXTAS)
  - Functional neurological disorders
  - Glut1 deficiency syndrome
  - Hereditary spastic parapaplegia (HSP) (complicated forms)
  - Hyperornithinemia–hyperammonemia–homocitrullinuria (HHH) syndrome and other disorders of glutamate and urea cycle metabolism
  - Chédiak–Higashi disease
  - Infections such as human immunodeficiency virus (HIV)-associated basal ganglia disease; Japanese encephalitis; Lyme neuroborreliosis (third stage); post-streptococcal autoimmune chorea (Sydenham's chorea); or Whiple's disease

- Mitochondrial disorders, including Leber hereditary optic atrophy (LHON) plus syndromes
- Monoclonal gammopathy of undetermined significance (MGUS)
- Moyamoya disease and syndrome
- Paraneoplastic brainstem encephalitis
- Presenilin-1 related familial Alzheimer's disease
- Sjogren's syndrome
- Spinocerebellar ataxia (SCA)
- Systemic lupus erythematosus (SLE)
- Wilson's disease

13.9 Headache

- Patients with MS have higher prevalence of migraine (21–36%) compared to general population (14–15%) [11].
- Several conditions that mimic MS may present with encephalopathy, headache, or aseptic pachymeningitis.
- Headache can be the primary symptom or present in a severe form in the following MS mimics:
  - Acute disseminated encephalomyelitis (ADEM), Baló concentric sclerosis, and Schilder's disease (may occur in prodromal phase)
  - Anti-phospholipid syndrome (often migraine)
  - Autoimmune or paraneoplastic encephalitis
  - Behçet's disease (focal lesions, vasculitis, pachymeningitis, cerebral venous thrombosis)
  - Brain tumors including primary CNS lymphomas (leptomeningeal involvement or mass lesions)
  - Cerebral amyloid angiopathy related inflammation
  - Cerebral autosomal dominant arteriopathy with subcortical infarcts and leukoencephalopathy (CADASIL)
  - Chiari malformation
  - Cogan's syndrome (particularly, in the case of systemic vasculitis)
  - Cytotoxic T lymphocyte antigen 4 (CTLA-4) haploinsufficiency
  - Giant cell arteritis
  - Chronic lymphocytic inflammation with pontine perivascular enhancement responsive to steroids (CLIPPERS; not common)
  - Churg–Strauss syndrome (pachymeningitis)
  - IgG4-related disease (pachymeningitis)
  - Inflammatory bowel disease (pachymeningitis)
  - Marburg's variant and tumefactive multiple sclerosis
  - Mitochondrial disorders
  - Moyamoya disease and syndrome
  - Myelin oligodendrocyte glycoprotein antibody-associated disease (MOGAD; may precede the onset of visual deficits)

- Neuroinfections
- Posterior reversible encephalopathy syndrome (PRES)
- Primary angitis of the CNS (PACNS)
- Reversible cerebral vasoconstriction syndrome
- Sarcoidosis (pachymeningitis, encephalopathy)
- Sjogren's syndrome (pachymeningitis)
- Some leukoencephalopathies
- Susac's syndrome and Vogt–Koyanagi–Harada disease
- Systemic connective tissue disorders such as: relapsing polychondritis, systemic sclerosis and localized scleroderma, rheumatoid arthritis, and systemic lupus erythematosus (SLE)
- Trochleitis
- Wilson's disease

13.10 Hearing Loss

- MS.
  - Around 4.5–6% of patients have hearing loss.
  - Sudden sensorineural hearing loss is defined as the loss of at least 30 decibels in three consecutive frequencies over 72 hours or more (0.7–1.7%; 2–12 times more frequent compared to the general population).
  - It is extremely rare as initial symptom of MS. However, a mild hearing loss is common in the general population.
  - Hearing symptoms may worsen with an increase in body temperature (Uhthoff's phenomenon) [12–15].
- Alternative diagnoses with hearing loss:
  - Anti-Kelch-like protein 11 encephalomyelitis (Autoimmune or paraneoplastic etiology; present anti-KLHL11 antibodies in serum and CSF; rhomboid encephalitis involves the brainstem and/or cerebellum; often associated with testicular germ cell tumors; poor response to immunotherapy).
  - Antiphospholipid antibody syndrome (due to microthrombosis affecting the inner ear or brainstem)
  - Behçet's disease
  - Biotinidase deficiency
  - Cathepsin A-related arteriopathy with strokes and leukoencephalopathy (CARASAL)
  - Charcot-Marie-Tooth Neuropathy
  - Cogan's syndrome
  - Fragile X-Associated Tremor/Ataxia Syndrome (FXTAS)
  - Friedreich's ataxia (FRDA)
  - Churg-Strauss syndrome and granulomatosis with polyangiitis
  - Mitochondrial disorders
  - Multiple system atrophy (MSA)
  - Ototoxic drugs

  - Sarcoidosis
  - Sjogren's syndrome
  - Spinocerebellar ataxia (SCA subtypes 31, 36 and DNMT1)
  - Superficial siderosis of CNS
  - Susac's syndrome
  - Traumatic brain injury
  - Vestibular schwannoma and other cerebellopontine angle neoplasms
  - Vogt-Koyanagi-Harada disease
  - Wernicke encephalopathy
  - Other infections (syphilis; tuberculosis; brucellosis; cytomegalovirus [CMV]; mumps; varicella zoster oticus known as Rumsay Hunt syndrome).

13.11 Multiple Cranial Neuropathies

- MS does not affect the peripheral nervous system, but brainstem lesions can involve brainstem nuclei (lower motor neurons) or nerve entry zones, mimicking peripheral cranial neuropathy.
- Isolated cranial nerve involvement is present in only a very small proportion of patients with MS.
- The trigeminal nerve is most frequently involved, followed by the facial, abducens, oculomotor, and cochlear nerves.
- Only a proportion of patients have focal brainstem pathology on MRI explaining the cranial neuropathy [16, 17].
- Multiple cranial neuropathies may be observed in the following MS mimickers:
  - Sarcoidosis (50–75% of patients with neurosarcoidosis)
  - Anti-GQ1b antibody syndrome (Bickerstaff's brainstem encephalitis, Miller–Fischer syndrome and Guillain–Barre syndrome)
  - Aseptic pachymeningitis in rheumatoid arthritis
  - Behçet's disease (rare)
  - Bell's palsy
  - Cogan's syndrome (rare)
  - Combined central and peripheral demyelination
  - Diabetic cranial neuropathy
  - Histiocytosis disorders (for example Erdheim–Chester disease) or
  - Churg–Strauss syndrome
  - IgG4-related disease
  - Ischemic cranial neuropathies related to vascular risk factors (atherosclerosis, diabetes, antiphospholipid syndrome)
  - Nitrous oxide-induced myeloneuropathy (rare)
  - Neuroinfections (acute flaccid myelitis; Epstein–Barr virus [EBV]; cat scratch disease; human immunodeficiency virus [HIV]; leptospirosis; rarely hepatitis E virus [HEV]; brucellosis; fungal meningitides ; herpes simplex virus [HSV]; human T-cell lymphotropic virus type 1 [HTLV-1]; leptospirosis; Lyme neuroboreliosis [43–67% of cases; facial nerve palsy is the most com-

mon]; Mycoplasma pneumonia; syphilis; tuberculous meningitis [29–38% of cases]; varicella-zoster virus (VZV); West Nile virus; Whiple's disease [7% of cases] etc.)
- Paraneoplastic neurologic disorders (rare), meningeal carcinomatosis, leptomeningeal metastasis, and radiation-induced cranial neuropathy
- Relapsing polychondritis
- Sjogren's syndrome
- Skull base anomalies (e.g., Chiari malformation or osteomyelitis)
- Systemic lupus erythematosus (SLE; rare)
- Systemic sclerosis and localized scleroderma
- Tumors

- Other disorders usually not considered in differential diagnosis of MS include:
  - Head trauma
  - Toxic etiology (a wide range of substances such as heavy metals (lead, arsenic), alcohol, chemotherapeutic drugs (cisplatin, vincristine), antibiotics (aminoglycosides), or environmental toxins (organophosphates, carbon monoxide)
- MS mimics affecting neuromuscular junction or the lower motor neurons in the brainstem, resembling peripheral cranial neuropathy include:
  - Amyotrophic lateral sclerosis (ALS)
  - Brainstem tumors and other mass lesions in brainstem
  - Chronic lymphocytic inflammation with pontine perivascular enhancement responsive to steroids (CLIPPERS)
  - Myasthenia gravis (disorder, but may simulate neuropathy)

13.12 Musculoskeletal Involvement

- MS is not associated with musculoskeletal pathology [2, 18].
- Arthritis/arthralgia are observed in the following conditions that may mimic MS:
  - Ankylosing spondylitis
  - Brucellosis (vertebral endplates and sacroiliac joints involvement)
  - Celiac disease
  - Cogan's syndrome
  - Fabry disease
  - Fibromyalgia
  - Infections (cat scratch disease; hepatitis C virus [HCV]; human parvovirus [B19V]; human T-cell lymphotropic virus type 1 [HTLV-1]; Lyme borreliosis; Mycoplasma pneumonie; syphilis; tuberculosis)
  - Inflammatory bowel disease
  - Relapsing polychondritis
  - Rheumatoid arthritis
  - Sjogren's syndrome
  - Systemic lupus erythematosus (SLE)
- Bone pathology may be observed in the following conditions that mimic MS:

- Brucellosis
- COL4A1-related disorders
- Friedreich's ataxia (FRDA)
- Histiocytosis disorders
- Lathyrism
- Vitamin E deficit

- Myopathy may be observed in the following conditions that mimic MS:
  - Aquaporin-4 (AQP4)-IgG seropositive neuromyelitis optica spectrum disorders (NMOSD)
  - Cerebral autosomal dominant arteriopathy with subcortical infarcts and leukoencephalopathy (CADASIL)
  - Infections (eg, HTLV-1)
  - Mitochondrial disorders (mitochondrial encephalomyopathy, lactic acidosis and stroke-like episodes [MELAS]; myoclonic epilepsy associated with ragged red fibers [MERRF]; coenzyme Q10 Deficiency and others)
  - Monoclonal gammopathy of undetermined significance (MGUS)
  - Pompe disease
  - Sarcoidosis
  - Sjögren's syndrome
  - Susac's syndrome
  - Systemic sclerosis and localized scleroderma
  - Whipple disease's

13.13 Optic Neuritis and Optic Neuropathy

- Optic neuritis in patients with MS is very often.
  - At disease onset (25–35%)
  - During disease course (70%) [21, 22]
- Optic nerve involvement may be observed in the following conditions that mimic MS:
  - Acute disseminated encephalomyelitis (ADEM)
  - Anterior non-arteritic ischemic optic neuropathy (NAION)
  - Anti-phospholipid syndrome
  - Autoimmune encephalitis with antibodies against neuronal surface
  - Autoimmune glial fibrillary acidic protein (GFAP) astrocytopathy
  - Autosomal recessive cerebellar ataxias (ARCA)
  - Baló concentric sclerosis
  - Behçet disease
  - Bickerstaff's brainstem encephalitis
  - Biotinidase deficiency
  - Cerebral autosomal dominant arteriopathy with subcortical infarcts and leukoencephalopathy (CADASIL, rare)
  - ClC-2 chloride channel deficiency leukoencephalopathy
  - Cobalamin and folate deficiency

- Cooper deficiency and zinc overload
- Combined central and peripheral demyelination
- Chronic relapsing inflammatory optic neuropathy (CRION)
- Churg-Strauss syndrome (Wegener granulomatosis)
- CTLA–4 haplo insufficiency (visual loss and optic atrophy)
- Giant cell arteritis
- Grave's disease (hyperthyroidism) associated with dysthyroid optic neuropathy, which occurs due to compression of the optic nerves caused by the enlargement of the extraocular muscles.
- Functional neurological disorders
- Hereditary spastic paraplegia (HSP)
- IgG4-related disease
- Infectious etiologies
  - Viral (A viral prodrome in children: varicella-zoster virus [VZV]; Epstein–Barr virus [EBV]; cytomegalovirus [CMV]; measles; mumps; influenza; human immunodeficiency virus [HIV]; hepatitis C virus [HCV]; brucellosis; human T-cell lymphotropic virus type 1 [HTLV-1]; Dengue fever)
  - Bacterial (syphilis; tuberculosis; Lyme disease; leptospirosis; cat scratch disease; Mycoplasma pnemumonie)
  - Parasitic (toxoplasmosis; cryptococcal meningitis; toxocarosis) or fungal (aspergillosis; candidiasis)
- Ischemic stroke (occlusion of retinal artery or hemispheric strokes)
- Mitochondrial disorders such as Leber hereditary optic atrophy (LHON), Dominant optic atrophy (DOA), but also other subtypes
- Marburg disease
- Myelin oligodendrocyte glycoprotein antibody-associated disease (MOGAD)
- Non-arteritic anterior ischemic optic neuropathy (NAION) (rare)
- Neuroretinitis
- Neuromyelitis optica spectrum disorders (NMOSD)
- Paraneoplastic optic neuropathy (CRMP-5) and paraneoplastic retinopathy, or optic nerve infiltration by lymphoma or leukemia
- Post- and para-infectious
- Retinal vasculopathy with cerebral leukoencephalopathy and systemic manifestations (RVCL-S)
- Rheumatoid arthritis
- Sarcoidosis
- Sjogren's syndrome
- Spinocerebellar ataxia (SCA 7)
- Susac's syndrome (microangiopathy affecting the retina)
- Systemic lupus erythematosus (SLE)
- Uveitis

13.14 Peripheral Nervous System Involvement

- Only a small proportion of examined nerves (14.2–16.5%) in patients with MS shows subtle subclinical pathological findings without evidence of small fiber pathology [19, 20]. A marked peripheral neuropathy is atypical for MS and is considered as a red flag [2, 18]. The following MS mimics are frequently associated with peripheral neuropathy:
  - Acute disseminated encephalomyelitis (ADEM, may occur sometime)
  - Acute intermittent porphyria
  - Adult polyglucosan body disease
  - Alpha-methylacyl-coA racemase deficiency
  - Autosomal recessive cerebellar ataxias (ARCA).
  - Bickerstaff's brainstem encephalitis and Guillain-Barré syndrome.
  - Cerebellar ataxia, neuropathy, and vestibular areflexia syndrome (CANVAS)
  - Cerebrotendinous xanthomatosis (CTX; often, but usually subclinical)
  - Charcot-Marie-Tooth Neuropathy
  - Cobalamin, folate, and cooper deficiency
  - Combined central and peripheral demyelination
  - Cree leukodystrophy
  - Fragile X-Associated Tremor/Ataxia Syndrome (FXTAS)
  - Hereditary spastic paraplegia (HSP) (some subtypes)
  - Homocysteine remethylation disorders
  - Churg–Strauss syndrome and other vasculitic neuropathies such as polyarteritis nodosa, microscopic polyangiitis, or cryoglobulinemia
  - Infections, such as hepatitis C virus (HCV), human immunodeficiency virus (HIV), or Lyme disease
  - Lysosomal storage and peroxisomal function disorders such as X-linked adrenoleukodystrophy, Krabbe disease, metachromatic leukodystrophy, and Fabry disease
  - Nitrous oxide-induced myeloneuropathy
  - Sarcoidosis
  - Sjogren's syndrome
  - Some mitochondrial disorders
  - Spinocerebellar ataxias (e.g., SCA 1, 2, 3, 4, 18, 25, 38, 43, 46)
  - Wernicke encephalopathy
- These MS mimics can be occasionally associated with peripheral neuropathy:
  - Autoimmune and paraneoplastic neuropathies/neuronopathies
  - Celiac disease
  - Fabry disease
  - Infections, such as brucellosis, human T-cell lymphotropic virus type 1 and 2 (HTLV-1 and 2), hepatitis B virus (HBV), or hepatitis E virus (HEV)
  - Lymphoma
  - Monoclonal gammopathy of undetermined significance (MGUS)
  - Rheumatoid arthritis
  - Systemic lupus erythematosus (SLE)
  - Systemic sclerosis and localized scleroderma

13.15 Simultaneous Upper and Lower Motor Neuron Syndrome

- MS is typically associated with upper motor neuron syndrome, but in cases of brainstem or spinal cord involvement, lower motor neuron involvement may occasionally occur, leading to lower motor neuron syndrome.
- Simultaneous involvement of upper and lower motor neuron may be observed in the following MS mimickers:
  - Adult polyglucosan body disease
  - Amyotrophic lateral sclerosis (ALS)
  - Cooper and cobalamin deficiency and zinc overload
  - Combined central and peripheral demyelination
  - Friedreich ataxia (FRDA) (subtype of autosomal recessive cerebelar ataxias; ARCA)
  - Hereditary spastic parapaplegia (HSP)
  - Infections such as human T-cell lymphotropic virus type 1 (HTLV-1), syphilis, or human immunodeficiency virus (HIV)
  - Mitochondrial disorders
  - Primary lateral sclerosis
  - Spinal dural arteriovenous fistula
  - Spinal Muscular Atrophy (SMA) and spinal and bulbar muscular atrophy (SBMA; also known as Kennedy's disease)
  - Spondylotic and other structural myelopathies such as spondylotic myelopathy or syringomyelia (lower motor neurons typically affected in lesser extent)
  - Lysosomal storage and peroxisomal function disorders (for example Tay-Sachs disease, Krabbe disease, or adrenomyeloneuropathy)

13.16 Skin Manifestations

- While MS itself does not involve skin pathology [4, 5], certain conditions that mimic MS may present with skin abnormalities:
  - Aicardi–Goutières syndrome
  - Anti-phospholipid syndrome
    - Livedo reticularis or racemosa; Raynaud phenomenon; oral ulcers; photosensitivity; patchy hair loss; Sneddon's syndrome
  - Autosomal recessive cerebellar ataxias (ARCA)
    - Refsum disease, xeroderma pigmentosum
  - Behçet's disease
    - Oral and genital aphthae/ulcers; acne-like lesions; erythema nodosum; papulopustular lesions; or pathergy reaction
  - Biotinidase deficiency
    - Alopecia, skin rash
  - Celiac disease
    - Dermatitis herpetiformis

- Cerebrotendinous xanthomatosis
  - Tendon xanthomas
- Chédiak-Higashi disease
  - Amyloid depositions, abnormal pigmentation
- Churg-strauss syndrom and other vasculitides such as polyarteritis nodosa, granulomatosis with polyangiitis, or microscopic polyangiitis
  - Palpable purpura and nodules
- Delta-1-pyrroline-5-carboxylase synthetase deficiency
  - Hyperelastic skin
- Fabry disease
  - Angiokeratomas, hypo/anhidrosis
- Histiocytosis disorders (Langerhans cell histiocytosis, juvenile xanthogranuloma)
- Homocysteine remethylation disorders, porphyria, and other metabolic/storage disorders such as Niemann–Pick disease type C or Gaucher disease (skin hyperpigmentation, xanthomas)
- IgG4-related disease
  - Cutaneous plasmacytosis; pseudolymphoma; inflammation of lacrimal and salivary glands; psoriasis-like lesions; unspecified maculopapular or erythematous lesions; purpura and urticarial vasculitis; ischaemic digit
- Inflammatory bowel disease
  - Erythema nodosum, pyoderma gangrenosum
- Infections (Cat scratch disease; cryptococcus; Dengue fever; herpes simplex virus [HSV; hepatitis E virus [HCV]; hepatitis E virus [HEV]; human Herpesvirus 6 [HHV-6]; human parvovirus B19 [B19V]; human T-cell lymphotropic virus type 1 [HTLV-1]; Lyme borreliosis [Erythema migrans, borrelial lymphocytoma, acrodermatitis atrophicans]; mediterranean spotted fever; Mycoplasma pneumonia; Rickettsia; schistosomiasis; syphilis; toxocarosis; tuberculosis; Varicella zoster virus [VZV]; West Nile virus)
- Pseudoxanthoma elasticum
  - Yellowish papules and plaques
- Relapsing polychondritis
- Rheumatoid arthritis
  - Palmar erythema; pyoderma gangrenosum; vasculitis; Leg ulcerations
- Sarcoidosis
  - Papules; subcutaneous nodules; erythema nodosum; bilateral hilar adenopathy; polyarthralgia; lupus pernio; scar sarcoidosis
- Sjogren's syndrome
  - Purpura; vasculitis; subacute cutaneous lupus; paniculitis; erythema nodosum; granuloma annulare; amyloidosis; mucosal ulcers
- Systemic lupus erythematosus (SLE)
  - Non-scaring alopecia; oral ulcers; subacute cutaneous or discoid lupus; acute cutaneous lupus etc.
- Susac's syndrome
  - Livedo reticularis or livedo racemosa (rare, only 5%)

- Systemic sclerosis, localized scleroderma, and dermatomyositis
- Systemic or intravascular lymphoma; paraneoplastic dermatomyositis; or acanthosis nigricans

13.17 Summary of Selected Clinical Red Flags of Multiple Sclerosis

Adopted [1, 2, 5] and modified.

13.17.1 Disease History

- Prominent family history (Mitochondrial disorders; spinocerebellar ataxia [SCA], adult-onset leukoencephalopathy with axonal spheroids and pigmented glia [ALSP]; X-linked adrenoleukodystrophy; Adult-onset autosomal dominant leukodystrophy; cerebral autosomal dominant arteriopathy with subcortical infarcts and leukoencephalopathy [CADASIL]; hereditary spastic paraplegia [HSP]; and many others genetic disorders).
- History of medical condition or drug treatment (tumor necrosis factor (TNF)-α inhibitors; immune checkpoint inhibitors and others) potentially affecting CNS.
- Recent head trauma (traumatic third, fourth, or sixth nerve palsy; traumatic axonal injury, X-linked adrenoleukodystrophy).
- Onset before age 11 years (for details, see chapter "Pediatric-onset multiple sclerosis [POMS]").
- Onset after age 50 years (for details, see chapter "Late-onset multiple sclerosis [LOMS]").

13.17.2 Disease Course

- Hyperacute presentation or stroke-like syndromes (all diseases associated with cerebral ischemia or hemorrhage; anti-phospholipid syndrome; biotinidase deficiency; CADASIL; cathepsin A-related arteriopathy with strokes and leukoencephalopathy [CARASAL]; cerebral autosomal recessive arteriopathy with subcortical infarcts and leukoencephalopathy [CARASIL]; Charcot–Marie–Tooth neuropathy; conditions associated with seizures; Glut1 deficiency; mitochondrial disorders [e.g., MELAS]; Moyamoya disease and syndrome; nonarteritic anterior ischaemic optic neuropathy [NAION]; autoimmune encephalitis (rarely); Sjögren's syndrome; systemic lupus erythematosus [SLE] (rarely); Susac's syndrome; or vasculitis).
- Brief or paroxysmal symptoms lasting minutes to hours (seizure; cerebral ischemia; presyncope; vestibular disorders; migraine; amyloid-related transient focal neurological episodes; functional neurological disorders).

- Acute onset with rapid worsening (Primary angiitis of central nervous system [PACNS]; intravascular lymphoma; gliomatosis cerebri; genetic and acquired cerebral hemophagocytic lymphohistiocytosis [HLH]; acute hemorrhagic leukoencephalitis; thrombotic thrombocytopenic purpura and many others).
- Persistently monofocal clinical manifestations (neoplasm; Moyamoya disease and syndrome; vascular malformation; structural CNS lesions; spinal cord compression etc.)
- Recurrent or stereotyped deficits (Myelin oligodendrocyte glycoprotein antibody-associated disease [MOGAD]; epilepsy; migraine; functional neurological disorder).

13.17.3 Supratentorial Manifestations

- Encephalopathy (for details, see chapter "Cognitive impairment").
- Insidious cognitive decline (for details, see chapter "Cognitive impairment").
- Psychosis or neuropsychiatric syndrome (SLE; autoimmune encephalitis; vasculitis or vasculopathy such as Susac's syndrome; encephalomyelitis with glial fibrillary acidic protein [GFAP] antibodies; Wilson's disease; GM2 gangliosidosis; metachromatic leukodystrophy; and others).
- Seizure (for details, see chapter "Epileptic seizures").
- Headache (for details, see chapter "Headache").
- Meningismus and meningeal syndrome (cerebral venous sinus thrombosis; encephalomyelitis with GFAP antibodies; hypertrophic cranial pachymeningitis and aseptic meningo-encephalitis; meningeal carcinomatosis; neuroinfections)
- Sarcoidosis; SLE; subarachnoid hemorrhage; vasculitis).
- Extrapyramidal movement disorders (for details see chapter "Extrapyramidal movement disorders").
- Giveaway weakness or other inconsistent or contradictory findings on neurological examination (functional neurological disorders).
- Narcolepsy (aquaporin-4 [AQP4]-IgG-positive neuromyelitis optica spectrum disorder [NMOSD], Ma2 paraneoplastic syndrome, DNMT1 subtype of spinocerebellar ataxia [SCA]).

13.17.4 Brainstem Manifestations

- Intractable nausea, hiccups, or vomiting (area postrema syndrome in NMOSD or less in MOGAD; lesions affecting area postrema in dorsal medulla oblongata).
- Primary or isolated brainstem syndrome (for details, see chapter "Prominent or isolated brainstem involvement").
- Multiple cranial neuropathies (for details, see chapter "Multiple cranial neuropathies").
- Hearing loss (for details, see chapter "Hearing loss").
- Bilateral seventh or eighth cranial neuropathy (riboflavin transporter deficiency).

- Paroxysmal dysarthria and ataxia (anti-contactin-associated protein-like 2 antibody-related autoimmune encephalitis; episodic ataxia).
- Myorhythmia (NMDAR-antibody encephalitis, Whipple's disease, Hashimoto's steroid-responsive encephalopathy associated with autoimmune thyroiditis).
- Ataxia (for details, see chapter "Cerebellar ataxia").
- Progressive ataxia without other neurological deficits (paraneoplastic or autoimmune ataxia [anti-GAD 65 and other antibodies]; celiac disease; neuroinfections such as syphilis, progressive multifocal leukoencephalopathy [PML], and others; Erdheim-Chester disease; SCA; vitamin E deficiency; POLG mutation; multiple system atrophy [MSA] etc.).

13.17.5 Spinal Cord Manifestations

- Acute attack-related severe bladder dysfunction (MOGAD, NMOSD).
- Progressive myelopathy without other neurological deficits (sarcoidosis; systemic rheumatological disease [SLE, Sjögren's syndrome]; paraneoplastic syndromes [antibodies to CRMP5 and CV2, or amphiphysin]; stiff person syndrome; neuroinfections [HTLV-1, HIV, brucellosis, syphilis, toxocarosis, schistosomiasis etc.]; neoplasms; metabolic [cobalamin or copper deficiency]; Leukoencephalopathy with brain stem and spinal cord involvement and lactate elevation [LBSL]; adrenomyeloneuropathy; hereditary spastic paraplegia [HSP]; amyotrophic lateral sclerosis [ALS]; primary lateral sclerosis; spinal xanthomatosis; dural AV fistula; syringomyelia; spinal cord compression; chemoradiation-induced demyelination).
- Complete myelopathy spanning the entire spinal cord transversely (AQP4-IgG-positive NMOSD; MOGAD; sarcoidosis; infectious myelitis; dural AV fistula; trauma; chemoradiation induced demyelination; rarely some metabolic myelopathies).
- Recurrent myelitis without involvement of other CNS regions (NMOSD etc.)
- Isolated pyramidal motor involvement (ALS, primary lateral sclerosis, HSP).
- Selective dorsal column involvement (syphilis; cobalamin and copper deficiency; posterior spinal artery ischemia; posterior spinal cord compression; intrathecal methotrexate) (for further details, see chapter "Dorsal or dorsal/lateral columns involvement [tractopathy lesions]").
- Episodic spasticity, hyperlordosis, axial rigidity, extremity rigidity and muscle spasms (stiff person syndrome spectrum disorders).

13.17.6 Peripheral Nervous System Manifestations

- Radiculopathy.
- Peripheral neuropathy (for further details, see chapter "Peripheral nervous system involvement").

- Muscle atrophy (for details, see chapter "Simultaneous upper and lower motor neuron syndrome").
- Peripheral neuropathy with optic nerve involvement (combined central and peripheral demyelination with or without Anti-neurofascin 155 antibody positivity).

13.17.7 Ophthalmological

- Acute-onset external ophthalmoplegia, ataxia (Bickerstaff brainstem encephalitis; infectious brainstem encephalitis).
- Hyperacute onset (anterior ischemic optic neuropathy [AION]; recurrent isolated optic neuritis [RION]; chronic relapsing inflammatory optic neuropathy [CRION]; central retinal artery occlusion [CRAO]; branch retinal artery occlusion [BRAO]).
- Progressive vision loss (>14 days) (sarcoidosis; anti-CRMP5 optic neuropathy; neoplasm; autosomal dominant optic atrophy; Leber hereditary optic neuropathy [LHON]; metabolic [Cobalamin and copper deficiency]; mitochondrial disorder; glaucoma; compressive optic neuropathy; lysosomal storage diseases, such as neuronal ceroid lipofuscinosis, Stargardt disease [genetic disorder affecting metabolism of vitamin A] and others).
- Bilateral simultaneous or sequential acute or subacute optic neuritis or optic neuropathy (for details see chapter "Bilateral visual loss").
- Optic neuritis with chiasm involvement (AQP4-IgG-positive NMOSD, MOGAD, sarcoidosis).
- Recurrent optic neuritis (MOGAD, NMOSD, RION, CRION etc.)
- Severe optic neuritis or optic neuropathy with acuity of 20/200 or worse (NMOSD, MOGAD, sarcoidosis, infections, LHON, toxic, or nutritional optic neuropathies).
- Altitudinal deficit (NMOSD; Arteritic, or non-arteritis ischemic optic neuropathy; CRAO or BRAO; retinal venous occlusion).
- Severe optic disc edema, with or without hemorrhages (MOGAD, neuroretinitis, infectious optic neuropathies, Ischemic optic neuropathy).
- Retinopathy (cherry red spot) (vasculitis or vasculopathy, such as Susac's syndrome; mitochondrial disorder; neuronal ceroid lipofuscinosis).
- Anterior or pan-uveitis (MOGAD; sarcoidosis; systemic rheumatological disease, such as SLE or Sjögren's syndrome); Behçet's disease; infections [tuberculosis, viral, parasitic]; lymphoma; Vogt–Koyanagi–Harada disease).
- Optic neuritis accompanied by normal brain and spinal cord MRI (NMOSD; MOGAD; sarcoidosis; systemic rheumatological disease; infections [Lyme borreliosis, cat scratch disease, syphilis]).
- Optic neuropathy with dry eye and dry mouth (Sjögren's syndrome).
- Positive visual phenomena (migraine, retinal detachment, vitreous detachment, epilepsy).

- Unilateral internuclear ophthalmoparesis with absence of clinical or MRI evidence of multiple sclerosis accompanied by comorbidities for vascular disease (ischemia).
- Complete gaze palsy (ischemia, primary ophthalmological disorder, mitochondrial disorder).
- Hemianopsia and cortical blindness (PML, neoplasm, mitochondrial disorder, ischemic stroke, posterior reversible encephalopathy syndrome [PRES]).
- Retro-orbital pain, worsened with eye movements, with no evidence of visual impairment (MOGAD; sarcoidosis; infections, such as tuberculosis; lymphoma; idiopathic trochleitis).
- Painless visual loss (ischemic optic neuropathy).
- Acute/subacute vision loss with red eye (uveitis).
- Acute/subacute vision loss with recurrent headaches (Susac's syndrome).
- Acute/subacute vision loss without afferent pupillary defect (RAPD) (functional neurological disorder).
- Asymptomatic optic disc edema (optic disc drusen that can be associated, e.g., with retinitis pigmentosa, angioid streaks, Usher syndrome, Noonan or Alagille syndrome).
- Painless acute vision loss (neuroretinitis).
- Symptomatic optic disc edema (intracranial hypertension, idiopathic, venous sinus thrombosis, neuroinfection, pachymeningitis).

13.17.8 Organ System Manifestations

- Gastrointestinal:
  - Area postrema syndrome with vomiting (NMOSD, MOGAD)
  - Anti-DPPX encephalitis
  - Anti-phospholipid syndrome
  - Autoimmune autonomic ganglionopathy
  - Behçet's disease
  - Celiac disease
  - Churg–Strauss syndrome
  - Cogan's syndrome
  - Hyperornithinemia–hyperammonemia–homocitrullinuria (HHH) syndrome and other disorders of glutamate and urea cycle metabolism
  - IgG4-related disease
  - Infections (acute flaccid myelitis, CMV, Dengue fever, hepatitis, Mycoplasma, Whipple's disease)
  - Inflammatory bowel disease
  - Malabsorptive states (gastric bypass or inflammatory bowel disease resulting in cobalamin, copper, or vitamin E deficiency)
  - Migraine
  - Mitochondrial Neurogastrointestinal Encephalopathy (MNGIE)
  - Paraneoplastic gastrointestinal dysmotility (ANNA-1 or anti-Hu)

- Porphyria
- Retinal vasculopathy with cerebral leukoencephalopathy and systemic manifestations (RVCL-S)
- Sarcoidosis associated small fibre neuropathy
- Systemic rheumatological diseases (SLE, rheumatoid arthritis etc.)

• Endocrine:
  - Adrenal insufficiency (X-linked adrenoleukodystrophy)
  - Autoimmune and paraneoplastic encephalitis associated with neuroendocrine tumors and ovarian teratomas
  - Autoimmune autonomic ganglionopathy (rarely)
  - FXTAS
  - Hypothalamic disturbance (for further details, see chapter "Diencephalic syndrome and hypophysitis")
  - Mitochondrial disorders
  - Ovarian dysgenesis (vanishing white matter disease)
  - Thyroiditis in HEV (rarely)
• Hematological:
  - Antiphospholipid syndrome
  - Behçet's disease, vasculitis, antiphospholipid syndrome, chronic meningitis (cerebral venous sinus thrombosis).
  - Celiac disease
  - CLIPPERS
  - Cobalamin, folate, cooper, or vitamin E deficiency
  - COL4A1-related disorders
  - Cytotoxic T lymphocyte antigen 4 haploinsufficiency (CTLA-4)
  - Histiocytosis disorders
  - Infections
  - Inflammatory bowel disease
  - Lymphoma
  - Malignancies with hypercoagulable state
  - Mitochondrial disorders
  - Monoclonal Gammopathy of undetermined significance (MGUS)
  - Retinal vasculopathy with cerebral leukoencephalopathy and systemic manifestations (RVCL-S)
  - Systemic rheumatological diseases
  - Wernicke encephalopathy
  - Wilson's disease
• Renal and Genitourinary:
  - Antiphospholipid syndrome
  - Behçet's disease
  - Central pontinne myelinolysis
  - Cerebrotendinous xanthomatos
  - Churg–Strauss syndrome
  - COL4A1-related disorders
  - Fabry disease

  - Infections
  - Inflammatory bowel disease
  - Mitochondrial disorders
  - Renal impairment
  - Rheumatoid arthritis and Sjögren's syndrome
  - SLE
  - Systemic vasculitis
  - Vitamin E deficiency
- Musculoskeletal (for details, see chapter "Musculoskeletal involvement")
- Skin (for details see chapter "Skin manifestations")
- Cardiovascular (for details, see chapter "Cardiovascular involvement")
- Respiratory (for details, see chapter "Cough and respiratory involvement")
  - Constitutional symptoms (for details, see chapter "Constitutional symptoms")

References

1. Hua LH, Solomon AJ, Tenembaum S, Scalfari A, Rovira À, Rostasy K, et al. Differential diagnosis of suspected multiple sclerosis in pediatric and late-onset populations: a review. JAMA Neurol. 2024;81:1210.
2. Solomon AJ, Arrambide G, Brownlee WJ, Flanagan EP, Amato MP, Amezcua L, et al. Differential diagnosis of suspected multiple sclerosis: an updated consensus approach. Lancet Neurol. 2023;22(8):750–68.
3. Petzold A, Fraser CL, Abegg M, Alroughani R, Alshowaeir D, Alvarenga R, et al. Diagnosis and classification of optic neuritis. Lancet Neurol. 2022;21(12):1120–34.
4. Solomon AJ, Hills W, Chen Z, Rosenbaum J, Bourdette D, Whitham R. Autoantibodies and Sjogren's syndrome in multiple sclerosis, a reappraisal. PLoS One. 2013;8(6):e65385.
5. Miller TM. Differential diagnosis of myotonic disorders. Muscle Nerve. 2008;37(3):293–9.
6. Uher T, Krasensky J, Sobisek L, Blahova Dusankova J, Seidl Z, Kubala Havrdova E, et al. Cognitive clinico-radiological paradox in early stages of multiple sclerosis. Ann Clin Transl Neurol. 2018;5(1):81–91.
7. Uher T, Blahova-Dusankova J, Horakova D, Bergsland N, Tyblova M, Benedict RH, et al. Longitudinal MRI and neuropsychological assessment of patients with clinically isolated syndrome. J Neurol. 2014;261(9):1735–44.
8. Benedict RHB, Amato MP, DeLuca J, Geurts JJG. Cognitive impairment in multiple sclerosis: clinical management, MRI, and therapeutic avenues. Lancet Neurol. 2020;19(10):860–71.
9. Ooi S, Kalincik T, Perucca P, Monif M. The prevalence of epileptic seizures in multiple sclerosis in a large tertiary hospital in Australia. Mult Scler J Exp Transl Clin. 2021;7(1):2055217321989767.
10. Mirmosayyeb O, Shaygannejad V, Nehzat N, Mohammadi A, Ghajarzadeh M. Prevalence of seizure/epilepsy in patients with multiple sclerosis: a systematic review and meta-analysis. Int J Prev Med. 2021;12:14.
11. Mrabet S, Wafa M, Giovannoni G. Multiple sclerosis and migraine: links, management and implications. Mult Scler Relat Disord. 2022;68:104152.
12. Furst M, Levine RA. Hearing disorders in multiple sclerosis. Handb Clin Neurol. 2015;129:649–65.
13. Atula S, Sinkkonen ST, Saat R, Sairanen T, Atula T. Association of multiple sclerosis and sudden sensorineural hearing loss. Mult Scler J Exp Transl Clin. 2016;2:2055217316652155.

14. Cianfrone G, Turchetta R, Mazzei F, Bartolo M, Parisi L. Temperature-dependent auditory neuropathy: is it an acoustic Uhthoff-like phenomenon? A case report. Ann Otol Rhinol Laryngol. 2006;115(7):518–27.
15. Leite HF, Leite Jda C, Melo MH, Vasconcelos CC, Alvarenga RM. Deafness in patients with multiple sclerosis. Audiol Neurootol. 2014;19(4):261–6.
16. Zadro I, Barun B, Habek M, Brinar VV. Isolated cranial nerve palsies in multiple sclerosis. Clin Neurol Neurosurg. 2008;110(9):886–8.
17. Thömke F, Lensch E, Ringel K, Hopf HC. Isolated cranial nerve palsies in multiple sclerosis. J Neurol Neurosurg Psychiatry. 1997;63(5):682–5.
18. Miller DH, Weinshenker BG, Filippi M, Banwell BL, Cohen JA, Freedman MS, et al. Differential diagnosis of suspected multiple sclerosis: a consensus approach. Mult Scler. 2008;14(9):1157–74.
19. Gartzen K, Katzarava Z, Diener HC, Putzki N. Peripheral nervous system involvement in multiple sclerosis. Eur J Neurol. 2011;18(5):789–91.
20. Anlar O, Tombul T, Kisli M. Peripheral sensory and motor abnormalities in patients with multiple sclerosis. Electromyogr Clin Neurophysiol. 2003;43(6):349–51.
21. Vidal-Jordana A, Rovira A, Arrambide G, Otero-Romero S, Río J, Comabella M, et al. Optic nerve topography in multiple sclerosis diagnosis: the utility of visual evoked potentials. Neurology. 2021;96(4):e482–e90.
22. Toosy AT, Mason DF, Miller DH. Optic neuritis. Lancet Neurol. 2014;13(1):83–99.

14 Demographic and Biochemical Red Flags and Key Features in the Differential Diagnosis of Multiple Sclerosis

14.1 Pediatric-Onset Multiple Sclerosis (POMS)

- Defined as the onset of the disease in patients under 18 years of age.
- The proportion of patients with POMS is only 2–10%, and the proportion of patients with disease onset before the age of 10 years is just 0.2–0.7%.
- A wide range of disorders can potentially imitate MS, but the most common mimics of POMS include (adapted from Hua et al., 2024) [1]:
- Optic neuritis.
  - Neuromyelitis optica spectrum disorder (NMOSD)
  - Myelin oligodendrocyte glycoprotein antibody-associated disease (MOGAD)
  - Isolated optic neuritis (seronegative)
  - Leber hereditary optic atrophy (LHON)
  - Parainfectious/postinfectious optic neuritis
  - Uveitis and other inflammatory eye diseases
- Supratentorial manifestations.
  - NMOSD
  - MOGAD
  - Acute disseminated encephalomyelitis (ADEM)
  - Hemophagocytic lymphohistiocytosis
  - Parainfectious/postinfectious encephalopathy
  - Migraine
- Brainstem and/or cerebellar manifestations.
  - NMOSD
  - MOGAD
  - Bickerstaff encephalitis
  - Hemophagocytic lymphohistiocytosis
  - Malignancy
  - Parainfectious/postinfectious cerebellitis/encephalitis
  - Mitochondrial disorders

T. Uher, *Mimics and Red Flags of Multiple Sclerosis*,
https://doi.org/10.1007/978-3-031-98945-2_14

- Myelitis.
  - NMOSD
  - MOGAD
  - Idiopathic acute transverse myelitis
  - Parainfectious/postinfectious transverse myelitis
  - Acute flaccid myelitis
  - Systemic rheumatological disorders

14.2 Late-Onset Multiple Sclerosis (LOMS)

- Defined as the onset of the disease in patients over 50 years of age.
- Given that the mean age of symptom onset in MS is 32 years (typically between 20 and 40 years) [2, 3], LOMS is considered as a red flag [4].
- The proportion of patients with LOMS is estimated to be around 5% [1, 5].
- The most often mimics of LOMS include (adapted and modified from Hua et al., 2024) [1].
- Optic neuritis
  - Neuromyelitis optica spectrum disorder (NMOSD)
  - Myelin oligodendrocyte glycoprotein antibody-associated disease (MOGAD)
  - Sarcoidosis and other granulomatous diseases
  - Anterior ischemic optic neuropathy (AION); non-arteritic anterior ischemic optic neuropathy (NAION); arteritic anterior ischemic optic neuropathy (AAION)
- Supratentorial manifestations
  - Stroke and cerebral small vessel disease (CSVD)
  - Vasculitis
  - Migraine
  - Autoimmune encephalitis
  - NMOSD
  - Sarcoidosis and other granulomatous diseases
  - Malignancy including primary CNS lymphoma
- Brainstem and/or cerebellar manifestations
  - Stroke and CSVD
  - NMOSD
  - Malignancies
  - Sarcoidosis and other granulomatous diseases
- Myelitis
  - Idiopathic acute transverse myelitis
  - NMOSD
  - MOGAD
  - Sarcoidosis and other granulomatous diseases

  - Vascular myelopathies
  - Parainfectious/postinfectious transverse myelitis
  - Spinal stenosis with compressive myelopathy
- Other less frequent alternative disorders to consider in older patients include:
  - Adult Polyglucosan Body Disease (genetic; combination of myelopathy and peripheral neuropathy; cognitive impairment; brain lesions on MRI)
  - Cerebellar ataxia, neuropathy, and vestibular areflexia syndrome (CANVAS)
  - Cerebral autosomal dominant arteriopathy with subcortical infarcts and leukoencephalopathy (CADASIL; typically presents between 30 and 50 years of age)
  - Cerebral amyloid angiopathy
  - Combined central and peripheral demyelination
  - Fragile X-Associated Tremor/Ataxia Syndrome (FXTAS)
  - Hashimoto's encephalopathy
  - Hereditary spastic parapaplegia (HSP; rarely)
  - Infections (brain absces; herpes simplex virus [HSV] encephalitis; human T-cell lymphotropic virus type 1 [HTLV-1] myelopathy; progressive multifocal leukoencephalopathy [PML]; varicella-zoster virus [VZV] herpes zoster)
  - Metabolic disorders (central pontinne myelopathy; cobalamin and folate deficiency; Marchiafava–Bignami disease; Wernicke encephalopathy)
  - Non-arteritic anterior ischemic optic neuropathy (NAION)
  - Paraneoplastic neurologic disorders
  - Primary angitis of the CNS (PACNS)
  - Rheumatoid arthritis
  - Sarcoidosis
  - Sjogren's syndrome
  - Superficial siderosis of CNS

14.3 Elevated Lactate Concentration in the Cerebrospinal Fluid (CSF)

- Although patients with MS tend to have higher lactate concentrations compared to healthy controls, their lactate levels generally remain within normal ranges. However, elevated lactate concentrations in the CSF (even within normal ranges, including during acute relapses) are associated with higher disease activity in MS [6, 7]. Abnormally high lactate levels in the CSF may be observed in the following conditions that mimic MS:
  - Bacterial and fungal (for example Cryptococcal) neuroinfections; only rarely mild elevation in viral infections
  - Biotinidase deficiency
  - Ischemic stroke in the CNS or cerebral venous sinus thrombosis

- Leukoencephalopathy with brainstem and spinal cord involvement and lactate elevation (nonmetabolic inherited leukoencephalopathy)
- Mitochondrial disorders
- Neuromyelitis optica spectrum disorder (NMOSD) and myelin oligodendrocyte glycoprotein antibody-associated disease (MOGAD)
  - Some patients may exhibit slightly increased lactate concentrations during attacks, but concentrations are much lower than those found in bacterial and fungal neuroinfections.
- Primary and secondary coenzyme Q10 deficiency (Only sometime)
- Sarcoidosis
- Malignancies (lymphoma, high-grade gliomas, metastase, meningeal carcinomatosis)

- Other disorders associated with elevated lactate levels in the CSF, which are typically not considered in the differential diagnosis of MS, include:
  - Severe hypoxia in the CNS
  - Severe epileptic seizure or status epilepticus
  - Subarachnoid hemorrhage

14.4 Eosinophils and/or Neutrophils in the CSF

- MS is typically associated with normal cytology or mild mononuclear pleocytosis [8–11].
- The presence of eosinophils in the CSF is atypical for MS and may be observed in the following conditions that mimic MS:
  - Churg–Strauss syndrome (Typically a high proportion of eosinophils in blood; but presence of eosinophils in CSF is uncommon)
  - Neuromyelitis optica spectrum disorder (NMOSD; 10%)
  - Sarcoidosis (rare)
  - Syphilis and tuberculosis (rare)
  - Toxocarosis and some other parasitic infections
- Other disorders usually not considered in differential diagnosis of MS include:
  - Drug-induced aseptic meningitis (nonsteroidal anti-inflammatory drugs, antibiotics, intrathecal drugs)
  - Fungal or viral infections (rare)
  - Idiopathic hyper-eosinophilic syndrome
  - Leptomeningeal carcinomatosis
- Neutrophils in the CSF of patients with MS are typically absent, or present in very small number [8–11]. On the other hand, neutrophils may be observed in the following conditions that mimic MS:
  - Behçet's disease (initially)
  - Fabry disease
  - Neuroinfections (bacterial, fungal, parasitic, and viral)

  - Myelin oligodendrocyte glycoprotein antibody-associated disease (MOGAD)
  - NMOSD
  - Paraneoplastic/autoimmune meningitis (rare)
  - Sarcoidosis (>30%)
- Other disorders usually not considered in differential diagnosis of MS include:
  - Leptomeningeal carcinomatosis
  - Chemical meningitis (Intrathecal drugs, contrast agents)
  - Traumatic meningitis (Traumatic lumbar puncture, CNS injury)

14.5 Cerebrospinal Fluid (CSF)-Restricted Oligoclonal Bands (OCB)

- CSF-restricted OCB IgG bands (Pattern II or III; ≥ 2–3 bands) are almost always present (90–95% of European and North American patients) [8, 12] and persist over time in the vast majority of patients, regardless of clinical disease activity or treatment [13].
- There is a reported lower prevalence of CSF-restricted OCB in Asia and South America, which has been explained or associated with differences in genetic susceptibility, latitude, and a high rate of misdiagnosis of MS [14, 15].
- Surprisingly, CSF-restricted OCB have also been found in a small proportion of healthy individuals (4%) and are relatively common in healthy siblings of patients with MS (19%) [16].
- The absence of CSF-restricted OCB has a high negative predictive value for the diagnosis of MS and is considered an important red flag for MS diagnosis [4, 8].
- However, some alternative diagnoses that may mimic MS can also be associated with CSF-restricted OCB.
- For several rare diagnoses that may mimic MS and are not presented in the figure, we lack data estimating the occurrence of CSF-restricted OCB (Fig. 14.1).

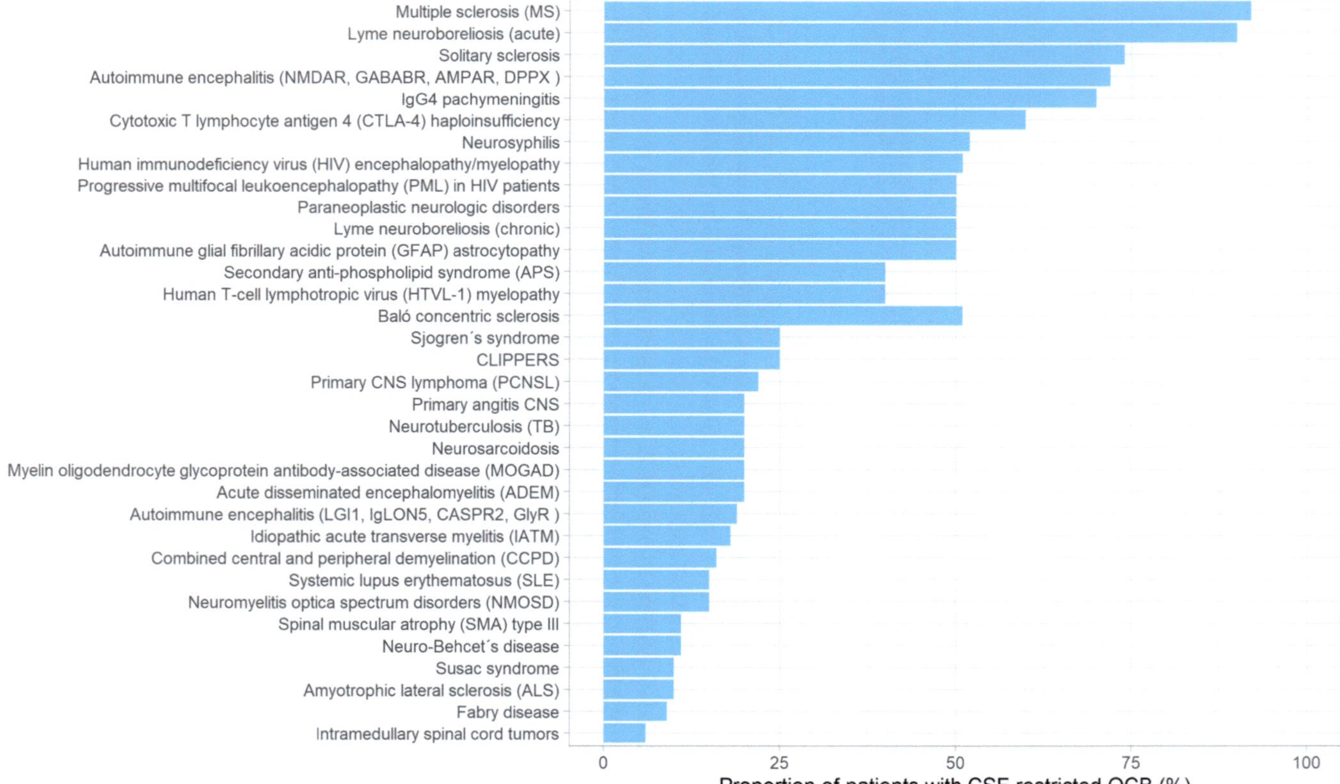

Fig. 14.1 Presence of CSF-restricted oligoclonal bands (OCB) in mimickers of multiple sclerosis

14.6 Transient Positivity of Cerebrospinal Fluid (CSF)-Restricted Oligoclonal Bands (OCB)

- The disappearance of CSF-restricted OCB in patients suspected of having MS should be considered a red flag. In MS patients, even with highly effective disease-modifying treatments, the disappearance of OCB from the CSF is uncommon (around 10%), even in patients on high-efficacy treatment [13, 17, 18].
- Disappearance of CSF-restricted OCB may be observed in the following conditions that mimic MS:
  - Acute disseminated encephalomyelitis (ADEM) (10–30%)
  - Balo concentric sclerosis (50%)
  - Behçet's disease
  - Combined central and peripheral demyelination
  - Myelin oligodendrocyte glycoprotein antibody-associated disease (MOGAD)
  - Neuromyelitis optica spectrum disorder (NMOSD; presence of CSF-restricted OCB may be only transient during an acute relapse, and their presence does not exclude a diagnosis of NMOSD)
  - Systemic lupus erythematosus (SLE)

References

1. Hua LH, Solomon AJ, Tenembaum S, Scalfari A, Rovira À, Rostasy K, et al. Differential diagnosis of suspected multiple sclerosis in pediatric and late-onset populations: a review. JAMA Neurol. 2024;81:1210.
2. Walton C, King R, Rechtman L, Kaye W, Leray E, Marrie RA, et al. Rising prevalence of multiple sclerosis worldwide: insights from the atlas of MS, third edition. Mult Scler. 2020;26(14):1816–21.
3. Romero-Pinel L, Bau L, Matas E, León I, Muñoz-Vendrell A, Arroyo P, et al. The age at onset of relapsing-remitting multiple sclerosis has increased over the last five decades. Mult Scler Relat Disord. 2022;68:104103.
4. Solomon AJ, Arrambide G, Brownlee WJ, Flanagan EP, Amato MP, Amezcua L, et al. Differential diagnosis of suspected multiple sclerosis: an updated consensus approach. Lancet Neurol. 2023;22(8):750–68.
5. Naseri A, Nasiri E, Sahraian MA, Daneshvar S, Talebi M. Clinical features of late-onset multiple sclerosis: a systematic review and meta-analysis. Mult Scler Relat Disord. 2021;50:102816.
6. Albanese M, Zagaglia S, Landi D, Boffa L, Nicoletti CG, Marciani MG, et al. Cerebrospinal fluid lactate is associated with multiple sclerosis disease progression. J Neuroinflammation. 2016;13:36.
7. Regenold WT, Phatak P, Makley MJ, Stone RD, Kling MA. Cerebrospinal fluid evidence of increased extra-mitochondrial glucose metabolism implicates mitochondrial dysfunction in multiple sclerosis disease progression. J Neurol Sci. 2008;275(1–2):106–12.
8. Deisenhammer F, Zetterberg H, Fitzner B, Zettl UK. The cerebrospinal fluid in multiple sclerosis. Front Immunol. 2019;10:726.
9. Zeman D, Adam P, Kalistová H, Sobek O, Anděl J, Anděl M. Cerebrospinal fluid cytologic findings in multiple sclerosis. A comparison between patient subgroups. Acta Cytol. 2001;45(1):51–9.

10. Vlad B, Reichen I, Neidhart S, Hilty M, Lekaditi D, Heuer C, et al. Basic CSF parameters and MRZ reaction help in differentiating MOG antibody-associated autoimmune disease versus multiple sclerosis. Front Immunol. 2023;14:1237149.
11. Stangel M, Fredrikson S, Meinl E, Petzold A, Stüve O, Tumani H. The utility of cerebrospinal fluid analysis in patients with multiple sclerosis. Nat Rev Neurol. 2013;9(5):267–76.
12. Franciotta D, Salvetti M, Lolli F, Serafini B, Aloisi F. B cells and multiple sclerosis. Lancet Neurol. 2008;7(9):852–8.
13. Ganapathy Subramanian R, Horakova D, Vaneckova M, Lorincz B, Krasensky J, Kubala Havrdova E, et al. Natalizumab induces changes of cerebrospinal fluid measures in multiple sclerosis. Diagnostics (Basel). 2021;11(12)
14. Correale J, Solomon AJ, Cohen JA, Banwell BL, Gracia F, Gyang TV, et al. Differential diagnosis of suspected multiple sclerosis: global health considerations. Lancet Neurol. 2024;23(10):1035–49.
15. Lechner-Scott J, Spencer B, de Malmanche T, Attia J, Fitzgerald M, Trojano M, et al. The frequency of CSF oligoclonal banding in multiple sclerosis increases with latitude. Mult Scler. 2012;18(7):974–82.
16. Haghighi S, Andersen O, Rosengren L, Bergström T, Wahlström J, Nilsson S. Incidence of CSF abnormalities in siblings of multiple sclerosis patients and unrelated controls. J Neurol. 2000;247(8):616–22.
17. Schlüter M, Oswald E, Winklmeier S, Meinl I, Havla J, Eichhorn P, et al. Effects of natalizumab therapy on intrathecal immunoglobulin G production indicate targeting of Plasmablasts. Neurol Neuroimmunol Neuroinflamm. 2021;8(5)
18. Harrer A, Tumani H, Niendorf S, Lauda F, Geis C, Weishaupt A, et al. Cerebrospinal fluid parameters of B cell-related activity in patients with active disease during natalizumab therapy. Mult Scler. 2013;19(9):1209–12.

15 Imaging Red Flags and Key Features in the Differential Diagnosis of Multiple Sclerosis

15.1 Brain Calcifications

- Calcifications in the brain are not associated with multiple sclerosis (MS) [1, 2]. Computed tomography (CT) is considered the most effective imaging method for detecting brain calcifications, as routine magnetic resonance imaging (MRI) often has difficulty reliably identifying them.
- Brain calcifications may be observed in the following conditions that mimic MS:
  - Aicardi–Goutières syndrome
  - Brain tumors (oligodendroglioma, astrocytoma, meningioma, pineoblastoma, ependymoma, and others)
  - Celiac disease (occipital lobe)
  - Cerebral amyloid angiopathy (rarely; in cortical gray matter of the occipital lobes)
  - Cerebrotendinous xantochromatosis (CTX)
  - Cogan's syndrome (in the vestibular labyrinth and the cochlea)
  - COL4A1-related disorders (frequent; punctate; in basal ganglia)
  - Hyperornithinemia-hyperammonemia-homocitrullinuria (HHH) syndrome and other disorders of glutamate and urea cycle metabolism (in basal ganglia)
  - Lysosomal storage and peroxisomal function disorders (rarely in Krabbe and Tay-Sachs disease; in thalamus).
  - Mitochondrial disorders (symmetric or asymmetric; in basal ganglia or less frequent in dentate nucleus and cerebellum)
  - Pseudoxanthoma elasticum
  - Retinal vasculopathy with cerebral leukoencephalopathy and systemic manifestations (RVCL-S) (in deep white matter; sparing basal ganglia; more than half of the cases)
  - Sarcoidosis (rare)
  - Systemic lupus erythematosus (SLE)
  - Systemic sclerosis and localized scleroderma

T. Uher, *Mimics and Red Flags of Multiple Sclerosis*,
https://doi.org/10.1007/978-3-031-98945-2_15

  - Adult-onset leukoencephalopathy with axonal spheroids and pigmented glia (ALSP)
  - Leukoencephalopathy with calcifications and cysts and cerebroretinal microangiopathy with calcification and cysts (Labrune syndrome)
- Other disorders usually not considered in differential diagnosis of MS include:
  - Fahr's syndrome/disease (bilateral striatopallidodentate calcinosis caused genetically or secondary due to a wide range of systemic diseases)
  - Genetic disorders (Down's syndrome; primary familial brain calcification).
  - Infections (fetal toxoplasmosis; congenital [CMV] infection; cystercosis).
  - Calcified embolus
  - Neurodegenerative diseases (Lewy body disease; Alzheimer's disease; Parkinson's disease; vascular dementia).
  - Phosphocalcic metabolism disorders (acquired or genetic disorders associated with elevated concentration of calcium)
  - Polycystic lipomembranous osteodysplasia with sclerosing leukoencephalopathy or Nasu-Hakola disease [3]

15.2 Brain Hemorrhages

- Macrohemorrhages (>5–10 mm in diameter) or microhemorrhages (<5–10 mm in diameter) are not associated with MS [1, 2] but sometime may be observed in the following conditions that mimic MS.
  - Arteriovenous malformations (cavernomas and others)
  - Autoimmune or paraneoplastic encephalitis
  - Acute hemorrhagic leukoencephalitis (AHLE)
  - Anti-phospholipid syndrome
  - Baló concentric sclerosis
  - Behçet's disease
  - Cerebral amyloid angiopathy
  - Cerebral autosomal dominant arteriopathy with subcortical infarcts and leukoencephalopathy (CADASIL)
  - Cerebral small vessel disease (CSVD)
  - COL4A1-related disorders
  - Fabry disease
  - Brain tumors and metastases
  - Infectious encephalitis (Dengue fever; Epstein–Barr virus [EBV]; hepatitis C virus [HCV]; herpes simplex virus [HSV]; leptospirosis; Listeria rhombencephalitis)
  - Churg-strauss syndrom
  - Marchiafava-Bignami disease (corpus callosum microbleeds)
  - Moyamoya disease and syndrome
  - Pontine autosomal dominant microangiopathy and leukoencephalopathy (PADMAL)
  - Posterior reversible encephalopathy syndrome (PRES)

- Primary angitis of the CNS (PACNS)
- Radiation-induced injury
- Rheumatoid arthritis
- Stroke
- Systemic lupus erythematosus (SLE)
- Traumatic axonal injury

15.3 Cauda Equina Involvement and Radiculopathy

- Involvement of the cauda equina is not seen in patients with MS but may be observed in the following conditions that mimic MS [4–6]:
  - Anti-GQ1b antibody syndrome (Bickerstaff's brainstem encephalitis; Miller–Fischer syndrome; Guillain–Barre syndrome)
  - Arachnoiditis
  - Degenerative spinal stenosis
  - Neoplasms (hematologic malignancies; solid tumors; meningeal carcinomatosis)
  - Chronic inflammatory demyelinating polyradiculoneuropathy (CIDP)
  - Infections:
    - Viral (Acute flaccid myelitis; cytomegalovirus [CMV]; Epstein–Barr virus [EBV]; herpes simplex virus [HSV] type 1 and type 2 (Elsberg Syndrome); human immunodeficiency virus [HIV]; tick-borne encephalitis; varicella-zoster virus [VZV]; West Nile virus).
    - Bacterial (brucellosis, Lyme neuroboreliosis, syphilis, tuberculosis).
    - Parasitic or Fungal (cysticercosis, hydatid cysts, cryptococcosis, nocardiosis, or schistosomiasis).
  - Myelin oligodendrocyte glycoprotein antibody-associated disease (MOGAD)
  - Primary angitis of the CNS (PACNS)
  - Radiation induced pathology
  - Sarcoidosis
  - Spine or intervertebral disc disease
  - Trauma

15.4 Cerebellar Peduncles Lesions

- The cerebral peduncles should not be confused with the cerebellar peduncles, that are located in the pons and medulla and connect the cerebellum to other parts of the brain. In contrast, the cerebral peduncles are white matter tracts that form the anterior part of the midbrain (mesencephalon) and connect the brainstem to the thalamus.
- Superior cerebellar peduncle (brachium conjunctivum).
  - Connect the cerebellum with the mesencephalon.
  - Lesions may cause neurotologic abnormalities and ataxia.

- Middle cerebellar peduncle (brachium pontis)
  - Larges peduncle which connects the cerebellum with the pons
  - Lesions in the middle cerebellar peduncles are characteristic of MS. However, other disorders can also cause unilateral or bilateral pathology in this area, typically in association with other brain abnormalities, rather than in isolation.
  - Involvement of the middle cerebellar peduncles may be observed in the following conditions that mimic MS:
  - Inflammatory and demyelinating diseases
    - Acute disseminated encephalomyelitis (ADEM)
    - Behçet's disease
    - Erdheim–Chester disease
    - Myelin oligodendrocyte glycoprotein antibody-associated disease (MOGAD)
    - Neuromyelitis optica spectrum disorder (NMOSD)
    - Progressive multifocal leukoencephalopathy (PML)
  - Metabolic and toxic etiology
    - Adrenoleukodystrophy
    - Cerebrotendinous xanthomatosis (CTX)
    - Extrapontine myelinolysis
    - Wilson's disease
    - Other disorders usually not considered in differential diagnosis of MS (acquired non-wilsonian hepatocerebral degeneration in patients with cirrhotic chronic liver disease; cyclosporin-A encephalopathy; heroin-induced leukoencephalopathy; hypoglycemic encephalopathy)
  - Neoplasms (brainstem glioma; leptomeningeal carcinomatosis; primary CNS lymphoma [PCNSL], and many others)
  - Neurodegenerative diseases
    - Neuronal intranuclear hyaline inclusion disease
    - Cerebral autosomal recessive arteriopathy with subcortical infarcts and leukoencephalopathy (CARASIL)
    - Charcot-Marie-Tooth Neuropathy
    - CLCN2-related leukoencephalopathy
    - Fragile X-associated tremor/ataxia syndrome (FXTAS)
    - Leukoencephalopathy with ataxia
    - Multiple systemic atrophy cerebellar type (MSA-C)
    - Spinocerebellar ataxia (e.g., SCA 17 or 34)
  - Infections (John Cunningham [JC] virus granule cell neuronopathy; human T-cell lymphotropic virus type 1 [HTLV-1]; human immunodeficiency virus [HIV] encephalopathy; Zika virus encephalitis in adults; and others).
  - Vascular disorders
    - Ischemic stroke
    - Wallerian degeneration secondary to pontine infarction
    - Posterior reversible encephalopathy syndrome (PRES) [7–11]

- Inferior cerebellar peduncle.
  - Connect the cerebellum to the medulla.
  - Pathology (encephalitis; ischemic stroke; demyelinative diseases of the CNS; tumors and others) can clinically mimic peripheral vestibular disorders [12].

15.5 Conus Medullaris Involvement

- Patients with MS typically have short-segment spinal cord lesions located in the cervical and upper thoracic regions. Involvement of the conus medullaris is seen in only a negligible proportion of patients (1.3%) [4–6].
- Pathology of the conus medullaris may be observed in the following conditions that mimic MS:
  - Biotinidase deficiency
  - Infections (schistosomiasis, West Nile virus)
  - Mitochondrial disorders
  - Myelin oligodendrocyte glycoprotein antibody-associated disease (MOGAD; 26–40%)
  - Neoplasms (hematologic malignancies; solid tumors; intramedullary spinal cord tumors; metastasis)
  - Neuromyelitis optica spectrum disorder (NMOSD; 6%)
  - Primary angitis of the CNS (PACNS)
  - Sarcoidosis
  - Vascular myelopathies (arteriovenous dural fistulas, spinal cord infarction)
  - Rarely, other conditions, including those associated with longitudinally extensive transverse myelitis (LETM), such as Behçet's disease, can lead to lesions in the conus medullaris.

15.6 Corpus Callosum Involvement

- More than half of the patients with MS have lesions in corpus callosum [13–15].
- Involvement of the corpus callosum lesion may be observed in the following conditions that mimic MS:
  - AARS2-related leukodystrophy
  - Anti-phospholipid syndrome
  - Bickerstaff's brainstem encephalitis (rarely)
  - Cerebral autosomal dominant arteriopathy with subcortical infarcts and leukoencephalopathy (CADASIL) (rarely)
  - Chronic lymphocytic inflammation with pontine perivascular enhancement responsive to steroids (CLIPPERS) (rarely)
  - Charcot-Marie-Tooth Neuropathy (splenium)
  - Churg-Strauss syndrome
  - Fragile X-Associated Tremor/Ataxia Syndrome (FXTAS) (splenium)
  - Hereditary diffuse leukoencephalopathy with spheroid cysts

- Hereditary spastic paraplegia (HSP) (usually atrophy without lesions)
- Leukoencephalopathy with brainstem and spinal cord involvement and lactate elevation
- Lysosomal storage and peroxisomal function disorders (Fabry disease [rarely]; Krabbe disease [splenium]; metachromatic leukodystrophy; Niemann-Pick disease type C; X-linked adrenoleukodystrophy)
- Marchiafava-Bignami disease (symmetrical T2 hyperintensity involving all or part of the corpus callosum, often associated with edema)
- Mitochondrial disorders
- Neoplasms (gliomas; primary CNS lymphoma [PCNSL] with typical subependymal extension and sometime crossing to the opposite side)
- Neuroinfections (Epstein–Barr virus [EBV]; Human parvovirus B19 [B19V]; Lyme neuroborreliosis; mediterranean spotted fever; progressive multifocal leukoencephalopathy [PML] (rarely); subacute sclerosing panencephalitis [SSPE])
- Neuromyelitis optica spectrum disorder (NMOSD; "cloud-like" poorly margined; often long or large; diffuse; heterogeneous or edematous)
- Schilder's disease
- Systemic lupus erythematosus (SLE; demyelinating syndrome)
- Susac's syndrome (rounded; centrally located; "snowball"-like lesions)
- Traumatic axonal injury
- Tumefactive MS (lesion may spread across the corpus callosum in a "butterfly" configuration and simulate an infiltrative astrocytoma or lymphoma)
- Wernicke encephalopathy (splenium)

15.7 Corticospinal Tract Involvement

Bilateral corticospinal tract abnormalities are not typical for MS and have a relatively broad differential diagnosis [16]. Conditions that may be associated with corticospinal tract hyperintensities on brain MRI include:

- Adult polyglucosan body disorder
- Adult-onset leukoencephalopathy with axonal spheroids and pigmented glia (ALSP)
- Alexander disease
- Amyotrophic lateral sclerosis (ALS) and primary lateral sclerosis
- Behçet's disease (usually unilateral pathology)
- Behr syndrome (genetic disorder characterized by early-onset optic atrophy, spinocerebellar degeneration with ataxia, pyramidal signs, peripheral neuropathy and developmental delay)
- Heroin leukoencephalopathy
- Infections (human T-cell lymphotropic virus type 1 [HTLV-1], human immunodeficiency virus [HIV], or Whipple's disease)

- Leukoencephalopathy with brainstem and spinal cord involvement and lactate elevation
- Lysosomal storage and peroxisomal function disorders (X-linked adrenoleukodystrophy [X-ALD]; Krabbe disease [globoid cell leukodystrophy]; metachromatic leukodystrophy)
- Myelin oligodendrocyte glycoprotein antibody-associated disease (MOGAD)
- Neuromyelitis optica spectrum disorder (NMOSD)
- Normal population (rare)
- Wilson's disease and sequela of liver transplantation
- X-linked Charcot-Marie-Tooth disease

15.8 Diencephalic Syndrome and Hypophysitis

- The diencephalon anatomically comprises the epithalamus, thalamus, metathalamus, subthalamus, and hypothalamus.
- Diencephalic syndrome is characterized by sleep disorders, autonomic dysfunction, failure to thrive in children, and endocrine abnormalities.
- The syndrome may be observed in the following conditions that mimic MS:
  - Neuromyelitis optica spectrum disorder (NMOSD)
  - Autoimmune and paraneoplastic encephalitis with diencephalic syndrome (Ma 1–2, IgLON5, DPPX)
  - Tumors (often causing rare diencephalic syndrome in children)
  - A variety of other diseases may occasionally be associated with diencephalic pathology (brain trauma; metabolic and genetic syndromes; neuroinfections; stroke).
- Inflammation of the pituitary gland (hypophysis), often leading to panhypopituitarism, headaches, and less commonly visual disturbances [17], can be caused by the following conditions that may mimic MS:
  - Autoimmune disorders (inflammatory bowel disease; polyglandular syndrome; primary biliary cirrhosis; Sjogren's syndrome; systemic lupus erythematosus [SLE]; thyroid disease; Type 1 diabetes mellitus)
  - Drug-induced (daclizumab; immune checkpoint inhibitors; interferon alpha; ustekinumab)
  - Granulomatosis with polyangiitis (Wegener's granulomatosis)
  - Histiocytosis disorders (Langerhans cell histiocytosis; Erdheim-Chester disease)
  - IgG4-related disease
  - Infections (syphilis; tuberculosis and others)
  - Sarcoidosis
  - Tumors (adenomas, craniopharyngiomas, or germinomas) and other focal pathologies (Rathke's cleft cysts or Pituitary apoplexy) can cause symptoms resembling hypophysitis.

15.9 Dominant Cortical/Subcortical Involvement

- Juxtacortical and cortical lesions in patients with MS are very common. However, the vast majority of these lesions remain undetected on standard MRI due to technical issues (e.g., low resolution of standard MRI), their pathological features (i.e., most of them involve only the more superficial, less myelinated layers of the cortex), and their small size.
- Juxtacortical lesions usually involve the U-fibers and can be located in all brain lobes, including the cerebellum.
- However, large cortical lesions in white matter and reaching the superficial cortical layers are atypical for MS. Cortical involvement may occur in the following conditions that mimic MS [18, 19]:
  - Genetic:
    - Adult-onset leukoencephalopathy with axonal spheroids and pigmented glia (ALSP; including Hereditary diffuse leukoencephalopathy with spheroids).
    - Cytotoxic T lymphocyte antigen 4 (CTLA-4) haploinsufficiency
    - Hyperornithinemia-hyperammonemia-homocitrullinuria (HHH) syndrome and other disorders of glutamate and urea cycle metabolism
    - Lysosomal storage and peroxisomal function disorders (Fabry disease; Tay-Sachs disease)
    - Mitochondrial diseases (MELAS)
    - Neuronal intranuclear inclusion disease
    - Spinal muscular atrophy type 4 (SMA4)
  - Infectious:
    - Cerebritis (before the development of a cerebral abscess)
    - Creutzfeldt-Jakob disease
    - Herpes simplex virus (HSV) encephalitis
    - Human immunodeficiency virus (HIV) encephalitis
    - Progressive multifocal leukoencephalopathy (PML)
    - Rabies encephalitis
    - Subacute sclerosing panencephalitis (SSPE)
    - Varicella-zoster virus (VZV)-associated vasculopathy and stroke
  - Inflammatory:
    - Autoimmune or paraneoplastic encephalitis (PCA-2, NMDAR, GABA A/B R, DPPX, MOG)
    - Churg–Strauss syndrome
    - IgG4-related disease (rarely)
    - Myelin oligodendrocyte glycoprotein antibody-associated disease (MOGAD; cerebral cortical encephalitis; FLAIR-hyperintense lesions in anti-MOG associated encephalitis with seizures [FLAMES]; with or without leptomeningeal contrast enhancement)

    - Neuromyelitis optica spectrum disorder (NMOSD; only rarely in acute stage [3%]; lesions tend to dissapear)
    - Sarcoidosis (rarely)
    - Vasculitis such as primary angiitis of the CNS (PACNS); systemic vasculitis associated with a wide range of systemic autoimmune diseases including systemic lupus erythematosus (SLE), Sjogren's syndrome; rheumatoid arthritis, and others.
  - Metabolic:
    - Hypoglycemic encephalopathy (only mild T2 hyperintensity)
    - Hepatic encephalopathy (in severe and acute hyperammonemia)
  - Structural:
    - Tumors (gliomatosis cerebri; glioblastoma; metastasis; rarely Primary CNS lymphoma [PCNSL])
    - Focal cortical dysplasia (developmental anomaly)
  - Status epilepticus and post-ictal changes (reversible)
  - Vascular pathology:
    - Cerebral amyloid angiopathy
    - Cerebral small vessel disease (CSVD)
    - Cerebral venous thrombosis
    - Hypoxic-ischemic encephalopathy
    - Ischemic strokes of different etiologies (often embolic)
    - Moyamoya disease and syndrome
    - Posterior reversible encephalopathy syndrome (PRES)
    - Primary or secondary antiphospholipid antibody syndrome with cortical infarctions
    - Reversible cerebral vasoconstriction syndrome [1, 18, 20, 21]

15.10 Dorsal or Dorsal/Lateral Columns Involvement (Tractopathy Lesions)

- Focal pathology with an increased T2 signal affecting the dorsal or both the dorsal and lateral columns of the spinal cord may occur in the following conditions that mimic MS [22–24].
  - Nutritional deficiency (Cobalamin, folic acid, zinc, cooper, vitamin E)
  - Autoimmune disorders (sarcoidosis)
  - Paraneoplastic syndromes
  - Mitochondrial disorders (ADLD, DARS2, LHON)
  - Toxic (intrathecal methotrexate, cytarabine, heroin, pyridoxine excess, inhalation of N_2O).
  - Infectious myelopathies (Coronavirus disease 2019 [COVID-19]; human immunodeficiency virus [HIV]; human T-cell lymphotropic virus type 1 [HTLV-1]; syphilis).

- Neurodegenerative hereditary diseases (autosomal recessive cerebellar ataxias [ARCA]; cerebrotendinous xantochromatosis [CTX]; spinocerebellar ataxia [SCA]; hereditary spastic paraplegia [HSP])
- Sensory ganglionopathy (Sjogren's syndrome, autoimmune autonomic ganglionopathy)
- Posterior spinal artery infarct

15.11 Ischemic Stroke and Microinfarctions

- Ischemic strokes are not associated with MS. If they do occur, vascular comorbidities are likely the cause. However, the incidence of ischemic stroke is higher in individuals with MS [25, 26]. The ischemic strokes may also occur in certain MS mimickers, some of which may also be associated with hemorrhagic strokes.
  - Anti-phospholipid syndrome
  - Behçet's disease (rarely vasculitis related-aneurysm, dissection or stenosis)
  - Cathepsin A-related arteriopathy with strokes and leukoencephalopathy (CARASAL)
  - Cerebral amyloid angiopathy
  - Cerebral autosomal dominant arteriopathy with subcortical infarcts and leukoencephalopathy (CADASIL)
  - Cerebral small vessel disease (CSVD)
  - COL4A1-related disorders
  - Fabry disease
  - Churg-strauss syndrom
  - Infections (brucellosis; Chagas disease; cryptococcal meningitis; Dengue fever; hepatitis E virus [HEV]; hepatitis C virus [HCV; rarely hemorrhage]; Human parvovirus B19 [B19V]; leptospirosis; Mycoplasma pneumoniae; toxocarosis; varicella-zoster virus [VZV]; secondary to infection-induced cerebral endarteritis in Lyme boreliosis, syphilis or tuberculosis)
  - Inflammatory bowel disease (caused by thromboembolism, hypercoagulation state, or vasculitis)
  - Intravascular lymphoma
  - Mitochondrial disorders
  - Moyamoya disease and syndrome
  - Primary angitis of the CNS
  - Pseudoxanthoma elasticum
  - Relapsing polychondritis
  - Retinal vasculopathy with cerebral leukoencephalopathy and systemic manifestations (RVCL-S)
  - Rheumatoid arthritis (caused by serum hyperviscosity from the elevated titers of circulating rheumatoid factor)
  - Sarcoidosis
  - Sjogren's syndrome

- Stroke-like lesions (alpha-methylacyl-coA racemase deficiency; hyperornithinemia–hyperammonemia-homocitrullinuria [HHH] syndrome; or mitochondrial disorders).
- Systemic lupus erythematosus (SLE)
- Susac's syndrome
- Vascular myelopathies
- Whiple's disease (secondary to endocarditis)

15.12 Lesion Resolution

- T2 lesions in MS may enlarge, shrink, or remain stable over time, but it is very rare for them to completely disappear.
- However, some lesions in certain MS mimickers may completely resolve, which can serve as a red flag for the diagnosis of MS. For example, T2 lesions in myelin oligodendrocyte glycoprotein antibody-associated disease (MOGAD) resolve more frequently than in neuromyelitis optica spectrum disorder (NMOSD) and MS.
- Complete or near-complete resolution of lesions may occasionally occur in the following conditions that mimic MS:
  - Acute disseminated encephalomyelitis (ADEM)
  - Atopic myelitis
  - Behçet's disease
  - Central pontine myelolinolysis
  - Charcot-Marie-Tooth Neuropathy
  - Chronic lymphocytic inflammation with pontine perivascular enhancement responsive to steroids (CLIPPERS)
  - Cytotoxic T lymphocyte antigen 4 haploinsufficiency (CTLA-4)
  - Human T-cell lymphotropic virus type 1 (HTLV1)-associated myelitis
  - Mitochondrial disorders
  - Susac's syndrome (especially punctate lesions)
  - Primary CNS lymphoma (PACNS) (following corticosteroids or cancer treatment)
  - Posterior reversible encephalopathy syndrome (PRES)
  - T2 lesions associated with some recent small subcortical infarcts ("acute lacunar infarcts") in cerebral small vessel disease (CSVD) may sometime completely disappear
  - MOGAD
  - Infections (Lyme neuroboreliosis; Toxocarosis; Viral encephalitis and other neuroinfections; Lesions may disappear spontaneously, or following antimicrobial treatment)
  - Spinal dural fistula (occasionally after a vascular intervention)
  - Sarcoidosis (rarely following treatment)
  - Systemic lupus erythematosus (SLE; rarely following treatment)

- Other disorders usually not considered in differential diagnosis of MS include:
  - Toxic and metabolic encephalopathies (e.g., acute carbon monoxide poisoning)
  - Radiation-induced brain injury [18, 27]

15.13 Leukodystrophy-like Pattern

- It refers to bilateral, often relatively symmetric, extensive confluent white matter changes, typically sparing the U-fibers, which resemble those seen in leukodystrophies (Table 15.1).
- A leukodystrophy-like pattern of brain lesions is atypical for MS but may rarely be observed in patients with very advanced stages of the disease.
- This MRI pattern of brain pathology may occur in the following conditions that mimic MS:
  - Acute disseminated encephalomyelitis (ADEM)
  - Autoimmune GFAP astrocytopathy (rarely)
  - Behçet's disease (advanced stages)
  - Brucellosis
  - Cerebral autosomal dominant arteriopathy with subcortical infarcts and leukoencephalopathy (CADASIL)
  - Celiac disease (rarely)
  - Central pontine myelinolysis (especially if affected supratentorial regions)
  - Cerebral small vessel disease (CSVD) (advanced stages)
  - Cerebrotendinous xanthomatosis (rarely)
  - Charcot-Marie-Tooth Neuropathy with CNS involvement
  - Chemoradiation induced demyelination
  - Cobalamin and folate deficiency (rarely)
  - COL4A1-related disorders
  - Combined central and peripheral demyelination
  - Cytotoxic T lymphocyte antigen 4 (CTLA-4) haploinsufficiency
  - Hereditary spastic paraplegia (HSP) (rarely SPG2)
  - Human immunodeficiency virus (HIV) leukoencephalopathy
  - Lysosomal storage and peroxisomal function disorders (Chédiak-Higashi disease; Fabry disease; Krabbe disease; metachromatic leukodystrophy; Niemann-Pick disease type C; Tay-Sachs disease; X-linked adrenoleukodystrophy)
  - Mitochondrial disorders
  - Myelin oligodendrocyte glycoprotein antibody-associated disease (MOGAD)
  - Neuromyelitis optica spectrum disorder (NMOSD; rarely)
  - Other rare inherited leukodystrophies and leukoencephalopathies (autosomal dominant leukodystrophy; Canavan disease; hereditary diffuse leukoencephalopathy with spheroid cysts; leukoencephalopathy with brainstem and spinal cord involvement and lactate elevation; Pelizaeus-Merzbacher disease)
  - Progressive multifocal leukoencephalopathy (PML) (advanced stages)

Table 15.1 Genetic leukodystrophies affecting predominantly WM [28–31]

Disease	Population	Onset	Clinical manifestations	MRI findings
Cree leukodystrophy (CLD)	Cree and Chippewayan descents	Infants (3–9 months) after infection or minor trauma	Severe rapid progression; letal within 2 years of age	Symmetric diffuse white matter involvement Deep gray matter pathology Little or no brain atrophy Can be restricted diffusion
Vanishing white matter disease (VWM), also known as childhood ataxia with central hypomyelination syndrome (CACH)	Northern European ancesters	Early childhood (later than CLD)	Considered as milder form of CLD (may be macrocephaly)	Symmetric diffuse white matter involvement Deep GM normal Without contrast enhancement
Canavan disease	Ashkenazi Jews	Infancy, rarely early childhood	Motor deficits, ataxia, macrocephaly	Multiple round cysts (dilated Virchow-Robin spaces) associated with spongiform degeneration Pathology of white matter is centripetal, begins in subcortical U-fibers (opposite to Krabbe or Alexander disease) Dominantly frontal distribution Restricted diffusion and brain atrophy
Alexander disease	Worldwide	Early childhood, less frequent juvenile and adult forms	Macrocephaly, growth failure, seizures, progressive neurological deficits	Atrophy and lesions in oblongata and upper cervical spinal cord Lesion in periventricular and deep white matter Periventricular frontal enhancement Brainstem lesions may be tumefactive and show contrast enhancement Can be restricted diffusion
Krabbe disease	Scandinavian descents	Infancy (1–7 months); late-onset forms in adulthood are very rare	Motor and cognitive deficit	Dominant symmetrical involvement of posterior and periventricular white matter and splenium of the corpus callosum U-fibers and subcortical white matter are spared Severe brain atrophy

  - Retinal vasculopathy with cerebral leukoencephalopathy and systemic manifestations (RVCL-S)
  - Syphilis (late stages)
- Other disorders usually not considered in differential diagnosis of MS include:
  - Radiation-induced leukoencephalopathy
  - Toxic leukoencephalopathy

15.14 Longitudinally Extensive Transverse Myelitis (LETM)

- Patients with MS typically have short-segment spinal cord lesions that are peripherally located. Long lesions are rare and, when present, usually result from the merging of adjacent short-segment lesions.
- LETM is a subtype of transverse myelitis characterized by a spinal cord lesion extending across three or more vertebral segments, as seen on MRI. The definition of transverse myelitis requires involvement of both sides of a specific section of the spinal cord [4, 18, 32].
- LETM, which is atypical for MS, may occur in the following conditions that mimic MS:
  - Acute disseminated encephalomyelitis (ADEM)
  - Anti-phospholipid syndrome (rarely)
  - Atopic myelitis (rarely)
  - Autoimmune autonomic ganglionopathy
  - Autoimmune glial fibrillary acidic protein (GFAP) astrocytopathy
  - Autoimmune myelitis with antibodies against neuronal surface (GABA-B-R, Glycine)
  - Behçet's disease
  - Biotinidase deficiency
  - Central pontine myelinolisis (rarely)
  - Cerebrotendinous xanthomatosis (CTX; rarely)
  - Cobalamin and folate deficiency
  - Cooper deficiency and zinc overload
  - Combined central and peripheral demyelination
  - Cytotoxic T lymphocyte antigen 4 (CTLA-4) haploinsufficiency
  - Idiopathic acute transverse myelitis
  - Infections
    - Viral (Acute flaccid myelitis; Dengue fever; Epstein–Barr virus [EBV]; hepatitis C virus [HCV]; herpes simplex virus [HSV]; human immunodeficiency virus [HIV]; human T-cell lymphotropic virus type 1 [HTLV−1]; varicella-zoster virus [VZV])
    - Bacterial (brucellosis; syphilis; tuberculosis; Whiple's disease; steptococcal pneumonia; Lyme borreliosis)
    - Shistosomiasis

- Inflammatory bowel disease (only case studies)
- Leukodystrophies (rarely)
- Marchiafava-Bignami disease (only case studies)
- Mitochondrial disorders
- Monoclonal gammopathy of undetermined significance (MGUS; only case studies)
- Myelin oligodendrocyte glycoprotein antibody-associated disease (MOGAD)
- Neuromyelitis optica spectrum disorder (NMOSD)
- Paraneoplastic myelitis (CV2/CRMP5, Amphiphysin, AQP4)
- Posterior reversible encephalopathy syndrome (PRES; rarely)
- Postradiation spinal cord injury
- Sarcoidosis
- Spinal cord tumors
- Spinal cord vasculopathy (spinal cord infarction; dural arteriovenous fistula; spondylosis with venous hypertension)
- Systemic rheumatological diseases, such as systemic lupus erythematosus (SLE) or Sjogren's syndrome

15.15 Normal Spinal Cord Imaging

- Normal spinal cord MRI findings in patient with spinal cord syndrome may occur in the following conditions that mimic MS:
  - Amyotrophic lateral sclerosis (ALS)
  - Biotinidase deficiency
  - Celiac disease associated myelopathy (rare)
  - Cerebrotendinous xanthomatosis (CTX)
  - Early phases of Myelin oligodendrocyte glycoprotein antibody-associated disease (MOGAD)
  - Early phases of spinal cord ischemic stroke (from 24 hours to few days)
  - Homocysteine remethylation disorders
  - Hereditary spastic paraplegia (HSP)
  - Human T-cell lymphotropic virus type 1 (HTLV-1) myelopathy
  - Idiopathic acute transverse myelitis
  - Lysosomal storage and peroxisomal function disorders (such as X-linked adrenoleukodystrophy)
  - Mild forms of spondylotic myelopathy
  - Nutritional myelopathy (cobalamin, folate, or vitamin E deficiency etc.)
  - Paraneoplastic myelopathy (amphyphysin, CRMP5/CV2, glycine etc.)
  - Spinocerebellar ataxia (SCA)
  - Syphilitic myelopathy

15.16 Persistent and Simultaneous Contrast Enhancement of Brain Lesions

- Contrast enhanceming lesions in MS is defined as a lesion with a diameter at least 3 mm and with a clear area of hyperintensity on T1-weighted images obtained at least 5 min after contrast agent administration.
- Duration of enhancement is typically around 2–8 weeks (typically less than 4 weeks). Contrast enhancement for longer than 3 months (persistent) is rare and is considered as a red flag for diagnosis of MS. However, very rarely also lesions in MS may demonstrate enhancement longer than 6 months [18, 33, 34].
- Persistent contrast enhancement of brain lesions may be observed in the following conditions that mimic MS:
  - Brain tumors (especially high-grade)
  - Crystal-storing histiocytosis
  - Histiocytosis disorders
  - Chronic neuroinfections (neurocysticercosis; tuberculosis and others)
  - Primary CNS lymphoma (PACNS)
  - Retinal vasculopathy with cerebral leukoencephalopathy and systemic manifestations (RVCL-S)
  - Sarcoidosis
  - Vascular abnormalities (developmental venous anomaly; capillary telangiectasia)
  - CNS vasculitis (e.g., Susac's syndrome and others)
- Persistent contrast enhancement of spinal cord lesions may be observed in the following conditions that mimic MS:
  - Sarcoidosis
  - Paraneoplastic myelitis
  - Tumors
  - Spondylotic myelopathy
  - Dural arteriovenous fistula
- Simultaneous contrast enhancement of the majority or almost all lesions indicates a similar pathological age of the lesions, which is highly atypical for MS. This phenomenon can occasionally be observed in the following MS mimickers:
  - ADEM
  - Sarcoidosis
  - Neoplasms and metastases
  - Primary CNS lymphoma (PCNSL)
  - Brain abscess
  - CNS vasculitis

15.17 Prominent or Isolated Brainstem Involvement

- It can occur in patients with MS, although it is not typical.
- Dominant brainstem involvement may be seen in a variety of diseases, but it is more commonly observed in the following MS mimickers:
  - Acute disseminated encephalomyelitis (ADEM)
  - Adul-onset Alexander disease
  - Anti-IgLON5 encephalitis (This is a rare autoimmune disease characterized by sleep disorders, bulbar syndrome, diencephalic syndrome, gait instability, cognitive impairment, and movement disorders. It typically presents with an insidious onset of symptoms and often results in irreversible neurological deficits. The condition is strongly associated with the HLA-DRB110:01-DQB105:01 haplotype, highlighting the involvement of genetic factors [35])
  - Behçet's disease
  - Bickerstaff's brainstem encephalitis
  - Cathepsin A-related arteriopathy with strokes and leukoencephalopathy (CARASAL)
  - Central pontinne myelopathy
  - Chronic lymphocytic inflammation with pontine perivascular enhancement responsive to steroids (CLIPPERS)
  - Infections (enterovirus 71; herpes simplex virus [HSV]; Listeria monocytogenes; Lyme boreliosis; progressive multifocal leukoencephalopathy [PML]; West Nile virus; Whipple's disease; rarely also Epstein–Barr virus [EBV] or human herpesvirus 6 [HHV-6])
  - Mitochondrial disorders (Leigh's disease and others)
  - Neoplasms
  - NMOSD (area postrema and periependymal surface of the fourth ventricle in the brainstem and cerebellum are often affected)
  - Nonmetabolic inherited leukodystrophies and leukoencephalopathies (adult-onset Alexander disease; leukoencephalopathy with brainstem and spinal cord involvement and lactate elevation)
  - Sarcoidosis
  - Solitary sclerosis
  - Superficial siderosis of CNS

15.18 Restricted Diffusion

- A high signal on diffusion weighted imaging (DWI) accompanied by a corresponding low signal on apparent diffusion coefficient (ADC) maps indicates cytotoxic edema (restricted diffusion). Conversely, a high signal on DWI images without a low signal on ADC images suggests the presence of vasogenic edema.
- Nine distinct diagnostic patterns of restricted diffusion in the brain have been defined, aiding in the differential diagnosis of lesions with restricted diffusion. For more details, please refer to the publication by Finelli et al. [36].

- Although most acute MS lesions do not exhibit restricted diffusion, approximately 14% of acute lesions may demonstrate this characteristic at the lesions' edge (periphery) over a period of several days to 2–3 weeks, with significant restriction occurring within the first 7 days of lesion formation. In these cases, restricted diffusion can precede the onset of contrast enhancement, potentially resembling ischemic lesions. In contrast, acute ischemic lesions typically show contrast enhancement later, during the days to weeks following the onset of infarction.
- High restricted diffusion may be observed in the following conditions that mimic MS:
  - This is typically seen in acute ischemic lesions, where there is restriction in the core. Acute ischemic strokes/lesions may occur in various conditions affecting blood vessels.
  - It is also observed in brain abscesses (restriction in the core).
  - Other diagnoses, which are usually not considered in the differential diagnosis of MS include: cytotoxic cerebral edema of various etiologies; chordoma; Creutzfeldt–Jakob disease (may be the only imaging pathology); some meningiomas).
- Variable or moderately high restricted diffusion may be observed in the following conditions that mimic MS:
  - Acute disseminated encephalomyelitis (ADEM; periphery).
  - Anti-phospholipid syndrome
  - Autoimmune encephalitis with antibodies against neuronal surface (rarely in the cortex)
  - Baló concentric sclerosis (periphery)
  - Cerebral autosomal dominant arteriopathy with subcortical infarcts and leukoencephalopathy (CADASIL)
  - Central pontine myelinolisis
  - ClC-2 chloride channel deficiency leukoencephalopathy
  - Cerebral vein thrombosis
  - Charcot-Marie-Tooth Neuropathy with CNS involvement
  - Fabry disease
  - Hyperornithinemia–hyperammonemia–homocitrullinuria (HHH) syndrome and other glutamate and urea cycle metabolism disorders
  - Churg-strauss syndrom
  - Infectious encephalitis (cytomegalovirus [CMV]; Dengue fever; Epstein–Barr virus [EBV]; herpes simplex virus [HSV]; infarctions in cryptococcal meningitis, progressive multifocal leukoencephalopathy [PML], tuberculous granulomas, West Nile virus)
  - Ischemic lesions in COL4A1-related disorders
  - Lysosomal storage and peroxisomal function disorders (metachromatic leukodystrophy; X-linked adrenoleukodystrophy)
  - Marchiafava–Bignami disease (corpus callosum)
  - Mitochondrial disorders (stroke-like lesions)
  - Necrotic brain tumors

- Neuronal intranuclear inclusion disease and hereditary diffuse leukoencephalopathy with spheroids (cortical or subcortical restriction)
- Neuromyelitis optica spectrum disorder (NMOSD; occasionally in acute large or symptomatic callosal lesions)
- Posterior reversible encephalopathy syndrome (PRES; only sometime)
- Primary angitis of the CNS (PACNS)
- Primary CNS lymphoma (PCNSL)
- Retinal vasculopathy with cerebral leukoencephalopathy and systemic manifestations (RVCL-S)
- Rheumatoid arthritis (rarely in the cortex)
- Schilder's disease
- Traumatic axonal injury
- Tumefactive MS
- Wallerian degeneration (acute; late acute)
- Wernicke encephalopathy (sometime)
- Wilson's disease

• Other conditions with restricted diffusion, which are usually not considered in differential diagnosis of MS include: brain radiation therapy; Canavan disease; carbon monoxide or methanol poisoning; choroid plexus cyst; hemangiopericytoma; hypoglycemia; hyperammonemia; inborn errors of metabolism (glutaric aciduria type I, maple syrup urine disease non-ketotic hyperglycemia, methylmalonic aciduria); intracranial germinoma; Japanese encephalitis; kuru; medulloblastoma; pineoblastoma; primitive neuroectodermal tumor (PNET); epileptic seizures [36–40].

15.19 Temporal Lobe Lesions

• Focal lesions in the temporal lobe, particularly in the inferior temporal lobe adjacent to the temporal horn of the lateral ventricle, are characteristic of MS [18, 41]. However, temporal lobe involvement can also be observed in other conditions that mimic MS:
  - Autoimmune or paraneoplastic limbic encephalitis (Hu, CRMP5/CV2, Ma2, NMDAR, AMPAR, LGI1, CASPR2, GAD65, GABABR, DPPX, mGluR5, AK5, Neurexin-3α)
  - Tumors
  - Cathepsin A-related arteriopathy with strokes and leukoencephalopathy (CARASAL)
  - Cerebral amyloid angiopathy (macrobleeds)
  - Cerebral autosomal dominant arteriopathy with subcortical infarcts and leukoencephalopathy Cerebral Small Vessel (CADASIL; confluent bilateral anterior temporal lobe T2 hyperintensities)
  - Cytotoxic T lymphocyte antigen 4 haploinsufficiency (CTLA-4)
  - Herpes simplex virus (HSV) encephalitis
  - Ischemic stroke

- Mitochondrial disorders (Stroke-like lesions)
- Other neuroinfections (Dengue fever; human Herpesvirus 6 [HHV-6]; West Nile virus; Whiple's disease)
- Posterior reversible encephalopathy syndrome (PRES; uncommon)
- Primary angitis of the CNS (PACNS; however, lesions are more commonly located in the frontal and parietal lobes)
- Traumatic axonal injury

- Lesions in the temporal lobe are typically absent in migraine and cerebral small vessel disease (CSVD). In contrast, status epilepticus may present with focal increases in T2 signal intensity and vasogenic edema on diffusion-weighted imaging (DWI). A variety of other diseases may occasionally be associated with nonspecific focal signal changes in the temporal lobes.

15.20 Tumefactive Lesions

- Except for the rare tumefactive variant, MS is typically characterized by relatively small lesions [1, 18, 42].
- Large tumefactive lesions in the brain may be observed in the following conditions that mimic MS (Fig. 15.1):
  - Acute disseminated encephalomyelitis (ADEM)
  - Acute hemorrhagic leukoencephalitis (AHLE)
  - Adult-onset Alexander disease (brainstem)

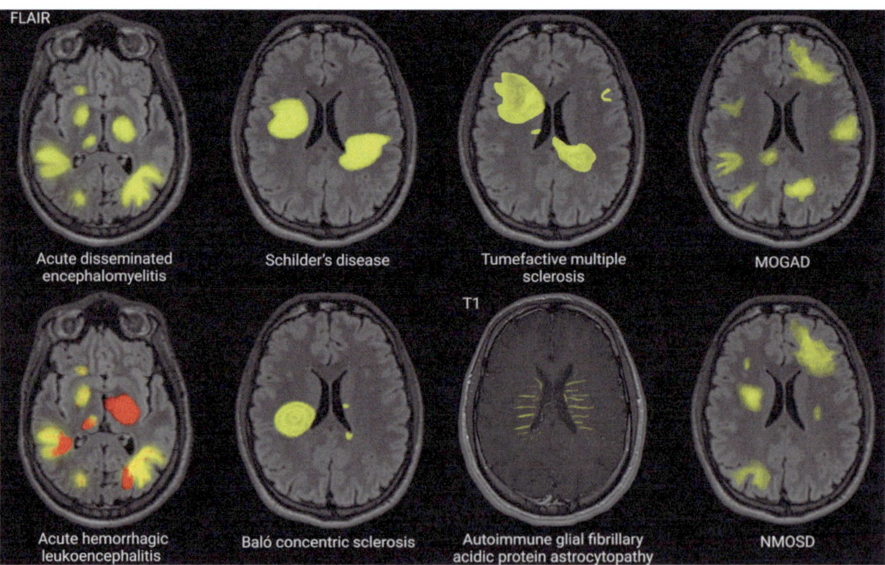

Fig. 15.1 Autoimmune demyelinating diseases that may be associated with tumefactive brain lesions

- Autoimmune encephalitis with antibodies against neuronal surface (e.g., with antibodies against N-methyl-D-aspartate receptor [NMDAR] and others)
- Autoimmune glial fibrillary acidic protein (GFAP) astrocytopathy (rarely)
- Baló concentric sclerosis
- Behçet's disease
- Central pontine myelinolisis
- Cerebral autosomal dominant arteriopathy with subcortical infarcts and leukoencephalopathy (CADASIL)
- CTLA-4 haploinsufficiency
- Gliomas and other brain tumors
- Histiocytosis disorders
- Ischemic stroke
- Marburg disease
- Mediterranean spotted fever
- Mitochondrial disorders
- Monoclonal gammopathy of undetermined significance (MGUS; rarely)
- Myelin oligodendrocyte glycoprotein antibody-associated disease (MOGAD)
- Neuromyelitis optica spectrum disorder (NMOSD)
- Posterior reversible encephalopathy syndrome (PRES)
- Primary CNS lymphoma (PCNSL)
- Progressive multifocal leukoencephalopathy (PML) and some other neuroinfections (Brain Abscess; Fungal infections; Neurocysticercosis; Syphilis; Tuberculosis)
- Radiation necrosis
- Retinal vasculopathy with cerebral leukoencephalopathy and systemic manifestations (RVCL-S)
- Sarcoidosis
- Schilder's disease
- SLE

15.21 U-Fibers Involvement

- MS is typically associated with juxtacortical lesions that affect the subcortical arcuate U-fibers, which are short association fibers connecting adjacent gyri in the brain, located within the subcortical white matter.
- U-fibers are myelinated the slowest and latest, with a reduced rate of myelin turnover; as a result, they are generally spared in most inherited leukodystrophies, except for Alexander and Canavan disease.
- Because U-fibers receive dual blood supply, their involvement is also uncommon in the early stages of cerebrovascular diseases.
- Apart from MS, subcortical U-fibers are commonly affected in the following diseases:
  - Progressive multifocal leukoencephalopathy (PML)
  - Acute disseminated encephalomyelitis (ADEM)

- Cerebral autosomal dominant arteriopathy with subcortical infarcts and leukoencephalopathy (CADASIL; anterior temporal and superior frontal regions)
- Two inherited metabolic leukodystrophies: Alexander disease (white matter of frontal lobe) and Canavan disease (early U-fiber involvement)
- Rare mitochondrial disorders (*TACO1* gene mutation)
- Glut1 deficiency syndrome (only in a small proportion of patients)
- Posterior reversible encephalopathy syndrome (PRES)
- Other disorders usually not considered in differential diagnosis of MS such as galactosemia, Salla disease, or van der Knaap disease

• Subcortical U-fibers can also be affected in the later stages of a wide range of brain diseases, including chronic neuroinfections, chronic small vessel disease, and metabolic or toxic leukoencephalopathies [18, 43–45].

15.22 Summary of Selected Imaging Red Flags of Multiple Sclerosis

Adopted [1, 46, 47] and modified.

15.22.1 Supratentorial

- Calcifications (for details, see chapter “Brain calcifications”)
- Cystic lesions (leukoenecephalopathy with intracranial calcifications and cysts [Labrune syndrome]; neoplasms; neuromyelitis optica spectrum disorder [NMOSD]; infections; congenital disorders)
- Dilation of the Virchow–Robin spaces (CNS vasculitis; cerebral small vessel disease [CSVD]; hyperhomocystinemia; cerebral amyloid angiopathy; mucopolysaccharidoses; Canavan disease; Glut1 deficiency syndrome; COL4A1-related disorders)
- Dominant cortical/subcortical involvement (for details, see chapter “Dominant cortical/subcortical involvement”)
- Edematous lesions with a typical marbled or “arch (NMOSD)
- Hemorrhages or microhemorrhages (for details, see chapter “Brain hemorrhages”)
- Hydrocephalus (sarcoidosis; NMOSD; neuroinfections; chronic meningitis; neoplasms; hereditary spastic paraplegia [HSP, subtype SPG1]; COL4A1-related disorders)
- Hypothalamic and/or pituitary stalk infiltration (for details, see chapter “Diencephalic syndrome and hypophysitis”)
- Lacunar infarcts (for details, see chapter “Ischemic stroke and microinfarctions”)
- Large lesions with absent or rare mass effect and absent contrast enhancement (progressive multifocal leukoencephalopathy [PML])
- Lesions across gray and white matter boundaries (stroke; cerebral autosomal dominant arteriopathy with subcortical infarcts and leukoencephalopathy [CADASIL]; systemic lupus erythematosus [SLE]; CNS vasculitis; PML etc.)

- Lesions in the deep gray matter (a wide range of conditions)
- Multifocal "snowball-like" lesions in the central corpus callosum (Susac's syndrome)
- Restricted diffusion (for details, see chapter "Restricted diffusion")
- Selective or predominant involvement of the anterior temporal lobe (CADASIL and cathepsin-A related arteriopathy with strokes and leukoencephalopathy [CARASAL]) (for details, see chapter "Temporal lobe lesions")
- Symmetrically distributed confluent white matter lesions (for details see chapter "Leukodystrophy-like pattern")
- Tumefactive lesions (> 2 cm in diameter) (for details, see chapter "Tumefactive lesions")
- T1 hyperintensity of the pulvinar (hepatic encephalopathy; manganese and calcium deposits; toxicity; rarely also Fabry disease)

15.22.2 Brainstem

- Central lesions along the transverse pontine fibers (stroke; ischemic lesions; or central pontine myelinolysis [MS lesions are usually located at the periphery of the pons])
- Fluffy lesions in the brain parenchyma, acute disseminated encephalomyelitis (ADEM)-like lesions, large lesions involving the brainstem in particular areas adjacent to the fourth ventricle and the cerebellar peduncles (myelin oligodendrocyte glycoprotein antibody-associated disease [MOGAD])
- Large and infiltrating brainstem lesions (Behçet's disease; Bickerstaff's brainstem encephalitis; CARASAL; central pontinne myelopathy; mitochondrial disorders; NMOSD; pontine glioma; and other neoplasms etc.) (for details, see chapter "Prominent or isolated brainstem involvement")
- Lesions in the periaqueductal area, area postrema (often as paired and discrete), and solitary tract (NMOSD, less frequent MOGAD)
- Regional atrophy of the brainstem (Behçet's disease, adult-onset Alexander's disease, multiple system atrophy etc.)

15.22.3 Spinal Cord

- Bright spotty T2-hyperintense lesions (NMOSD)
- Central lesion with hypointense core and hyperintense rim with or without contrast enhancement on axial view ("bagel sign") in longitudinal myelopathy (Behçet's disease)
- Central spinal cord lesions that involving >50% of the cross-sectional spinal cord area (NMOSD, MOGAD, and wide range of other diagnoses)
- Centrally located lesions, involving grey and white matter (NMOSD, MOGAD, venous hypertension from vascular or spondylitic process)
- Complete transverse myelopathy (wide range of conditions other than MS)
- Conus and cauda equina involvement (for details, see chapter "Conus medullaris involvement")

- Disappearance of T2-hyperintense lesions on follow up imaging (for details, see chapter "Lesion resolution")
- Flow voids or tortuous contrast enhancement in the CSF (dural AV fistula)
- Lesions in the anterior two-thirds of the spinal cord ("snake eye" or "owl's eye" sign), bilateral hyperintensities of the anterior gray matter horns (spinal infarction and spinal cord compression in spondylotic myelopathy)
- Linear dorsal subpial enhancement combined with central canal enhancement on axial view (trident sign) (sarcoidosis)
- Long and selective involvement of the white matter columns/tracts (metabolic or paraneoplastic etiology)
- Longitudinally extensive lesion extending into the brainstem (NMOSD, MOGAD, cobalamin deficiency, Alexander disease etc.)
- Longitudinally extensive myelitis extending over three or more vertebral segments (for details, see chapter "Longitudinally extensive transverse myelitis [LETM]")
- Micro or macro-bleeds in the spinal cord (dural AV fistula; spinal infarction, neoplasms; infections [e.g., varicella-zoster virus (VZV) infection, schistosomiasis]; cavernoma)
- Myelopathy in the absence of spinal cord lesions (stiff person syndrome; human immunodeficiency virus [HIV]; amyotrophic lateral sclerosis [ALS]; HSP; adrenomyeloneuropathy; dynamic compressive myelopathy; early spinal cord ischemia; functional neurological disorders; MOGAD etc.) (For details, see chapter "Normal spinal cord imaging")
- Nerve-root enhancement (for further details, see chapter "Cauda equina involvement and radiculopathy")
- Persistent enhancement of T2-hyperintense lesion (>3 months): (For details, see chapter "Persistent and simultaneous contrast enhancement of brain lesions," which is applicable also to the spinal cord lesions)
- Predominant corticospinal tract involvement (for details, see chapter "Corticospinal tract involvement")
- Prominent involvement of the central gray matter and spinal cord swelling (NMOSD, MOGAD)
- Ring enhancement with ill-defined triangular extension at the top and/or th bottom of the lesion ("Flame sign") (intramedullary spinal cord metastasis)
- Ring enhancement (NMOSD; infections [e.g., neurocysticercosis or abscess]; metastases; radiation necrosis)
- Selective and extensive anterior spinal cord or anterior horn cell involvement (NMOSD; infections [West Nile virus, enterovirus D68]; anterior spinal artery ischemia)
- Selective and extensive involvement of the dorsal or lateral columns (paraneoplastic syndrome; Sjögren's syndrome; infections [HIV, HTLV-1, syphilis]; cobalamin and copper deficiency; leukoencephalopathy with brainstem and spinal cord involvement and lactate elevation [LBSL]; cerebrotendinous xanthomatosis [CTX]; posterior spinal artery ischemia; intrathecal methotrexate)
- Spinal cord cavities (NMOSD, syringohydromyelia, neoplasms)
- T1-hypointense lesions restricted to GM (NMOSD, infection, ischemia)

- T2 hyperintensity in the anterior horns (acute flaccid myelitis, spinal cord infarction)
- T2 hyperintensity restricted to grey matter (H-sign) (MOGAD; infection [e.g., Enterovirus D68, West Nile virus]; ischemia; Hirayama disease; myelomalacia from spondylosis)
- Transverse band of enhancement with the width greater than or equal to the height on sagittal view (pancake-like sign), just below the site of maximal stenosis, involving white matter and sparing gray matter on axial view (spondylotic myelopathy)
- Vertebral body infarct (spinal cord infarct)
- Patchy/punctate or large ring enhancement in the spinal cord (NMOSD)

15.22.4 Optic Nerve

- Absence of an acute T2-hyperintense optic nerve lesion (ischemic and toxic optic neuropathies; Leber's hereditary optic neuropathy hyperintensity [LHON])
- Bilateral simultaneous optic neuritis (for details, see chapter "Bilateral visual loss")
- Extension of enhancement to orbital fat (MOGAD, IgG4-related disease)
- Longitudinally extensive anterior segment enhancing optic nerve lesion, which can extend to the chiasm (MOGAD)
- Longitudinally extensive posterior segment enhancing optic nerve lesions with or without involvement of the chiasm or optic tract (NMOSD; sarcoidosis; less frequent biotinidase deficiency; or mitochondrial disorders)
- Optic nerve sheath enhancement (peri-neuritis) (MOGAD; sarcoidosis; IgG4-related disease; granulomatosis with polyangiitis; infection; neoplasms [lymphoma, meningioma]; idiopathic orbital inflammatory syndrome [orbital pseudotumor])
- Optic neuritis/neuropathy with normal brain MRI (MOGAD, NMOSD, mitochondrial disorders)
- Persistent (>3 months) optic nerve enhancement (sarcoidosis, glioma, lymphoma, meningioma) (for details, see chapter "Persistent and simultaneous contrast enhancement of brain lesions")
- Soft tissue enhancement extrinsic to the optic nerve affecting the orbit, orbital apex, or cavernous sinus (granulomatous disease, tumor, infection, MOGAD)

15.22.5 Contrast Enhancement in the Brain

- Band-like brain lesion enhancement (Baló concentric sclerosis)
- Cloud-like brain lesion enhancement (NMOSD, MOGAD)
- Complete ring contrast enhancement (infections; CNS abscess; glioblastoma; metastases; less frequently in autoimmune demyelinating diseases)

- Linear radial perivascular enhancement (encephalomyelitis with GFAP antibodies; sarcoidosis; primary or secondary CNS vasculitis; lymphomatoid granulomatosis)
- Pachymeningeal, leptomeningeal, or cranial nerve enhancement
  - Antineutrophil cytoplasmic antibodies (ANCA) vasculitis
  - Aseptic meningitis
  - Behçet's disease
  - Chronic meningitis
  - CNS vasculitis
  - IgG4-related disease
  - Infectious meningitis [e.g., in Lyme borreliosis]
  - Leptomeningeal carcinomatosis
  - Low CSF pressure
  - Lymphomatosis
  - MOGAD
  - Neoplasm (e.g., lymphoma)
  - Rheumatoid arthritis
  - Sarcoidosis
  - Susac's syndrome
  - Syphilis
- Patchy and persistent enhancement (>3 months) with no or minimal corresponding T2 hyperintensity, often located in the pons (capillary telangiectasia)
- Pencil-thin ependymal enhancement (NMOSD)
- Persistent contrast enhancement of lesion (>3 months) (for details see chapter "Persistent and simultaneous contrast enhancement of brain lesions")
- Punctiform or miliary parenchymal contrast enhancement
  - Behçet's disease
  - CLIPPERS
  - CNS vasculitis
  - Erdheim–Chester disease
  - Lymphoma
  - Metastatic disease
  - Neuroinfections (Lyme borreliosis, candidiasis, tuberculosis, histoplasmosis, PML)
  - NMOSD
  - Sarcoidosis
  - Susac's syndrome
  - Cobalamin deficiency
- Punctiform parenchymal contrast enhancement confined to the pons (but can also be in the peduncles, hemispheres, and cervical spinal cord) (CLIPPERS)
- Purely cortical enhancement (vasculitis, ischemia)
- Simultaneous contrast enhancement of all or almost all lesions (for details see chapter "Persistent and simultaneous contrast enhancement of brain lesions")
- Vessel wall or perivascular enhancement (vasculitis, sarcoidosis, intravascular lymphoma)

15.22.6 Summary of Selected Myelopathy Patterns [4, 22, 48–53] (Figs. 15.2, 15.3 and 15.4)

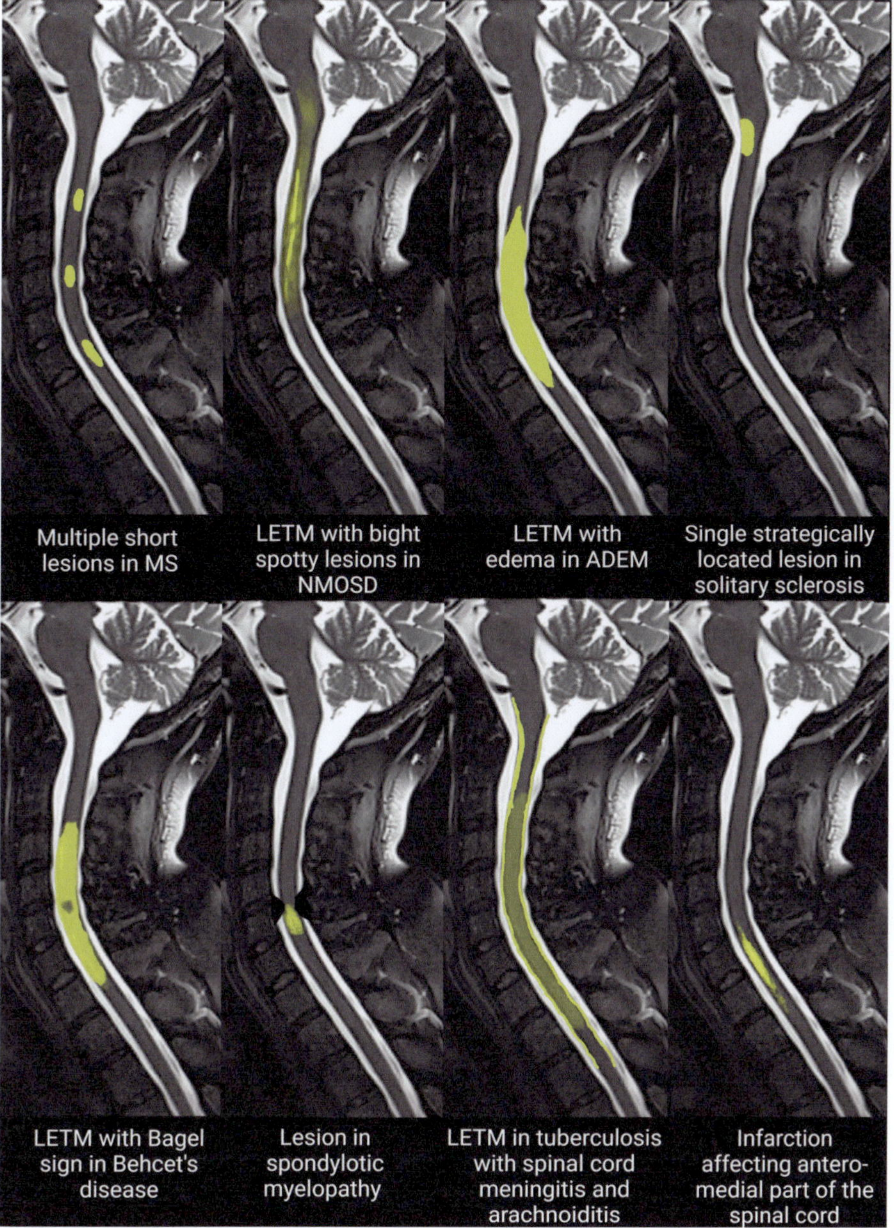

Fig. 15.2 Myelopathy patterns on sagittal spinal cord MRI

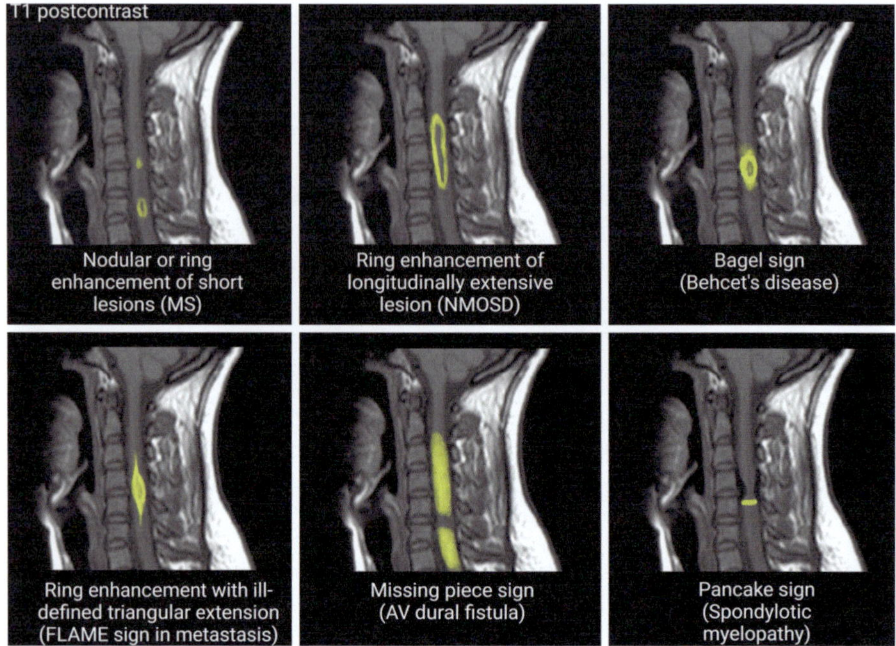

Fig. 15.3 Contrast enhancement patterns on sagittal spinal cord MRI

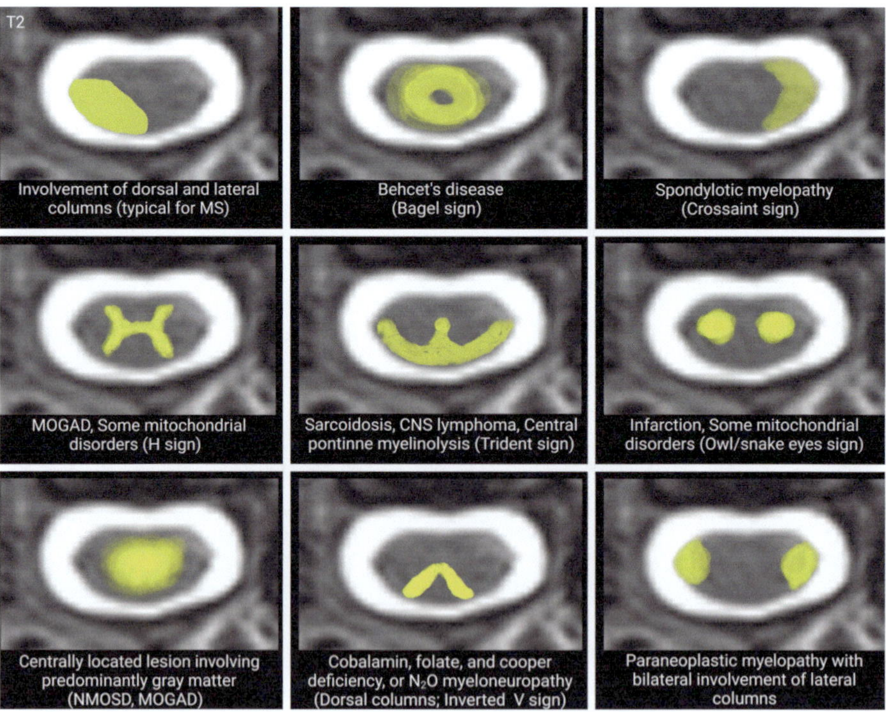

Fig. 15.4 Selected patterns of spinal cord involvement on axial MRI

References

1. Solomon AJ, Arrambide G, Brownlee WJ, Flanagan EP, Amato MP, Amezcua L, et al. Differential diagnosis of suspected multiple sclerosis: an updated consensus approach. Lancet Neurol. 2023;22(8):750–68.
2. Miller DH, Weinshenker BG, Filippi M, Banwell BL, Cohen JA, Freedman MS, et al. Differential diagnosis of suspected multiple sclerosis: a consensus approach. Mult Scler. 2008;14(9):1157–74.
3. Ayrignac X, Nicolas G, Carra-Dallière C, Hannequin D, Labauge P. Brain calcifications in adult-onset genetic leukoencephalopathies: a review. JAMA Neurol. 2017;74(8):1000–8.
4. Ciccarelli O, Cohen JA, Reingold SC, Weinshenker BG. Spinal cord involvement in multiple sclerosis and neuromyelitis optica spectrum disorders. Lancet Neurol. 2019;18(2):185–97.
5. Diehn FE, Krecke KN. Neuroimaging of spinal cord and cauda Equina disorders. Continuum (Minneap Minn). 2021;27(1):225–63.
6. Etemadifar M, Salari M, Kargaran PK, Sigari AA, Nouri H, Etemadifar F, et al. Conus medullaris involvement in demyelinating disorders of the CNS: a comparative study. Mult Scler Relat Disord. 2021;54:103127.
7. Lee HI, Kwon E, Oh E, Jeong SH. Antisaccades in spinocerebellar ataxia type 17 with middle cerebellar peduncle hyperintensities without hot-cross-bun sign. J Clin Neurol. 2024;20(3):342–4.
8. Ozaki K, Doi H, Mitsui J, Sato N, Iikuni Y, Majima T, et al. A novel mutation in ELOVL4 leading to spinocerebellar ataxia (SCA) with the hot cross bun sign but lacking erythrokeratodermia: a broadened Spectrum of SCA34. JAMA Neurol. 2015;72(7):797.
9. Guo Z, Lu T, Peng L, Cheng H, Peng F, Li J, et al. CLCN2-related leukoencephalopathy: a case report and review of the literature. BMC Neurol. 2019;19(1):156.
10. Sone J, Mori K, Inagaki T, Katsumata R, Takagi S, Yokoi S, et al. Clinicopathological features of adult-onset neuronal intranuclear inclusion disease. Brain. 2016;139(Pt 12):3170–86.
11. Gaillard F, Sharma R, Ibrahim D et al. Bilateral middle cerebellar peduncle lesions. Radiopaedia.org; 2011. Available from: https://radiopaedia.org/articles/13017
12. Choi JH, Seo JD, Choi YR, Kim MJ, Kim HJ, Kim JS, et al. Inferior cerebellar peduncular lesion causes a distinct vestibular syndrome. Eur J Neurol. 2015;22(7):1062–7.
13. Caligiuri ME, Barone S, Cherubini A, Augimeri A, Chiriaco C, Trotta M, et al. The relationship between regional microstructural abnormalities of the corpus callosum and physical and cognitive disability in relapsing-remitting multiple sclerosis. Neuroimage Clin. 2015;7:28–33.
14. Simon JH, Holtås SL, Schiffer RB, Rudick RA, Herndon RM, Kido DK, et al. Corpus callosum and subcallosal-periventricular lesions in multiple sclerosis: detection with MR. Radiology. 1986;160(2):363–7.
15. Garg N, Reddel SW, Miller DH, Chataway J, Riminton DS, Barnett Y, et al. The corpus callosum in the diagnosis of multiple sclerosis and other CNS demyelinating and inflammatory diseases. J Neurol Neurosurg Psychiatry. 2015;86(12):1374–82.
16. Wallach A, Stember D, Valentine D, Howard J. Differential Diagnosis of MRI Corticospinal Tract Abnormalities (P2201). 2017;88(16_suppl):P2.201.
17. Langlois F, Varlamov EV, Fleseriu M. Hypophysitis, the growing Spectrum of a rare pituitary disease. J Clin Endocrinol Metab. 2022;107(1):10–28.
18. Filippi M, Preziosa P, Banwell BL, Barkhof F, Ciccarelli O, De Stefano N, et al. Assessment of lesions on magnetic resonance imaging in multiple sclerosis: practical guidelines. Brain. 2019;142(7):1858–75.
19. Bouman PM, Steenwijk MD, Pouwels PJW, Schoonheim MM, Barkhof F, Jonkman LE, et al. Histopathology-validated recommendations for cortical lesion imaging in multiple sclerosis. Brain. 2020;143(10):2988–97.
20. Sheerin F, Pretorius PM, Briley D, Meagher T. Differential diagnosis of restricted diffusion confined to the cerebral cortex. Clin Radiol. 2008;63(11):1245–53.

21. Baba Y, Botz B. Cerebral cortical T2 hyperintensity: Radiopaedia.org; 2021. Available from: https://doi.org/10.53347/rID-86421
22. Mariano R, Flanagan EP, Weinshenker BG, Palace J. A practical approach to the diagnosis of spinal cord lesions. Pract Neurol. 2018;18(3):187–200.
23. Montalvo M, Flanagan EP. Paraneoplastic/autoimmune myelopathies. Handb Clin Neurol. 2024;200:193–201.
24. Desai AB, Agarwal A, Mohamed AS, Mohamed KH, Middlebrooks EH, Bhatt AA, et al. Motor neuron diseases and central nervous system tractopathies: clinical-radiologic correlation and diagnostic approach. Radiographics: a review publication of the Radiological Society of North America, Inc. 2025;45(1):e240067.
25. Stefanou MI, Giannopapas V, Kitsos DK, Chondrogianni M, Theodorou A, Kosmidou M, et al. Prevalence and epidemiology of stroke in patients with multiple sclerosis: a systematic review and meta-analysis. J Neurol. 2024;271(7):4075–85.
26. Palladino R, Marrie RA, Majeed A, Chataway J. Evaluating the risk of macrovascular events and mortality among people with multiple sclerosis in England. JAMA Neurol. 2020;77(7):820–8.
27. Sechi E, Krecke KN, Messina SA, Buciuc M, Pittock SJ, Chen JJ, et al. Comparison of MRI lesion evolution in different central nervous system demyelinating disorders. Neurology. 2021;97(11):e1097–e109.
28. Harder S, Gourgaris A, Frangou E, Hopp K, Huntsman R, Lowry N, et al. Clinical and neuroimaging findings of Cree leukodystrophy: a retrospective case series. AJNR Am J Neuroradiol. 2010;31(8):1418–23.
29. Weisfeld-Adams JD, Katz Sand IB, Honce JM, Lublin FD. Differential diagnosis of Mendelian and mitochondrial disorders in patients with suspected multiple sclerosis. Brain. 2015;138(Pt 3):517–39.
30. Sedel F, Tourbah A, Fontaine B, Lubetzki C, Baumann N, Saudubray JM, et al. Leukoencephalopathies associated with inborn errors of metabolism in adults. J Inherit Metab Dis. 2008;31(3):295–307.
31. Ayrignac X, Carra-Dallière C, Marelli C, Taïeb G, Labauge P. Adult-onset genetic central nervous system disorders masquerading as acquired neuroinflammatory disorders: a review. JAMA Neurol. 2022;79(10):1069–78.
32. Trebst C, Raab P, Voss EV, Rommer P, Abu-Mugheisib M, Zettl UK, et al. Longitudinal extensive transverse myelitis--it's not all neuromyelitis optica. Nat Rev Neurol 2011;7(12):688–698.
33. Guttmann CR, Ahn SS, Hsu L, Kikinis R, Jolesz FA. The evolution of multiple sclerosis lesions on serial MR. AJNR Am J Neuroradiol. 1995;16(7):1481–91.
34. He J, Grossman RI, Ge Y, Mannon LJ. Enhancing patterns in multiple sclerosis: evolution and persistence. AJNR Am J Neuroradiol. 2001;22(4):664–9.
35. Ramanan VK, Crum BA, McKeon A. Subacute encephalitis with recovery in IgLON5 autoimmunity. Neurol Neuroimmunol Neuroinflamm. 2018;5(5):e485.
36. Finelli PF. Diagnostic approach to restricted-diffusion patterns on MR imaging. Neurol Clin Pract. 2012;2(4):287–93.
37. Hyland M, Bermel RA, Cohen JA. Restricted diffusion preceding gadolinium enhancement in large or tumefactive demyelinating lesions. Neurol Clin Pract. 2013;3(1):15–21.
38. Abou Zeid N, Pirko I, Erickson B, Weigand SD, Thomsen KM, Scheithauer B, et al. Diffusion-weighted imaging characteristics of biopsy-proven demyelinating brain lesions. Neurology. 2012;78(21):1655–62.
39. Eisele P, Szabo K, Griebe M, Rossmanith C, Förster A, Hennerici M, et al. Reduced diffusion in a subset of acute MS lesions: a serial multiparametric MRI study. AJNR Am J Neuroradiol. 2012;33(7):1369–73.
40. Mudgal P, Weerakkody Y, Hacking C, et al. Cerebral restricted diffusion 2024.; https://doi.org/10.53347/rID-26903(Radiopaedia.org).
41. Thompson AJ, Banwell BL, Barkhof F, Carroll WM, Coetzee T, Comi G, et al. Diagnosis of multiple sclerosis: 2017 revisions of the McDonald criteria. Lancet Neurol. 2018;17(2):162–73.
42. Hardy TA, Reddel SW, Barnett MH, Palace J, Lucchinetti CF, Weinshenker BG. Atypical inflammatory demyelinating syndromes of the CNS. Lancet Neurol. 2016;15(9):967–81.

43. Gaillard F, Ranchod A, Rasuli B et al. Subcortical U-fibers: Radiopaedia.org; 2024. Available from: https://doi.org/10.53347/rID-32173
44. Sferruzza G, Del Bondio A, Citterio A, Vezzulli P, Guerrieri S, Radaelli M, et al. U-fiber leukoencephalopathy due to a novel mutation in the TACO1 gene. Neurol Genet. 2021;7(2):e573.
45. Riley KJ, O'Neill DP, Kralik SF. Subcortical U-fibers: signposts to the diagnosis of white matter disease. Neurographics. 2018;8(4):234–43.
46. Hua LH, Solomon AJ, Tenembaum S, Scalfari A, Rovira À, Rostasy K, et al. Differential diagnosis of suspected multiple sclerosis in pediatric and late-onset populations: a review. JAMA Neurol. 2024;81:1210.
47. Miller TM. Differential diagnosis of myotonic disorders. Muscle Nerve. 2008;37(3):293–9.
48. Zalewski NL, Flanagan EP, Keegan BM. Evaluation of idiopathic transverse myelitis revealing specific myelopathy diagnoses. Neurology. 2018;90(2):e96–e102.
49. Mustafa R, Zalewski NL, Flanagan EP, Kumar N. Challenging myelopathy cases. Semin Neurol. 2022;42(6):723–34.
50. Flanagan EP, Krecke KN, Marsh RW, Giannini C, Keegan BM, Weinshenker BG. Specific pattern of gadolinium enhancement in spondylotic myelopathy. Ann Neurol. 2014;76(1):54–65.
51. Zalewski NL. Vascular myelopathies. Continuum (Minneap Minn). 2021;27(1):30–61.
52. Lopez Chiriboga S, Flanagan EP. Myelitis and other autoimmune myelopathies. Continuum (Minneap Minn). 2021;27(1):62–92.
53. Flanagan EP. Autoimmune myelopathies. Handb Clin Neurol. 2016;133:327–51.

Index

T. Uher, *Mimics and Red Flags of Multiple Sclerosis*, https://doi.org/10.1007/978-3-031-98945-2

C

D

N

O

T

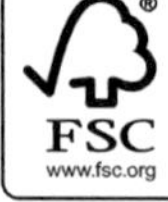

MIX
Papier aus verantwortungsvollen Quellen
Paper from responsible sources
FSC® C105338

If you have any concerns about our products,
you can contact us on
ProductSafety@springernature.com

In case Publisher is established outside the EU,
the EU authorized representative is:
Springer Nature Customer Service Center GmbH
Europaplatz 3, 69115 Heidelberg, Germany

Printed by Libri Plureos GmbH
in Hamburg, Germany